INTRODUCTORY TEXTBOOK
OF PSYCHIATRY

INTRODUCTORY TEXTBOOK OF PSYCHIATRY

Nancy C. Andreasen, M.D., Ph.D.
Professor of Psychiatry
Director, Mental Health Clinical Research Center

Donald W. Black, M.D.
Assistant Professor
Director of Residency Training

Department of Psychiatry
The University of Iowa College of Medicine
Iowa City, Iowa

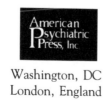

Washington, DC
London, England

Library of Congress Cataloging-in-Publication Data

Andreasen, Nancy C.
   Introductory textbook of psychiatry / Nancy C. Andreasen, Donald W. Black — 1st ed.
      p.   cm.
   Includes bibliographical references.
   Includes index.
   ISBN 0-88048-112-9 (alk. paper). — ISBN 0-88048-114-5 (pbk. : alk. paper)
   1. Psychiatry.   I. Andreasen, Nancy C., 1938–   .   II. Black, Donald
W., 1956–   .   III. Title.
   [DNLM: 1. Mental Disorders.   WM 100 A557i]
RC454.A427   1990
616.89—dc20
DNLM/DLC
for Library of Congress   90-530
                                                                        CIP

British Library Cataloguing in Publication Data

A CIP record is available from the British Library.

Table of Contents

Section III
Special Topics

Section IV
Treatments

Preface

Students sometimes begin working in psychiatry with a set of preconceptions about what it is, preconceptions shaped by the fact that information about psychiatry is omnipresent in popular culture. Taxi drivers, CEOs, teachers, and ministers often feel qualified to offer information and advice about how to handle "psychiatric problems," even though they may be unaware of distinctions as fundamental as the difference between psychiatry and psychology. These two disciplines are blurred together in the popular mind, and the term *psychiatry* evokes a potpourri of associations—Freud's couch, Jack Nicholson receiving electroconvulsive therapy in *One Flew Over the Cuckoo's Nest*, or Dr. Ruth discussing sexual adjustment on television. These images and associations tend to cloak psychiatry with an aura of vagueness, imprecision, muddleheadedness, and mindless coercion. It is unfortunate that such preconceptions are so pervasive, but fortunate that most of them are in fact in error, as students who use this book in conjunction with studying psychiatry in a clinical setting will soon discover.

What is psychiatry? It is the branch of medicine that focuses on the diagnosis and treatment of mental illnesses. Some of these illnesses are very serious, such as schizophrenia, Alzheimer's disease, or the various mood disorders. Others may be less serious, but still very significant, such as adjustment disorders or personality disorders. Psychiatry differs from psychology by virtue of its medical orientation. Its primary focus is illness or abnormality, as opposed to normal psychological functioning; the latter is the primary focus of psychology. Of course, abnormal psychology is a small branch within psychology, just as understanding normality is necessary for the psychiatrist to recognize and treat abnormal functioning. As a discipline within medicine, the primary purposes of psychiatry are to define and recognize illnesses, to identify methods for treating them, and ultimately to develop methods for discovering their causes and implementing preventive measures.

Psychiatry during the last decade of the 20th century may be the most exciting discipline within medicine. Contemporary psychiatry is exciting for a variety of reasons. First, psychiatrists are specialists who work with the most interesting organ within the body, the brain. The brain is intrinsically fascinating because it controls nearly all aspects of functioning within the rest of the body, as well as the way people interact with and relate to one another. Psychiatry has received enormous support during recent years through the burgeoning of neuroscience, which has provided psychiatrists with the tools by which they can understand brain anatomy, chemistry, and physiology, thereby gradually developing a scientific base that will permit them to understand human emotion and behavior and to develop methods for treating abnormalities in these domains.

Yet, as psychiatry evolves into a relatively high-powered science, it remains a very clinical and human branch within medicine, and therefore a very rewarding field for students who have chosen medicine because they wish to have contact with patients. The clinician working in psychiatry must spend time with his or her patients and learn about them as human beings as well as as individuals who have illnesses or problems. Learning the life stories of individual people is fun and interesting; as one colleague once said, "It amazed me when I realized that I would get paid for asking people things that everybody always wants to know about anyway!"

Finally, psychiatry has enormous breadth. As a scientific discipline, it ranges from the highly detailed facts of molecular biology to the abstract concepts of the mind. As a clinical discipline, it ranges from the absorbingly complex disturbances that characterize illnesses such as schizophrenia to the understandable fearfulness shown by young children when they must separate from their parents and attend school or be left with a baby-sitter. It can be very scientific and technical, as in the frontier-expanding research currently occurring in molecular genetics or neuroimaging; but it can also be very human and personal, as when a clinician listens to a patient's story and experiences the pleasure of being able to offer help by providing needed insights or even simple encouragement and support.

This book is intended as a tool to help you learn from your patients and from your teachers. We have tried to keep it simple, clear, and factual. References are provided for students who want to explore in more depth the topics covered in the various chapters. We have written this book primarily for medical students and residents during the first several years of their training, although we anticipate that it may also be useful to individuals seeking psychiatric training from the perspectives of other disciplines such as nursing or social work. We hope that, using this book as a tool, students of all ages and types will learn to enjoy working with psychiatric patients and with the art and science of contemporary psychiatry as much as we do.

Section I
Background

Chapter 1
History of Psychiatry

What curiosity, that delicate little plant needs more than anything, besides stimulation, is freedom.

Albert Einstein

To understand some of the conceptual tensions in modern psychiatry, as well as the somewhat confused attitudes of contemporary society toward the mentally ill, it is helpful to examine current situations and thinking in the light of their historical background. Over many centuries, a complicated and conflicting array of attitudes have been built up, and many of these still affect our current perceptions and ideas.

Mental Illness in Biblical and Classical Times

Mental illnesses are among the first diseases to have been recognized as discrete illnesses. The concept of cancer or even congestive heart failure is relatively new compared to the concept of mental illness. Perhaps the oldest medical document in existence, the Ebers papyrus (probably composed in 1900 B.C.), contains references to specific syndromes such as depression. Biblical writings also contain descriptions of individuals suffering from major mental illnesses; for example, in 1 Samuel, Saul is portrayed as falling into a serious depression, for which he is treated with soothing music.

By classical times, a full classification of mental illnesses had been developed. These included melancholia (depression), mania (various psychotic states), delirium (mental confusion accompanied by fever), and hysteria (sudden unexplained

3

episodes of somatic illness involving pain, drop attacks, paralysis, etc.). Although Greek and Roman physicians generally recognized these as major classes of mental illness, they could not agree on their specific causes. Hippocrates, for example, argued that mental illnesses, as well as all other cognitive and emotional functions, derived principally from the brain. Galen and his followers believed that mental illnesses were due to imbalances in quantities of body fluids. Melancholia, for example, was due to an excess of black bile, and other abnormalities arose from imbalances in the other three main fluids, or humors, of the body (blood, phlegm, and yellow bile). Still others argued for an "organ theory" of disease and believed that specific dysfunctions could be attributed to abnormalities in specific organs; delirium or mania, for example, were brain abnormalities, whereas hysteria was due to a wandering uterus.

Although physicians in classical times had their major or minor differences about both the nosology and pathophysiology of major mental illnesses, they rather consistently shared the belief that these illnesses were physical in nature. Although the Greeks developed highly sophisticated theories about the nature of the spirit, soul, or mind, they nevertheless believed that illnesses such as mania or melancholia were due to aberrations in the body rather than the soul or spirit. This led in turn to humane practices for the treatment of serious mental illnesses, involving rest and peaceful surroundings.

Medieval and Renaissance Attitudes

As Roman civilization declined and finally fell, enlightened attitudes about mental illness declined as well. The Barbarian tribes that conquered Rome had no interest in maintaining learning or education, leading to massive destruction of the libraries that summarized classical knowledge about science and literature. Europe gradually struggled out of the Dark Ages, largely through the influence of the Christian church, but the new prevailing worldview was not conducive to enlightenment about human illness in general or mental illness in particular. The emphasis was on saving souls, not bodies.

In this environment, the mentally ill were often believed to be possessed by the devil rather than to be suffering from some form of illness. Witches, warlocks, and demons in disguise were very real to the people of the Middle Ages. Various types of misfortune or suffering were often perceived as just punishments meted out through divine intervention as a consequence of sinful behavior. Thus, it was easy to believe that a person who fell into the deep despondency of depression, and who was experiencing a delusion of sin and guilt, was spiritually rather than physically ill. A person suffering from the agitation and mental confusion that often accompanies severe psychosis could easily be seen as possessed by diabolical forces. Such individuals were often "treated" through the church rather than through medicine, and many were tortured or burned at the stake. The church published texts, such as the *Malleus Maleficarum* ("Hammer of Witches") to explain how such possessed individuals could be identified and killed, since they were considered to be dangerous to society. As late as the 17th century, the reigning monarch in England, James I, wrote a book on this topic, *Demonologie*. The last witch was hung in England in 1684, but witch trials continued in the United States in Salem, Massachusetts, into the 18th century.

The Renaissance, the rebirth of interest in classical learning that began in Italy in the 15th century and spread throughout the rest of Europe during the next 100 years, brought a refreshing new light to this rather dim atmosphere. Artists redis-covered the study of anatomy, forbidden by the church, in order to better depict the human body. Authoritarian teachings were questioned. The new physics of Copernicus and Galileo displaced man and the earth from the center of the universe. Doctors began to believe what their eyes and their inferences taught them, in contrast to arbitrary dogma that was obviously in error.

A few brave voices began to suggest that mental illnesses were diseases rather than forms of possession and bewitchment. In 1584, Reginald Scot published *The Discoverie of Witchcraft*, in which he argued that individuals accused of witchcraft were not in fact possessed by demons, but were instead mentally ill, and that their own descriptions of being possessed represented false products of their fevered imaginations and thus should be considered as delusions. Two years later, in 1586, a physician, Timothy Bright, published the first textbook about mental illness to appear in English, *The Treatise of Melancholie*. In this book, he described the classic symptoms of depression and their tendency to alternate with periods of being "high" in a way that anticipated later descriptions of manic-depressive illness and argued that the symptoms of mental illness were "naturall perturbations" that "altered either brayne or hart." Although these revolutionary ideas did not instantly gain wide acceptance, the foundations of modern psychiatry were being laid.

The Dawn of Scientific Psychiatry

Serious mental illnesses tended to be relatively chronic and incapacitating, espe-cially in an era when no good treatments were available. If the mentally ill were not burned at the stake, some other disposition had to be made. Hospitals or asylums were an alternative solution. To refer to the institutions created for the mentally ill during the 17th and 18th centuries as hospitals or asylums is, however, by and large a misnomer. Patients were in fact typically incarcerated, and many were not only locked in, but were also locked up in chains. Making matters worse, often distinctions were not clearly made between the mentally ill, the criminal, the mentally retarded, and the economically unfortunate. The desire to spare the rich from being forced to observe the suffering of the poor, the handicapped, or the seriously ill seems to be a persistent human failing, although hardly an appealing one.

The seeds of skepticism and doubt sown during the Renaissance flowered into rebellion and revolution during the era of the enlightenment in the 18th century. All over the world, the weak, deprived, and powerless sought to take back their rights and to seize authority from the rich and powerful. The United States led the way with the first revolution of modern times, declaring all men to be created equal. Benjamin Rush, a physician who signed the Declaration of Independence, was also a specialist in the care of the mentally ill who founded the Pennsylvania Hospital, the first psychiatric facility in the United States. The revolutionary movement in America sparked others in France, Italy, and elsewhere.

Phillipe Pinel, a leader of the French Revolution, is usually considered to be the founding father of modern psychiatry. In 1793, he was named director of the Bicêtre, the hospital in Paris for insane men. Soon afterward, he instituted a grand, symbolic change by removing the chains that bound the patients to the walls at the Bicêtre and instituted a new type of treatment that he referred to as "moral treatment." (This meant treating patients in ways that were morally and ethically sensitive, rather than attempting to teach them "morality.") He was later made director of the corresponding hospital for women, the Salpêtrière. In addition to attempting to treat patients with kindness and decency, Pinel also tried to approach the study of the mentally ill scientifically. As he described his efforts in his *Treatise on Insanity* (1806), he said:

> I, therefore, resolved to adopt that method of investigation which has invariably succeeded in all the departments of natural history, viz. To notice successively every fact, without any other object than that of collecting materials for future use; and to endeavor, as far as possible, to divest myself of the influence, both of my own re-possessions and the authority of others. (p. 2)

The *Treatise on Insanity* contains detailed case histories of individual patients so clearly described that they are instantly diagnosable as "classic cases" of what we now call schizophrenia or manic-depressive illness 200 years later.

In addition to introducing psychotherapy, in the form of moral treatment, and stressing the importance of empirical observation, Pinel also applied scientific method to the study of psychiatry. He established epidemiological methods for recording numbers of cases, instituted follow-up studies so that the natural history of diseases could be observed, and used whatever scientific technology he had at hand to understand the pathophysiology of mental diseases. His approaches became the standard methods in most enlightened psychiatric facilities throughout Europe and the United States in the 19th century.

Thus, a new specialty within medicine was created consisting of those doctors who chose to specialize in the care of the mentally ill. They became known as *psychiatrists*, which means literally "physicians who heal the mind." Psychiatry was one of the first disciplines within medicine to identify itself as a specialty. This was no doubt a consequence of both the many patients suffering from mental illness and the special needs and challenges that they presented.

The First Era of Neuroscience

While psychiatry was establishing itself as a medical specialty, a new subdivision within science was also emerging. During the 19th century, clinical observations

Table 1-1.   Major discoveries in the first era of neuroscience

Year	Discovery
1837	Dax: Lateralization of language
1861	Broca: Identification of Broca's area
1868	Harlow: Description of Phineas Gage and the role of the frontal cortex
1870	Fritsch and Hitzig: Lateralization of motor function
1876	Wernicke: Localization of language comprehension
1909	Brodmann: Maps of cortical cytoarchitecture
1920s	Penfield: Mapping of cognitive and motor functions with microelectrodes
1921	Foix: Localization of Parkinson's in the substantia nigra
1937	Papez: Description of the limbic system

and technological developments converged to create an era when the brain was studied scientifically for the first time.

Some of the landmark achievements of the first era of neuroscience are summarized in Table 1-1. One major aspect was the mapping of specific cortical functions in the human brain. The initial observations focused on the specificity of language systems in the brain, beginning in 1837 with the observation of Marc Dax that left-sided injury tended to be associated with aphasia and right hemiparesis. A steady progression of discoveries ensued. More specific language functions were mapped as Pierre-Paul Broca observed that posterior frontal lesions led to impaired speech but intact comprehension, and Carl Wernicke observed that more posterior lesions in the parietal cortex (now recognized as language association regions) led to impaired comprehension with fluent but garbled and incomprehensible speech. Well-defined motor and sensory regions were subsequently recognized as well. The vast area of the frontal cortex, anterior to the central sulcus, was observed to mediate various higher cognitive and emotional functions that distinctly differentiate human personality and behavior, such as social judgment, long-term planning, and the capacity to form close emotional attachments.

These various observations about human cerebral specialization were achieved through a combination of clinical observation and developments in the basic sciences. Most of the observations about language function were made through the study of stroke patients, whereas the role of the prefrontal cortex in governing human personality was first identified through the famous case of Phineas Gage, who suffered a major lesion to his frontal lobes in an accident. The motor cortex was mapped through the developing science of neurophysiology.

Basic neuroscience was also making major strides, as the brain was studied systematically for the first time—anatomically, microscopically, and functionally. A variety of staining techniques were developed that permitted scientists to examine the cellular structure of the brain and begin to explore the neural networks that connected various regions. Nissl, Golgi, and Welgert provided methods for visualizing neuronal cell bodies, axons, and dendrites. Subsequently, Brodmann used these staining techniques to systematically map structural differentiation within the brain and to relate it to specific types of cortical function. His detailed maps of differentiations in cell layers and structures permitted the identification of the

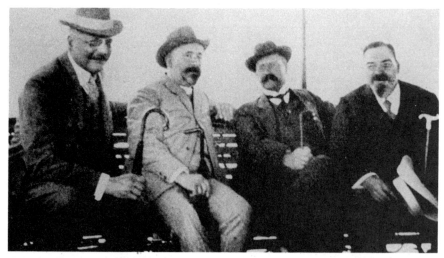

Figure 1-1. Emil Kraepelin, seated with other members of his department of psychiatry, near the Starnberger lake. From *left to right*: Alzheimer, Kraepelin, Gaupp, and Nissl (circa 1908). Reprinted with permission from Hippius H: Kraepelin's Memoirs. New York, Raven, 1989, p 257.

more primitive paleocortex (such as is found in the limbic system) from the neocortex and also permitted the identification of different types of cell layers in cortical regions specialized for different functions such as sensory perception versus motor activity.

These advances did not escape the notice of forward-looking individuals in the new discipline of psychiatry. While still a student and trainee, young Sigmund Freud attempted to develop a new staining technique for nerve cells that was never successful; later he wrote a treatise on aphasia in children and worked in pharmacology by examining the potential therapeutic effects of cocaine.

One of the greatest departments of psychiatry of all time was assembled in Munich at the turn of the century under the leadership of Emil Kraepelin, who joins Phillipe Pinel as a major founding father of modern psychiatry.

Emil Kraepelin and some of the members of his department of psychiatry in Munich are shown in Figure 1-1. Brodmann, also a member of this department for a time, is not in this particular picture. The assemblage of Kraepelin, Alzheimer, Brodmann, and Nissl within a single department of psychiatry was a remarkable achievement.

Kraepelin sought to combine careful clinical description with good basic neuroscience. Kraepelin himself was a superb clinician and teacher who provided us with the classification of major mental illnesses that we still use. Combining information about age at onset with the natural history and longitudinal course of disorders, he differentiated dementia praecox (now referred to as schizophrenia) from dementia in the elderly (now referred to as Alzheimer's disease), paranoia (now referred to as delusional disorder), and manic-depressive illness (now referred to as bipolar affective disorder). He did this by observing that some individuals develop intellectual deterioration at a young age and fail to recover, whereas others develop this deterioration relatively late in life; he decided the former individuals had a discrete illness that he referred to as dementia praecox, whereas the latter had a very different illness because of their long period of intact functioning before the onset of dementia. He distinguished between dementia praecox and manic-depressive illness because the former had a relatively chronic course leading to deterioration, whereas the latter was typically episodic with full remission between episodes of psychosis.

As Kraepelin and others within his department laid out this nosological structure, they then applied the techniques of neuroscience to the study of postmortem brain specimens from patients whom they had known during life. Alzheimer observed that the elderly demented patients had characteristic neuropathological lesions, consisting of plaques and tangles; these became the neuropathological indicator of what we now know as Alzheimer's disease. Similar characteristic lesions were sought in schizophrenia and manic-depressive illness, but none were found, though occasional abnormalities were noted in frontal and temporal regions. Kraepelin and his group were convinced that the major mental illnesses would ultimately be understood in terms of aberrations in neural functions. The goals that they set for themselves at the turn of the 19th century remain those that we have set for ourselves at the turn of the 20th century.

In this era, achievements were also being made for the first time in the domain of somatic therapy. Working in Vienna, another contemporary of Freud and Kraepelin, Julius Wagner-Jauregg, accidentally observed in 1887 that infection with malaria had a beneficial effect on patients suffering from psychosis. This eventually led him to conduct a formal set of experiments 20 years later in which he infected with malaria a group of patients suffering from syphilis, a disorder largely under the care of psychiatrists because of its severe cognitive, behavioral, and emotional symptoms. The treatment was so effective that Wagner-Jauregg was later awarded a Nobel prize for this discovery in 1927. Malarial treatment for syphilis remained a standard part of the therapeutic armamentarium until the discovery of penicillin.

In the early 20th century, other relatively crude and nonspecific treatments were also developed. These included the introduction of insulin shock therapy as a treatment for psychosis by Manfred Sakel in 1927 and the later development of electroshock therapy by Ugo Cerletti and Lucio Bini in 1938. Although most of the older forms of somatic therapy have now been supplanted by more specific methods of modulating brain chemistry through medications (see Chapter 24), electroconvulsive therapy is still widely used and highly effective in a small subgroup of psychiatric patients suffering primarily from severe mood disorders.

The Development of Psychoanalysis

Psychoanalysis was developed in the late 19th and early 20th centuries as well. Because of its widespread popular appeal, the history of psychoanalysis is much better known than that of the neuroscience traditions of psychiatry. It is important to realize, however, that psychoanalysis actually had its beginnings within the tradition of neuroscience. Sigmund Freud, the founder of the psychoanalytic method, spent his early career thinking about cerebral specialization, higher cortical functions, and their relationship to the symptoms of mental illness. He embodied this thinking in a treatise, *A Project for a Scientific Psychology*, in which he suggested that most specific symptoms of mental illness could be understood in terms of brain mechanisms.

Methods for investigating brain-behavior relationships were still relatively limited in the early 20th century, however, consisting largely of neuroanatomy and neuropathology, with only a modest amount of neuropharmacology and neurophysiology. Thus, Freud himself turned to another fruitful avenue, the observation of clinical phenomena combined with speculations and hypotheses about their underlying psychic mechanisms. Unlike Kraepelin and his group, Freud was less interested in symptoms of psychosis and more interested in the symptoms referred to as conversion or hysterical phenomena. These symptoms consisted of peculiar, unexplained pains and paralyses that afflicted many individuals in the early 20th century.

Freud's earliest thoughts on this subject, contained in *Studies on Hysteria* (co-authored with Josef Breuer), contained the fundamental ideas that were the basis for what was later to become the extensive field of psychoanalysis. Based on his own experience in treating patients who suffered from the sudden onset of paralyses or seizures with no obvious physical cause, Freud speculated that these symptoms could be due to some type of trauma that occurred early in life and remained embedded in the psyche and caused irritation: "The memory of the trauma acts like a foreign body which long after its entry must continue to be regarded as an agent that is still at work." He observed that releasing these embedded memories, either through hypnosis or through free association, sometimes led to the remission of symptoms. This led to Freud and Breuer's famous pronouncement: "Hysterics suffer mainly from reminiscences" (p. 7).

These early ideas led to the extensive development of theories of psychological structure and function, such as the id, ego, and superego, as well as various methods of psychotherapy for manipulating psychological structures and functions and reducing symptomatology. Psychoanalysis also extensively explored human sexuality, a courageous step at a time when most people were bound by rigid Victorian inhibitions about what they were allowed to say, think, or do. Because of its imagination and courage, the work of Freud and his disciples gained widespread respect. The methods that he developed for clinical management of milder psychiatric syndromes gained popularity and are still in use today, mostly in modified form.

The Second Era of Neuroscience

The term *neuroscience* did not in fact exist during the 19th or early 20th century. Kraepelin, Alzheimer, Nissl, and Brodmann would have described themselves as "brain scientists." By the early to mid-20th century, however, a new array of techniques had been developed that have permitted brain scientists to go far beyond the simple processes of looking at neurons under the microscope or studying the gross structure of the brain. Developments in neuropharmacology, neurochemistry, molecular biology and molecular genetics, and various other related fields have been extraordinary. These developments led to the founding of a society of neuroscience in 1970, so that scientists working in the diverse areas related to the nervous system could meet and communicate with one another. By 1989, the Society for Neuroscience had gained approximately 15,000 members, making it one of the largest scientific organizations in the United States.

The vast array of techniques now available for studying the nervous system has rekindled the strong connections between psychiatry and neuroscience. Many psychiatrists believe that the dream (shared by Kraepelin and Freud) of understanding mental phenomena in terms of neural mechanisms now lies within our reach.

The growth of knowledge and expertise in neuroscience can be easily summarized by examining the history of Nobel prize awards since their inception (Table 1-2). Early awards were given for microscopic techniques and for clinical achievements. Two awards, to Wagner-Jauregg for malarial treatment of syphilis, and to Moniz for the development of prefrontal leukotomy to treat schizophrenia, have been purely clinical. Others have been given more recently in basic areas that have laid important foundations for clinical applications, such as Axelrod's studies of neurotransmission within the catecholamine system. The listing in Table 1-2 indicates that there has been a steady increase in prizes awarded in the area of neuroscience during the past several decades.

For any Nobel prize given in any single year, there are of course dozens of other equally deserving individuals who have made major contributions to science and clinical practice. For example, Nobel prizes have not been awarded for positron-emission tomography, a far more powerful imaging technique than computerized tomography, nor for neuroleptic drugs or antidepressants, which have been far more lasting and powerful ameliorators of human suffering than prefrontal leukotomy. Nevertheless, this list of Nobel laureates indicates that our knowledge base in neuroscience and in its clinical applications has been steadily advancing.

Within psychiatry as a specialized discipline, the major sources of impact from neuroscience have been neuropharmacology and neurochemistry. Coupled with the overall development in neuroscience, the discovery of relatively potent pharmacologic treatments for major mental illnesses has also served to reawaken interest in clinical neurobiology. The discovery of chlorpromazine by Delay and Deniker in 1952 indicated that drugs could be developed that would have a powerful calming effect on psychotic and agitated patients. This discovery led rapidly to the development of a variety of neuroleptic drugs that are used for the treatment of psychosis. By the late 1950s, a second new specific class of medications had been developed, the antidepressants, the prototype of which is imipramine. Antianxiety drugs such as meprobamate were also developed. By the early 1960s, it had become clear to psychiatrists that an entire new discipline, psychopharmacology, was at their feet, and that this discipline provided a powerful alternative to the techniques of psy-

Table 1-2. Nobel prizes awarded in neuroscience and psychiatry

Year	Investigators	Discovery
1906	Camillo Golgi and Santiago Ramón y Cajal	Work on structure of the nervous system
1927	Julius Wagner-Jauregg	Discovery of the therapeutic importance of malaria inoculation in dementia paralytica
1932	Edgar D. Adrian and Sir Charles Scott Sherrington	Discoveries regarding function of the neurons
1936	Sir Henry H. Dale and Otto Loewi	Discoveries relating to the chemical transmission of nerve impulses
1944	Joseph Erlanger and Herbert S. Gasser	Research on the differentiated function of single nerve fibers
1949	Walter Rudolf Hess	Discovery of the functional organization of the midbrain as coordinator of the activities of the internal organs
1949	Antonio Egas Moniz	Discovery of the therapeutic value of leukotomy in certain psychoses
1963	Sir John C. Eccles, Sir Alan Lloyd Hodgkin, and Andrew F. Huxley	Study of the transmission of nerve impulses along a nerve fiber (or relationship between inhibition of nerve cells and repolarization of a cell's membrane)
1970	Julius Axelrod, Sir Bernard Katz, and Ulf von Euler	Discoveries concerning the chemistry of nerve transmission
1971	Earl Wilbur Sutherland, Jr.	Study of hormones, the chemical substances that regulate virtually every body function
1977	Rosalyn S. Yalow	Radioimmunoassay
1977	Roger C.L. Guillemin and Andrew V. Schally	Production of peptide hormones in the brain
1979	Earl Hounsfield and Sir Allan M. Cormack	Development of computerized tomography
1981	Roger W. Sperry, David H. Hubel, and Tosten N. Wiesel	Studies on the function of the corpus callosum (split brain research, functions of left and right hemispheres). Discoveries on the organization of the visual system
1986	Rita Levi-Montalcini and Stanley Cohen	Discovery of nerve growth factor

chotherapy that had been their major means of treating patients up to this point. Psychopharmacology (also referred to as *neuropharmacology* or *neuropsychopharmacology*) was clearly not only a tool for treatment, but also a tool for studying brain chemistry and for developing new classifications of diseases based on their responses to specific drugs that manipulated specific classes of chemicals within the brain.

These developments have placed psychiatry in the 1990s squarely within the traditions of medicine and neuroscience. To an interest in neuropharmacology have been added neuroimaging and molecular biology. The modern student of psychiatry must simultaneously view patients on multiple planes: as human beings suffering from particular symptoms (psychological), as individuals living within a social and cultural context (social), as products of the genetic endowments given them by their parents and coded in their chromosomes (genetic-molecular), and as individuals whose ideas and emotions are both the product and the producers of a complex set of chemical events in their brains (neurochemical-neuroanatomical).

The Mind/Body Problem in Psychiatry

As this brief summary of the history of psychiatry indicates, people have not consistently agreed about the origins of mental illness or the appropriate areas of expertise for the clinicians who treat mental illness. Although the historical origins of psychiatry are clearly biological, in that the first individuals to identify and define mental illness in classical times believed that these illnesses were physical in origin, for many centuries people have also believed mental illnesses to be caused by a disease of the "spirit" or "psyche." From the Middle Ages up through the 18th or 19th century, the mentally ill were perceived as spiritually or morally diseased. Although the bulk of contemporary psychiatrists no longer hold this belief, there are literally centuries of misunderstanding that must be forgotten or eliminated. Old ideas do not die easily, and consequently, mental illnesses tend to be stigmatized or misunderstood. The role of psychiatry is confused as well. Many lay people still view psychiatrists as literally "doctors of the mind, or soul."

Part of this misunderstanding is also contributed by a long-standing controversy about the relationship between the mind and the body. Many religions teach that there is a soul or spirit that exists independently of the body and that survives it after death. People who think concretely and metaphorically tend to see soul or spirit as a tiny ghost sitting somewhere in the body (usually in the brain in modern thinking) and moving or guiding its actions. The existence of the spirit or soul is fundamentally a philosophical or religious issue, not a scientific or medical one. There is simply no way to prove or disprove the existence of the soul and its continuing existence after death. That is a matter of faith.

It is clear that, on at least one level, what is commonly referred to as the "mind" is simply the summation of a variety of electrical and chemical events occurring in the brain. Thinking, believing, remembering, feeling, tasting, and all the other cognitive, sensory, and behavioral functions that humans experience are fundamentally determined at the molecular level, within a context of neural networks. These events do not exist independently of external environmental influences, but rather are influenced by and react to them. Head injuries damage neurons and cause new networks to be developed. Perceptions and experiences are encoded and "remembered," and this learning and memory affects later cognitive events. Thus, mental phenomena, often referred to as "mind," can and must be understood in terms of the brain.

The study of psychiatry, the branch of medicine devoted to the study of mental illnesses, is, therefore, a discipline dedicated to the investigation of abnormalities in brain function. The clinical appearance of these abnormalities may be florid and obvious, as in the case of psychosis. They may be subtle and mild, as in the case of personality disorders. Ultimately, the drive of modern psychiatry is to develop a comprehensive understanding of normal brain function at levels that range from mind to molecule, and to determine how aberrations in these normal functions (produced either endogenously through genetic coding, or exogenously through environmental influences) lead to the development of symptoms of mental illnesses.

Bibliography

Ackerknecht EH: Short History of Psychiatry. New York, Hafner, 1968

Alexander FG, Selesnick ST: The History of Psychiatry: An Evaluation of Psychiatric Thought and Practice From Prehistoric Times to the Present. New York, Harper & Row, 1966

Andreasen NC: The Broken Brain: The Biological Revolution in Psychiatry. New York, Harper & Row, 1984

Freud S, Breuer J: Studies on Hysteria. Translated by Strachey J. New York, Basic Books, 1957

Gilman SL: Seeing the Insane. New York, John Wiley, 1982

Kraepelin E: Lectures on Clinical Psychiatry. London, Bailliere, Tindall & Cox, 1904

Pichot P: A Century of Psychiatry. Paris, Editions Roger Dacosta, 1983

Pinel P: A Treatise on Insanity. London, Messrs Cadell and Davies, 1806

Rush B: Two Essays on the Mind. Philadelphia, PA, Charles Cist, 1786

Zilboorg G: A History of Medical Psychology. New York, WW Norton, 1941

Self-assessment Questions

1. Describe Greek attitudes toward mental illness. What were the four humors?
2. Describe attitudes toward the mentally ill during the Middle Ages. How long ago was the last witch known to be tormented or burned at the stake?
3. Describe the ideas and accomplishments of Phillipe Pinel.
4. Who was Emil Kraepelin? Name two eminent neuroscientists who were members of his department.
5. Wagner-Jauregg and Moniz received Nobel prizes for clinical achievements. What were they? Describe two more recent achievements that received Nobel prizes and that provide a link between neuroscience and psychiatry.

Chapter 2
Diagnosis and Classification

Knowledge keeps no better than fish.

Alfred North Whitehead

Beginning students of psychiatry are often puzzled as to what is expected of them when they are asked to make a diagnosis. This is because two major traditions for observing and understanding patients coexist within psychiatry: the biological model and the psychodynamic model. The biological model is closely allied with general medicine and stresses an orientation that involves identifying discrete disorders that a patient is experiencing. The psychodynamic model, on the other hand, stresses the importance of understanding the patient's complaints and behavior in terms of their underlying dynamics. A psychiatrist applying the biological or medical model attempts to determine whether the patient has one of the group of commonly recognized disorders, such as schizophrenia or bipolar illness, and then plans the care of the patient accordingly. A psychiatrist applying the psychodynamic model attempts to understand why patients present with a particular complaint, often in terms of relationships with parents or early life experiences, and then seeks to help patients change maladaptive behavior or reduce psychological pain by helping them understand and readjust these dynamics. Both of these approaches are legitimate and appropriate in particular circumstances. The second is a highly specialized field within psychiatry, however, and is outside the general range of this volume. Thus the focus of this chapter, and the remainder of this book, is primarily on diagnosis in the first sense: the recognition of discrete disorders, their relationship to one another, and their implications for patient care.

Fundamental Purpose of Diagnosis and Classification

The fundamental purpose of diagnosis and classification is to isolate a group of discrete disease entities, each of which is characterized by a distinct pathophysiology and/or etiology. Ideally, all diseases in medicine would be defined in terms of etiology. For most illnesses, however, we do not know or understand the specific etiology. By and large, a full understanding of etiology is limited to the infectious diseases, where the etiology is due to exposure to some infectious agent to a degree sufficient that the body's immune mechanisms are overwhelmed (and even in this instance, our knowledge of immune mechanisms is incomplete). Other diseases for which we understand the etiology are various hereditary metabolic diseases, such as phenylketonuria (PKU). We have been able to define these diseases in terms of a specific metabolic defect (e.g., failure to metabolize phenylalanine) and have traced that metabolic defect to a specific genetic locus that produces an abnormal protein. The case of PKU, however, illustrates how complex the search for causes can actually be. We now know that there are two forms of PKU; both are characterized by failure to metabolize phenylalanine, but they involve two different enzymes within the metabolic pathway. Thus, even for a simple disease with a recognized metabolic defect, increasing knowledge can also increase complexity. Now this simple disease must be understood as two different diseases with two different specific causes at the molecular level.

For most diseases, however, our understanding is at the level of pathophysiology rather than etiology. Diseases are defined in terms of the mechanisms that produce particular symptoms, such as infarction in the myocardium, inflammation in the joints, or abnormal regulation of insulin production.

In the areas of pathophysiology and etiology, psychiatry lags even farther behind than the rest of medicine. Most of the disorders or diseases diagnosed in psychiatry are simply syndromes—collections of symptoms that tend to occur together and that appear to have a characteristic course and outcome. The research community in psychiatry is working hard toward the goal of defining specific mental illnesses in terms of pathophysiology and etiology, but this goal has been achieved for only a few disorders (Alzheimer's disease, multi-infarct dementia, Huntington's chorea, and substance-induced syndromes such as amphetamine psychosis or the Wernicke-Korsakoff syndrome).

Purposes of Diagnosis in Psychiatry

Even though they do not contain information about specific mechanisms or causes for an identified group of symptoms, diagnoses in psychiatry serve a variety of important purposes. Thus, making a careful diagnosis is as fundamental in psychiatry as it is in the remainder of medicine.

Diagnosis helps to simplify our thinking and reduce the complexity of clinical phenomena in psychiatry. Psychiatry is a very diverse field, and symptoms of mental illness encompass a broad range of emotional, cognitive, and behavioral

Table 2-1. DSM-III-R classification

Disorders usually first evident in infancy, childhood, or adolescence
  Developmental disorders
    Mental retardation
    Pervasive developmental disorders
    Specific developmental disorders
  Disruptive behavior disorders
  Anxiety disorders of childhood or adolescence
  Eating disorders
  Gender identity disorders
  Tic disorders
  Elimination disorders
  Speech disorders not elsewhere classified
  Other disorders of infancy, childhood, or adolescence
Organic mental disorders
  Dementias arising in the senium and presenium
  Psychoactive substance–induced organic disorders
  Organic mental disorders associated with Axis III physical disorders or conditions, or
    disorders whose etiology is unknown
Psychoactive substance use disorders
Schizophrenia
Delusional (paranoid) disorder
Psychotic disorders not elsewhere classified
Mood disorders
  Bipolar disorders
  Depressive disorders
Anxiety disorders
Somatoform disorders
Dissociative disorders
Sexual disorders
  Paraphilias
  Sexual dysfunctions
Sleep disorders
  Dyssomnias
  Parasomnias
Factitious disorders
Disorders of impulse control not elsewhere classified
Adjustment disorders
Psychological factors affecting physical conditions
Personality disorders

---

abnormalities. The use of diagnoses introduces order and structure to this complexity. Disorders are divided into broad classes, based on common features (e.g., psychosis, substance abuse, dementia, anxiety). The overall structure of the current psychiatric classification system used in this text is summarized in Table 2-1. Within each of the major classes, specific syndromes are then further delineated (e.g., dividing substance abuse in terms of the type of substance involved, dividing the dementias into Alzheimer's disease and multi-infarct dementia). The existence of broad groups of diagnostic categories, subdivided into specific disorders, creates a structure within the apparent chaos of clinical phenomena and makes mental illnesses easier to learn about and understand. Although diagnoses are not necessarily defined in terms of etiology or pathophysiology, they are typically defined in terms of clinical features. Thus, this creation of order out of chaos does not misrepresent reality in the process of facilitating understanding.

Psychiatric diagnoses facilitate communication between clinicians. When a physician gives a patient a specific diagnosis, such as bipolar affective disorder, he or she is making a specific statement about the clinical picture with which that particular patient presents. A diagnosis concisely summarizes information for all other clinicians who subsequently examine the patient's records, or to whom the patient is referred. A diagnosis of bipolar affective disorder, for example, indicates that the patient has suffered from at least one episode of mania; during that episode of mania the patient will have experienced a characteristic group of symptoms such as elated mood, increased energy, racing thoughts, rapid speech, grandiosity, and poor judgment; the patient has probably had episodes of depression as well, characterized by sadness, insomnia, decreased appetite, feelings of worthlessness, and other typical depressive symptoms. The use of diagnostic categories gives clinicians a kind of "shorthand" through which they can summarize large quantities of information relatively easily.

Diagnoses help to predict the outcome of the disorder. Many psychiatric diagnoses are associated with a characteristic course and outcome. For example, bipolar illness is usually episodic with periods of relatively severe abnormalities in mood interspersed with periods of near normality or complete normality. Most patients with bipolar affective disorder have a relatively good outcome. Some other types of disorders, such as schizophrenia or personality disorders, typically run a more chronic course. Diagnoses are a useful way of summarizing the clinician's expectations about the patient's course of illness in the future.

Diagnoses are often used to decide on an appropriate treatment. As psychiatry has advanced clinically and scientifically, relatively specific treatments for particular disorders or groups of symptoms have been developed. For example, neuroleptic drugs are typically used to treat psychoses. Thus, they will be used for disorders such as schizophrenia, in which psychosis is typically prominent, as well as forms of affective disorder in which psychotic symptoms occur. A diagnosis of mania suggests the use of medications such as lithium carbonate or carbamazepine. Some relatively targeted medications are now available, such as clomipramine for obsessive-compulsive disorder or alprazolam for panic disorder.

Diagnoses are used to assist in the search for pathophysiology and etiology. Clinical researchers use diagnoses to reduce heterogeneity in their samples and to separate groups of patients who may share a common mechanism or cause that produces their symptoms. Patients who share a relatively specific set of symptoms, such as severe schizophrenia characterized by negative symptoms, are often hypothesized to have a disorder that is mechanistically or etiologically distinct. Knowledge about specific groupings of clinical symptoms can be related to knowledge about brain specialization and function in order to formulate hypotheses about the neurochemical or anatomical substrates of a particular disorder. Ideally, the use of diagnoses defined on the basis of clinical picture will lead ultimately to diagnoses that serve the fundamental purpose of identifying causes.

Development of the *Diagnostic and Statistical Manual of Mental Disorders*

The process of diagnosis in psychiatry is partially simplified because the national professional organization to which most psychiatrists belong, the American Psychiatric Association (APA), has formulated a manual that summarizes all the diagnoses used in psychiatry, specifies the symptoms that must be present to make a given diagnosis, and organizes these diagnoses together into a classificatory system. This handbook is referred to as the *Diagnostic and Statistical Manual of Mental Disorders* (DSM). Over the years, it has gone through two major revisions (DSM-II and DSM-III) and a more recent minor revision (DSM-III-R). Currently, diagnoses in psychiatry are based on DSM-III-R. A third major revision, DSM-IV, is currently in progress and will be available in 1993.

Psychiatry is the only specialty in medicine that has so consistently and comprehensively formalized the diagnostic processes for the disorders within its domain. This precision and structure is particularly important in psychiatry because it lacks recognized etiologies for most disorders, and it lacks specific laboratory diagnostic tests as well. Consequently, diagnosis relies largely on the patient's presenting symptoms and past history. Without such structure, the diagnostic process could become confused and fuzzy.

The impetus to organize DSM began during World War II. For the first time, psychiatrists from all over the United States were brought together in clinical settings that required them to communicate clearly with one another. It became apparent that diagnostic practices varied widely throughout the United States, no doubt reflecting a diversity of training. After the second World War, the Veterans Administration attempted to design a relatively comprehensive diagnostic system for its own use. Shortly thereafter, the APA convened a task force to develop a diagnostic manual for use in all of American psychiatry. The product was DSM-I, which was published in 1952. The first revision, DSM-II, was published in 1968.

Compared with DSM-III and DSM-III-R, the more recent manuals, DSM-I and DSM-II were relatively simple. The definitions of disorders and the overall classification system were designed by a small group of clinicians who convened, discussed their clinical experiences, and decided together on appropriate categories and defining features. Definitions tended to be brief, descriptive, and relatively vague. For example, the definition of manic-depressive illness in DSM-II was as follows:

Manic-depressive illnesses (Manic-depressive psychoses)

These disorders are marked by severe mood swings and a tendency to remission and recurrence. Patients may be given this diagnosis in the absence of a previous history of affective psychosis if there is no obvious precipitating event. This disorder is divided into three major subtypes: manic type, depressed type, and circular type. (p. 8)

These handbooks were both relatively small. DSM-I contained 132 pages, and DSM-II contained only 119 pages.

DSM-III, by contrast, represented a major change and, most clinicians would concur, a major improvement. Because of their vagueness and imprecision, the definitions in DSM-I and DSM-II did not adequately fulfill many of the purposes summarized above. In particular, the descriptions were not specific enough to facilitate communication among clinicians and to delineate one disorder from another. Although the purpose of DSM-I and DSM-II was to ensure that a psychiatrist in Peoria, Illinois, meant the same thing by a diagnosis of schizophrenia as a psychiatrist on Park Avenue in New York City or in Laguna Beach, California, this was clearly not the case.

Numerous research investigations had examined diagnostic agreement between clinicians. They had made it clear that, using DSM-I or DSM-II guidelines, different clinicians would give different diagnoses to the same patient. Naturally, this lack of consensus and agreement about how to diagnose patients called the credibility of psychiatry into question. These research studies of poor agreement, completed during the 1960s, coincided with the development of relatively specific new medications such as neuroleptics and antidepressants. When relatively specific treatments for particular disorders became available, it was clearly important to define the disorders well so appropriate treatment would be prescribed.

When the DSM-III task force was appointed in 1972, its members decided to set a new agenda for the development of the DSMs. Many members of this task force were eminent researchers with expertise in disciplines such as pharmacology or genetics. Thus, they were especially aware of the importance of diagnostic precision. At their first meetings, they decided to formulate a set of rules by which they would abide: they would attempt to formulate specific diagnostic criteria that would be as objective as possible in order to define each of the disorders included in the manual; they would make their decisions about defining criteria and overall organizational structure based on existing research data whenever possible; they would not resort to anecdotal approaches or simple clinical opinion if at all possible; they would include a glossary to define terms used in the text; in addition to the criteria, they would provide clinicians with information that would assist them in understanding specific disorders better, such as population frequency, sex ratio, or longitudinal course; and they would provide a set of references that would support their decisions. Apart from the last rule, which was not feasible because of the large quantity of references that would have been needed, these rules were followed relatively closely.

When DSM-III finally appeared in 1980, it was widely recognized as a major innovation. Although some clinicians complained that it was "boring" or "dull," most appreciated its objectivity. For the first time, the methods by which a psychiatric diagnosis could be made were relatively clear. The process has been somewhat facetiously referred to as the "Chinese menu approach" to diagnosis. Most of the time, the criteria require that a specified subset from a listed group of symptoms be required in order to make a diagnosis (e.g., four out of eight). For example, in contrast to the rather vague definition of manic-depressive illness above, the DSM-III definition of major depressive disorder is as follows:

Diagnostic criteria for Major Depression

A. One or more major depressive episodes
B. Has never had a manic episode

Diagnostic criteria for major depressive episode

A. Dysphoric mood or loss of interest or pleasure in all or almost all usual activities and pastimes. The dysphoric mood is characterized by symptoms such as the following: depressed, sad, blue, hopeless, low, down in the dumps, irritable. The mood disturbance must be prominent and relatively persistent, but not necessarily the most dominant symptom, and does not include momentary shifts from one dysphoric mood to another dysphoric mood, e.g., anxiety to depression to anger, such as are seen in states of acute psychotic turmoil. (For children under 6, dysphoric mood may have to be inferred from a persistently sad facial expression.)
B. At least four of the following symptoms have been present nearly every day for a period of at least 2 weeks (in children under 6, at least three of the first four).
   (1) poor appetite or significant weight loss (when not dieting) or increased appetite or significant weight gain (in children under 6, consider failure to make expected weight gains)
   (2) insomnia or hypersomnia
   (3) psychomotor agitation or retardation (but not merely subjective feelings of restlessness or being slowed down) (in children under 6, hypoactivity)
   (4) loss of interest or pleasure in usual activities, or decrease in sexual drive not limited to a period when delusional or hallucinating (in children under 6, signs of apathy)
   (5) loss of energy; fatigue
   (6) feelings of worthlessness, self-reproach, or excessive or inappropriate guilt (either may be delusional)
   (7) complaints or evidence of diminished ability to think or concentrate, such as slowed thinking, or indecisiveness not associated with marked loosening of associations or incoherence
   (8) recurrent thoughts of death, suicidal ideation, wishes to be dead, or suicide attempt
C. Neither of the following dominates the clinical picture when an affective syndrome is absent (i.e., symptoms in criteria A and B above):
   (1) preoccupation with a mood-incongruent delusion or hallucination
   (2) bizarre behavior
D. Not superimposed on either schizophrenia, schizophreniform disorder, or a paranoid disorder

E. Not due to any organic mental disorder or uncomplicated bereavement (pp. 213–214, 218)

Shortly after DSM-III appeared, minor errors and inconsistencies were noted—an inevitable consequence of the first effort to provide a comprehensive and detailed diagnostic manual. (In contrast to its predecessors, DSM-III was 494 pages long.) Various minor revisions were introduced, leading to the publication of DSM-III-R (i.e., a revised version of DSM-III) in 1987.

Advantages of the DSM Approach

The DSM-III approach has many advantages.

DSM-III substantially improved the reliability of diagnosis. Reliability, a biometric concept, refers to the ability of two observers to agree on what they see. It is measured by various statistical methods, such as percent agreement, correlation coefficients, or the kappa statistic, which corrects for chance agreement. The reliability of DSM-III was assessed in field trials and found to be relatively good. The original field-trial data for some diagnostic categories, based on kappa, are summarized in Table 2-2. A kappa of 0.8 or greater is considered very good, and

Table 2-2. Kappa coefficients of agreement for DSM-III Axes I and II diagnostic classes for adults (18 and older)

	Phase 1 (*n* = 339)		Phase 2 (*n* = 331)	
	Kappa	**% of sample**	**Kappa**	**% of sample**
Axis I				
Disorders usually first evident in infancy, childhood, or adolescence	.65	5.3	.73	3.6
Organic mental disorders	.79	11.8	.76	10.0
Substance use disorders	.86	21.2	.80	21.2
Schizophrenic disorders	.81	17.7	.81	23.3
Paranoid disorders	.66	1.2	.75	1.5
Psychotic disorders not elsewhere classified	.64	11.2	.69	6.7
Mood disorders	.69	43.1	.83	38.7
Anxiety disorders	.63	9.1	.72	8.8
Somatoform disorders	.54	3.8	.42	3.3
Dissociative disorders	.80	0.9	− .003	0.6
Psychosexual disorders	.92	2.1	.75	1.5
Factitious disorders	.66	1.2	− .005	0.9
Disorders of impulse control not elsewhere classified	.28	1.8	.80	1.8
Adjustment disorders	.67	12.1	.68	8.5
Psychological factors affecting physical condition	.62	3.2	.44	2.1
Overall kappa for Axis I	.68		.72	
Axis II				
Specific developmental disorders			.40	1.2
Personality disorders	.56	59.9	.65	49.8
Overall kappa for Axis II	.56		.64	

a kappa between 0.5 and 0.8 is considered acceptable. The kappas in Table 2-2 are generally in this range. By contrast, percent agreements (which are not even corrected for chance agreement) for disorders such as depression or schizophrenia had been estimated as low as 20–30% in several studies before DSM-III was published.

DSM-III clarified the diagnostic process and facilitated history taking.   Because DSM-III specifies exactly which symptoms must be present to make a diagnosis and the characteristic course of disorders whenever this is appropriate, it is highly objective. Because of the prevalence of psychodynamic training, which de-emphasized a medical approach to diagnosis, many clinicians during the 1970s received minimal training in the recognition of signs and symptoms; instead, they developed psychodynamic formulations. DSM-III provided an alternative approach to making a medical diagnosis based on signs and symptoms, because it lists systematically which signs must be observed and which symptoms must be inquired about. This structured approach also makes it an excellent teaching tool for medical students and residents.

DSM-III clarified and facilitated the process of differential diagnosis.   Again, because it is so explicit, it helps clinicians decide which symptoms must be present to rule in or rule out a particular diagnosis. For example, it specifies that a diagnosis of schizophrenia cannot be made if a full affective syndrome is present. Likewise, a diagnosis of schizophrenia cannot be made if some type of "organic" factor such as amphetamine abuse has led to the presence of psychotic symptoms. Not only are differential diagnostic issues embedded in the criteria, but the text of DSM-III also contains a relatively detailed discussion of the differential diagnosis for each disorder.

Disadvantages of the DSM Approach

Every paradise has its serpent and poisoned apple. Thus, DSM-III and DSM-III-R also have certain problems and disadvantages.

The increased precision has given clinicians and researchers a false sense of certainty about what they are doing.   The DSM-III criteria are simple provisional agreements, arrived at by a group of experts, on what characteristic features must be present to make a diagnosis. Although the criteria were based on data whenever possible, often inadequate data were available to build the criteria totally on a scientific data base. Thus, the selection of signs and symptoms was often relatively arbitrary. The diagnoses themselves are certainly arbitrary. They will remain arbitrary as long as we are ignorant about pathophysiology and etiology. Medical students and residents often crave certainty (as do many physicians long out of training), and so they want very much to believe that a given DSM-III or DSM-III-R diagnosis refers to some "real thing." Thus, DSM sometimes leads clinicians to lapse into petty and pointless debates about whether a patient "really" is depressed if he or she does or does not meet DSM-III criteria. The criteria should be seen for what they are: a useful tool that introduces structure, but is arbitrary in essence. They should be applied with a healthy sense of skepticism.

DSM-III may sacrifice validity to reliability. Whereas reliability refers to the capacity of individuals to agree on what they see, validity refers to the capacity to make useful predictions. In particular, the validity of a medical diagnostic system refers to the ability to predict prognosis and outcome, response to treatment, and ultimately etiology. Put simply, reliability refers to whether something can be measured precisely, whereas validity refers to whether it is worth measuring at all. Psychodynamically oriented clinicians have objected that DSM has sacrificed some of psychiatry's most clinically important concepts, because psychodynamic explanations and descriptions are by and large excluded from DSM. More biologically oriented psychiatrists have objected to the lack of validity in DSM as well. In this instance, they point to the arbitrary nature of the definitions, which are not rooted in information about biological causes. Some descriptions of disorders have excluded clinically important symptoms because they are more difficult to define reliably; an excellent example is the minimal inclusion of the negative symptoms of schizophrenia (e.g., apathy, amotivation) in DSM-III and DSM-III-R.

Overview of DSM-III-R Nosology

As Table 2-1 indicates, the various diagnoses that can be given to psychiatric patients are divided among a substantial number of main categories or headings. A more detailed description of the various diagnoses under these headings appears in Section II of this book, where specific diagnoses are discussed in detail.

Disorders usually first evident in infancy, childhood, or adolescence include a large variety of conditions that typically begin before adulthood, although some (e.g., the eating disorders such as anorexia nervosa) are included here even though they often occur in adults as well. Likewise, some disorders that are often observed in children and adolescents, such as depression or schizophrenia, are not classified here because the preponderance of individuals with these diagnoses are adults, and the clinical syndromes are essentially the same in both children and adults. The developmental disorders include mental retardation, pervasive developmental disorder (autism), and specific developmental disorders (specific learning disabilities such as developmental arithmetic disorder). The disruptive behavior disorders include some of the most common conditions seen in children, such as attention-deficit (hyperactivity) disorder and the various conduct disorders. The anxiety disorders include conditions such as separation anxiety, and the eating disorders include anorexia nervosa, bulimia nervosa, and pica. The gender identity disorders include conditions such as transsexualism. The tic disorders include Tourette's disorder and other tic syndromes. The elimination disorders include encopresis and enuresis. Speech disorders include conditions such as stuttering.

Organic mental disorders include the various dementias such as Alzheimer's disease, multi-infarct dementia, Huntington's chorea, and Creutzfeldt-Jakob disease. The psychoactive substance–induced disorders include the various syndromes that occur as a consequence of substance abuse. These vary depending on the substance. For example, the alcohol-induced disorders include intoxication, withdrawal, hallucinosis, amnestic disorder, and dementia associated with alcoholism (i.e., Wernicke-Korsakoff syndrome). The syndromes produced by cocaine include intoxication, withdrawal, delirium, and delusional disorder. Finally, a group of syndromes are specified that often occur in association with specific medical conditions ("organic mental disorders associated with Axis III physical disorders"). These refer to syndromes that occur secondary to medical illness, such as delirium, dementia, amnestic disorder, delusional disorder, etc. For example, delirium frequently occurs as a consequence of metabolic disorders, surgical or other trauma, and/or sensory deprivation occurring in an intensive care unit. Amnestic disorders or organic personality disorders often occur as the long-term consequence of head injury or seizure disorders.

Psychoactive substance use disorders include the various conditions that occur as a consequence of substance abuse, such as alcohol dependence or abuse, amphetamine dependence or abuse, cannabis dependence or abuse, etc. When these affect cognition, an organic disorder may be diagnosed as well (e.g., Wernicke-Korsakoff syndrome).

Schizophrenia is a severe psychotic disorder that is among the most common psychiatric disorders. It is characterized by a variety of psychotic symptoms, such as delusions or hallucinations, and social withdrawal and intellectual impoverishment; patients often have a chronic and deteriorating course.

Delusional (paranoid) disorder is a relatively rare condition in which patients display delusions in the context of a well-preserved personality and normal cognition. Patients with delusional disorder typically do not deteriorate.

Psychotic disorders not elsewhere classified includes various conditions related to schizophrenia, such as schizophreniform disorder (similar to schizophrenia, but of briefer duration), brief reactive psychosis, and schizoaffective disorder.

Mood disorders are also among the most common conditions seen in psychiatry. They are divided into two broad groups. The bipolar conditions are characterized by at least one episode of mania (and typically episodes of depression as well), whereas the depressive disorders involve only depression (and therefore are sometimes referred to as "unipolar" disorders).

Anxiety disorders also include a variety of very common conditions, such as panic disorder, agoraphobia, social phobia, simple phobia, obsessive-compulsive disorder, posttraumatic stress disorder, and generalized anxiety disorder.

Somatoform disorders represent a category in which the patient has a variety of physical complaints for which no specific etiology can be found. They include conversion disorder (unexplained paralyses, seizures, etc.), hypochondriasis, somatization disorder (a disorder characterized by multiple somatic complaints and sometimes referred to as Briquet's syndrome), and somatoform pain disorder (single, unexplained pains).

Dissociative disorders are a grouping of conditions that are relatively rare. They include multiple personality disorder, psychogenic fugue, psychogenic amnesia, and depersonalization disorder. Unlike the somatoform disorders, the essential feature of these disorders is a disturbance in identity, memory, or consciousness that cannot be explained on a physical basis.

The sexual disorders include conditions often referred to as sexual deviations (paraphilias), such as exhibitionism, pedophilia, sexual masochism, or sexual sadism. They also include specific sexual dysfunctions, such as difficulty in achieving erection or orgasm, premature ejaculation, or dyspareunia.

Sleep disorders are divided into dyssomnias and parasomnias. The dyssomnias are disorders of initiating or maintaining sleep, such as insomnia, or hypersomnia. The parasomnias include conditions more "psychological" in nature, such as nightmares, sleep terrors, and sleepwalking. These conditions are particularly common in children, but are grouped with the sleep disorders to maintain consistency.

Factitious disorders are feigned disorders in which the patient produces the symptoms intentionally; either physical or psychological symptoms may be feigned.

Disorders of impulse control not elsewhere classified include various conditions involving poor impulse control such as kleptomania, pathological gambling, or pyromania.

Adjustment disorders include a group of disorders involving a painful or maladaptive reaction to some specific stress, such as divorce, marital discord, loss of a job, etc. The adjustment disorders are further subdivided according to the type of symptomatology that the patient experiences, such as anxiety, depression, physical complaints, etc.

"Psychological factors affecting physical conditions" is a rather loose and poorly defined category that permits clinicians to note that some psychological factor contributes to the development or exacerbation of some physical problem, such as obesity, headaches, or ulcers.

Personality disorders refer to conditions in which personality traits become maladaptive. The personality disorders are divided into three "clusters." Cluster A consists of personality disorders that are symptomatically (and perhaps etiologically) related to psychotic disorders, such as paranoid personality, schizoid personality, and schizotypal personality. Cluster B includes personality disorders sometimes referred to as "acting out." People with these personality disorders are often somewhat difficult to deal with because they are erratic, unpredictable, overemotional, and self-centered. They include antisocial, borderline, histrionic, and narcissistic personality disorders. Cluster C consists of personality disorders characterized by fearfulness and anxiety. They include avoidant, dependent, obsessive-compulsive, and passive-aggressive personality disorders.

The DSM classification system is multiaxial. The term *multiaxial* refers to a system that characterizes patients in multiple ways so that the clinician is encouraged to evaluate all aspects of the patient's health and social background. The five axes used to code patient characteristics are summarized in Table 2-3.

Axis I is used to indicate the major syndromes, such as schizophrenia, bipolar disorder, or panic disorder. If several diagnoses are present, all can be noted.

Axis II is used to code disorders that arise relatively early in life and persist; specifically, developmental disorders and personality disorders are coded on this

Table 2-3. Multiaxial system of DSM-III-R

Axis I	Clinical syndromes
Axis II	Developmental disorders/personality disorders
Axis III	Physical disorders and conditions
Axis IV	Severity of psychosocial stressors
Axis V	Global assessment of functioning

axis. This is seen as a way of calling the clinician's attention to these conditions, which are often ignored (particularly the personality disorders). Patients may of course have both Axis I and Axis II diagnoses (e.g., major depressive disorder and borderline personality disorder).

Axis III is used to code the various medical conditions from which the patient suffers, such as hypertension, diabetes, or thyroid disease, that may be relevant to the patient's care. Axis III is an important component of diagnosis because it calls the clinician's attention to medical conditions that might interact with the various psychiatric disorders from which the patient suffers. It also alerts the clinician to the fact that the patient might be on medications to treat these conditions that could interact with any psychoactive drugs prescribed.

Axis IV codes the severity (i.e., none, mild, moderate, severe, extreme, catastrophic) of psychosocial stressors. Whenever possible, the clinician notes the specific stressor. Because stressors sometimes exacerbate various psychiatric con-

Table 2-4. DSM-III-R Severity of Psychosocial Stressors Scale: Adults

		Examples of stressors	
Code	Term	Acute events	Enduring circumstances
1	None	No acute events that may be relevant to the disorder	No enduring circumstances that may be relevant to the disorder
2	Mild	Broke up with boyfriend or girlfriend; started or graduated from school; child left home	Family arguments; job dissatisfaction; residence in high-crime neighborhood
3	Moderate	Marriage; marital separation; loss of job; retirement; miscarriage	Marital discord; serious financial problems; trouble with boss; being a single parent
4	Severe	Divorce; birth of first child	Unemployment; poverty
5	Extreme	Death of spouse; serious physical illness diagnosed; victim of rape	Serious chronic illness in self or child; ongoing physical or sexual abuse
6	Catastrophic	Death of child; suicide of spouse; devastating natural disaster	Captivity as hostage; concentration camp experience
0	Inadequate information, or no change in condition		

Table 2-5.   DSM-III-R Global Assessment of Functioning (GAF) Scale

Consider psychological, social, and occupational functioning on a hypothetical continuum of mental health–illness. Do not include impairment in functioning due to physical (or environmental) limitations.

Note: Use intermediate codes when appropriate, e.g., 45, 69, 72.

Code

90 | **Absent or minimal symptoms** (e.g., mild anxiety before an exam), **good functioning in all areas, interested and involved in a wide range of activities, socially effective, generally satisfied with life, no more than everyday problems or concerns** (e.g., an occasional argument with family members).
81

80 | **If symptoms are present, they are transient and expectable reactions to psychosocial stressors** (e.g., difficulty concentrating after family argument); **no more than slight impairment in social, occupational, or school functioning** (e.g., temporarily falling behind in schoolwork).
71

70 | **Some mild symptoms** (e.g., depressed mood and mild insomnia) **OR some difficulty in social, occupational, or school functioning** (e.g., occasional truancy, or theft within the household), **but generally functioning pretty well, has some meaningful interpersonal relationships.**
61

60 | **Moderate symptoms** (e.g., flat affect and circumstantial speech, occasional panic attacks) **OR moderate difficulty in social, occupational, or school functioning** (e.g., few friends, conflicts with co-workers).
51

50 | **Serious symptoms** (e.g., suicidal ideation, severe obsessional rituals, frequent shoplifting) **OR any serious impairment in social, occupational, or school functioning** (e.g., no friends, unable to keep a job).
41

40 | **Some impairment in reality testing or communication** (e.g., speech is at times illogical, obscure, or irrelevant) **OR major impairment in several areas, such as work or school, family relations, judgment, thinking, or mood** (e.g., depressed man avoids friends, neglects family, and is unable to work; child frequently beats up younger children, is defiant at home, and is failing at school).
31

30 | **Behavior is considerably influenced by delusions or hallucinations OR serious impairment in communication or judgment** (e.g., sometimes incoherent, acts grossly inappropriately, suicidal preoccupation) **OR inability to function in almost all areas** (e.g., stays in bed all day; no job, home, or friends).
21

20 | **Some danger of hurting self or others** (e.g., suicide attempts without clear expectation of death, frequently violent, manic excitement) **OR occasionally fails to maintain minimal personal hygiene** (e.g., smears feces) **OR gross impairment in communication** (e.g., largely incoherent or mute).
11

10 | **Persistent danger of severely hurting self or others** (e.g., recurrent violence) **OR persistent inability to maintain minimal personal hygiene OR serious suicidal act with clear expectation of death.**
1

0 | **Inadequate information.**

ditions, this particular axis serves to alert the clinician to any personal factors that might be relevant to the patient's diagnosis (e.g., the exacerbation of depression produced by living with an alcoholic spouse). The coding for the severity of psychosocial stressors in adults and children is summarized in Table 2-4.

Axis V provides a global assessment of the overall level of functioning and "psychological health" of the patient. It includes various indices of social, psychological, and occupational functioning. These are coded on the Global Assessment of Functioning (GAF) Scale, which ranges from 1 to 90, with 90 representing absent or minimal symptoms. The GAF Scale is summarized in Table 2-5. The use of this scale provides the clinician with some indication of the patient's overall prognosis, because high-functioning individuals typically have a better outcome.

How to Become Familiar With the DSM-III-R System

The DSM-III-R system is obviously large and complex. Beginning clinicians should not attempt to master everything at once. Rather, they should focus on the major and common conditions that are frequently seen either in psychiatric practice or primary-care settings. They should become very familiar with the diagnostic criteria for a few common conditions such as schizophrenia, major depression, dementia, anxiety disorders, and personality disorders. A few sets of symptom criteria (e.g., major depression) should be committed to memory, simply because they are used so often in so many different clinical settings. The system is too vast to commit all of it to memory, however, and so the clinician should not feel concerned about the need to refer back to the criteria frequently when evaluating patients and making diagnoses.

Bibliography

American Psychiatric Association: Diagnostic and Statistical Manual of Mental Disorders. Washington, DC, American Psychiatric Association, 1952

American Psychiatric Association: Diagnostic and Statistical Manual of Mental Disorders, 2nd Edition. Washington, DC, American Psychiatric Association, 1968

American Psychiatric Association: Diagnostic and Statistical Manual of Mental Disorders, 3rd Edition. Washington, DC, American Psychiatric Association, 1980

American Psychiatric Association: Diagnostic and Statistical Manual of Mental Disorders, 3rd Edition, Revised. Washington, DC, American Psychiatric Association, 1987

Andreasen NC: The clinical assessment of thought, language, and communication disorders, I: the definition of terms and evaluation of their reliability. Arch Gen Psychiatry 36:1315–1321, 1979

Andreasen NC: The clinical assessment of thought, language, and communication disorders, II: diagnostic significance. Arch Gen Psychiatry 36:1325–1330, 1979

Feighner JP, Robins E, Guze SB, et al: Diagnostic criteria for use in psychiatric research. Arch Gen Psychiatry 26:57–63, 1972

Goodwin DW, Guze SB: Psychiatric Diagnosis, 4th Edition. New York, Oxford University Press, 1989

King LS: Medical Thinking: A Historical Preface. Princeton, NJ, Princeton University Press, 1982

Spitzer RL, Endicott J, Robins E: Research Diagnostic Criteria: rationale and reliability. Arch Gen Psychiatry 35:773–782, 1978

Tischler GL (ed): Diagnosis and Classification in Psychiatry: A Critical Appraisal of DSM-III. Cambridge, Cambridge University Press, 1987

Wing JK, Cooper JE, Sartorius N: The Measurement and Classification of Psychiatric Symptoms. Cambridge, Cambridge University Press, 1974

Self-assessment Questions

1. What is the overall purpose of diagnosis and classification in medicine generally? Give several examples of diseases for which this purpose has been achieved. Describe the extent to which it has been achieved in psychiatry.
2. Describe some of the specific purposes of psychiatric diagnosis.
3. Describe some of the changes introduced by DSM-III.
4. Define the concepts of reliability and validity.
5. Describe the advantages of DSM-III and DSM-III-R. What are their disadvantages?
6. What is meant by the term *multiaxial*? List the five axes that are included in DSM-III-R.

Chapter 3
Interviewing and Assessment

Festina lente
Make haste slowly

A Latin proverb

Because so much of psychiatric diagnosis depends at present on clinical history, the ability to interview and to take an accurate history is one of the most fundamental skills in psychiatry. Demands placed on the interviewer will vary, depending on the type of illness from which the patient suffers and its severity. Patients with milder syndromes, such as anxiety disorders or personality disorders, are usually more capable of describing their symptoms and past history clearly and articulately. The severely ill depressed, manic, or psychotic patient represents a real challenge. These patients may speak in a disorganized manner, be very distractible, or be uninterested or uncooperative, or even mute. Clinicians may have to depend on informants, such as family members or friends, in addition to the patient.

Interviewing Techniques

Although the demands of the interview may vary depending on the patient and his or her illness, some techniques are common to most interview situations.

Establish rapport as early in the interview as possible. It is often best to begin by asking the patient about himself—what kind of work he does, where he goes to school, what he is studying, how old he is, whether he is married or single, etc. Questions about these topics should not be asked in a manner that seems to "grill" the patient, but rather in a way that indicates that the interviewer is genuinely interested in getting to know the patient. The overall tone of the opening of the interview should, therefore, convey warmth and friendliness. After rapport has been established, the interviewer should then inquire about what kind of problem the patient has been having, what brought him to the clinic, or why he came into the hospital.

Determine the patient's "chief complaint." Sometimes this will be helpful and explicit (e.g., "I've been feeling very depressed," or "I've been having a pain in my head that other doctors can't explain"); other times the chief complaint may be relatively vague and require a number of follow-up questions (e.g., "I don't know why I'm here—my family brought me," "I've been having trouble at work"). When the replies are not particularly explicit, the interviewer will need to follow up initial questions with others that will help in determining the nature of the patient's problem (e.g., "What kinds of things have been bothering your family?" "What kind of trouble at work?"). The initial portion of the interview, devoted to eliciting the chief complaint, should take as long as is necessary to determine the patient's primary problem. When the patient is a clear, logical informant, let him tell his story as freely as possible without interruption. When he is a relatively poor informant, the interviewer will need to be active and directive.

Use the chief complaint to develop a provisional differential diagnosis. As in the rest of medicine, once the patient's primary problem has been determined, the interviewer begins to construct in his or her mind a range of explanations as to the specific diagnosis that might lead to that particular problem. For example, if the patient indicates that he has been hearing voices, the differential diagnosis includes various disorders that produce this type of psychotic symptom, such as schizophrenia, schizophreniform disorder, psychotic mania, substance abuse involving hallucinogens, or alcoholic hallucinosis. Being able to develop a differential diagnosis, of course, requires some knowledge of the various types of psychiatric disorders and their characteristic symptoms. As in the rest of medicine, skill in making a differential diagnosis increases with knowledge and experience. Overall, however, it may be comforting to realize that the fundamental process of interviewing and diagnosing is the same in psychiatry as it is in internal medicine or neurology.

Rule the various diagnostic possibilities out or in by using more focused and detailed questions. The existence of DSM-III-R is particularly helpful in this regard. If the patient's chief complaint has suggested three or four different possible diagnoses, the interviewer can determine which is most relevant by referring to the diagnostic criteria for those disorders. Thus, the interviewer will determine what additional symptoms have been present besides those already enumerated when the chief complaint was elicited. The interviewer will inquire about the course and onset of the symptoms, or the existence of physical or psychological precipitants such as use of drugs or alcohol or personal losses.

Follow up vague or obscure replies with enough persistence to accurately determine the answer to the question. Some patients, particularly psychotic patients, have great difficulty answering questions clearly and concisely. They may answer "yes" or "no" to every question asked. When a pattern of this sort is observed, the patient should be repeatedly asked to describe his experiences as explicitly as possible. For example, if the patient says that he hears voices, he should be asked to describe them in more detail—whether they are male or female, what they say, and how often they occur. The greater the level of detail the patient is able to provide, the more confident the clinician can feel that the symptom is truly present. Because making a diagnosis of schizophrenia or other major psychiatric disorder has important prognostic implications, the clinician should not hastily accept an answer that suggests vaguely that the patient may have a particular symptom of a disorder.

Let the patient talk freely enough to observe how tightly his thoughts are connected. Most patients should be allowed to talk for at least 3 or 4 minutes in the course of any psychiatric interview without interruption. The very laconic patient will not, of course, be able to do this, but most can. The coherence of the pattern with which the patient's thoughts are presented may provide major clues to the type of problem that he is experiencing. For example, patients with mania, schizophrenia, and depression may have any one of various types of "formal thought disorder" (see the definition of common symptoms later in this chapter). Coherence of thought may also be helpful in making a differential diagnosis between dementia or depression.

Use a mixture of open-ended and closed questions. Interviewers can learn a great deal about the patient by mixing up their types of questions, just as a good pitcher mixes up pitches. Open-ended questions permit the patient to ramble and become disorganized, whereas closed questions determine whether the patient can come up with the specifics when pressed. These are important indicators as to whether the patient is conceptually disorganized or confused, whether he is being evasive, or whether he is answering randomly or falsely. The content of the questions should be mixed as well. For example, at some point in the interview, the interviewer will probably want to drop his or her objective style of interviewing and focus on some personal topic that is affect laden, such as sexual or interpersonal relationships. These questions will give the interviewer important clues about the patient's capacity to show emotional responsiveness. Evaluating the patient's mood and affect is a fundamental aspect of the psychiatric evaluation, just as is evaluating the coherence of his thinking and communication.

Don't be afraid to ask about topics that you or the patient might find difficult or embarrassing. Beginning interviewers, in particular, find it hard to ask about topics such as sexual relationships, sexual experiences, or even use of alcohol or drugs. Yet all this information is part of a complete psychiatric interview and must be included. Nearly all patients expect doctors to ask these questions and are not offended. Likewise, beginning interviewers are sometimes embarrassed to ask about symptoms of psychosis, such as hearing voices. To the interviewer, these symptoms seem so "crazy" that the patient might be insulted by being asked about them. Again, however, information of this type is basic and cannot be avoided. If John Hinckley, Jr.'s psychiatrist had been more aggressive in inquiring about delusions, a diagnosis of schizophrenia might have been made before a presidential assassination attempt and a great deal of misery avoided. If the patient seems "obviously" not psychotic, questions about psychotic symptoms should still be asked, and in an unapologetic manner. If the patient seems amused or annoyed, then the interviewer can explain the necessity of covering all kinds of questions to provide a comprehensive evaluation of each patient.

Don't forget to ask about suicidal thoughts. This is another topic that may seem to fall into the "embarrassing" category. Nevertheless, suicide is a common outcome of many psychiatric illnesses, and it is incumbent on the interviewer to ask about it. The subject can be broached quite tactfully by a question such as, "Have you ever felt life isn't worth living?" The topic of suicide can then be approached gradually, leading to questions such as, "Have you ever thought about taking your life?" Further tips on interviewing the suicidal patient are presented in Chapter 20.

Give the patient a chance to ask questions at the end of the interview. From the patient's point of view, there is nothing more frustrating than being interviewed for an hour and then ushered out of the office or examining room with his own questions unanswered. The questions that patients ask often tell a great deal about what is on their mind (or not on their mind). Thus, these questions may be quite helpful in the differential diagnostic process. Even if not helpful, they are important to the patient and therefore are intrinsically important.

Conclude the initial interview by conveying a sense of confidence and, if possible, of hope. Thank the patient for providing so much information. Compliment him, in whatever way it can be done sincerely, on having told his story well. Indicate that you now have a much better understanding of his problems, and conclude by indicating that you will do what you can to help him. If you already have a relatively good idea that his problem is one that is amenable to treatment, explain that to him. At the end of the initial interview, if you are uncertain about diagnosis or treatment, indicate that you have learned a great deal, but that you need to think about his problem some more and perhaps gather more information before arriving at a recommendation.

Components of a Psychiatric Interview and Assessment

An initial psychiatric evaluation serves several purposes. One is to formulate an impression as to the patient's diagnosis or differential diagnosis and to begin to generate a treatment plan. The second purpose is to produce a written document for the patient's record that contains information organized in a standard, readable, and easily interpreted way. The initial interview is often therapeutic as well, in that it permits the clinician to establish a relationship with the patient and to reassure her that help will be provided.

The outline of that written record is summarized in Table 3-1. As Table 3-1 indicates, a standard psychiatric evaluation is very similar to those used in the rest of medicine, with some minor modifications. The content of the present illness and past history focuses primarily on psychiatric symptoms, and the family history will include more information about psychiatric illnesses in the family. Family

Table 3-1. Outline of the psychiatric evaluation

Identification of patient and informants	General medical history
Chief complaint	Mental status examination
History of present illness	General physical examination
Past history	Neurological examination
Family history	Diagnostic impression
Social history	Treatment and management plan

history and social history will also include more sociodemographic and personal information than is recorded in the standard medical history. The mental status examination is typically only included in psychiatric and neurological evaluations.

Identification of Patient and Informants

Identify the patient by stating her age, handedness, race, sex, marital status, and occupational status. Indicate whether the patient acted as her own informant, or whether additional history was obtained from family members or previous psychiatric records. Indicate whether the patient was self-referred, was brought in at the request of family members, or was referred by a physician; if either of the latter two, specify which family members or physician. In addition, indicate how reliable the informants appear to be.

Chief Complaint

Begin by stating the patient's chief complaint in her own words. An additional sentence or two of amplifying information may also be provided, particularly if the patient's chief complaint is relatively vague.

History of Present Illness

Provide a concise history of the illness or problem that brought the patient in for treatment. Begin by describing the onset of the symptoms. If this is the patient's first episode, first psychiatric evaluation, or first hospital admission, this should be stated early in the "present illness." Indicate how long ago the first symptoms began, the nature of their onset (acute, insidious, etc.), and whether the onset was precipitated by any particular life events or problems, which should be described in some detail if present. Likewise, medical conditions that may have served as precipitants should be described. If drug or alcohol abuse was a potential precipitant, this should also be noted. The evolution of the patient's various symptoms should be described. A systematic summary of all symptoms present, in a form useful for making a differential diagnosis of the present illness, should be provided. This listing of symptoms should reflect the criteria included in DSM-III-R and should specify both which symptoms are present and which symptoms are absent. The description of symptoms should not be limited to those included in the DSM-III-R diagnostic criteria, however, because these typically do not provide a full description of the range of symptoms that patients have (i.e., they are minimal, not comprehensively descriptive). The description of the present illness should also indicate the degree of incapacity that the patient is experiencing as a consequence of her symptoms, as well as their influence on her personal and family life. Any treatments that the patient has received for the present illness should be noted, including dosages, time, and effectiveness of the specific medications, because this will often dictate what the next step will be.

Past History

The past history has two main components: history of past psychiatric illness and personal history.

The *history of past psychiatric illness* provides a summary of past illnesses, problems, and their treatment. In patients with complex histories and chronic psychiatric illnesses, this portion of the history will be quite extensive. It should begin by noting the number of past hospitalizations or episodes, and the age at which the patient was first seen for psychiatric evaluation. Thereafter, past episodes should be described in chronological order, with some information about duration of episodes, types of symptoms present, severity of symptoms, treatments received, and response to treatment. If some characteristic pattern is present (e.g., episodes of mania are always followed by episodes of depression, or past depressive episodes have consistently responded to a particular medication), this should be noted because it provides useful prognostic information. If the patient's memory for past symptoms is relatively poor, this should also be noted. If the bulk of the past history is obtained from old records rather than from the patient herself, this should be recorded. Confirmation by family members of types and patterns of symptoms and number of episodes should also be noted.

Personal history provides a narrative description of the patient's life history in a concise manner. It includes information about where the patient was born, where she grew up, and the nature of her early life adjustment. If she had problems during childhood, such as temper tantrums, school phobia, or delinquency, these should be noted. Her relationship to her parents and siblings should be described. Psychosexual development, such as age at first sexual experience, should also be described. Information about familial religious or cultural attitudes that are relevant to the patient's condition should be noted. Educational history should be summarized, including information about how far the patient went in school, how well she performed, and what her academic interests were. Some description should be provided of her interest and participation in extracurricular activities and her interpersonal relationships during adolescence and early adulthood. Work history and military history should also be summarized. Certain areas may need more emphasis and detail, depending on the chief complaint and diagnostic formulation.

Family History

The age and occupation of both parents and all siblings should be noted, as should the age and education or occupation (if applicable) of all children. If any of these first-degree relatives has a history of any mental illness, the specific illness should be mentioned, along with information about treatment, hospitalization, and long-term course and outcome. It may be necessary to run through specific disorders, because many patients will not recognize alcoholism or criminality, for example, as "emotional problems": "Do any blood relatives have a history of alcoholism, criminality, drug abuse, severe depression, or suicide attempts or suicide? Have any ever had psychiatric hospitalization or institutionalization? Have any ever taken 'nerve pills,' or seen psychiatrists, psychologists, or counselors?" The interviewer should obtain as much information as possible about mental illness in second-degree relatives as well. Any relevant information about the family's social, cultural, or educational background may also be included in this section of the interview. It is often helpful to draw pedigrees in complicated cases.

Social History

This section of the history contains a summary of the patient's current social situation. It summarizes marital status, occupation, and income. The location of her residence should be described, as well as the specific family members who live with her. This section of the history should provide information about the various social supports currently available to the patient. Record habits as well (e.g., smoking, use of alcohol).

General Medical History

The patient's current and past state of health should be summarized. Any existing illness for which the patient is currently being treated should be noted, as well as the types of treatments, medications, and their dosages. Past surgeries, traumatic injuries, or other serious illnesses should be summarized. Head injuries, headaches, seizures, and other problems involving the central nervous system are particularly relevant.

Mental Status Examination

The mental status examination is the psychiatric equivalent to the physical examination in medicine. It includes a comprehensive evaluation of the patient's appearance, thinking and speech patterns, etc.

The components of the mental status examination are summarized in Table 3-2. Some portions of mental status are determined simply by observing the patient (e.g., appearance, affect). Others are determined by asking the patient relatively specific questions (e.g., mood, abnormalities in perception). Still others are assessed

Table 3-2.   Mental status examination

Appearance and attitude	General information
Motor activity	Calculations
Thought and speech	Capacity to read and write
Mood and affect	Visuospatial ability
Perception	Attention
Orientation	Abstraction
Memory	Judgment and insight

through asking the patient a specified set of questions (e.g., memory, general information). For those portions of the mental status examination that assess functions such as memory, general information, or calculation, the interviewer should develop his or her own repertoire of techniques for assessment and should consistently use this same repertoire for all patients so that he or she develops a good sense of the range of normal and abnormal responses in a variety of individuals of various ages, educational levels, and psychopathological states.

Appearance and attitude.   Describe the patient's general appearance, including grooming, hygiene, and facial expression. Note whether the patient looks his stated age, younger, or older. Note type and appropriateness of dress. Describe whether the patient's attitude is cooperative, guarded, angry, or suspicious.

Motor activity.   Note the patient's level of motor activity. Does he sit quietly, or is he physically agitated? Note any abnormal movements, tics, or mannerisms. If relevant, evaluate for and note any indications of catatonia such as waxy flexibility (see below). Determine whether any indications of tardive dyskinesia or any other abnormal movements are present.

Thought and speech.   Psychiatrists often speak about "thought disorder" or "formal thought disorder." This concept refers to the patient's pattern of speech, from which abnormal patterns of thought are inferred. It is, of course, not possible to evaluate thought directly. Note the rate of the patient's speech—whether it is normal, slowed, or pressured. Indicate whether his speech indicates a pattern of thought that is logical and goal oriented, or whether any abnormalities in form of thought are present (e.g., derailment, incoherence, poverty of content of speech). Summarize the content of thought, noting in particular any delusional thinking that is currently observed. If delusions are present, they should be described in detail (if this has already been done in the present illness, this can be noted with a simple statement such as, "Delusions were present as described above.").

Mood and affect.   The term *mood* refers to an emotional attitude that is relatively sustained; it is typically determined through the patient's own self-report, although some inferences can be made from the patient's facial expression. Note whether the patient's mood is neutral, euphoric, depressed, anxious, or irritable.

Affect refers to brief emotional responses, usually triggered by some stimulus.

Affect is how the patient conveys his emotional state and is observed. Mood refers to a more persistent emotional state and is reported by the patient. The examiner watches the response of the patient's face to smiling, determines whether the patient shows appropriate or inappropriate emotional reactions, and notes the degree of reactivity of emotion. Affect is typically described as full, flat, blunted, or inappropriate. Flat or blunted affect is inferred when the patient shows very little emotional response and seems emotionally dulled, whereas inappropriate affect refers to emotional responses that are not appropriate to the content of the discussion, such as silly laughter for no apparent reason.

Perception.   Note any abnormalities in perception. The most common perceptual abnormalities are hallucinations—abnormal sensory perceptions in the absence of an actual stimulus. Hallucinations may be auditory, visual, tactile, or olfactory. Sometimes hypnagogic or hypnopompic hallucinations occur when the patient is falling asleep or waking from sleep; these are not considered to be true hallucinations.

Orientation.   Describe the patient's level of orientation. Normally, this includes orientation to time, place, and person. This is assessed by asking the patient to describe the day, date, year, time, and place where he is currently residing, and his name and identity.

Memory.   Memory is divided into very short term, short term, and long term. All three should be described. Very short-term memory involves the immediate registration of information, usually assessed by having the patient repeat back immediately a series of digits or three pieces of information (e.g., the color green, the name Mr. Williams, and the address 1915 High Street). The examiner determines whether the patient can recall these immediately after told them. If the patient has difficulty, he should be given the items repeatedly until he is able to register them. If he is unable to register after three or four trials, this should be noted. The patient should then be warned that he will be asked to recall these in 3–5 minutes. His ability to remember them after that time interval is an indication of his short-term memory. Remote memory is assessed by asking the patient to recall events that occurred in the past several days, as well as events occurring in the more remote past, such as months or years ago.

General information.   This is assessed by asking the patient a specific set of questions covering topics such as who were the last five presidents, current events, or information about history or geography. The patient's fund of general information should be noted in relation to his level of educational achievement. This is particularly important in assessing the possibility of dementia.

Calculations.   The standard test is "serial 7s." This involves having the patient subtract 7 from 100, then 7 from that result, and so on for at least five subtractions. Some chronic patients become relatively well trained on this, so it is a good idea to have other tools in one's repertoire. One that is quite useful involves asking the patient to make calculations necessary in daily living (e.g., If I went to the store and bought six oranges, priced at three for a dollar, and gave the clerk a 10-dollar bill, how much change would I get back?). Calculations can be modified for the patient's educational level. Poorly educated patients may need to calculate "serial 3s." Likewise, "real-life" calculations can be simplified or made more complicated.

Capacity to read and write. The patient should be given a simple text and asked to read it aloud. He should also be asked to write down some specific sentence, either of the examiner's choice or his own.

Visuospatial ability. The patient should be asked to copy a figure. This can be quite simple, such as a square inside a circle. An alternative task is to ask the patient to draw a clock face and set the hands at some specified time, such as 20 minutes to three.

Attention. Attention is, in part, assessed by a number of the tasks above, such as calculations or clock setting. Additional tests of attention can be used, such as asking the patient to spell a word backward (e.g., *world*). The patient can also be asked to name five things that start with some specific letter, such as the letter *d*. The latter is also a good test of cognitive and verbal fluency.

Abstraction. The patient's capacity to think abstractly can be assessed in various ways. One favorite method is asking the patient to interpret proverbs, such as "A rolling stone gathers no moss" or "Don't cry over spilt milk." Alternatively, the patient can be asked to identify commonalities between two items (e.g., How are an apple and an orange alike? How are a fly and a tree alike?).

Judgment and insight. Assess the patient's overall judgment and insight by noting how realistically he has assessed his illness and his various life problems.

General Physical Examination

The general physical examination should follow the standard format used in the rest of medicine, covering organ systems of the body from head to foot. Examinations of patients of the opposite sex (e.g., male physician examining a female patient) should be chaperoned.

Neurological Examination

Likewise, a standard neurological examination should be recorded. A detailed neurological evaluation is particularly important in psychiatric patients to rule out focal signs that might explain the patient's symptoms.

Diagnostic Impression

The diagnostic impression section of the history indicates the clinician's diagnostic impression. Whenever possible, diagnoses should be made using all five DSM-III-R axes. When appropriate, more than one diagnosis should be made. When the diagnosis is uncertain, the qualifier "provisional" should be added. Not infrequently, it will be difficult to make a definitive diagnosis at the time of the index evaluation. When this situation occurs, a listing of differential diagnostic possibilities should be made.

Treatment and Management Plan

The section of the history on the treatment and management plan will vary, depending on the level of diagnostic certainty. If the diagnosis is quite uncertain, the first step in treatment and management will involve additional assessments to determine the diagnosis with more certainty. Thus, the treatment and management plan may include a list of laboratory tests appropriate to assist in the differential diagnosis listed above. Alternatively, when the diagnosis is straightforward, it will be possible to outline a specific treatment plan, including a proposed medication regimen, plans for vocational rehabilitation, a program for social skills training, marital counseling, or other ancillary treatments appropriate to the patient's specific problems.

Definitions of Common Signs and Symptoms and Methods for Eliciting Them

A vast panoply of signs and symptoms can characterize major mental illnesses. The following are some of the more common signs and symptoms that are seen in relatively severe psychopathology. They include symptoms seen in psychotic states, affective syndromes, and anxiety states. Where appropriate, some suggested questions are provided that can be used to probe for these symptoms. Those in parentheses are follow-up questions.

Psychotic Symptoms

Psychotic symptoms are often divided into two broad groups: positive and negative. Positive symptoms include delusions, hallucinations, bizarre behavior, positive formal thought disorder, and inappropriate affect. The first two are evaluated by questioning and the final three by observation. Negative symptoms, which are common in psychosis but may also occur in nonpsychotic illnesses such as depression, include alogia, affective blunting, avolition-apathy, anhedonia-asociality, and attentional impairment. The first two are evaluated primarily by observation and the final three by interview.

Delusions

Delusions represent an abnormality in content of thought. They are false beliefs that cannot be explained on the basis of the subject's cultural background. Although delusions are sometimes defined as "fixed false beliefs," in their mildest form delusions may persist only for weeks to months, and the subject may question her beliefs or doubt them. The subject's behavior may or may not be influenced by her delusions. The assessment of severity of individual delusions and of the global severity of delusional thinking should take into account their persistence, their complexity, the extent to which the subject acts on them, the extent to which the subject doubts them, and the extent to which the beliefs deviate from the ones that normal people might have.

Persecutory delusions.   People suffering from persecutory delusions believe that they are being conspired against or persecuted in some way. Common manifestations include the belief that one is being followed, that one's mail is being opened, that one's room or office is bugged, that the telephone is tapped, or that police, government officials, neighbors, or fellow workers are harassing the subject. Persecutory delusions are sometimes relatively isolated or fragmented, but sometimes the person has a complex system of delusions involving both a wide range of forms of persecution and a belief that there is a well-designed conspiracy behind them: for example, that his house is bugged and that he is being followed because the government wrongly considers him a secret agent of a foreign government; this delusion may be so complex that it explains almost everything that happens to him.

Have you had trouble getting along with people?

Have you felt that people are against you?

Has anyone been trying to harm you in any way?

(Do you think people have been plotting against you?)

Delusions of jealousy.   The patient believes that her mate is having an affair with someone. Miscellaneous bits of information are construed as "evidence." The person usually goes to great effort to prove the existence of the affair, searching for hair in the bedclothes, the odor of perfume or smoke on clothing, or receipts or checks indicating a gift has been bought for the lover. Elaborate plans are often made to trap the two together.

Have you worried that your (husband, wife, boyfriend, girlfriend) might be unfaithful to you?

(What evidence do you have?)

Delusions of sin or guilt. The patient believes that he has committed some terrible sin or done something unforgivable. Sometimes the patient is excessively or inappropriately preoccupied with things he did wrong as a child, such as masturbating. Sometimes the patient feels responsible for causing some disastrous event, such as a fire or accident, with which he in fact has no connection. Sometimes these delusions have a religious flavor involving the belief that the sin is unpardonable and that the subject will suffer eternal punishment from God. Sometimes the patient simply believes that he deserves punishment by society. The patient may spend a good deal of time confessing these sins to whomever will listen.

Have you felt that you have done some terrible thing?

(Is there anything that is bothering your conscience?)

(What is it?)

(Do you feel you deserve to be punished for it?)

Grandiose delusions. The patient believes that he has special powers or abilities. He may think he is actually some famous person, such as a rock star, Napoleon, or Christ. He may believe he is writing some definitive book, composing a great piece of music, or developing some wonderful new invention. The patient is often suspicious that someone is trying to steal his ideas, and he may become quite irritated if his abilities are doubted.

Do you have any special powers, talents, or abilities?

Do you feel you are going to achieve great things?

Religious delusions. The patient is preoccupied with false beliefs of a religious nature. Sometimes these exist within the context of a conventional religious system, such as beliefs about the Second Coming, the Antichrist, or possession by the Devil. At other times, they may involve an entirely new religious system or a pastiche of beliefs from a variety of religions, particularly Eastern religions, such as ideas about reincarnation or Nirvana. Religious delusions

Are you a religious person?

Have you had any unusual religious experiences?

(What was your religious training as a child?)

may be combined with grandiose delusions (if the subject considers himself a religious leader), delusions of guilt, or delusions of being controlled. Religious delusions must be outside the range considered normal for the patient's cultural and religious background.

Somatic delusions. The patient believes that somehow her body is diseased, abnormal, or changed. For example, she may believe that her stomach or brain is rotting, that her hands have become enlarged, or that her facial features are unusual (dysmorphophobia). Sometimes somatic delusions are accompanied by tactile or other hallucinations, and when this occurs, both should be considered to be present. (For example, the patient believes that she has ball bearings rolling about in her head, placed there by a dentist who filled her teeth, and can actually hear them clanking against one another.)

Is there anything wrong with the way your body is working?

Have you noticed any change in your appearance?

Ideas and delusions of reference. The patient believes that insignificant remarks, statements, or events refer to her or have some special meaning for her. For example, the patient walks into a room, sees people laughing, and suspects that they were just talking about her and laughing at her. Sometimes items read in the paper, heard on the radio, or seen on television are considered to be special messages to the subject. In the case of ideas of reference, the patient is suspicious, but recognizes her idea may be erroneous. When the patient actually believes that the statements or events refer to her, then this is considered a delusion of reference.

Have you walked into a room and thought people were talking about you or laughing at you?

Have you seen things in magazines or on TV that seem to refer to you or contain a special message for you?

Have you received special messages in any other ways?

Delusions of being controlled. The patient has a subjective experience that his feelings or actions are controlled by some outside force. The central requirement for this type of delusion is an actual strong subjective experience of being controlled. It does not include simple beliefs or ideas, such as that the subject is acting as an agent of God or that friends or parents are trying to coerce him into something. Rather, the patient must describe, for example, that his body has been occupied by some alien force that is making it move in peculiar ways, or that messages are being sent to his brain by radio waves and causing him to experience feelings that he recognizes are not his own.

Have you felt that you were being controlled by some outside force?

Do you feel that any person is controlling you?

Delusions of mind reading. The patient believes that people can read her mind or know her thoughts. This is different from thought broadcasting (see below) in that it is a belief without a percept, that is, the patient subjectively experiences and recognizes that others know her thoughts, but she does not think that they can be heard out loud.

Have you had the feeling that people could read your mind or know what you are thinking?

Thought broadcasting/audible thoughts. The patient believes that his thoughts are broadcast so that he or others can hear them. Sometimes the patient experiences his thoughts as a voice outside his head; this is an auditory hallucination as well as a delusion. Sometimes the subject feels his thoughts are being broadcast, although he cannot hear them himself. Sometimes he believes that his thoughts are picked up by a microphone and broadcast on the radio or television.

Have you heard your own thoughts out loud, as if they were a voice outside your head?

Have you felt your thoughts were broadcast so other people could hear them?

Thought insertion. The patient believes that thoughts that are not her own have been inserted into her mind. For example, the patient may believe that a neighbor is practicing voodoo and planting alien sexual thoughts in her mind. This symptom should not be confused with experiencing unpleasant thoughts that the patient recognizes as her own, such as delusions of persecution or guilt.

Have you felt that thoughts were being put into your head by some outside force or person?

Thought withdrawal. The patient believes that thoughts have been taken away from his mind. He is able to describe a subjective experience of beginning a thought and then suddenly having it removed by some outside force. This symptom does not include the mere subjective recognition of alogia.

Have you felt your thoughts were taken away by some outside force or person?

Hallucinations

Hallucinations represent an abnormality in perception. They are false perceptions occurring in the absence of some identifiable external stimulus. They may be experienced in any of the sensory modalities, including hearing, touch, taste, smell, and vision. True hallucinations should be distinguished from illusions (which involve a misperception of an external stimulus), hypnagogic and hypnopompic experiences (which occur when a patient is falling asleep or waking up, respectively), or normal thought processes that are exceptionally vivid. If the hallucinations have a religious quality, then they should be judged within the context of what is normal for the patient's social and cultural background. The patient should always be requested to describe the hallucination in detail. The term *pseudohallucinations* refers to hallucinations that the patient reports, but that have no identifiable percept (e.g., the patient says that she "sees things that aren't there," but is unable to describe any actual specific perceptions).

Auditory hallucinations. The patient has reported voices, noises, or sounds. The most common auditory hallucinations involve hearing voices speaking to the patient or calling him names. The voices may be male or female, familiar or unfamiliar, and critical or complimentary. Typically, patients suffering from schizophrenia experience the voices as unpleas-

Have you heard voices or other sounds when no one is around, or when you couldn't account for them?

(What did they say?)

ant and negative. Hallucinations involving sounds other than voices, such as noises or music, should be considered less characteristic and less severe.

Voices commenting. These hallucinations involve hearing a voice that makes a running commentary on the patient's behavior or thought as it occurs.

Have you heard voices commenting on what you are thinking or doing?

(What do they say?)

Voices conversing. These hallucinations involve hearing two or more voices talking with one another, usually discussing something about the patient.

Have you heard two or more voices talking with each other?

(What do they say?)

Somatic or tactile hallucinations. These hallucinations involve experiencing peculiar physical sensations in the body. They include burning sensations, tingling, and perceptions that the body has changed in shape or size.

Have you had burning sensations or other strange feelings in your body?

(What were they?)

Olfactory hallucinations. The patient experiences unusual smells which are typically quite unpleasant. Sometimes the patient may believe that he himself smells. This belief should be considered a hallucination if the patient can actually smell the odor himself, but should be considered a delusion if he believes that only others can smell the odor.

Have you experienced any unusual smells or smells that others don't notice?

(What were they?)

Visual hallucinations. The patient sees shapes or people that are not actually present. Sometimes these are shapes or colors, but most typically they are figures of people or humanlike objects. They may also be characters of a religious nature, such as the Devil or Christ. As always, visual hallucinations involving religious themes should be judged within the context of the patient's cultural background.

Have you had visions or seen things that other people cannot see?

(What did you see?)

(Did this occur when you were falling asleep or waking up?)

Bizarre Behavior

The patient's behavior is unusual, bizarre, or fantastic. The information for this symptom will sometimes come from the patient, sometimes from other sources, and sometimes from direct observation. Bizarre behavior due to the immediate effects of intoxication with alcohol or drugs should not be considered to be a symptom of psychosis. Social and cultural norms must be considered in making the determination of bizarre behavior, and detailed examples should be elicited and noted.

Clothing and appearance. The patient dresses in an unusual manner or does other strange things to alter his appearance. For example, he may shave off all his hair or paint parts of his body different colors. His clothing may be quite unusual; for example, he may choose to wear some outfit that appears generally inappropriate and unacceptable, such as a baseball cap backward with rubber galoshes and long underwear covered by denim overalls. He may dress in a fantastic costume representing some historical personage or a man from outer space. He may wear clothing completely inappropriate to the climatic conditions, such as heavy wools in the midst of summer.

Has anyone made comments about the way you look?

Social and sexual behavior. The patient may do things that are considered inappropriate according to usual social norms. For example, he may masturbate in public, urinate or defecate in inappropriate receptacles, walk along the street muttering to himself, or begin talking to people whom he has never before met about his personal life (as when riding on a subway or standing in some public place). He may drop to his knees praying and shouting, or suddenly sit in an unusual position when in the midst of a crowd. He may make inappropriate sexual overtures or remarks to strangers.

Have you done anything that others might think unusual or that has called attention to yourself?

(Has anyone complained or commented about your behavior?)

Aggressive and agitated behavior. The patient may behave in an aggressive, agitated manner, often quite unpredictably. He may start arguments inappropriately with friends or members of his family, or he may accost strangers on the street and begin haranguing them angrily. He may write letters of a threatening or angry nature to government officials or others with whom he has some quarrel. Occasionally, patients may perform violent acts such as injuring or tormenting animals, or attempting to injure or kill humans.

Have you been unusually angry or irritable with anyone?

(How did you express your anger?)

(Have your done anything to try to harm animals or people?)

Ritualistic or stereotyped behavior. The patient may develop a set of repetitive actions or rituals that she must perform over and over. Sometimes she will attribute some symbolic significance to these actions and believe that they are either influencing others or preventing herself from being influenced. For example, she may eat jelly beans every night for dessert, assuming that different consequences will occur depending on the color of the jelly beans eaten. She may have to eat foods in a particular order or wear particular clothes or put them on in a certain order. She may have to write messages to herself or to others over and over, sometimes in an unusual or occult language.

Are there any things you do over and over?

Are there any things that you have to do in a certain way or in a particular order?

(Why do you do it?)

(Does it have any special meaning or significance?)

Positive Formal Thought Disorder

Positive formal thought disorder is fluent speech that tends to communicate poorly for various reasons. The patient tends to skip from topic to topic without warning, to be distracted by events in the nearby environment, to join words together because they are semantically or phonologically alike, even though they make no sense, or to ignore the question asked and answer another. This type of speech may be rapid, and it frequently seems quite disjointed. It has sometimes been referred to as "loose associations." Unlike alogia (negative formal thought disorder) (see below), a wealth of detail is provided, and the flow of speech tends to have an energetic rather than an apathetic quality to it.

To evaluate thought disorder, the patient should be permitted to talk without interruption for as long as 5 minutes. The interviewer should observe closely the extent to which the patient's sequencing of ideas is well connected. He or she should also pay close attention to how well the patient can reply to a variety of different types of questions, ranging from simple (When were you born?) to more complicated (Why did you come to the hospital?). If the ideas seem vague or incomprehensible, the interviewer should prompt the patient to clarify or elaborate.

Derailment (loose associations). A pattern of spontaneous speech in which the ideas slip off the track onto another that is clearly but obliquely related, or onto one completely unrelated. Things may be said in juxtaposition that lack a meaningful relationship, or the patient may shift idiosyncratically from one frame of reference to another. At times, there may be a vague connection between the ideas, and at others, none will be apparent. This pattern of speech is often characterized as sounding "disjointed." Perhaps the most common manifestation of this disorder is a slow, steady slippage, with no single derailment being particularly severe, so that the speaker gets farther and farther off track with each derailment without showing any awareness that her reply no longer has any connection with the question that was asked. This abnormality is often characterized by lack of cohesion between clauses and sentences and by unclear pronoun references.

Example: *Interviewer: Did you enjoy college? Patient: Um-hm. Oh hey well I, I oh, I really enjoyed some communities. I tried it, and the, and the next day when I'd be going out, you know, um, I took control like uh, I put, um, bleach on my hair in, in California. My roommate was from Chicago and she was going to the junior college. And we lived in the YWCA, so she wanted to put it, um, peroxide on my hair, and she did, and I got up and I looked at the mirror and tears came to my eyes. Now do you understand it—I was fully aware of what was going on but why couldn't I, I . . . why the tears? I can't understand that, can you?*

Tangentiality. Replying to a question in an oblique, tangential, or even irrelevant manner. The reply may be related to the question in some distant way, or the reply may be unrelated and seem totally irrelevant.

Example: *Interviewer: What city are you from? Patient: Well, that's a hard question to answer because my parents . . . I was born in Iowa, but I know that I'm white instead of black, so apparently I came from the North somewhere and I don't know where, you know, I really don't know whether I'm Irish or Scandinavian, or I don't, I don't believe I'm Polish, but I think I'm, I think I might be German or Welsh.*

Incoherence (word salad, schizophasia).
A pattern of speech that is essentially incomprehensible at times. Incoherence is often accompanied by derailment. It differs from derailment in that in incoherence the abnormality occurs within the level of the sentence or clause, which contains words or phrases that are joined incoherently. The abnormality in derailment involves unclear or confusing connections between larger units, such as sentences or clauses. This type of language disorder is relatively rare. When it occurs, it tends to be severe or extreme, and mild forms are quite uncommon. It may sound quite similar to Wernicke's aphasia or jargon aphasia, and in these cases the disorder should only be called incoherence definitively when history and laboratory data exclude the possibility of a past stroke and clinical testing for aphasia is negative.

Example: *Interviewer: What do you think about current political issues like the energy crisis? Patient: They're destroying too many cattle and oil just to make soap. If we need soap when you can jump into a pool of water, and then when you go to buy your gasoline, my folks always thought they should, get pop but the best thing to get, is motor oil, and, money. May, may as, well go there and, trade in some, pop caps and, uh, tires, and tractors to grup, car garages, so they can pull cars away from wrecks, is what I believed in.*

Illogicality. A pattern of speech in which conclusions are reached that do not follow logically. This may take the form of *non sequiturs* ("it does not follow"), in which the patient makes an inference between two clauses that is unwarranted or illogical. It may take the form of faulty inductive inferences. It may also take the form of reaching conclusions based on faulty premises without any actual delusional thinking.

Example: *Parents are the people that raise you. Anything that raises you can be a parent. Parents can be anything—material, vegetable, or mineral—that has taught you something. Parents would be the world of things that are alive, that are there. Rocks— a person can look at a rock and learn something from it, so that would be a parent.*

Circumstantiality. A pattern of speech that is very indirect and delayed in reaching its goal ideas. In the process of explaining something, the speaker brings in many tedious details and sometimes makes parenthetical remarks. Circumstantial replies or statements may last for many minutes if the speaker is not interrupted and urged to get to the point.

No example is provided because it would require too much space!

Interviewers will often recognize circumstantiality on the basis of needing to interrupt the speaker in order to complete the process of history taking within an allotted time. When not called circumstantial, these people are often referred to as "long-winded."

Although it may coexist with instances of poverty of content of speech or loss of goal, it differs from poverty of content of speech in containing excessive amplifying or illustrative detail and from loss of goal in that the goal is eventually reached if the person is allowed to talk long enough. It differs from derailment in that the details presented are closely related to some particular goal or idea and that the particular goal or idea must, by definition, eventually be reached (unless the patient is interrupted by an impatient interviewer).

Pressure of speech.   An increase in the amount of spontaneous speech as compared with what is considered ordinary or socially customary. The patient talks rapidly and is difficult to interrupt. Some sentences may be left uncompleted because of eagerness to get on to a new idea. Simple questions that could be answered in only a few words or sentences are answered at great length so that the answer takes minutes rather than seconds, and indeed may not stop at all if the speaker is not interrupted. Even when interrupted, the speaker often continues to talk. Speech tends to be loud and emphatic. Sometimes speakers with severe pressure will talk without any social stimulation and talk even though no one is listening. When patients are receiving neuroleptics or lithium, their speech is often slowed down by the medication, and then it can be judged only on the basis of amount, volume, and social ap-

No example is provided because the abnormality is manifested by rate, loudness, and amount of speech.

propriateness of speech. If a quantitative measure is applied to the rate of speech, then a rate greater than 150 words per minute is usually considered rapid or pressured. This disorder may be accompanied by derailment, tangentiality, or incoherence, but it is distinct from them.

Distractible speech. During the course of a discussion or interview, the patient stops talking in the middle of a sentence or idea and changes the subject in response to a nearby stimulus, such as an object on a desk, the interviewer's clothing or appearance, etc.

Example: *"Then I left San Francisco and moved to . . . Where did you get that tie? It looks like it's left over from the 50s. I like the warm weather in San Diego. Is that a conch shell on your desk? Have you ever gone scuba diving?"*

Clanging. A pattern of speech in which sounds rather than meaningful relationships appear to govern word choice, so that the intelligibility of the speech is impaired and redundant words are introduced in addition to rhyming relationships. This pattern of speech may also include punning associations so that a word similar in sound brings in a new thought.

Example: *"I'm not trying to make a noise. I'm trying to make sense. If you can make sense out of nonsense, well, have fun. I'm trying to make sense out of sense. I'm not making sense [cents] any more. I have to make dollars."*

Inappropriate Affect

Inappropriate affect appears in factor analytic studies to be poorly correlated with blunted affect and more related to positive thought disorder. Therefore, it is sometimes considered a positive symptom.

Affect expressed is inappropriate or incongruous, not simply flat or blunted. Most typically, this manifestation of affective disturbance takes the form of smiling or assuming a silly facial expression while talking about a serious or sad subject. Occasionally, patients may smile or laugh when talking about a serious subject that they find uncomfortable or embarrassing. Although their smiling may seem inappropriate, it is due to anxiety and therefore should not be rated as inappropriate affect.

Catatonic Motor Behavior

These symptoms are not common and should only be considered present when they are obvious and have been directly observed by the clinician or some other professional.

Stupor. Marked decrease in reactivity to environment and reduction of spontaneous movements and activity. The patient may appear to be aware of the nature of his surroundings.

Rigidity. Patient exhibits signs of motor rigidity, such as resistance to passive movement.

Waxy flexibility. Patient maintains postures into which she is placed for at least 15 seconds.

Excitement. Apparently purposeless and stereotyped excited motor activity not influenced by external stimuli.

Posturing and mannerisms. Voluntary assumption of inappropriate or bizarre posture. Manneristic gestures or tics may also be observed. These involve movements or gestures that appear artificial or contrived, are not appropriate to the situation, or are stereotyped and repetitive. (Subjects with tardive dyskinesia may have manneristic gestures or tics, but these should not be considered to be manifestations of catatonia.)

Alogia

Alogia is a general term coined to refer to the impoverished thinking and cognition that often occur in patients with schizophrenia (Greek *a* = "no," *logos* = "mind, thought"). Subjects with alogia have thinking processes that seem empty, turgid, or slow. Because thinking cannot be observed directly, it is inferred from the patient's speech. The two major manifestations of alogia are nonfluent empty speech (poverty of speech) and fluent empty speech (poverty of content of speech). Blocking and increased latency of response may also reflect alogia.

Poverty of speech. Restriction in the *amount* of spontaneous speech, so that replies to questions tend to be brief, concrete, and unelaborated. Unprompted additional information is rarely provided. Replies may be monosyllabic, and some questions may be left unanswered altogether. When confronted with this speech pattern, the interviewer may find himself frequently prompting the patient in order to encourage elaboration of replies. To elicit this finding, the examiner must allow the patient adequate time to answer and to elaborate his answer.

Example: *Interviewer: Can you tell me something about what brought you to the hospital? Patient: A car.*

Interviewer: I was wondering about what kinds of problems you've been having. Can you tell me something about them? Patient: I dunno.

Poverty of content of speech. Although replies are long enough so that speech is adequate in amount, it conveys little information. Language tends to be vague, often overabstract or overconcrete, repetitive, and stereotyped. The interviewer may recognize this finding by observing that the patient has spoken at some length but has not given adequate information to answer the question. Alternatively, the patient may provide enough information but require many words to do so, so that a lengthy reply can be summarized in a sentence or two.

This abnormality differs from circumstantiality in that the circumstantial patient tends to provide a wealth of detail.

Example: *Interviewer: Why is it, do you think, that people believe in God? Patient: Well, first of all because He uh, He are the person that is their personal savior. He walks with me and talks with me. And uh, the understanding that I have, um, a lot of people, they don't readily, uh, know their own personal self. Because, uh, they ain't, they all, just don't know their personal self. They don't, know that He uh—seemed like to me, a lot of 'em don't understand that He walks and talks with 'em.*

Blocking. Interruption of a train of speech before a thought or idea has been completed. After a period of silence, which may last from a few seconds to minutes, the person indicates that she cannot recall what she has been saying or meant to say. Blocking should only be judged to be present if a person voluntarily describes losing her thought or if, on questioning by the interviewer, the person indicates that was her reason for pausing.

Example: *Patient: So I didn't want to go back to school so I . . . (1-minute silence while the patient stares blankly). Interviewer: What about going back to school? What happened? Patient: I dunno. I forgot what I was going to say.*

Increased latency of response. The patient takes a longer time to reply to questions than is usually considered normal. He may seem "distant," and sometimes the examiner may wonder if he has heard the question. Prompting usually indicates that the patient is aware of the question, but has been having difficulty in formulating his thoughts in order to make an appropriate reply.

Example: *Interviewer: When were you last in the hospital? Patient: (30-second pause) A year ago.*

Interviewer: Which hospital was it? Patient: (30-second pause) This one.

Perseveration. Persistent repetition of words, ideas, or phrases so that once a patient begins to use a particular word, she continually returns to it in the process of speaking.

Exclusions: This differs from "stock words" in that the repeated words are used in ways inappropriate to their usual meaning. Some words or phrases are commonly used as pause-fillers, such as *you know* or *like*. These should not be considered perseverations.

Example: *Interviewer: Tell me what you are like—what kind of person you are. Patient: I'm from Marshalltown, Iowa. That's 60 miles northwest, northeast of Des Moines, Iowa. And I'm married at the present time. I'm 36 years old, my wife is 35. She lives in Garwin, Iowa. That's 15 miles southeast of Marshalltown, Iowa. I'm getting a divorce at the present time. And I am at present in a mental institution in Iowa City, Iowa, which is a 100 miles southeast of Marshalltown, Iowa.*

Affective Flattening or Blunting

Affective flattening or blunting manifests itself as a characteristic impoverishment of emotional expression, reactivity, and feeling. Affective flattening can be evaluated by observation of the patient's behavior and responsiveness during a routine interview. The evaluation of some items may be affected by drugs, because the parkinsonian side effects of neuroleptics may lead to masklike facies and diminished associated movements. Other aspects of affect, such as responsivity or appropriateness, will not be affected, however.

Unchanging facial expression. The patient's face does not change expression, or changes less than normally expected, as the emotional content of discourse changes. It appears wooden, mechanical, frozen. Because neuroleptics may partially mimic this effect, the interviewer should be careful to note whether the patient is on medication, but should not try to "correct" his assessment accordingly.

Decreased spontaneous movements. The patient sits quietly throughout the interview and shows few or no spontaneous movements. He does not shift position, move his legs, or move his hands, or does so less than normally expected.

Paucity of expressive gestures. The patient does not use her body as an aid in expressing her ideas through such means as hand gestures, sitting forward in her chair when intent on a subject, or leaning back when relaxed. This may occur in addition to decreased spontaneous movements.

Poor eye contact. The patient avoids looking at others or using his eyes as an aid in expression. He appears to be staring into space even when he is talking. Consider the quality of eye contact as well as quantity.

Affective nonresponsivity. Failure to smile or laugh when prompted may be tested by smiling or joking in a way that would usually elicit a smile from a normal individual.

Lack of vocal inflections. While speaking, the patient fails to show normal vocal emphasis patterns. Speech has a monotonic quality, and important words are not emphasized through changes in pitch or volume. The patient also may fail to change volume with changes of content, so that he does not drop his voice when discussing private topics or raise it as he discusses things that are exciting or for which louder speech might be appropriate.

Avolition-Apathy

Avolition manifests itself as a characteristic lack of energy and drive. Patients are unable to mobilize themselves to initiate or persist in completing many different kinds of tasks. Unlike the diminished energy or interest of depression, the avolitional symptom complex in schizophrenia is usually not accompanied by saddened or depressed affect. The avolitional symptom complex often leads to severe social and economic impairment.

Grooming and hygiene. The patient displays less attention to grooming and hygiene than normal. Clothing may appear sloppy, outdated, or soiled. Subject may bathe infrequently and not care for hair, nails, or teeth—leading to such manifestations as greasy or uncombed hair, dirty hands, body odor, or unclean teeth and bad breath. Overall, the appearance is dilapidated and disheveled. In extreme cases, the patient may even have poor toilet habits.

Impersistence at work or school. The patient has difficulty in seeking or maintaining employment (or schoolwork) as appropriate for her age and sex. If a student, she does not do homework and may even fail to attend class. Grades will tend to reflect this. If a college student, she may have registered for courses, but dropped several or all of them. If of working age, the patient may have found it difficult to work at a job because of inability to persist in completing tasks and apparent irresponsibility. She may go to work irregularly, wander away early, fail to complete expected assignments, or complete them in a disorganized manner. She may simply sit around the house

Have you been able to (work, go to school) during the past month?

Have you been attending vocational rehabilitation or occupational therapy sessions (in the hospital)?

What have you been able to do?

Do you have trouble finishing what you start?

What kinds of problems have you had?

and not seek any employment or seek it only in an infrequent or desultory manner. If a homemaker or a retired person, the patient may fail to complete chores, such as shopping or cleaning, or complete them in an apparently careless and half-hearted way. If in a hospital or institution, she does not attend or persist in vocational or rehabilitative programs effectively.

Physical anergia.   The patient tends to be physically inert; he may sit in a chair for hours at a time and not initiate any spontaneous activity. If encouraged to become involved in an activity, he may participate only briefly and then wander away or disengage himself and return to sitting alone. He may spend large amounts of time in some relatively mindless and physically inactive task such as watching television or playing solitaire. His family may report that he spends most of his time at home "doing nothing except sitting around." Either at home or in an inpatient setting, he may spend much of his time sitting in his room.

How have you been spending your time?

Do you have any trouble getting yourself going?

Anhedonia-Asociality

This symptom complex encompasses the patient's difficulties in experiencing interest or pleasure. It may express itself as a loss of interest in pleasurable activities, an inability to experience pleasure when participating in activities normally considered pleasurable, or a lack of involvement in social relationships of various kinds.

Recreational interests and activities.
The patient may have few or no interests, activities, or hobbies. Although this symptom may begin insidiously or slowly, there will usually be some obvious decline from an earlier level of interest and activity. Patients with relatively milder loss of interest will engage in some activities that are passive or nondemanding, such as watching television, or will show only occasional or sporadic inter-

What do you do for enjoyment?

How often do you do that (those things)?

Have you been attending recreational therapy?

What have you been doing?

Do you enjoy it?

ests. Patients with the most extreme loss will appear to have a complete and intractable inability to become involved in or enjoy activities. The evaluation in this area should take both the quality and quantity of recreational interests into account.

Sexual interest and activity. The patient may show a decrement in sexual interest and activity or enjoyment as would be judged normal for the patient's age and marital status. Individuals who are married may manifest disinterest in sex or may engage in intercourse only at the partner's request. In extreme cases, the patient may not engage in sex at all. Single patients may go for long periods of time without sexual involvement and make no effort to satisfy this drive. Whether married or single, patients may report that they subjectively feel only minimal sex drive or they take little enjoyment in sexual intercourse or in masturbatory activity even when they engage in it.

What has your sex drive been like?

Have you been able to enjoy sex lately?

(What is your usual sexual outlet?)

(When was the last time?)

Ability to feel intimacy and closeness. The patient may display an inability to form close and intimate relationships of a type appropriate for his age, sex, and family status. In the case of a younger person, this area should be evaluated in terms of relationships with the opposite sex, and with parents and siblings. In the case of an older person who is married, the relationship with spouse and with children should be evaluated, whereas older unmarried individuals should be judged in terms of relationships with the opposite sex and any family members who live nearby. Patients may display few or no feelings of affection to available family members, or they may have arranged their lives so that

Do you feel close to your family (husband, wife, children)?

Is there anyone outside your family that you feel especially close to?

How often do you see (them, him, her)?

they are completely isolated from any intimate relationships, living alone and making no effort to initiate contacts with family or members of the opposite sex. If the patient is homosexual, then relationships with members of the same sex may be evaluated as indications of ability to feel intimacy and closeness.

Relationships with friends and peers. Patients may also be relatively restricted in their relationships with friends and peers of either sex. They may have few or no friends, make little or no effort to develop such relationships, and choose to spend all or most of their time alone.

Do you have many friends?

Are you very close to them?

How often do you see them?

(What do you do together?)

Have you gotten to know any patients in the hospital?

Do you spend much time with them?

Attentional Impairment

Attention is often poor in psychotic patients. The patient may have trouble focusing her attention, or she may only be able to focus sporadically and erratically. She may ignore attempts to converse with her, wander away while in the middle of an activity or task, or appear to be inattentive when engaged in formal testing or interviewing. She may or may not be aware of her difficulty in focusing her attention.

Social inattentiveness. While involved in social situations or activities, the patient appears inattentive. He looks away during conversations, does not pick up the topic during a discussion, or appears uninvolved or disengaged. He may abruptly terminate a discussion or a task without any apparent reason. He may seem "spacey" or "out of it." He may seem to have poor concentration when playing games, reading, or watching television.

Inattentiveness during mental status testing. The patient may perform poorly on simple tests of intellectual functioning despite adequate education and intellectual ability. This should be assessed by having the patient spell *world* (or some equivalent five-letter word) backward and by serial 7s (for patients with at least a 10th-grade education) or serial 3s (for patients with at least a 6th-grade education) for a series of five subtractions. A perfect score is 10.

Manic Symptoms

Euphoric mood. The patient has had one or more distinct periods of euphoric, irritable, or expansive mood, not due to alcohol or drug intoxication.

Have you been having any periods when you felt extremely good or high—clearly different from your normal self?

Did your friends or family think this was more than just feeling good?

What about periods when you felt irritable and easily annoyed?

How long did this mood last?

Increase in activity. Patient shows an increase in involvement or activity level associated with work, family, friends, sex drive, new projects, interests, or activities (e.g., telephone calls, letter writing).

Was there a time when you were more active or involved in things compared with the way you usually are?

(How about at work, at home, with your friends, or with your family?)

(What about your involvement in hobbies or other interests?)

Were there times when you were unable to sit still or you always had to be moving, or pacing up and down?

Racing thoughts/flight of ideas. Patient has the subjective experience that thinking is markedly accelerated. Example: "My thoughts are ahead of my speech."

Were there times when your thoughts raced through your mind?

Did you have more ideas than usual?

Inflated self-esteem. Patient displays increased self-esteem and appraisal of his worth, contacts, influence, power, or knowledge (may be delusional) as compared with his usual level. Persecutory delusions should not be considered evidence of grandiosity unless the patient feels persecution is due to some special attributes (e.g., power, knowledge, contacts).

Have you felt more self-confident than usual?

(What about special plans?)

Have you felt you are a particularly important person or that you have special talents or abilities?

Decreased need for sleep. Patient needs less sleep than usual to feel rested (this rating should be based on the average of several days rather than a single severe night).

Have you needed less sleep than usual to feel rested?

(How much sleep do you ordinarily need?)

(How much sleep do you need now?)

Distractibility. Patient's attention is too easily drawn to unimportant or irrelevant external stimuli. For example, the patient gets up and inspects some item in the room while talking or listening, shifts her topic of speech, etc.

Have you found that things around you tend to distract you?

Poor judgment. Patient shows excessive involvement in activities that have a high potential for painful consequences that are not recognized, e.g., buying sprees, sexual indiscretions, foolish business investments, reckless giving.

Have you done anything that caused trouble for you or your family or friends?

Looking back now, was there anything you did that showed poor judgment?

Did you do anything foolish with money?

Did you do anything sexually that was unusual for you?

Depressive Symptoms

Dysphoric mood. The patient feels sad, despondent, discouraged, or unhappy; significant anxiety or tense irritability should also be rated as a dysphoric mood. The evaluation should be made irrespective of length of mood.

Have you been having periods of feeling depressed, sad, or hopeless? When you didn't care about anything or couldn't enjoy anything?

Have you felt tense, anxious, or irritable?

(How long did this last?)

Change in appetite or weight. Patient has had significant weight loss. This should not include dieting, unless the dieting is associated with some depressive belief that approaches delusional proportions.

Did you have any changes in your appetite—either increase or decrease?

Did you lose or gain much more weight than is usual for you?

Insomnia or hypersomnia. Insomnia may include waking up after only a few hours of sleep, as well as difficulty getting to sleep. Patterns of insomnia include *middle* (waking in the middle of the night, but eventually falling asleep again), *initial* (trouble going to sleep), and *terminal* (waking early—e.g., 2–5 A.M.—and remaining awake).

Have you had trouble sleeping?

(What was it like?)

(Do you have trouble falling asleep?)

(Do you wake up too early in the morning?)

Have you been sleeping more than usual?

How much sleep do you get in a typical 24-hour period?

Psychomotor agitation. Patient is unable to sit still, with a need to keep moving. Do not include mere subjective feelings of restlessness. Objective evidence should be present (e.g., hand-wringing, fidgeting, pacing).

Have you felt restless or agitated? Do you have trouble sitting still?

Psychomotor retardation. Patient feels slowed down and experiences great difficulty moving. Do not include mere subjective feelings of being slowed down. Objective evidence (e.g., slowed speech) should be present.

Have you been slowed down?

Loss of interest or pleasure. Patient has loss of interest or pleasure in usual activities, or a decrease in sexual drive. This may be similar to the anhedonia seen in psychosis. In the depressive syndrome, loss of interest or pleasure is invariably accompanied by intense, painful affect, however, whereas in psychosis the affect is often blunted.

Have you noticed a change in your interest in things?

What kinds of things do you normally enjoy?

Loss of energy. This symptom includes loss of energy, becoming easily fatigued, or feeling tired. These energy comparisons should be based on the person's usual activity level whenever possible.

Have you had a tendency to feel more tired than usual?

(Have you been feeling as if all your energy is drained?)

Feelings of worthlessness. In addition to feelings of worthlessness, patient may report feeling self-reproach, or excessive or inappropriate guilt. (Either may be delusional.)

Have you been feeling down on yourself?

Have you been feeling guilty about anything?

(Could you tell me about some of the things for which you feel guilty?)

Diminished ability to think or concentrate. Patient complains of diminished ability to think or concentrate, such as slowed thinking or indecisiveness; not associated with marked derailment or incoherence.

Have you had trouble thinking?

What about your concentration?

Have you had trouble making decisions?

Recurrent thoughts of death or suicide. Patient has thoughts about death and suicide, plus possible wishes to be dead and/or suicide attempts.

Have you been thinking about death, or about taking your own life?

(How often have these thoughts occurred?)

If yes, inquire for more details.

Distinct quality to mood. The patient's depressed mood is experienced as distinctly different from the kind of feelings experienced after the death of a loved one. If the patient has not lost a loved one, ask him to compare the feelings to those after some significant personal loss appropriate to his age and experience.

The feelings of (sadness) you are having now—are they the same as the feelings you would have had when someone close to you died, or are they different?

How are they similar or different?

Nonreactivity of mood. Doesn't feel much better even temporarily, when something good happens.

Do your feelings of depression go away or get better when you do something you enjoy—like talking with friends, visiting your family, or [mention some favorite recreation]?

Diurnal variation. The mood shifts during the course of the day. Some patients feel terrible in the morning, but steadily better as the day goes on, and even near normal in the evening. Others feel good in the morning and worse as the day progresses.

Is there any time of the day that is especially bad for you?

(Do you feel worse in the morning?) (In the evening?)

(Or is it about the same all the time?)

Anxiety Symptoms

Panic attacks.   These are discrete episodes of intense fear or discomfort, in which a variety of symptoms occur such as shortness of breath, dizziness, palpitations, or shaking.

Have you ever experienced a sudden attack of panic or fear, in which you felt extremely uncomfortable?

How long did it last?

Did you notice any other symptoms occurring at the same time?

Did you feel as if you were going to die?

Agoraphobia.   This is a fear of going outside (literally "a fear of the marketplace"). In many patients, however, the fear is more generalized and involves being afraid of being in a place or situation from which escape might be difficult.

Have you ever been afraid of going outside, so that you tended to just stay home all the time?

Have you been afraid of getting caught or trapped somewhere, so that you would be unable to escape?

Social phobia.   The patient has a fear of being in some social situation where she will be seen by others and may do something that she might find to be humiliating or embarrassing. Some common social phobias include fear of public speaking, fear of eating in front of others, or fear of using public bathrooms.

Do you have any specific fears, such as a fear of public speaking?

Of eating in front of others?

Simple phobia.   The patient is afraid of some specific circumscribed stimulus. Simple phobias often involve animals, such as snakes or insects; they also involve seeing blood, being at high places, or fear of flying on airplanes.

Do you have any other specific fears?

Are you afraid of snakes?

The sight of blood?

Air travel?

Obsessions.   The patient experiences persistent ideas, thoughts, or impulses that he sees as ego alien and that he finds unpleasant. He tends to ruminate and worry about them. He may try to ignore or suppress them, but typically finds this difficult. Some common ob-

Are you ever bothered by persistent ideas that you can't get out of your head?

Can you give me some specific example?

sessions include repetitive thoughts of performing some violent act or becoming contaminated by touching other people or public objects.

Compulsions. The patient finds she has to perform specific acts over and over in a way that she recognizes to be useless or inappropriate. Usually, the compulsions are performed to ease some worry or obsession, or prevent some feared event from occurring. For example, a patient may worry that she has left the door unlocked and have to return over and over to check it. Obsessions about contamination may lead to repetitive hand washing. Obsessions about thoughts of violence may lead to ritualistic behavior designed to prevent injury to the person about whom violence has been imagined.

Do you have any acts you have to perform over and over?

Can you give me some examples?

Interviews and Rating Scales for Research

To standardize research assessments, various interviews and rating scales have been developed. Typically, these interviews and rating scales have been rigorously evaluated to document that they have excellent reliability, making them relatively precise instruments for measurement and assessment.

Structured Interviews

There are six major structured interviews currently available for psychiatric research (Table 3-3). Each of these has various strengths and weaknesses. All use a structured or systematic approach to eliciting information about the patient's current and past history.

Table 3-3.   Structured interviews

Present State Examination (PSE)
Schedule for Affective Disorders and Schizophrenia (SADS)
Diagnostic Interview Schedule (DIS)
Structured Clinical Interview for DSM-III-R (SCID)
Comprehensive Assessment of Symptoms and History (CASH)
Structured Clinical Interview for DSM-III-R—Personality Disorders (SCID-II)

The *Present State Examination* (PSE), developed by John Wing in England in the 1960s, is the oldest of the structured psychiatric interviews. Its time frame is limited to symptoms present during the past month, making it unsatisfactory for lifetime diagnoses. It cannot be used to make DSM-III diagnoses without substantial adaptations and additions. Consequently, it is used infrequently in American research.

The *Schedule for Affective Disorders and Schizophrenia* (SADS) was the first well-developed American structured interview, becoming available in the 1970s. It includes two sections, one evaluating the current condition and a second evaluating symptoms occurring during the patient's lifetime. Thus, it gives a broader coverage of symptoms and past history. It was developed before DSM-III, however, and cannot be used to make DSM-III diagnoses. It has its own set of diagnostic criteria, the Research Diagnostic Criteria (RDC).

The *Diagnostic Interview Schedule* (DIS) was designed largely for epidemiological field studies of large samples of patients. Unlike the PSE or the SADS, it does not require interviewers with prior experience working with psychiatric patients. It can be used to make DSM-III diagnoses. Although it is well suited for large-scale epidemiological studies, its coverage is relatively sparse for working with actual patients suffering from relatively severe psychiatric syndromes.

The *Structured Clinical Interview for DSM-III-R* (SCID) was the first interview designed to apply DSM-III-R criteria to psychiatrically ill patients. Its focus is largely on making diagnoses. It includes only information listed in DSM-III-R diagnostic criteria. It is concise and "user friendly," but incomplete in its coverage of clinical symptoms.

The *Comprehensive Assessment of Symptoms and History* (CASH) is the most recent of the structured interviews, developed in the 1980s. Because diagnostic criteria have been changing rapidly during the past few years, the CASH was designed to provide a broad coverage of symptoms so that investigators would have a comprehensive data base that could be adapted to various different diagnostic systems. It includes a current and a past section. It also includes structured sections to assess sociodemographic history, handedness, memory impairment, negative symptoms, and various other aspects of clinical description that are not included in the structured interviews listed above.

The *Structured Clinical Interview for DSM-III-R—Personality Disorders* (SCID-II) was developed as a complement to the other structured interviews designed to make Axis I diagnoses. The SCID-II provides a structured interview that permits clinicians and investigators to make assessments for diagnoses of personality syndromes according to DSM-III-R criteria.

Rating Scales

Rating scales typically are designed to provide a rapid and concise assessment of a specific aspect of psychopathology. Most rating scales have been developed for use in clinical drug trials, or other situations in which investigators wish to assess a change in the patient's status by taking repeated measurements over time (usually

Table 3-4.   Rating scales

Brief Psychiatric Rating Scale (BPRS)
Scale for the Assessment of Negative Symptoms (SANS)
Scale for the Assessment of Positive Symptoms (SAPS)
Hamilton Rating Scale for Depression (HRSD)
Beck Depression Inventory (BDI)
Hamilton Anxiety Rating Scale
Abnormal Involuntary Movement Scale (AIMS)
Simpson-Angus Scale
Mini-Mental State Exam (MMSE)
Global Assessment Scale (GAS)

at weekly intervals). Table 3-4 summarizes some of the rating scales that are commonly used in psychiatric research of this type. Copies of each of these scales, except the Beck Depression Inventory, appear in the Appendix.

The *Brief Psychiatric Rating Scale* (BPRS) is the oldest of the rating scales. It was developed in the 1960s and used factor analysis to sift through a broad array of symptoms seen in psychiatric patients and to generate a relatively small number of factors. These include things such as conceptual disorganization, hostility, or social withdrawal. The BPRS is still widely used, although most of the items rated are relatively abstract when compared with the specific symptoms currently used to assess psychopathology.

The *Scale for the Assessment of Negative Symptoms* (SANS) and the *Scale for the Assessment of Positive Symptoms* (SAPS) were designed to provide a more complete coverage of the symptoms of psychosis than is provided by the BPRS. The SANS is the only scale currently in wide use that assesses negative symptoms. These scales rate the phenomena that clinicians are accustomed to assessing, such as delusions, hallucinations, positive formal thought disorder, etc.

The *Hamilton Rating Scale for Depression* (HRSD) is also among the oldest rating scales. It was specifically designed to provide a quantitative measurement of symptoms of depression that would be sensitive to change. Like the BPRS, it was developed shortly after the discovery of psychoactive drugs and was a standard instrument used to assess the efficacy of new antidepressants as they were developed. Although a number of other rating scales for depression have been developed, none has supplanted the HRSD in general use.

The *Beck Depression Inventory* (BDI) is also very commonly used. Unlike the HRSD, the BDI focuses on cognitive or psychological symptoms of depression.

The *Hamilton Anxiety Rating Scale* performs a similar function to the HRSD for assessing anxiety. It is also widely used in clinical drug trials, and as an overall assessment instrument.

The *Abnormal Involuntary Movement Scale* (AIMS) was developed to determine whether patients had developed abnormal movements characteristic of tardive dyskinesia. It is currently widely used in neuroleptic trials.

The *Simpson-Angus Scale* is also widely used and is similar to the AIMS, but it focuses more specifically on the side effects of neuroleptics, such as parkinsonian symptoms or akathisia.

The *Mini-Mental State Exam* (MMSE) is a brief instrument designed to assess cognitive status. It provides quantitative measurements of orientation, memory, calculations, and other aspects of the systematic mental status examination. It is a quantitative scale with a perfect score of 30 points. It is now widely used as a simple, rapid method for assessing abnormalities in mental status.

The *Global Assessment Scale* (GAS) is a 100-point scale that is included in various structured interviews, such as the SADS or the CASH. It is very similar to the Global Assessment of Functioning (GAF) Scale (described in Chapter 2), which was derived from the GAS. This scale provides a brief, simple way of assessing the patient's level of functioning and severity of psychopathology. Because it is quite sensitive to change, it is frequently used as an overall index of the patient's improvement over time.

Bibliography

Andreasen NC: Thought, language, and communication disorders, I: clinical assessment, definition of terms, and evaluation of their reliability. Arch Gen Psychiatry 36:1315–1321, 1979

Andreasen NC: Thought, language, and communication disorders, II: diagnostic significance. Arch Gen Psychiatry 36:1325–1330, 1979

Andreasen NC: Negative symptoms in schizophrenia: definition and reliability. Arch Gen Psychiatry 39:784–788, 1982

Andreasen NC: The Scale for the Assessment of Negative Symptoms (SANS). Iowa City, The University of Iowa, 1983

Andreasen NC: The Scale for the Assessment of Positive Symptoms (SAPS). Iowa City, The University of Iowa, 1984

Andreasen NC: Comprehensive Assessment of Symptoms and History (CASH). Iowa City, The University of Iowa, 1985

Beck AT: Depression Inventory. Philadelphia, PA, Philadelphia Center for Cognitive Therapy, 1978

Endicott J, Spitzer RL: A diagnostic interview: the Schedule for Affective Disorders and Schizophrenia (SADS). Arch Gen Psychiatry 35:837–844, 1978

Endicott J, Spitzer RL, Fleiss JL, et al: The Global Assessment Scale: a procedure for measuring overall severity of psychiatric disturbance. Arch Gen Psychiatry 33:766–771, 1976

Folstein MF, Folstein SE, McHugh PR: "Mini Mental State": a practical method for grading the cognitive state of patients for the clinician. J Psychiatr Res 12:189–198, 1975

Guy W: ECDEU: assessment manual for psychopharmacology (DHEW Publ No 76-338). Washington, DC, Department of Health, Education, and Welfare, Psychopharmacology Research Branch, 1976, pp 534–537

Hamilton M: The assessment of anxiety states by rating. Br J Med Psychol 32:50–55, 1959

Hamilton M: A rating scale for depression. J Neurol Neurosurg Psychiatry 23:56–62, 1960

Overall JE: The Brief Psychiatric Rating Scale (BPRS): recent developments in ascertainment and scaling. Psychopharmacol Bull 24:97–99, 1988

Robins LN, Helzer JE, Croughan J, et al: National Institute of Mental Health Diagnostic

Interview Schedule: its history, characteristics, and validity. Arch Gen Psychiatry 38:381–389, 1981

Simpson GM, Angus JWS: A rating scale for extrapyramidal side effects. Acta Psychiatr Scand [Suppl] 212:11–19, 1970

Spitzer RL, Williams JBW, Gibbon M, et al: Structured Clinical Interview for DSM-III-R (SCID). Washington, DC, American Psychiatric Press, 1990

Spitzer RL, Williams JBW, Gibbon M, et al: Structured Clinical Interview for DSM-III-R—Personality Disorders (SCID-II). Washington, DC, American Psychiatric Press, 1990

Stangl D, Pfohl B, Zimmerman M, et al: A structured interview for DSM-III personality disorder. Arch Gen Psychiatry 42:591–596, 1985

Wing JK: A standard form of psychiatric Present State Examinations (PSE) and a method for standardizing the classification of symptoms, in Psychiatric Epidemiology. Edited by Hare EH, Wing JK. London, Oxford University Press, 1970, pp 93–108

Self-assessment Questions

1. Describe the way in which the patient's chief complaint can be used to take a history and to develop a differential diagnosis.
2. Describe several techniques that are important for concluding the initial interview with a patient.
3. Enumerate the components of a standard psychiatric history, giving each of the main headings of the overall outline.
4. Summarize the major components of the mental status examination.
5. List the five positive symptoms of psychosis. Give examples of some typical kinds of delusions and hallucinations.
6. List the five common negative symptoms of psychosis.
7. Enumerate and define some of the symptoms observed in depression.
8. Enumerate and define some of the symptoms observed in mania.
9. Enumerate and define some of the symptoms observed in anxiety disorders.

Chapter 4
Laboratory Tests

There is no observer outside the experiment.

Heisenberg

Although psychiatry places a greater emphasis on careful history taking and assessment than do most other medical specialties, laboratory tests are also growing in importance. The capacity to develop laboratory tests that will assist in making a specific diagnosis will depend heavily on the continuing growth of a neuroscience base within psychiatry, a topic that is discussed in more detail in Chapter 5. Psychiatry is just beginning to have specific "diagnostic tests" with reasonable sensitivity and specificity. Tests of this type are only available for a few disorders (e.g., Alzheimer's disease), and even in these few instances their diagnostic validity is still not firmly established. Research efforts are, however, developing a strong scientific base that will very likely lead to a growing number of useful laboratory tests in the future, particularly in the area of neuroimaging.

Some type of laboratory workup will be appropriate for all inpatient admissions to a psychiatric unit, although the laboratory workup may be quite simple. The need for laboratory evaluations among outpatients will vary, depending on the age of the patient, the type of symptoms with which he or she presents, and the type of treatment plan. Young healthy individuals who have received a medical evaluation within the past few years and who have relatively mild psychiatric symptoms will probably need nothing. On the other hand, even among outpatients, some laboratory assessments may be necessary in patients who are elderly or who present with severe or complex problems, particularly if there is a differential diagnosis that suggests some medical cause for the presenting symptoms.

Most laboratory procedures conducted with psychiatric patients are done for one of four purposes:

1. To complete a general medical workup of the sort done routinely for any hospital admission
2. To rule out some nonpsychiatric cause of the presenting symptoms
3. To conduct a specific workup appropriate for a specific treatment that has been planned (e.g., a workup before conducting electroconvulsive therapy [ECT])
4. To conduct clinical research

Each of these purposes and the relevant laboratory procedures are discussed in more detail below. The first three have a direct clinical applicability. The fourth purpose is also worth discussing in some detail because research applications are growing quickly toward clinical applications.

The General Medical Workup

Standards as to what is considered an appropriate general medical workup may vary in different hospital settings. The list of procedures that are considered appropriate or required may tend to decrease as increasing cost constraints are applied by third-party payers. In general, however, most patients admitted to a hospital receive a set of screening laboratory evaluations. Typically, these consist of a complete blood count (CBC), urinalysis, serum electrolytes, liver enzymes (i.e., serum glutamic-oxaloacetic transaminase [SGOT] and serum glutamic pyruvic transaminase [SGPT]), serum creatinine, blood urea nitrogen (BUN), and sometimes a chest film or electrocardiogram (ECG) (the relevance of the latter two depend in part on the patient's age, smoking history, and overall physical condition). Female patients need a Pap smear, and most gynecologists believe that women over age 45 should be evaluated with mammography at periodic intervals.

The psychiatrist should assume responsibility for ensuring that an appropriate laboratory screen is obtained, taking into account whether the patient has had any of these evaluations recently. A psychiatrist who is seeing outpatients at regular intervals should also attempt to assume responsibility for ensuring that these patients receive annual general medical workups, including appropriate histories, physicals, and laboratory tests. In many cases, the psychiatrist assumes the role of a primary-care physician, being the physician whom the patient sees most frequently. Depending on regional mores, the psychiatrist may or may not assume responsibility for conducting physical and neurological examinations, ordering the tests, and interpreting them.

Laboratory Tests to Rule Out Nonpsychiatric Causes of Symptoms

Many diagnoses in psychiatry are diagnoses of exclusion. That is, they are typically made after it has been determined that the symptoms the patient manifests are not due to some other specific medical or neurological disorder. Historically, psychi-

Table 4-1. Conditions commonly considered in the differential diagnosis of major mental illnesses

---

Multi-infarct dementia
Subdural hematoma
Normal pressure hydrocephalus
Tumors
AIDS dementia
Temporal lobe epilepsy
Endocrine/metabolic disorders
Exposure to toxins
Vitamin deficiency syndromes (e.g., pernicious anemia)
Other central nervous system infections (e.g., syphilis)
Substance-induced symptoms
Neuropsychiatric effects of medical treatment (e.g., potassium deficiency from diuretics, fatigue from propranolol, digitalis toxicity, phenytoin [Dilantin] toxicity)

---

atrists used to say that they were ruling out "organic" causes of the symptoms. This phraseology is somewhat outdated, because diseases such as schizophrenia or manic-depressive illness (i.e., bipolar affective disorder) almost certainly have a specific organic cause, rooted in aberrations in brain chemistry or circuitry. Identifying the pathophysiology and etiology of serious mental illnesses is one of the major goals of most current psychiatric research.

Table 4-1 lists various conditions commonly considered in the differential diagnosis of serious mental illnesses such as the dementias, schizophrenia, bipolar disorder, or the various anxiety disorders. In general, when DSM-III-R states that "it cannot be established that an organic condition initiated or maintained the disorder," one of the group of disorders in Table 4-1 is to be ruled out. These various disorders are discussed in more detail under the differential diagnosis of the various conditions presented in Section II ("Psychiatric Disorders") of this volume. Because the majority of the conditions listed in Table 4-1 are nonpsychiatric conditions, methods for evaluating them and ruling them out are more properly the province of other medical disciplines apart from psychiatry. Nevertheless, they are discussed briefly here for the convenience of the student. A more detailed description of some of the specific laboratory tests is provided later in this chapter, under the various relevant headings (e.g., neurophysiological techniques, neuroimaging).

Multi-infarct dementia, subdural hematoma, normal pressure hydrocephalus, tumors, and acquired immunodeficiency syndrome (AIDS) dementia may all present with confusion, memory impairment, personality change, poor attention and drive, tearfulness and depression, or suspiciousness and even frank delusions. The most common psychiatric conditions that must be differentiated from these "organic disorders" include Alzheimer's disease, schizophrenia and related psychotic conditions (e.g., schizophreniform disorder, delusional disorder), and the various mood disorders.

Neuroimaging provides the most efficient method for ruling out the majority of these conditions. A simple computerized tomography (CT) scan may be sufficient.

Magnetic resonance imaging (MRI) is more effective because it permits the identification of small focal lesions, which may represent old infarcts, and which typically appear as areas of increased signal intensity. The white matter lesions of multiple sclerosis are also readily seen with MRI, and AIDS dementia may show similar small focal lesions. Because of its excellent resolution and three-dimensional capacity, MRI is particularly useful for identifying tumors. Tumors typically appear bright on MRI, when T2 weighted sequences (specific scanning sequences that are especially sensitive for detecting abnormal tissue, but poorer for seeing structure) are used.

As is described in more detail later in this chapter, Alzheimer's disease represents a "special case" in neuroimaging evaluations. With functional imaging techniques such as single photon emission computer tomography (SPECT) or positron-emission tomography (PET), 70–80% of patients with Alzheimer's disease show a characteristic decrease in metabolic function or cerebral blood flow in posterior temporoparietal regions. Alzheimer's disease appears at present to be the only major mental illness that shows this characteristic pattern of hypometabolic function; thus, functional imaging techniques such as SPECT or PET may be particularly useful in differentiating Alzheimer's disease from other disorders that present with confusion and intellectual deterioration. Other laboratory tests, such as electroencephalography or neuropsychological assessment, may also be useful in evaluating this particular group of "rule outs."

Temporal lobe epilepsy (TLE) typically presents with dissociative-like episodes or personality changes such as hyperreligiosity, hypergraphia (writing prolifically), hyposexuality, temper outbursts, and, occasionally, mood or psychotic-like symptoms. Thus, its differential diagnosis includes the various dissociative disorders, obsessive-compulsive personality disorder, antisocial personality disorder, conduct disorders, and the mood and psychotic disorders. Because TLE is due to an electrical and functional disturbance in the brain, it is best evaluated by the laboratory tests that employ the methods of neurophysiology or functional neuroimaging. The electroencephalogram (EEG) is the "test of choice" because of its noninvasive nature, inexpensiveness, and ease of administration. Nevertheless, the focal lesion in TLE may be deeply embedded inside the brain in the anterior poles of the temporal lobes or even the medial aspects of the temporal lobes. Because EEG uses surface electrodes, it may not pick up seizure foci in these deep brain regions. Consequently, the assessment of TLE may require additional techniques, even when EEG is used. Sleep deprivation may bring out focal abnormalities not noticed with routine EEG, and nasopharyngeal leads are particularly appropriate if a diagnosis of TLE is being considered. PET may also pick up focal regions of hypometabolic function, but this neuroimaging technique is not widely available.

Endocrine disorders, exposure to toxins, vitamin deficiency syndromes (e.g., pernicious anemia), and other central nervous system infections apart from AIDS (e.g., syphilis) may present with fatigue, weakness, decreased drive, memory impairment, intellectual confusion, and personality change. Again, the most common psychiatric differential diagnoses are the various dementias, psychotic conditions, mood disorders, and a few anxiety or personality disorders. Hyperthyroidism is a common mimic of anxiety conditions, and myxedema is a common mimic of mood disorders. The other "rule outs" are considerably less common. These conditions are evaluated by various specific assessment techniques, including serum T_3 and T_4, CBC, serum assays for toxins, or a VDRL test for syphilis.

Finally, the clinician must attempt to determine whether the patient's presenting symptoms are due to various "street drugs" that are all too readily available, or to various medications prescribed by physicians that are often also all too readily available. "Street drugs" such as amphetamines, cocaine, or phencyclidine (PCP) are special culprits in producing psychotic-like syndromes that resemble schizophrenia. Marijuana abuse leads to lethargy and withdrawal that may mimic depression, the negative symptoms of schizophrenia, or personality syndromes such as schizoid or schizotypal personality. These drugs may also produce periods of feeling "high" that may mimic mood disorders. Use of street drugs, which is often denied by patients on interview, can be assessed though routine urine drug screens. Because of the substantial prevalence of substance abuse in contemporary American society, a urine drug screen should be very nearly a routine diagnostic test for patients admitted as inpatients to psychiatric facilities.

Iatrogenic psychiatric disorders are also not uncommon. Patients who have received large quantities of prescribed drugs may also present with a variety of symptoms that mimic psychiatric disorders. Patients being treated with diuretics for hypertension may have a potassium deficiency that produces fatigue and that mimics depression. Propranolol may have similar effects. Digitalis toxicity and phenytoin (Dilantin) toxicity can produce fatigue and intellectual confusion that may mimic depression, psychosis, or dementia. Particularly in elderly patients, the clinician should maintain a high index of suspicion that symptoms that present as possible "psychiatric disorder" are in fact due to prescribed medications. Anxiolytics and hypnotics, which are frequently prescribed by nonpsychiatric physicians, can also produce various symptoms that mimic classic psychiatric disorders, such as confusion, lethargy, or withdrawal. Frequently, the diagnosis of a psychiatric condition due to prescribed drugs can be made simply from the history. Sometimes, however, laboratory tests are also needed, as in establishing low serum potassium levels, or obtaining quantitative blood levels for prescribed medications such as benzodiazepines.

Workups Pertaining to Specific Types of Psychiatric Treatments

In addition to using laboratory evaluations to assist in diagnosis and differential diagnosis, some laboratory procedures may be necessary before instituting a particular treatment. Some treatments, such as ECT, have a modest risk associated with them. Therefore, it is desirable to obtain laboratory assessments to determine and document the patient's physical condition before the treatment, to rule out conditions that might be adversely affected by the treatment, and to establish baseline values for the patient before instituting treatment.

Electroconvulsive therapy (ECT). As is discussed in more detail in Chapter 24, "Somatic Treatments," ECT is a relatively safe and highly effective treatment for some psychiatric disorders, such as severe depression. The actual physical convulsion involved is typically attenuated through the use of succinylcholine, but there is nevertheless a very modest risk for fractures if the initial dose of succinylcholine is not correctly established. Spine films may be indicated in elderly or arthritic patients before instituting ECT. Noticing signs of osteoporosis on spine films does not necessarily rule out the use of ECT, if it is clinically appropriate, but it may suggest that a somewhat higher dose of succinylcholine would be desirable.

An ECG is usually obtained before ECT to determine baseline cardiac status, because arrhythmias may occur during or after a treatment. Some clinicians also like to obtain an EEG on patients before ECT because any EEG obtained after ECT has been initiated would be uninterpretable because ECT can produce EEG changes that may last for months. Thus, if an elderly depressed patient has questionable signs of dementia before ECT, it is best to obtain a full dementia workup before ECT, because ECT itself may produce memory impairment. Neuropsychological tests obtained within several months after ECT may also be uninterpretable.

Lithium treatment. Lithium carbonate (used in the treatment of bipolar disorder) occasionally has adverse effects on both the thyroid gland and the kidney. Thus, it is desirable to obtain a urinalysis, serum electrolytes, BUN, serum creatinine, and serum T_3 and T_4 before instituting lithium treatment. Because lithium produces ECG changes that are nonspecific in nature and do not reflect cardiotoxicity, many clinicians often consider it worthwhile to obtain an ECG before prescribing lithium as well.

Determining whether the patient is on a therapeutic level of lithium is also assessed through a simple laboratory test to measure lithium blood levels. These are usually obtained twice weekly during the first few weeks of lithium treatment. Thereafter, they are typically obtained at regular intervals, such as every 6 months or every year on an outpatient basis as long as the patient remains on lithium. Serum electrolytes, BUN, serum creatinine, and serum T_3 and T_4 are also typically rechecked at similar intervals. An elevated serum creatinine should be followed up with a 24-hour creatinine clearance.

Tricyclic antidepressants. These medications do not necessarily require any specific laboratory workup before instituting treatment. This decision will depend on the age and physical condition of the patient. Typically, no tests are needed for healthy young adults. Because tricyclics also produce ECG changes, however, an ECG should be obtained before prescribing tricyclics if there is any question that it may be needed later. Older patients or patients in whom there is any possible cardiac abnormality should definitely be evaluated with an ECG before being prescribed tricyclics, because the major adverse effects of tricyclics involve the cardiac conduction system.

Blood levels may be monitored for tricyclics. Their use to monitor treatment may serve several purposes. A few tricyclics, such as nortriptyline, have a definite "therapeutic window." Blood level determinations may also be ordered in instances when the clinician is wondering whether the patient is taking the medication at all (to determine the presence of some blood level), when the clinician is concerned that the patient appears to be toxic, or when the patient is failing to respond to established therapeutic doses. (See Chapter 24, "Somatic Treatments," for a more complete discussion of management of dosages of psychoactive medications.)

All patients treated with tricyclics should receive an annual physical examination with close attention to cardiac function and evaluation of blood pressure every 3–6 months, because the primary adverse effects of tricyclics are on cardiac conduction and baroreceptors. Tricyclics can also produce changes in liver enzymes, which should be checked annually.

Antipsychotics. Like tricyclics, antipsychotics may need no special workup before prescription. Typically, no tests are needed. Blood levels are more difficult to monitor for neuroleptics because many produce active metabolites. Assays are currently available for several antipsychotics, but they are of questionable value because research has not definitely shown a relationship between blood level and clinical response. The main reasons for ordering blood level determinations of neuroleptic drugs are similar to those just described above for tricyclics.

The major adverse effects of neuroleptics appear to be on the extrapyramidal system in the brain. The development of tardive dyskinesia is the single most important serious long-term side effect. No laboratory tests are currently available to test for this side effect, although neuroimaging may eventually provide such tests. At present, the development of tardive dyskinesia is best monitored through regular physical examinations with careful attention to the development of abnormal movements using the Abnormal Involuntary Movement Scale (AIMS) (described in Chapter 3).

Laboratory Procedures Used in Clinical Research

Laboratory tests are frequently used in clinical research. Although research applications may not be relevant to medical students or residents in most other branches of clinical medicine, they are highly relevant in psychiatry. Many laboratory assessments currently in use in clinical research are being studied because they are felt to have potential clinical applications. Thus, the student or resident will often want to familiarize himself or herself with a variety of these techniques, because they are rapidly growing toward clinical application. Many are used for clinical assessment in some situations (e.g., CT or MRI to rule out an "organic" condition), whereas they are research tools in other applications (e.g., attempting to determine whether structural brain abnormalities occur in major mental illnesses and whether they progress over time). Some of these laboratory tests, such as CT, have such a well-established research base that many clinicians feel that they should be ordered routinely in patients who present with a first episode of a relatively severe mental illness.

Overview of Laboratory Tests Frequently Used in Psychiatry

Neurophysiological Techniques

Electroencephalogram (EEG).   This is one of the oldest laboratory tests available to psychiatrists. Hans Berger, a psychiatrist who pioneered the development of EEG, was the first person to record the electrical activity of the brain. Until the advent of structural imaging techniques, such as CT and MRI, EEG was the major method for evaluating abnormalities in brain activity produced by disorders such as tumors, head injuries, or seizures. CT and MRI now offer relatively benign methods for studying the brain in vivo to rule out the presence of diseased regions of tissue, but EEG remains the simplest, most noninvasive method for evaluating seizures and metabolic dysfunctions.

EEG measures electrical activity using a montage of electrodes scattered over the surface of the brain. An example of a typical montage appears in Figure 4-1. Electrical activity is recorded from leads connected to these surface electrodes; a typical modern EEG uses 16 leads. The electrical activity is then recorded on a polygraph, much like an ECG, and the pattern of activity is evaluated. Although computerized methods have been developed for reading EEGs, the best computer continues to be the human brain connected to the human eye.

EEG characteristics are described in terms of the frequency of the waveforms observed (measured in cycles per second). The normal human brain typically shows activity in either the beta (>12) or alpha (8–12) range during the waking state. As individuals become drowsy, theta (4–8) and delta (<4) are observed. In the

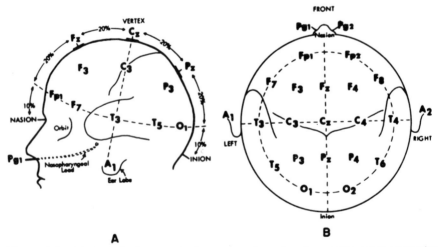

Figure 4-1.   Typical electroencephalogram montage. Leads are arrayed to cover the entire brain, ranging from frontal to occipital.

waking state, both theta and delta activity are considered to be abnor[mal]
healthy human brain. (Diffuse theta activity is sometimes seen in elderly i[n]
while awake, however.) Delta activity in the waking state is clearly abno[rmal]
represents sick or dying tissue.

Abnormalities observed on EEG include spike and wave patterns, focal s[lowing,]
and diffuse slowing. Spike and wave patterns are typically seen in brains susc[eptible]
to seizures. The location of the spike may indicate the primary focus from [which]
the seizure derives. The spikes of a brain predisposed to produce epileptic at[tacks]
are less often seen during the waking state. Consequently, EEGs are best obta[ined]
while the patient is asleep; sedation is often prescribed to induce sleep during [the]
EEG so that abnormal seizure foci can be observed.

Encephalographers believe that a seizure disorder cannot be ruled out throug[h]
a simple waking EEG. In addition, nasopharyngeal leads may be needed to identif[y]
a deep seizure focus. The tendency to manifest spike activities is suppressed by
anticonvulsant medications, such as phenytoin (Dilantin). Thus, a patient with
epilepsy may have a normal EEG if appropriately medicated, particularly if only a
waking EEG is obtained. A normal EEG does not rule out the existence of a seizure
disorder because the identification of spike and wave activity requires catching the
brain during the elusive moments when spikes are occurring. Nevertheless, serial
normal EEGs obtained in sleeping, unmedicated individuals do make the diagnosis
of a seizure disorder unlikely.

The EEG is very sensitive to metabolic dysfunctions and to the effects of various
drugs. In the case of metabolic dysfunctions, an EEG may be the simplest of methods
for determining that the patient's cognitive symptoms are due to some type of
metabolic disorder. Various psychoactive drugs affect the EEG: lithium, for example, produces an increase in theta activity, and benzodiazepines produce rapid,
fast activity (i.e., beta activity). Sometimes the EEG provides a clinician with the
first clue that a patient has been taking unprescribed medications, or even medications prescribed by another physician. In a few rare instances, the EEG can serve
as a useful test for ruling out psychiatric disorders that represent conversion phenomena or malingering. For example, the presence of photic driving (visual stimulation with flashes of bright lights) on EEG will rule out hysterical blindness.

Sleep EEG (polysomnography) is a special type of EEG involving the collection
of electrical brain activity data during all-night sleep. During a normal full night's
sleep, individuals go through a sleep cycle characterized by drowsiness (indicated
with theta activity on the EEG), leading into alternating periods of rapid eye
movement (REM) sleep and deep dreamless sleep (delta sleep). The normal individual passes through approximately five such cycles during the course of a night's
sleep. Polysomnography can be used to monitor various sleep disorders that are
often characterized by abnormal sleep patterns such as depression. A short REM
latency and reduced delta sleep are frequently observed in patients suffering from
depression. This abnormality occurs so frequently in depression that some investigators consider it a "biological marker," but it is too time-consuming and expensive to be widely used in this way.

Brain electrical activity mapping (BEAM).   This technique extends the capacity of EEG by generating computerized maps of brain electrical activity to produce images or pictures of it. BEAM techniques start from a basic 20-lead montage of electrodes. Clinicians and investigators can work either with the basic EEG information, or they can study evoked potentials (large waveforms that stand out from the background of the EEG and are produced by giving the individual a specific stimulus to evoke a large burst of activity, such as is produced by an auditory click). A computer is used to average electrical activity over some specified period. Information about electrical activity can be summarized by superimposing a grid matrix (typically 64 × 64) over the summarized numerical data generated by a computer (using a fast Fourier transformation). The numerical values contained in the matrix can then be converted to a color scale, with red typically representing high activity and blue representing low activity (or fast versus slow), and a picture of the brain's electrical activity is thereby generated.

BEAM techniques have no established clinical diagnostic utility in psychiatry. Abnormal electrical patterns have been reported in some mental illnesses, such as increased frontal delta in schizophrenia, but these findings have not been consistently replicated and are not diagnostic of the disorder. Brain mapping techniques may have importance as investigative tools, however, for several reasons. First, unlike most neuroimaging techniques such as CT, SPECT, or PET, this neurophysiological technique does not involve any radiation exposure and is noninvasive. Therefore, it is potentially valuable for studying brain activity in special populations, such as children. Second, it is the only "functional" imaging technique (i.e., technique that permits visualization of the brain performing particular functions or tasks) that has very fine temporal resolution. It can record events that occur in milliseconds.

Structural Neuroimaging Techniques

Structural neuroimaging techniques include computerized tomography (CT) and magnetic resonance imaging (MRI).

CT.   This technique has been available since the early 1970s and was the first in vivo brain imaging technique to become widely used. Before CT, brain structure could be visualized only through the use of crude and invasive techniques such as pneumoencephalography.

The development of CT only became possible after the invention of efficient, high-speed computers. CT provides the prototype for most of the other neuroimaging techniques currently in use. In CT, an X-ray beam is passed through serial slices of the brain, and the degree of attenuation is measured when it emerges through to the other side. The brain slice is divided into a series of tiny cubes (voxels, or volume elements), and a number reflecting the degree of attenuation can be assigned to each of the voxels. These numerical codes are then assigned a shade of gray, reflecting the degree of X-ray attenuation, which gives a visual picture of brain structure. Cerebrospinal fluid, which attenuates least, appears darkest, whereas white matter, which attenuates most, appears lightest. When MRI scans first became available in the 1970s, their level of resolution seemed astonishing. Now, in an era when MRI is widely available, CT seems extremely crude by comparison. Examples of CT scans appear in Figure 4-2.

CT is now used as both a clinical and a research tool to assess a wide variety of psychiatric conditions. It is well recognized that abnormalities can be seen on a CT scan in many mental disorders, including dementia, schizophrenia, alcoholism, anorexia nervosa, and perhaps some mood disorders. The most typical findings are ventricular enlargement or cortical atrophy. In general, these findings, when present, do not absolutely confirm a specific diagnosis because the same types of abnormalities may be present in many different disorders. Further, in interpreting CT scans, the age of the individual must be taken into consideration. Neuronal loss and the development of ventricular enlargement and cortical atrophy appear to occur in normal individuals as a part of the aging process. Thus, in interpreting CT scans in elderly individuals, in order to make a diagnosis of dementia, it can often be difficult to decide whether the atrophy and ventricular enlargement seen with CT are within normal limits for an individual's age or whether they represent a pathological process. In spite of these disclaimers, assessment with CT scanning can be useful in a variety of ways.

Schizophrenia is the psychiatric illness that has been most extensively studied with CT. By now, more than 50 controlled CT studies have been conducted (Figure 4-3). As Figure 4-3 indicates, the vast majority of these studies have shown that schizophrenic patients as a group tend to have an increase in ventricular size when compared with normal control subjects. Among the positive studies, the prevalence of extreme degrees of abnormality varies from study to study, ranging from as low as 5% to as high as 40%.

It is quite clear that ventricular enlargement is not seen in all schizophrenic patients. When present, ventricular enlargement appears to be correlated with various other characteristics. Thus, a CT scan may provide the clinician with some information about long-term clinical course and prognosis. Schizophrenic patients with ventricular enlargement tend to have a lower level of educational achievement, often a more insidious onset, and indications of cognitive impairment when assessed neuropsychologically. They may also respond less well to neuroleptic medication, and some appear to even be worsened by it. Thus, their treatment should be managed somewhat more cautiously than patients whose CT scans indicate normal brain structure.

It has recently been observed that ventricular enlargement in schizophrenia probably does not represent a progressive neuronal loss, as occurs in Alzheimer's disease. Although very few studies have included a single cohort of patients with serial scans over a 5- to 10-year period, ventricular size in a large group of schizophrenic patients covering a broad age range has been observed. The results of these studies are summarized in Figures 4-4 through 4-6.

As these figures indicate, ventricular size does increase in normal individuals, with some differences across the sexes. Ventricular enlargement appears to begin in normal males approximately 10 years earlier than in normal females. In this

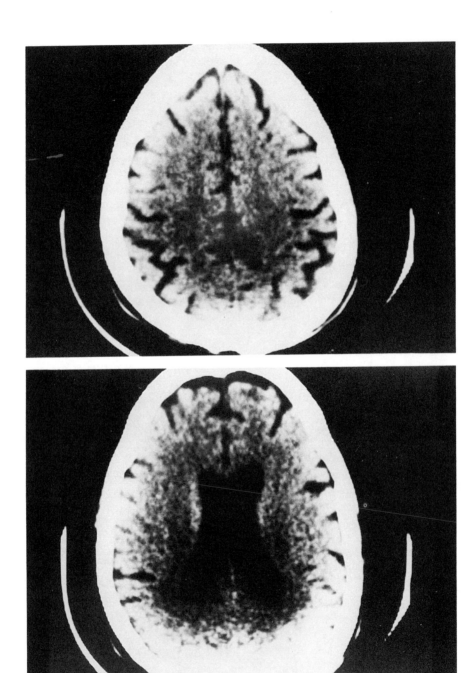

Figure 4-2. Computerized tomography scan from an individual suffering from schizophrenia. The slice on the *bottom* passes through the body of the ventricles and shows ventricular enlargement. Sulcal prominence is noted as well. The slice on the *top* is obtained from a higher level in the same individual brain and also shows prominent cortical sulci.

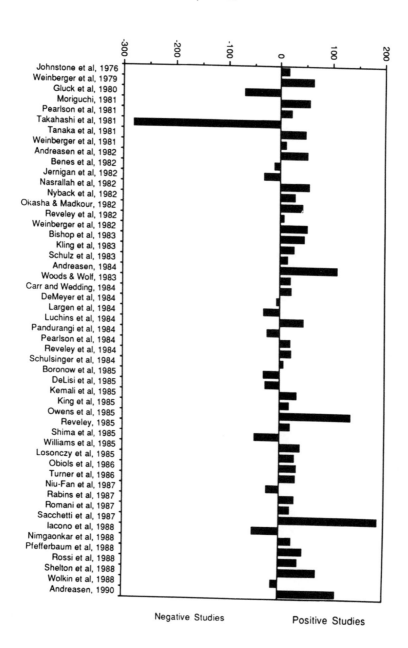

Figure 4-3. Summary of 51 controlled computerized tomography studies evaluating the presence of ventricular enlargement in schizophrenia. The majority of the studies have demonstrated ventricular enlargement.

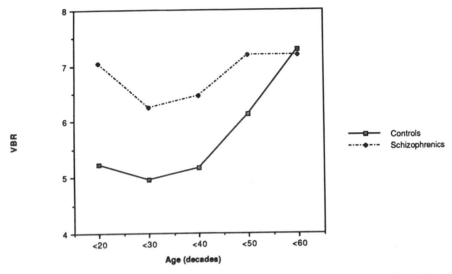

Figure 4-4.   Mean ventricle-to-brain ratio (VBR) compared at different ages in schizophrenic patients and normal control subjects. Note that the schizophrenic patients under age 20 have a mean VBR greater than 7, compared to a VBR of 5.3 in the normal control subjects. Curves remain more or less similar throughout life.

study, ventricular enlargement is in fact not seen in the female patients at all. The finding is instead limited to the male patients, and it is already present in young males when they present with schizophrenia in their teenage years. Because males are known to be much more vulnerable to birth injuries and developmental defects (i.e., males have a higher rate of learning disability, hyperactivity, spontaneous abortion, etc.), it seems likely that the finding of ventricular enlargement in young male schizophrenic patients presenting for their first episode reflects some type of cerebral injury that occurred relatively early in life and created a cerebral substrate that was more vulnerable to the development of schizophrenia in later years. Once the ventricular enlargement is present in these young males, however, it does not progress at a more rapid rate than occurs in normal males.

Studies of mood disorders have been more equivocal (Figure 4-7). As these figures indicate, some studies have been positive, whereas others have been negative. In general, sample sizes have been too small to evaluate age and sex effects. The existing data appear to suggest that there is also a sex effect in the presence of ventricular enlargement in bipolar depressed patients, with males being more vulnerable as well. The ventricular enlargement seen in depressed patients may not exceed that which is normal for the aging process, making it appear that ventricular enlargement is not statistically increased in depression when age is controlled for. This does not, of course, mean that ordering a CT scan is inappropriate in an elderly depressive patient, because the differential diagnosis of dementia and depression is often a difficult one in this age-group; a finding of

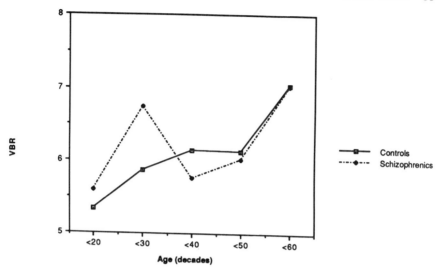

Figure 4-5. Ventricle-to-brain ratio (VBR) in female schizophrenic patients compared with normal control subjects at different ages. Note that VBR in females is approximately the same as for the control subjects throughout life, with the exception of increased VBR in the schizophrenic cohort between the ages of 20 and 30. (The explanation for this is not clear.)

substantial cortical atrophy and ventricular enlargement would definitely tip the balance in the direction of diagnosing dementia.

Starvation, as occurs in anorexia nervosa and alcoholism, also often shows characteristic abnormalities on CT. Anorexic patients who have fallen substantially below their normal weight typically have cortical atrophy, which reverses with adequate nutrition. Younger alcoholic patients, who also suffer from malnutrition and dehydration, may also have reversible CT abnormalities. On the other hand, long-term, severe alcohol abuse is likely to produce irreversible abnormalities.

MRI. This technique has a substantial number of advantages over CT. The images produced through MRI are developed by placing the patient's brain or body in a magnetic field, which causes their hydrogen protons to be aligned and concentrates the force of the magnetic moment produced so that it is large enough to be measurable. Thereafter, the protons can be raised to a higher energy level through stimulation with a radiofrequency signal targeted to their own Larmor frequency; the relaxation, or decay, to the original energy state can then be measured as a signal that is produced from tissue voxels, much as in the case of CT.

Only a few risks are involved in the use of MRI. Because of the presence of the magnetic field, patients whose bodies contain metal objects, such as aneurysm clips or metal plates in their skulls, cannot be imaged. Patients with pacemakers must also be excluded. Because patients must be placed inside a tubelike metal cavity

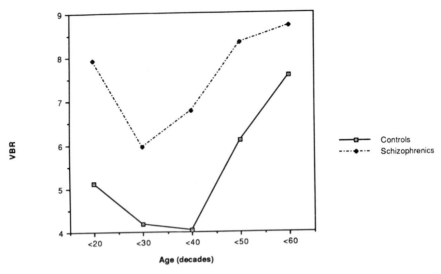

Figure 4-6. Ventricle-to-brain ratio (VBR) in male schizophrenic patients and normal control subjects, compared across various age decades. Note that the separation of the males from the females demonstrates prominently that male schizophrenic patients consistently have a larger VBR throughout life. The profiles of the schizophrenic patients and control subjects are similar, but the male schizophrenic patients start with larger VBRs and continue to have larger ones throughout their lives.

to be scanned, there is some risk of experiencing claustrophobia. This can usually be minimized or eliminated with adequate patient preparation, however.

In addition to being relatively risk free, MRI has numerous other advantages. Unlike CT, whose images are limited to the transverse or transaxial plane, MRI permits reconstruction of images from the brain in all planes. Because of the complex three-dimensional structure of the brain, multiple perspectives are very useful. Coronal cuts, in particular, are especially valuable for visualizing small subcortical structures of great interest to psychiatry, such as the caudate nucleus, the putamen, the amygdala, and the hippocampus. Resolution is superb with MRI, producing "slices" of brain that look as if they were obtained in a pathology lab at postmortem. With CT, it is difficult to see the posterior fossa because of the great density of bone in that region, but bone artifacts are not a problem with MRI, and posterior fossa structures are well visualized.

MRI is somewhat more difficult to use than CT, however. One major difficulty arises because many different imaging options are available. The technician can substantially change the type of pictures produced by altering imaging parameters such as repetition time (TR) or echo time (TE). The actual image signal is a mixture of four components: flow velocity, proton density, and relaxation of the protons in different three dimensional planes (T1 and T2 relaxation times). Depending on the scanning sequence used, images can be weighted by enhancing the

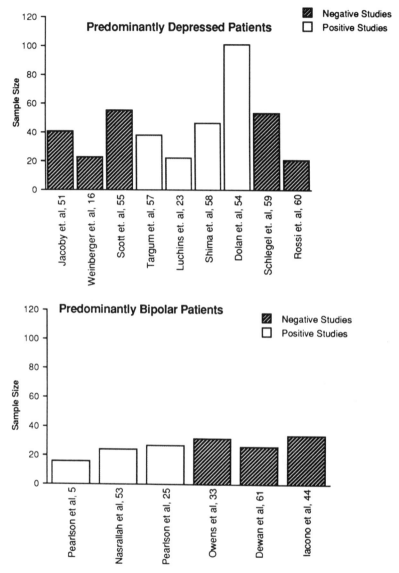

Figure 4-7. Summary of controlled computerized tomography studies of ventricle-to-brain ratio of patients suffering from bipolar and unipolar affective disorder. Note that these studies are much less consistent than those conducted with patients suffering from schizophrenia.

proton density component, the T1 component, or the T2 component. A scanning sequence may be selected to produce impressive anatomical resolution (e.g., a proton density image or a T1 weighted image), or a sequence may be selected that shows very poor anatomical resolution, but displays clearly specific areas of tissue abnormality (e.g., T2 weighted images with a long TE and TR). Examples of types of MRI scans appear in Figure 4-8.

Clinicians need to be aware of what they may be looking for when deciding to order MRI. If they are looking for a tumor, multiple sclerosis plaques, or areas of microinfarction, a T2 weighted image may be preferred. If seeking a clear picture of the size and shape of the ventricles, or the amygdala-hippocampus, a T1 weighted image will be preferred. The question to be answered should, therefore, clearly be stated on the order form used to request an MRI scan, so that the radiologist and technicians can choose the appropriate sequence.

Because MRI is a relatively new technique in neuroimaging, generalizations about its usefulness cannot be supported at this point with the same array of evidence that is available for CT. As might be expected, the presence of ventricular enlargement in schizophrenia has also been repeatedly confirmed with MRI. Various other specific anomalies, seen with the higher resolution of MRI, have also been reported, such as partial agenesis of the callosum or decreased temporal lobe size. Cerebellar abnormalities have been reported in children with autism. Some patients with bipolar disorder have been reported to have an increased number of small regions of high signal intensity (referred to colloquially as "unidentified bright objects" [UBOs]). The clinical significance of UBOs is uncertain, both in bipolar illness and in other disorders in which they are seen, such as the dementias, but they almost certainly represent tiny areas of tissue loss, due to microinfarctions in at least some cases.

The indications for ordering a structural imaging technique such as CT or MRI are summarized in Table 4-2. In general, clinicians will want to order one of these procedures when they need to rule out an "organic" cause for the patient's symptoms, such as a tumor or multiple sclerosis. Because of the rather substantial literature supporting the presence of structural abnormalities in schizophrenia, as well as their prognostic significance, it is probably appropriate to obtain a CT or MRI scan in a young individual presenting with his or her first episode of psychosis. These techniques may also be used to monitor progressive loss of tissue in the dementias and to observe the reversibility of structural changes in conditions such as anorexia nervosa or alcoholism.

As MRI has become increasingly available, physicians are faced with a decision as to whether to order CT or MRI first. Until recently, the choice was almost invariably CT, largely because of its wide availability and inexpensiveness. Because MRI is a much superior imaging technique, however, it is ultimately likely to supplant CT. Table 4-3 compares these two imaging techniques.

Functional Neuroimaging Techniques

Functional neuroimaging includes two major modalities: single photon emission computer tomography (SPECT), and positron-emission tomography (PET). Both techniques are used to observe regional metabolic functions and dysfunctions in the brain. At the moment, SPECT is used primarily to measure regional cerebral

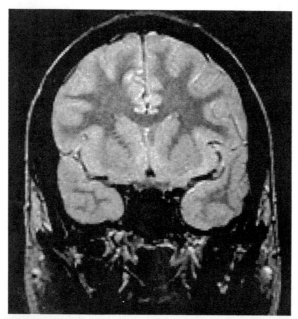

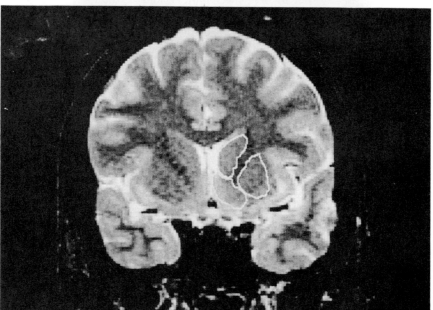

Figure 4-8. Two types of magnetic resonance imaging scans. A proton density scan is seen *above,* and a T2 weighted image *below*. Both scans are coronal slices through a central region of the brain and show the ventricular system, caudate, and putamen/ globus pallidus. This individual has prominent ventricular enlargement, consistent with the diagnosis of schizophrenia, but no prominent sulcal enlargement. Note that cerebrospinal fluid in the ventricles appears bright white on the T2 weighted image, but considerably darker on the proton density image. In general, gray-white resolution is superior on the proton density image.

Table 4-2. Indications for ordering computerized tomography or magnetic resonance imaging

Confusion and/or dementia of unknown cause
First episode of a psychotic disorder of unknown etiology
First episode of a major affective disorder after age 50
Marked personality change after age 50
History of recent head trauma
Anorexia nervosa with marked weight loss
Alcoholism or other substance abuse disorder with signs or symptoms of cognitive
  deterioration

blood flow, although future applications are currently being developed in order to visualize and measure densities of neuroreceptors. PET at present can be used to measure regional blood flow, metabolic function through the measurement of glucose utilization, and density of neuroreceptors.

The characteristics, strengths, and limitations of these two functional imaging techniques are summarized in Table 4-4. The basic principles of both techniques are the same, in that they involve imaging the regional localization of radioactive isotopes that localize in an area of high functional activity in the brain. For examples of typical SPECT and PET scans, see Andreasen's book *Brain Imaging: Applications in Psychiatry* (1989).

SPECT. In the case of SPECT, the isotopes are single photon emitters, whereas in PET, the isotopes are positron emitters. The isotopes used in SPECT include technetium, xenon-133, and iodine-123; each of these is stable, with a relatively long half-life, making them convenient for long-term storage and relatively handy to use. On the other hand, these molecules are not normally present in the human body, and they are relatively difficult to attach to informative compounds to make them suitable as imaging agents; when they are attached, there is some risk that the biological activity of the compound will be changed because of the introduction of the "foreign"

Table 4-3. Comparison of computerized tomography (CT) versus magnetic resonance imaging (MRI)

	CT	MRI
Resolution	1 cm	1–3 mm
Imaging planes	Transaxial only	Transaxial, sagittal, coronal
Imaging time	1–5 minutes	5–60 minutes
Contraindications	None apart from those associated with radiation exposure	Pacemakers, metal plates in skull, aneurysm clips, claustrophobia, very restless patient
Strengths	Visualizing recent infarcts, bone	Visualizing small focal lesions, posterior fossa lesions, fine anatomical detail, no radiation exposure
Cost	$100–$200	$400–$800

Table 4-4. Comparison of single photon emission computer tomography (SPECT) versus positron-emission tomography (PET)

	SPECT	PET
Resolution	0.8–2 cm	0.3–1.2 cm
Imaging time	10–60 minutes	10–60 minutes
Contraindications	None apart from those associated with radiation exposure	None apart from those associated with radiation exposure
Strengths	Uses commercially available tracers, low in cost, widely available	Superior resolution, very flexible in applications (e.g., blood flow, glucose metabolism, neuroreceptors)
Weaknesses	Generally poor resolution, difficult to quantify	Technically very difficult, very expensive
Cost	$300–$500	$300–$5000

isotope. Thus, the types of imaging agents currently available for SPECT are limited to tracers suitable for measuring blood flow, which include xenon-133 (typically inhaled) and technetium-labeled HMPAO (Ceretek). Compounds to study the cholinergic and dopaminergic systems are in development and just becoming available, but these are not likely to reach clinical use for several years.

SPECT studies can be done either with dedicated head units or with a single-headed rotating gamma camera of the sort available in most nuclear medicine departments. The dedicated head units tend to give greater flexibility and improved resolution. Because the blood flow agents such as HMPAO are commercially available and because the imaging equipment is available in most hospitals, SPECT is currently available for evaluating psychiatric patients as needed.

Studies done using xenon as a tracer differ from those using iodinated or technetium-labeled compounds. Xenon, a noble gas, clears relatively quickly, lending itself to serial back-to-back studies. In addition, a washout curve can be obtained, permitting the measurement of blood flow in absolute units (millimeters per minute per gram of tissue). Xenon-133 has a relatively low energy, however, a characteristic that produces pictures of lower resolution than can be obtained with higher-energy tracers such as iodine-123 or technetium. The pros and cons of using xenon-133 (a "dynamic" tracer), as opposed to the so-called static tracers (iodinated and technetium-labeled compounds) to measure blood flow are summarized in Table 4-5. The dynamic characteristics and short half-life of xenon make it an ideal tracer for mapping the changes in blood flow that occur in response to some type of physiological or cognitive challenge.

Blood flow is typically diverted to brain regions that are more active. For example, SPECT scanning, using xenon as a tracer, can show diversion of blood flow to the occipital cortex produced through visual stimulation. Mapping the responses of the brain to cognitive and emotional challenges, such as solving abstract puzzles or performing language tasks, is somewhat more difficult because of the various brain regions that may be recruited in such tasks. Nevertheless, functional neuroimaging techniques such as SPECT and PET give the modern neuroscientist an opportunity

Table 4-5.   Comparison of dynamic (xenon-133) versus static (HMPAO) tracers

	Xenon-133	HMPAO
Clearance	30 minutes	1–2 days
Duration of scanning time	5 minutes	30 minutes
Measurements	Absolute (mm/100 g/minute)	Relative (ratio of flow in one region versus another)
Resolution	2 cm	0.8–1.2 mm
Imaging planes	Transaxial	All planes
Strengths	Study of dynamic functions such as cognitive activation	Static images of blood flow (may be adapted to study cognitive activation with some difficulty)

to map the brain functionally and develop a "Brodmann's map" based on blood flow and metabolism. Although xenon is the ideal SPECT tracer for such applications, methods are currently in development for adapting static agents to the study of physiological and cognitive activation in order to take advantage of their capacities for producing higher-resolution images.

At present, the clinical applications of SPECT as a laboratory test are limited to several areas. SPECT is well suited to documenting the occurrence of stroke because it provides a direct measure of cerebral blood flow. In addition, SPECT is often diagnostically useful in the differential diagnosis of depression versus dementia in elderly patients. Patients with Alzheimer's disease have a relatively characteristic decrease in cerebral blood flow in posterior temporoparietal regions; this abnormality occurs in 70–80% of patients suffering from Alzheimer's disease. No specific blood-flow abnormality has been observed consistently in depression, although some patients display a generalized decrease in flow, whereas others show more focal left anterior decreases. In any case, however, the flow patterns observed in Alzheimer's disease are relatively distinctive. Thus, when making this particular differential diagnosis, SPECT may provide useful information that is more specific than that obtained from structural images (CT or MRI), because ventricular enlargement and cortical atrophy occur relatively often in normal elderly individuals as part of the aging process.

Other types of abnormalities occurring in other mental illnesses are currently under study. Patients suffering from AIDS appear to begin to develop patchy areas of decreased perfusion as the symptoms of dementia begin. Caffeine and nicotine produce generalized decreases in cerebral perfusion, and anxiety appears to produce a generalized increase. Some patients with schizophrenia display difficulty in activating their prefrontal cortex when given "frontal" cognitive challenges developed in neuropsychology, such as the Tower of London, the Continuous Performance Test, or the Wisconsin Card Sorting Test. At present, these various findings are not supported by a sufficiently broad data base to make them definitive or useful diagnostic tests, but it is likely that SPECT will eventually be used diagnostically for at least some other major mental illnesses in addition to Alzheimer's disease.

PET.   This is the second major functional imaging technique. Because of the great expense involved in conducting PET studies, it is not widely available either as a clinical or a research tool. Its cost is based on the fact that the tracers used consist of positrons (positively charged electrons), which must be generated in an on-site cyclotron, and which tend to have short half-lives (2 minutes for oxygen-15, 30 minutes for carbon-11, approximately 2 hours for fluorine-18). Nevertheless, because the nonradioactive forms of these tracers are widely present in biological substances, they can more readily be attached to informative molecules and used to study various metabolic, neurochemical, and physiological processes, making PET an extremely powerful research tool, and perhaps ultimately a powerful clinical tool as well.

PET scanning became available in a few centers in the middle to late 1970s. Its first applications were to the study of glucose utilization in the brain. Many of the early years of PET work were devoted to developing models for quantitatively measuring glucose utilization using fluorodeoxyglucose (FDG), which is trapped in the brain in the midst of its metabolic pathway, thereby permitting efficient study. Abnormal metabolic patterns of glucose utilization have been observed in various disorders, such as seizures, tumors, stroke, Alzheimer's disease, schizophrenia, bipolar disorder, and obsessive-compulsive disorder. In addition, FDG has been used to map cognitive function and cognitive activation. FDG already has clear clinical applications in the presurgical evaluation of intractable seizures, because it provides more specific focal localization than EEG. The decreased cerebral blood flow in posterior temporoparietal regions observed in Alzheimer's disease with SPECT can also be seen as decreased glucose utilization with PET, making this another current clinical application of PET. However, because of the expense involved in doing PET studies, as well as their limited availability, SPECT is likely to be used more frequently for this differential diagnosis.

Other abnormalities have also been observed with PET, using either FDG or other ligands and tracers. As in the case of SPECT, these findings are promising, but not definitive. Schizophrenic patients show difficulty activating their frontal lobes, bipolar patients show switches from high glucose utilization during mania to low glucose utilization during depression, and obsessive-compulsive patients have hypermetabolic activity in both their prefrontal cortex and their basal ganglia. Increased areas of cerebral blood flow have been observed in the hippocampal regions in individuals suffering from panic attacks. Schizophrenic patients suffering from tardive dyskinesia may have hypermetabolic activity in their basal ganglia, and patients with Parkinson's disease show decreased activity. When these various findings, now typically reported from a single research center, have been consistently replicated, PET may also move into the diagnostic arena in psychiatry.

A major application of PET is to the study of the neurochemical systems within the brain. To date, this has primarily involved the labeling of neuroreceptors. Because this application of PET is somewhat more technically difficult, most of the developmental work in this area occurred after the FDG model had been well established. Thus, the study of neurotransmitter systems in the human brain with

PET is a young, but rapidly growing, field. This application of PET can be used both to study the distribution of neurochemical systems in the human brain and to seek specific abnormalities (either increases or decreases in function) in specific disorders.

In addition, quantitative models can be developed to measure receptor density (B_{max}). For example, methods have already been developed to measure the B_{max} of D_2 receptors using either raclopride or spiperone. Although methods for studying transmitter synthesis and metabolism are technically more difficult, these too are in the process of development. Thus, during the next decade, PET will almost certainly be applied extensively to the visualization and measurement of neurochemical systems in the normal human brain and in the brains of patients suffering from major mental illness and neurological diseases.

Neuroendocrine Techniques

Some mental illnesses, such as depression or the anxiety disorders, have a variety of symptoms that suggest some type of neuroendocrinologic abnormality. Just as frontal lobe tumor or temporal lobe epilepsy are important in the differential diagnosis of schizophrenia (thereby suggesting the importance of frontal and temporal abnormalities in that illness), so too adrenal and thyroid diseases provide important differential diagnoses for depression and anxiety disorders. Depression, in particular, has many symptoms suggestive of chronobiological dysregulation: insomnia, anorexia, and disrupted diurnal variation.

This recognition has been supported by nearly two decades of research in neuropsychoendocrinology. This research necessarily confronted many difficult methodological problems, because of the well-recognized effects of stress on the endocrine system, and the resultant difficulty in separating cause from effect. Nevertheless, a picture has emerged suggesting that some patients with major mental illnesses show clear neuroendocrine abnormalities.

One specific laboratory test that has developed out of this research is the *dexamethasone suppression test* (DST) to assist in the diagnosis of depression. When the DST is used as a "laboratory test," typically 1 mg of dexamethasone is given at 11 P.M., and blood samples are drawn the next day at 8 A.M., 4 P.M., and 11 P.M. If the patient "breaks through" the dexamethasone suppression, displaying a serum cortisol level above 5 μg/dl, the test is considered to be positive. Approximately 40% of depressed patients have a positive ("abnormal") DST; unfortunately, positive DSTs are seen in various other conditions, such as anorexia nervosa and other disorders characterized by weight loss. Thus, although psychiatrists for a time hoped that they might have a relatively sensitive and specific laboratory test for severe depression, this is clearly not the case. Nevertheless, a DST may at times be useful to the psychiatrist confronting a difficult differential diagnosis, particularly when other causes of an abnormal DST have been excluded, such as weight loss.

Other neuroendocrine challenge tests are also currently under exploration. Perhaps the most widely studied at present is the *thyrotropin-releasing hormone (TRH) challenge.* In this test, the patient is given 500 μg of TRH, and thereafter thyroid-stimulating hormone (TSH) is measured at 15-, 30-, 60-, and 90-minute intervals. A blunted TSH response has been observed in depression, but it has also been observed in various other disorders, such as bulimia or anxiety disorders. Like the DST, the TRH stimulation test needs further research before it is moved into the clinical arena and treated as a diagnostic test.

IQ Testing

IQ testing is a relatively simple "laboratory test" that has been used in psychiatry for many years. By and large, IQ testing is done with one of two standard tests: the Wechsler Adult Intelligence Scale—Revised (WAIS-R), and the Wechsler Intelligence Scale for Children—Revised (WISC-R). Both of these tests are revisions developed in 1981 and 1974, respectively, based on earlier tests developed by David Wechsler in the 1940s and 1950s.

These tests consist of 11 subscales, summarized in Table 4-6. Six of these tests measure verbal abilities, whereas five are considered to be "performance" tests. These tests are well normed, and the scoring has been devised so that the average individual will achieve a score of 100.

Although the WAIS and WISC are frequently referred to as intelligence tests and are indeed used to generate verbal, performance, and full-scale IQs, their most powerful application is to observe the patterning of intellectual abilities that is reflected on the 11 subscales. Most "normal" individuals tend to have similar scores on all tests. Individuals suffering from various psychopathological conditions can show various deviations from this pattern. For example, with normal aging, scores on the verbal items tend to remain relatively high, whereas scores on the performance items tend to decline; these are sometimes referred to as "hold" and "don't hold" tests because of their characteristic changes with aging. If an elderly individual shows very poor performance on both the verbal and the performance tests, to a degree inconsistent with his or her past education, this pattern of findings is consistent with the diagnosis of dementia. Because motivation, attention, and effort are an important part of IQ testing, however, poor performance may be relatively nonspecific. A depressed individual may also perform poorly on the verbal tests due to disinterest and apathy, although typically these tests are affected less by depression than the performance tests.

Table 4-6. Subscales of the Wechsler Adult Intelligence Scale—Revised

Verbal tests	Performance tests
Information	Picture completion
Digit span	Picture arrangement
Vocabulary	Block design
Arithmetic	Object assembly
Comprehension	Digit symbol
Similarities	

IQ testing can also be quite helpful in evaluating children and adolescents. It may provide some index to specific intellectual deficits that may be interfering with the child's capacity to perform well in school. Again, erratic patterns are particularly helpful in assessment. For example, children with specific learning disabilities may be performing very poorly in school and yet have normal or even high intelligence, indicating that the child has the basic intellectual capacity to perform at a normal or high level if the specific learning handicaps can be minimized (e.g., reading disability, mathematics disability). Children with conduct disorders typically have higher scores on the performance tests than on the verbal tests.

Personality Testing

The most widely used personality test is the Minnesota Multiphasic Personality Inventory (MMPI), developed in the 1940s. The MMPI generates scores on nine scales: hypochondriasis, depression, hysteria, psychopathic deviance, masculinity/ femininity, paranoia, psychasthenia (or anxiety), schizophrenia, and mania.

This test was developed empirically, with the original intent of creating a measure of psychopathology. A list of symptom items was generated and then given to individuals diagnosed as suffering from the various conditions that the scales tap. Normal individuals were also assessed. If groups of patients suffering from a specific condition such as paranoia assented to specific items to a degree that differentiated them significantly from normal subjects, those items were considered to tap that diagnosis. For example, patients diagnosed as schizophrenic often scored "yes" on the item "I sometimes think about things too terrible to mention."

Although the MMPI was originally developed to aid in diagnosis, its widest use at present is more descriptive than diagnostic. As in the case of the WAIS, clinicians can learn much more by looking at profiles and patterns than they can by looking at a single peak. Thus, for example, a patient who is depressed may indeed score high on the depression scale, but a high score on the psychasthenia scale may suggest that the patient's depressive symptoms are largely neurotic and likely to be chronic. High scores on Scales 1 and 3 (hypochondriasis and hysteria) coupled with a low score on depression (Scale 2), are consistent with "acting-out" personality disorders that are likely to be difficult to treat psychotherapeutically because the patient lacks the capacity to feel depression. Patients who score high on hysteria, psychopathic deviance, and mania are also likely to have difficult personality problems that may be consistent with borderline personality.

Although the MMPI is the most widely used personality inventory, several others have also been developed. The Cattell-16 PF was developed as a more "pure" personality test, because it did not attempt to base its profiles on individuals with diagnosed psychopathology. Rather, a variety of normal individuals were evaluated with a preselected set of items, and subsequently the items were subjected to factor analysis, yielding a profile consisting of 16 personality factors.

The Eysenck Personality Questionnaire, a somewhat more modest instrument, was also developed through factor analysis. It taps the dimensions of introversion, extraversion, and neuroticism. Although the Cattell-16 PF and the Eysenck Personality Questionnaire are sometimes used in personality research, the MMPI remains the most widely used instrument in clinical settings.

Neuropsychological Testing

Neuropsychological testing was developed as a method for assessing cognitive deficits believed to be neurally based. Originally, as was the case for the MMPI or the Wechsler intelligence tests, batteries were developed in the hope that they would assist in making a specific diagnosis. The premier example of this is the Halstead-Reitan Neuropsychological Test Battery, originally developed to assist in the differential diagnosis of dementia and specific neurological conditions. Again, it has become increasingly clear that no single test can bear the burden of making specific diagnoses that clinicians themselves find difficult to make. Thus, the area of neuropsychology has also turned recently toward the goal of examining profiles and patterns and attempting to identify specific kinds of abnormality.

Increasingly, neuropsychology attempts to assess a variety of specific cognitive functions, such as memory, attention, and fluency of thinking. A clinician assessing patients neuropsychologically will tailor the assessment to the types of problems that the specific patient is having, to try to identify whether a specific area of deficit is present.

For example, a group of tests are available to assess aphasia. These evaluate the patient's capacity to comprehend verbal and written information, to follow commands, to process syntactically versus semantically, and to speak fluently. When a comprehensive assessment for aphasia is completed, the clinician can define the patient's specific areas of deficit. For example, the clinician will be able to indicate that the patient has impaired fluency of expression and poor syntactic expression, but with intact syntactic comprehension, a pattern consistent with a posterior frontal lesion.

Other tests have been developed to tap frontal functions. One widely used test is the Wisconsin Card Sorting Test, in which individuals are asked to sort cards according to some abstract principle, such as color, shape, or number. After they have completed a specified number of sortings, they are arbitrarily corrected and told that they are sorting wrong; the "test" involved is individuals' ability to recognize that they must begin to sort by another principle, i.e., if they have been sorting by color, they must now switch and sort according to shape or number. Patients with frontal lobe lesions tend to perseverate and use the same sorting strategy repeatedly, even after they have been corrected. Because the capacities to abstract and to shift response set are considered to be frontal functions, this test is considered a reasonable one of frontal lobe capacity; individuals with lesions in the frontal lobes have been found to perform poorly on it.

Memory is often assessed with the Wechsler Memory Scale—Revised, which evaluates various aspects of memory. For example, one component is "logical memory," which involves having the subject listen to a coherent story and then recall as many details of the story as possible. Both immediate and delayed recall can be assessed. Another widely used test of verbal memory is the Rey Auditory

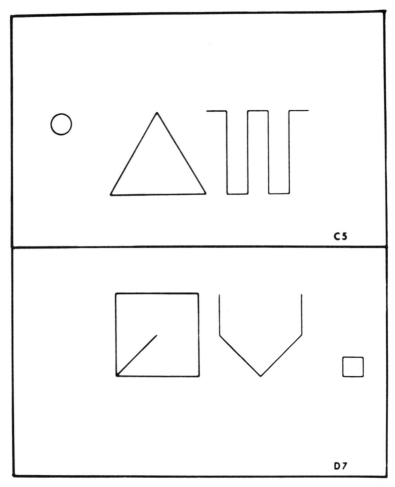

Figure 4-9. Examples of figures that patients are asked to copy and recall using the Benton Visual Retention Test.

Verbal Learning Test (RAVLT), which assesses the subject's capacity to learn a list of words by rote. Yet another widely used verbal memory test is paired associate learning, a more complicated memory test that asks a subject to learn a list of words associated with a cue set of words (e.g., metal-iron, baby-cries).

Tests have also been developed to assess visual memory. Two of the most widely used are the Benton Visual Retention Test (BVRT) and Rey-Osterreith Complex Figure. The BVRT examines the ability to copy and to later recall a variety of figures and shapes. Examples appear in Figure 4-9. The Rey-Osterreith Complex Figure is a much larger and more complicated figure that the subject is asked to copy, to draw from memory immediately, and then to draw again after a delay.

When a grouping of neuropsychological tests, such as those described above, is administered to an individual, the clinician obtains some sense of the person's overall patterns of abilities and deficits. Patients suffering from psychosis or depression often have a generalized impairment on all tests, although patients with schizophrenia may have specific regional deficits (e.g., frontal deficits) depending on their symptoms. Tests of verbal versus visual memory can be used to compare left versus right hemisphere function and to isolate patterns of abnormality within a single hemisphere. Tests of memory are particularly useful in evaluating dementia versus depression. Although depressed patients may score somewhat poorly on all tests due to a lack of interest and motivation, they typically do not have highly selective memory deficits.

Bibliography

American Psychiatric Association Task Force on Laboratory Tests in Psychiatry: The dexamethasone suppression test: an overview of its current status in psychiatry. Am J Psychiatry 144:1253–1262, 1987

Anastasi A: Psychological Testing. London, Macmillan, 1968

Andreasen NC: Brain imaging: applications in psychiatry. Science 239:1381–1388, 1988

Andreasen NC (ed): Brain Imaging: Applications in Psychiatry. Washington, DC, American Psychiatric Press, 1989

Carroll BJ: The dexamethasone suppression test for melancholia. Br J Psychiatry 140:292–304, 1982

Elster AD (ed): Magnetic Resonance Imaging: A Reference Guide and Atlas. Philadelphia, PA, JB Lippincott, 1986

Gold PW, Goodwin FK, Chrousos GP: Clinical and biochemical manifestations of depression: relation to the neurobiology of stress, Part 1. N Engl J Med 319:348–353, 1988

Gold PW, Goodwin FK, Chrousos GP: Clinical and biochemical manifestations of depression: relation to the neurobiology of stress, Part 2. N Engl J Med 319:413–420, 1988

Heilman KM, Valenstein E: Clinical Neuropsychology. New York, Oxford University Press, 1979

Kooi KA: Fundamentals of Electroencephalography. New York, Harper & Row, 1971

Krishnan KRR, Manepalli AN, Ritchie JC, et al: Growth hormone-releasing factor stimulation test in depression. Am J Psychiatry 145:90–92, 1988

Kupfer DJ, Thase ME: The use of the sleep laboratory in the diagnosis of affective disorders. Psychiatr Clin North Am 5:3–25, 1983

Lavine RA: Neurophysiology: The Fundamentals. Lexington, MA, DC Heath, 1983

Lezak MD: Neuropsychological Assessment. New York, Oxford University Press, 1983

Nemeroff CB: The role of corticotropin-releasing factor in the pathogenesis of major depression. Pharmacopsychiatry 21:76–82, 1988

Phelps ME, Mazziotta JC, Schelbert HR: Positron Emission Tomography and Autoradiography Principles and Applications for the Brain and Heart. New York, Raven, 1986

Reynolds CF, Kupfer DJ: Sleep research in affective illness: state of the art circa 1987. Sleep 10:199–215, 1987

Salamon G, Huang YP: Computed Tomography of the Brain. Berlin, Springer-Verlag, 1980

Self-assessment Questions

1. What are some of the conditions that must be considered in the differential diagnosis of serious mental illnesses? Describe ways in which laboratory tests can be used in ruling out these disorders.
2. Describe the workup usually required before ECT.
3. Describe some special techniques that may be necessary to enhance the power of EEG, particularly to detect seizure foci deep within the brain. What is polysomnography? What is BEAM?
4. Describe some applications of structural imaging techniques such as CT or MRI to the study of mental illnesses such as schizophrenia. Why must the clinician carefully specify the question that he or she is asking before ordering MRI?
5. What is functional neuroimaging? Describe some applications of functional neuroimaging to the evaluation of psychiatric patients.
6. What is the most widely used test to assess personality? What are its major clinical applications?
7. What is neuropsychological testing? Enumerate four different neuropsychological tests, and describe the cognitive functions that they are designed to evaluate.

Chapter 5

The Neurobiology
of Mental Illness

*Men ought to know that from the brain, and from the
brain only, arise our pleasures, joys, laughter, and jests, as
well as our sorrows, pains, griefs, and fears. Through it, in
particular, we think, see, hear . . .*

Hippocrates

Both historically and conceptually, psychiatry grows from the soil of neurobiology.
Its fruits are the improved understanding and treatment of the aberrations in
thinking, behavior, and emotions that characterize mental illnesses. These fruits
are only able to mature, however, as they reach back to their roots in neuroscience.
We will only be able to understand how and why we think, hear, and feel if we
understand how our brains work.

Thus, psychiatry as a discipline begins with abnormal behavior. Its understanding
of abnormal behavior is dependent on the understanding of the mechanisms of
normal behavior. Normal behavior must be understood in turn as a consequence
of functional brain systems that mediate language, perception, memory, attention,
and other cognitive systems. These functional brain systems are more or less "hard
wired" in the normal adult brain, although they are plastic and dynamic in the
young developing brain. The functional systems are the product of a set of neural
systems or networks that communicate with one another electrically and chemically. Although the circuits within these neural networks may also be more or less
"hard wired" in the mature adult brain in that long tracts and connections are

101

established, the neurochemical circuits of the brain appear to be highly adaptable and subject to multiple modulatory influences and feedback loops. These neural circuits are in turn composed of cells, and the cells communicate with one another through chemical messengers such as dopamine. Instructions for synthesizing and metabolizing the molecular messengers of the mind are coded in the neuron's DNA within its nucleus. Thus, psychiatry stretches from mind to molecule and from clinical neurobiology to molecular neurobiology, as it attempts to understand how aberrations in behavior are rooted in underlying biological mechanisms. Abnormalities in DNA can be studied directly through the developing techniques of molecular biology and molecular genetics, whereas the genetic transmission of illnesses within families must be determined through clinical assessment of affected and unaffected individuals, thus bringing us back full circle from the molecule to the mind and from the laboratory to the clinic.

Functional and Anatomic Brain Systems

The human brain may be divided into various systems that mediate many different cognitive, emotional, and perceptual functions, such as the motor system, the visual system, the auditory system, or the somatosensory cortical system. The systems that are of special interest to psychiatry are those that represent functions that are particularly disturbed in mental illnesses. These systems, which tend to represent the "last frontiers" in the human brain, include the prefrontal system, the limbic system, the basal ganglia system, the memory system, and the language system. Consequently, the student of psychiatry should be particularly familiar with these five systems.

As will become more apparent as these five systems are discussed, any method for dividing the brain into parts or systems is somewhat arbitrary. The three anatomic systems (prefrontal, limbic, and basal ganglia) are all interconnected with one another and work interactively. The two more purely functional systems, subserving memory and language, are also highly interdependent with one another and with the prefrontal, limbic, and basal ganglia systems as well. Further, the division of the brain into functional and anatomic systems and neurochemical systems is also arbitrary. These oversimplifications are introduced purely for conceptual convenience, providing a strategy for reducing the overwhelming complexity of the central nervous system (CNS) to a level that permits discussion and analysis. Ultimately, however, a full understanding of the brain can only occur by an ongoing process of analysis (or breakdown and simplification) as well as synthesis (or rebuilding and unifying).

To the above words of caution about the temptations of oversimplification, a word of caution about our existing level of ignorance must be added. We do not as yet have a complete map of the human brain, summarizing accurately its various neural circuits, chemical anatomy, or functional specialization and interaction. Just as molecular biologists are striving to map the human genome, neuroscientists are working to map the human brain. This process is ongoing and not likely to be complete for many years.

The Prefrontal System

The prefrontal system, or prefrontal cortex, is one of the largest cortical subregions in the human brain. Brodmann estimated that it constitutes 29% of the cortex in humans, as compared to 17% in chimpanzees, 7% in dogs, and 3.5% in cats. The relative development of the prefrontal cortex in various animal species is shown in Figure 5-1.

Because of the extraordinary development of the prefrontal cortex in humans, its function has been a focus of speculation and investigation for many years. An early landmark in our understanding of the prefrontal cortex was the case of Phineas Gage, a quarry worker who was accidentally injured by an explosion that drove an iron bar through his left frontal lobe. Gage survived the bizarre accident, but sustained major personality changes that were originally described by Harlow. Before the accident, Gage was conscientious, serious, and hardworking, but after the accident he became immature, childlike, socially inappropriate, and irresponsible. This early initial report has been supplemented by a substantial literature based on studies of patients with frontal tumors, traumatic injuries to the frontal lobes, and surgical treatments for epilepsy, psychosis, or obsessive-compulsive disorder. This work clearly indicates that substantial damage to the prefrontal cortex typically produces a syndrome quite similar to that of Gage. Although gross intelligence is not necessarily impaired by frontal lesions (and actually may be improved in patients suffering from severe psychosis), individuals with substantial frontal injury lose other capacities such as volition, the ability to plan, and social judgment.

These clinical studies in humans have been supplemented during recent years by substantial neurophysiological studies of nonhuman primates with techniques of neurophysiology, neuroanatomy, and neurochemistry. Primate studies have reinforced the conclusions from the earlier clinical work, indicating that the prefrontal cortex subserves a variety of major functions that permit us to integrate information from various sources, to plan and make decisions, and to generate new thoughts and ideas.

The prefrontal cortex is a massive association cortex receiving connections from all over the brain. Its multiple connections are shown schematically in Figure 5-2. Although the prefrontal cortex has been defined in various ways, perhaps the most widely accepted is based on its thalamic connections. According to this definition, the prefrontal cortex is defined as the anterior (or rostral) brain region that receives projections from the mediodorsal nucleus of the thalamus. This definition identifies more or less homologous brain regions across a variety of species. In primates, the morphological boundaries are the arcuate sulcus, the inferior precentral sulcus, and the anterior cingulate gyrus. The cortical region thus defined typically has six layers, with pyramidal cells in layers 3 and 5 and granular cortex

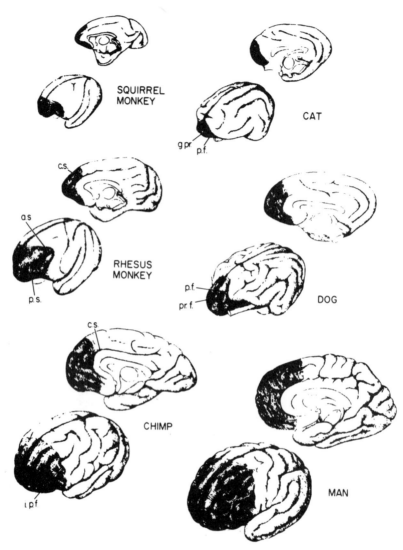

Figure 5-1. Phylogenetic development of the prefrontal cortex. a.s. = arcuate sulcus. c.s. = cingulate sulcus. g.pr. = gyrus proreus. i.p.f. = inferior precentral fissure. p.f. = presylvian fissure. pr.f. = proreal fissure. p.s. = principal sulcus. Reprinted with permission from Fuster JM (ed): The Prefrontal Cortex: Anatomy, Physiology, and Neuropsychology of the Frontal Lobe, 2nd Edition. New York, Raven, 1989.

in layer 4. In the more posterior (or caudal) portions of the prefrontal cortex, however, layer 4 becomes transitional.

The interconnections of the prefrontal cortex provide some clues as to its functions. The medial dorsal thalamic projections have two components: magnocellular and parvocellular. The magnocellular component projects principally to the orbital and medial portions of the prefrontal cortex, whereas the parvocellular component

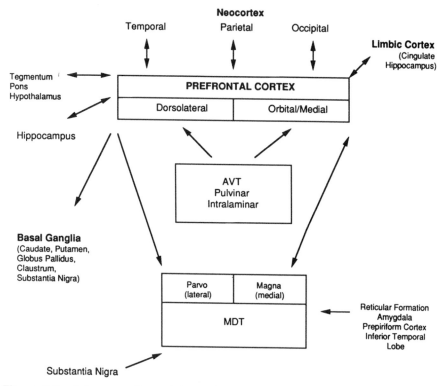

Figure 5-2. Interconnections of the prefrontal cortex. AVT = anterior ventral thalamus. MDT = medial dorsal thalamus.

projects the dorsolateral portion of the prefrontal cortex. These different projections appear to be related to differences in function in these two parts of the prefrontal cortex. Two quite different types of "frontal syndromes" have been observed. Lesions to the orbital region of the prefrontal cortex tend to produce euphoria, hyperkinesis, and inappropriate social behavior, whereas lesions to the dorsolateral portion produce apathy, hypokinesis, and impairment in cognitive performance.

The prefrontal cortex has reciprocal connections with most other parts of the neocortex, including somatic, auditory, and visual regions, suggesting that the prefrontal cortex is responsible for integrating information from various sensory modalities. It also has direct reciprocal connections with the hippocampus and amygdala, indicating some role in integrating learning and memory. It also has reciprocal connections with three other thalamic nuclei (anterior ventral, intralaminar, and pulvinar), and to the tegmentum, pons, substantia nigra, and septal area. Although these connections are reciprocal, the prefrontal cortex is the only cortical region that sends direct projections to the hypothalamus and septal regions, suggesting a major role for the prefrontal cortex in the regulation of limbic functions (whatever they may be!). In addition, the orbitomedial portion of the prefrontal cortex sends direct, and unreciprocated, projections to the basal ganglia (caudate nucleus, putamen, globus pallidus, claustrum, and substantia nigra). These projections appear to be excitatory (i.e., glutaminergic); because of the possible importance of the dopamine-rich basal ganglia in mediating the symptoms of psychosis, and in developing side effects to long-term neuroleptic treatment such as tardive dyskinesia, this particular set of efferent fibers may suggest the mechanism by which the prefrontal cortex could interact with the basal ganglia to produce psychotic symptoms.

The above survey of anatomic connections suggests some of the functions of the prefrontal cortex. It is clearly a huge association region in the brain that integrates input from much of the neocortex, limbic regions, hypothalamic and brain stem regions, and (via the thalamus) most of the rest of the brain. Its high degree of development in humans suggests that it may mediate a variety of specifically human functions such as high-order abstract thought, creative problem solving, and social interrelatedness and responsibility.

Lesion and trauma studies, supplemented by experimental studies in nonhuman primates, have substantially added to this view of the function of the prefrontal cortex. It is now clear that the prefrontal cortex mediates a large variety of functions, including attention and perception, motility, temporal integration, and affect and emotion. Lesions to the prefrontal cortex can produce lowering of awareness, sensory neglect, distractibility, disorders of visual search and gaze control, difficulty in concentrating, hyperkinesis or hypokinesis (depending on the site of the lesion), difficulty in planning and completing sequential acts, difficulty in organizing speech, defective memory, defective control of interference, defective planning, and abnormalities in affect (apathy or euphoria).

Depending on the site of the lesion, some features may predominate, suggesting some specialization in the organization of the prefrontal cortex. Orbitomedial lesions produce a "euphoric syndrome" characterized by sporadically hypomanic affect, hyperactivity, distractibility, emotional shallowness, childish humor, antisocial behavior, and disinhibition of sex drive and other basic instinctual drives. Dorsolateral lesions, on the other hand, tend to produce an "apathetic syndrome" characterized by impoverished affect, hypokinesis, inattentiveness, decreased drive and initiative, impoverished speech, "pseudodepression," and impaired capacity to generate abstract concepts. Within both of these syndromes, however, lies a common core: impairment in the capacity to pursue goal-directed behavior, based on the integration of environmental and internal cues. Most investigators believe that this function is the basic one pursued in the prefrontal cortex.

The intactness of the prefrontal cortex can be assessed by various cognitive tasks, and it has been explored through neuroimaging as well. The Wisconsin Card Sorting Test, which assesses the capacity to think abstractly and to shift response set, and the Tower of London or Porteus Mazes, which assess the capacity to plan ahead, are three standard "frontal lobe" tests in neuropsychology. The Continuous Performance Test is a measure of attention that is also thought to tap prefrontal cortical functioning.

Several of these tests have been explored with neuroimaging and shown (at least

in some individuals) to produce frontal lobe activation. Because of the close resemblance between the apathetic syndrome and the negative symptoms of schizophrenia, investigators have proposed that some patients with schizophrenia might
suffer from "hypofrontality," a finding that has been supported in numerous studies,
but not all, using both single photon emission computer tomography (SPECT) and
positron-emission tomography (PET). Patients with obsessive-compulsive disorder,
which is characterized by excessive planning and overabstractness of thought, have
been shown in PET studies to be "hyperfrontal" (see Chapter 11 for further details).

The Limbic System

The word *limbic* means "border" in Latin. This term was first used by Broca to
refer to the circular ring of tissue that appears to "hem" the prefrontal, parietal,
and occipital neocortex when the brain is viewed from a midsagittal perspective.
(He also called it the "great lobe of the hem.") Because the olfactory nerve is
connected to both the superior (septal region) and inferior (uncus, amygdala)
portions of this reverse-C-shaped group of structures in the center of the brain, it
was also known for a time as the *rhinencephalon*, or "nose brain." Cytoarchitectonic
maps also revealed that the cellular structure in these regions was paleocortex rather
than neocortex.

The function of this "primitive" central brain region was assumed to be related
to olfaction until the 1930s, when James Papez proposed another alternative. He
introduced the idea of the "Papez circuit," which is illustrated in Figure 5-3. He
suggested that the major input to this circuit was not the olfactory portion of the
brain, but rather a group of association cortices that collected information from
various neocortical regions and then relayed this information on to the Papez circuit
in the limbic system. Papez suggested that the major function of this brain region
was to experience and to regulate emotion. Within the circuit, messages would
flow from higher cortical regions to the cingulate gyrus, hippocampus, amygdala,
mammillary bodies, and anterior thalamus. Papez suggested that emotions were
concentrated in deeper structures such as the hippocampus, whereas awareness of
them occurred in the cingulate gyrus.

The work of Papez has subsequently been supplemented by that of Paul MacLean,
Walle Nauta, and many others. There is still no consensus as to what constitutes
a clear definition of the limbic system, or of its components. As in other brain
systems, boundaries can be defined on the basis of cytoarchitectonics, interconnections, or inputs. Nauta has proposed, as a unifying concept, that the various
structures in the limbic system share circuitry that connects them to the hypothalamus. He points out that the interconnections between the hypothalamus (via
the mammillary bodies), the amygdala, the hippocampus, and the cingulate gyrus
are reciprocal. The hypothalamus collects visceral sensory signals from the spinal
cord and brain stem, whereas input also comes to this circuit through two major
neocortical association regions, the prefrontal cortex and the inferior temporal
association cortex.

The functions of the limbic system are also uncertain, although clearly of great

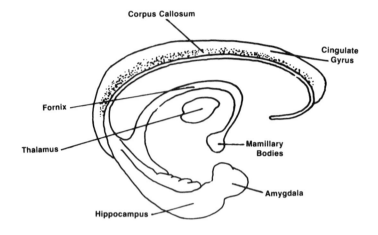

Anatomic Structures

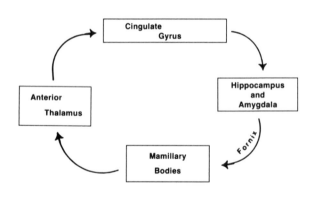

The Papez Circuit

* *

Figure 5-3. The limbic system as conceptualized by Papez. Reprinted with permission from Andreasen NC: The Broken Brain: The Biological Revolution in Psychiatry. New York, Harper & Row, 1984, p 101. Copyright 1984 Nancy C. Andreasen.

importance to the understanding of human emotion and psychological experience. The various interconnections suggest functions related to integrating visceral sensation and the experience of the external environment through multiple modalities (visual, sensory, auditory, etc.). It is well recognized that the amygdala and hippocampus serve as storage centers for memory. Thus, references to past experiences may also occur within the limbic system.

The symptoms and subjective experiences of patients suffering from temporal lobe epilepsy (TLE) provide some clues as to the functions of this region. Such patients experience a variety of phenomena, including olfactory or gustatory hallucinations, déjà-vu, derealization, and depersonalization. They also perform repetitive motoric acts that may be highly complex and that appear to rely on stored memories. Patients with TLE have an increased rate of psychosis, and TLE is often considered to be a crude "neurological model" for the psychotic syndromes.

Lesion studies and electrical stimulation studies of limbic substructures such as the hippocampus and amygdala confirm the role of these structures in recording and interpreting memories, as well as in interpreting experiences and emotions; amygdala lesions in particular appear to lead to fearfulness and suspiciousness, suggesting that this region may play some role in the development of paranoia.

The Basal Ganglia

The structure, functions, and interconnections of the basal ganglia are relatively simple compared with the prefrontal cortex or the limbic system. At first impression, it might seem that this brain region has no relevance to psychiatry. The usual concept of the basal ganglia is that they primarily regulate and mediate motor activity. For various reasons, however, it appears increasingly likely that the basal ganglia may also play a major role in the expression and regulation of emotion and cognition.

The major structures of the basal ganglia include the caudate, putamen, and globus pallidus, which are shown schematically in Figure 5-4. A coronal section of these structures, as seen on magnetic resonance imaging (MRI), is shown in Figure 5-5. The substantia nigra, located in the midbrain, is not visualized. The caudate is a C-shaped mass of gray matter tissue that has its head at the lateral anterior borders of the frontal horns of the ventricles. It arches back posteriorly in a circular fashion and then curls forward again, ending in the amygdala bilaterally. Separated from it, and lateral to it, is the lentiform nucleus, so called because it is shaped like a lens. The medial portion of the lentiform nucleus, which is darker and more densely full of gray matter, is the putamen, and the globus pallidus is lateral to it. The caudate is separated from the lentiform nucleus by the anterior limb of the internal capsule, but MRI shows clearly that bands of gray matter interconnect these two nuclei; posteriorly, the lentiform nucleus is separated from the thalamus by the posterior limb of the internal capsule. Because these structures contain an intermixture of gray and white matter, they have a striped appearance in postmortem brains and on MRI scan, causing them to be referred to as the *corpus striatum* (striped body).

The basal ganglia brain region is of possible importance to the understanding of mental illness for several reasons. First, there are several major syndromes involving abnormalities in this region that manifest psychiatric symptoms. Huntington's chorea, characterized by severe atrophy in the caudate nucleus, typically presents with a variety of mental symptoms that are similar to those seen in psychosis. Patients with Huntington's chorea often develop delusional thinking, depression,

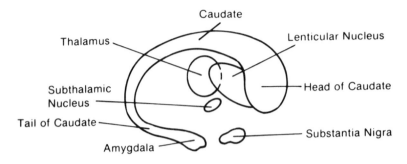

Anatomic Structures

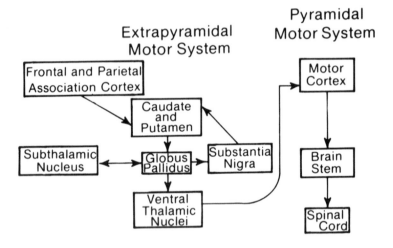

Connections

Figure 5-4. Interconnections of the basal ganglia. Reprinted with permission from Andreasen NC: The Broken Brain: The Biological Revolution in Psychiatry. New York, Harper & Row, 1984, p 105. Copyright 1984 Nancy C. Andreasen.

or inappropriate impulsive behavior. They also, of course, develop severe dementia, occurring in the context of a previously normal personality. Parkinson's disease is another syndrome affecting the basal ganglia; it is due to neuronal loss in the substantia nigra, the midbrain region of the basal ganglia that sends projections to the caudate, using dopamine as its primary neurotransmitter. Loss of dopaminergic input produces various symptoms similar to the negative symptoms of schizophrenia, including affective blunting and loss of volition. A mild dementia may also occur.

A second reason for thinking that the basal ganglia may be of some relevance to the development of symptoms of major mental illnesses derives from their chemical anatomy. The caudate and putamen contain a very high concentration of dopamine receptors, particularly D_2 receptors. The efficacy of antipsychotic

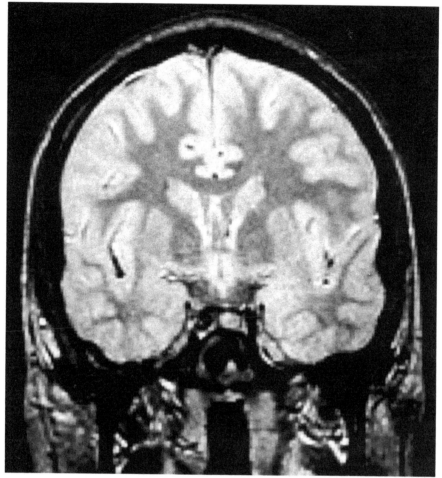

Figure 5-5.   Basal ganglia as seen with magnetic resonance imaging.

medications has been shown to be highly correlated with their ability to block D_2 receptors (see Chapter 24, "Somatic Treatments"). Because the density of D_2 receptors in these regions appears to be greater than anywhere else in the brain, it is possible that the site of antipsychotic action might be occurring within the caudate and putamen, suggesting that these regions could somehow mediate psychotic symptoms. Because antipsychotics are particularly effective for ameliorating positive symptoms, the caudate and putamen might be acting as trigger sites for positive symptoms such as delusions and hallucinations.

The Memory System

The memory system is a major functional brain system that may be impaired in some patients suffering from major mental illnesses. Deficits in learning and memory are the hallmark of the dementias. Although patients with psychoses do not typically have severe memory deficits, some investigators have speculated that the neural mechanisms of psychotic phenomena such as delusions and hallucinations might be based, at least in part, on either abnormal excitability or abnormal "wiring" in brain subregions dedicated to the storage and interpretation of memories, such as the amygdala or hippocampus. Within psychoanalytic theory, it has long been believed that the various "neuroses," such as anxiety disorders or hysteria (i.e., somatization disorder), might represent the painful stimulus of repressed memories that have not been psychologically integrated. The process of psychotherapy certainly involves the process of learning, which is based in turn on memory; patients who successfully complete a course of psychotherapy have learned new ways of thinking about themselves, understanding their past experiences, and relating to other people. Thus, the treatment of mental illnesses probably also involves the memory system in the brain.

It is a truism that we still have a great deal to learn about learning and memory. Nevertheless, we have also learned a great deal during recent decades. For many years, cognitive psychologists have dedicated themselves to identifying the site or sites where memories are encoded, sometimes referred to as the "search for the engram." For example, Karl Lashley of Harvard spent much of his career placing lesions in various parts of the brain in experimental animals, demonstrating that no specific lesion could produce memory deficits, thereby suggesting that the brain was equipotential in its capacity for learning and memory. This situation changed radically, however, as the result of a single informative and very famous case, that of H.M. H.M. was treated surgically for intractable epilepsy by removal of the anterior temporal poles bilaterally. Afterward, he was observed to have totally lost the capacity to remember any new information that he was given, although his memory for information learned before the surgery was completely intact. This famous case focused attention on the gray matter structures located in the anterior poles of the temporal lobes, the amygdala and hippocampus, and on the possible importance of bilateral as opposed to unilateral lesions.

We now know, based on the case of H.M., as well as a large quantity of other human and animal evidence, that unilateral lesions do not typically produce memory deficits, but that bilateral lesions in certain specific locations can completely destroy learning and memory.

We now suspect that the functions of learning and memory occur primarily in two brain regions, the hippocampus and amygdala. Because the memory system appears to depend on the presence of multiple "backup files," dissecting the specific and interdependent roles of these brain regions has not been simple. For example, it was thought for a number of years that the hippocampus was a primary site for encoding memory, with the amygdala serving very little function, based on evidence that bilateral removal of the amygdala alone did not impair learning and memory. Later, however, it was observed by Mishkin that similar bilateral lesions to the hippocampus also did not impair the performance of macaques on visual recognition memory tasks. Thus, most recently, it has been concluded that both these brain regions work together to store memories. Loss of both produces massive memory defects, whereas loss of one or the other produces relatively restricted, or even no, abnormalities.

It is very likely, however, that the functions of the amygdala and hippocampus are not simply duplicative. Current evidence suggests that the amygdala may work primarily to integrate memories learned from different modalities. For example, monkeys who have lesions in the amygdala cannot visually recognize objects that they have examined only by touch, whereas monkeys with lesions in the hippocampus can do so. The amygdala also plays an important role in social behavior, at least in nonhuman primates, because animals with lesions in the amygdala have difficulty in recognizing social hierarchies, expressing aggression, experiencing fear, or demonstrating normal maternal behavior. It seems likely that the amygdala plays an important role in facial recognition and facial perception.

Just as the brain regions that encode memories do not appear to be homogeneous or equipotential, so too memory itself is probably a diverse set of functions that are mediated in different ways. Typically, memory is now thought of as a two-stage process. The first stage involves short-term memory, or recognition and short-term recall memory. This type of memory is relatively brief. It is the form that we use when we "learn" a telephone number long enough to dial it, or a driver's license number long enough to write it down. Sometimes this type of memory is also referred to as "working" memory because it is accessible in some type of short-term storage. Long-term memory, on the other hand, consists of information that we have learned and retained for periods greater than a few minutes. This type of memory is sometimes referred to as "consolidated" memory. This type of memory is currently being used by the students reading this textbook.

Normal human experience, as well as research in neuroscience, indicates that a variety of techniques can be used to facilitate learning, or consolidation of memory. These include such things as repetition, rehearsal, or mnemonic devices. This type of memory is probably mediated by a different set of mechanisms that lead to long-term storage of information. Once such information is stored, some of it may be slowly lost.

The mechanisms mediating short-term versus long-term memory are not clear, although an increasing consensus is developing that short-term memories are coded through different mechanisms than long-term memories. Current research suggests that short-term memory probably involves activating short synaptic circuits through neurochemical transmission; this type of neural activity is both rapidly implemented and rapidly reversed. On the other hand, long-term memory probably involves a more permanent process, most likely through the development of a sequence of molecules that encode information. Substantial work in this area has been conducted by Eric Kandel, using the Gill withdrawal reflex in *Aplysia* as a model. Kandel has suggested that long-term memory may depend on the synthesis of proteins and RNA in neurons that are synaptically connected during the time that short-term learning has been occurring; this type of process would represent a molecular consolidation of memory that could be permanently stored.

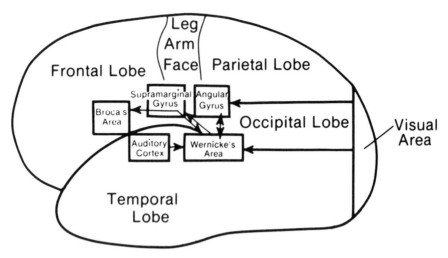

Figure 5-6. Interconnections of the language system. Reprinted with permission from Andreasen NC: The Broken Brain: The Biological Revolution in Psychiatry. New York, Harper & Row, 1984, p 113. Copyright 1984 Nancy C. Andreasen.

The Language System

As far as we know, the capacity to communicate in a highly developed and complex language is limited to humans. Although porpoises, dolphins, and a few other creatures are believed to communicate specific messages to one another, humans alone appear to have a syntactically complex language that exists in both oral and written forms. The ability to record our history and to communicate scientifically and culturally has permitted us to repeatedly build complex civilizations and social systems, and perhaps to destroy them as well.

The capacity to communicate in oral and written language is coded in dedicated brain regions that probably occur only in humans. These language systems are localized in the neocortex. A schematic diagram of them appears in Figure 5-6. This system is located almost totally in the left hemisphere in most individuals, although about one-third of left-handers use either their right hemisphere or both hemispheres to perform language functions.

Although the history of our understanding of the language system reaches back to the 19th century, and specifically to the work of Broca and Wernicke (each of whom has a neocortical region that bears his name), much of our understanding of the specialized detail of the language system derives from the work of Norman Geschwind and his colleagues in Boston. Geschwind was one of the earliest neuroscientists to reawaken interest in hemispheric specialization and asymmetry, observing that the functional specialization in the brain is reflected at least partially in its anatomic structure. He observed that the planum temporale (the flat plane of the temporal lobe that is seen from the top when the cortex above is removed through dissection) is larger on the left side, reflecting the specialized development of the left hemisphere for language.

Within the left hemisphere are three major language regions, as well as some subsidiary ones. Broca's area is the region dedicated to the production of speech. It contains information about the syntactical structure of language, provides the "little words" such as prepositions that tie the fabric of language together, and is the generator for fluent speech. Lesions to Broca's area, which occur in stroke victims (often with an accompanying right hemiparesis), lead to halting, stammering, and ungrammatical speech.

Wernicke's area is often referred to as the "auditory association cortex." It encodes the information that permits us to "understand" or "interpret" information that is presented to us in auditory form. The perception of sound waves, which encode speech, occurs through transducers in the ear that convert the information to neural signals. The signals are received in the auditory cortex, but the meaning of the specific signals cannot be understood (i.e., perceived as constituting words with specific meanings—as opposed, for example, to the wordless music of a symphony) without being compared with "templates" in Wernicke's area. An analogous process occurs when we understand written language. In this case, the information is collected through our eyes, relayed via the optic tracts back to the primary visual cortex in the occipital lobe, and then forwarded on to the angular gyrus, a visual association cortex that contains the information or templates that permit us to recognize language presented in visual form.

Various stroke syndromes have been described that represent specific damage to these various specialized brain regions. For example, Wernicke's aphasia occurs as a result of damage to Wernicke's area and leaves the individual without the ability to understand what is said; this is a direct consequence of loss of the auditory association cortex, which attributes meaning to the sound waves heard. In addition, individuals with Wernicke's aphasia lose the ability to speak coherently because they have lost the "meaning" of language; they produce fluent, disorganized speech that is sometimes referred to as word salad or jargon aphasia. Wernicke's aphasia is sharply distinguished from Broca's aphasia; in the latter case, individuals can comprehend what is said, but have a marked deficit in ability to express themselves, a situation that typically leads to great frustration. Damage to the angular gyrus leads to loss of the ability to read and write, the two forms of language that are visually mediated, with no loss of auditory comprehension or spontaneous speech.

Patients suffering from major mental illnesses have a variety of disruptions in their capacity to communicate in language. Some of these incapacities are similar to those that are observed in the aphasias produced by stroke, but none is precisely identical. Some patients with schizophrenia have very impoverished speech that is reminiscent of Broca's aphasia, but it lacks the halting, ungrammatical quality of Broca's aphasia. Likewise, some patients suffering from schizophrenic or manic psychosis produce very disorganized abundant speech similar to Wernicke's aphasia, but (unlike the patient with Wernicke's aphasia) they appear to have intact comprehension. Auditory hallucinations ("hearing voices") is abnormal auditory perceptions of language; that is, the individual perceives auditory speech when none

Table 5-1.   Criteria for a "classic" neurotransmitter

1. It is synthesized in the neuron.
2. It is present in the presynaptic terminal and is released in an amount sufficient to exert a particular effect on a receptor neuron.
3. When applied exogenously (as drug) in reasonable concentrations, it mimics exactly the action of the endogenously released neurotransmitter.
4. A specific mechanism exists for removing it from its site of action, the synaptic cleft.

is present. The reasons for these various disruptions and aberrations in language function in psychosis (and in many of the dementias as well) are not clear. They may represent specific abnormalities in specialized language regions in the brain, but more likely they represent a disorganization at some "higher" or "lower" integrative level.

Neurochemical Systems

In addition to the functional and anatomic systems described above, the brain also consists of a grouping of neurochemical systems. These systems provide the "fuel" that permits the functional and anatomic systems to run (or run poorly, when an abnormality occurs). The neurochemical systems are not isomorphic with the anatomic and functional systems. Rather, they are interwoven and interdependent. Any anatomic subsystem within the brain usually "runs" on multiple classes of neurotransmitters. Clearly, this complexity of anatomic and neurochemical organization permits much greater "fine-tuning" of the entire system.

Neuron, Synapse, Receptor, and Second Messenger

Neurons may have varying configurations depending on the function they perform. They all consist of a cell body containing the nucleus and at least one axon of variable length that transfers from the cell body the propagation of electrical excitation that ultimately leads to the release of neurotransmitters that are located in terminals at the synapses. The cell body is surrounded by dendrites that enlarge the capacity of the cell body to receive information through synaptic input from other neurons. Likewise, axons may branch as they terminate, and then produce multiple synaptic contacts.

Although the initial propagation of messages is electrical, communication at the synapse is chemical. It is mediated through various substances that are recognized to be chemical messengers between neurons, or *neurotransmitters*. Neuroscientists have agreed for several decades on a set of criteria that are used to define "classic" neurotransmitters (Table 5-1). For a substance to be accepted as a neurotransmitter, investigators must establish that it is contained within the neuron, synthesized by the neuron, and released at the synapse and that it causes a reproducible physiological response. The classic neurotransmitters that meet these criteria are prin-

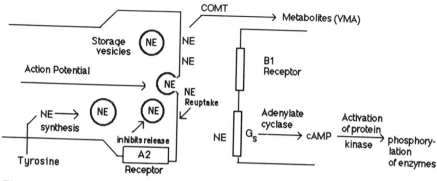

Figure 5-7. Cascade of events occurring during synaptic transmission, beginning with neurotransmitter release, stimulated through an action potential, and leading to occupation of a receptor and subsequent activation of second-messenger systems. COMT = catechol-O-methyl-transferase. VMA = vanillylmandelic acid. NE = norepinephrine.

cipally catecholamines and amino acids, such as dopamine, serotonin, acetylcholine, gamma-aminobutyric acid (GABA), glutamic acid, aspartic acid, glycine, homocysteine, and taurine.

In addition to these classic neurotransmitters, chemical communication between regions also occurs through other neurotransmitters that have not yet been proved to meet all of the above criteria. It has now been recognized for nearly two decades that peptides are also synthesized in the CNS. Although the earliest peptides to be recognized were those that were clearly hormonal in nature (e.g., adrenocorticotropic hormone [ACTH]), the discovery of endogenous opioid peptide neurotransmitters (endorphins) substantially expanded interest in peptide transmitters within the CNS. Because they are proteins (i.e., have their synthesis directed by nuclear DNA), the peptide neurotransmitters must be synthesized in the neuronal cell body rather than in the synapse. They are carried down to the synapse through storage vesicles, where they can then be released. Whereas some peptide neurotransmitters function in much the same way as the classic neurotransmitters, others serve as "co-transmitters."

Although the belief in a "single neuron–single neurotransmitter" used to be universal, it is now recognized that many neurons contain at least two neurotransmitters. Often, a classic neurotransmitter and a neuropeptide are coupled. For example, cholecystokinin (CCK) serves as a co-transmitter with the dopamine neurons that project to the cortex and limbic system (but not those that project to the basal ganglia). The peptide co-transmitters are generally thought to be modulatory or regulatory.

A schematic representation of a synapse appears in Figure 5-7. The classic neurotransmitters are synthesized at the neuronal synapse from precursor molecules (e.g., tyrosine). The neurotransmitter molecules must be sequestered in vesicles to prevent breakdown from enzymes contained within the neuronal cytosol (e.g., by monoamine oxidase [MAO]). Adequate quantities of neurotransmitter are maintained at the synapse through various regulatory factors. Short-term monitoring to determine whether adequate quantities of the neurotransmitter are contained in vesicular storage is done through end-product inhibition. For example, tyrosine hydroxylase is the rate-limiting enzyme for the synthesis of dopamine and norepinephrine. If adequate supplies of norepinephrine are available at the terminal, these inhibit the activity of tyrosine hydroxylase, preventing further synthesis.

On the other hand, if the synapse is very active, leading to depletion of neurotransmitter, protein kinases stimulate phosphorylation of tyrosine hydroxylase, a process that is triggered by persistent membrane depolarization. Increased quantities of tyrosine hydroxylase can also be produced in the neuronal cell body, under the supervision of nuclear DNA, a response that occurs in response to long-term neuronal hyperactivity and synaptic depletion.

Finally, at least for neurons that possess presynaptic receptors, the release of neurotransmitter can also be "downregulated" through these presynaptic receptors. For example, noradrenergic neurons contain alpha$_2$-receptors at their terminals, which decrease the amount of norepinephrine released at the terminal when activated either by an increased production in overall adrenergic activity, or by exogenous alpha$_2$ agonists such as clonidine. The presynaptic receptors work principally to decrease firing rate of the neuron and thereby vesicular release of neurotransmitter. Thus, the regulation of neurotransmitter synthesis and release is governed by a complex set of interactive mechanisms that can adapt neuronal responsiveness to rapidly varying conditions.

After a neurotransmitter is released, it can experience various fates. In the free-floating world of intersynaptic connections, enzymes, such as catechol-O-methyl-transferase (COMT), hover there and can lead to its metabolic inactivation or breakdown. The neurotransmitter may saturate presynaptic receptors, thereby telling the transmitter neuron that it is time to "slow down." It may cross the synapse and occupy a postsynaptic receptor, thereby actually succeeding in sending a message to another neuron. Finally, because nature often loves efficiency and abhors waste, it may be returned to the original transmitter neuron and again stored in the vesicles, eventually to be subsequently released again.

Medications used to treat mental illness often exert their primary effects through acting on one of these aspects of neural communication. For example, the MAO inhibitors, which prevent the breakdown of norepinephrine, enhance noradrenergic transmission by blocking the action of MAO. The classic antidepressants, such as imipramine, also facilitate noradrenergic transmission by blocking the uptake mechanisms. Clonidine decreases anxiety by blocking presynaptic alpha$_2$-receptors, thereby producing downregulation. Classic antipsychotics are thought to decrease the symptoms of psychosis by diminishing hyperdopaminergic activity through blocking postsynaptic dopamine receptors, principally D$_2$ receptors.

If a neurotransmitter succeeds in making its way across the synapse and affixing itself to a receptor, it then initiates a series of events that are at present only poorly understood, but that represent the consequences of sending this particular type of message. The receptors to which it complexes are large protein molecules that are

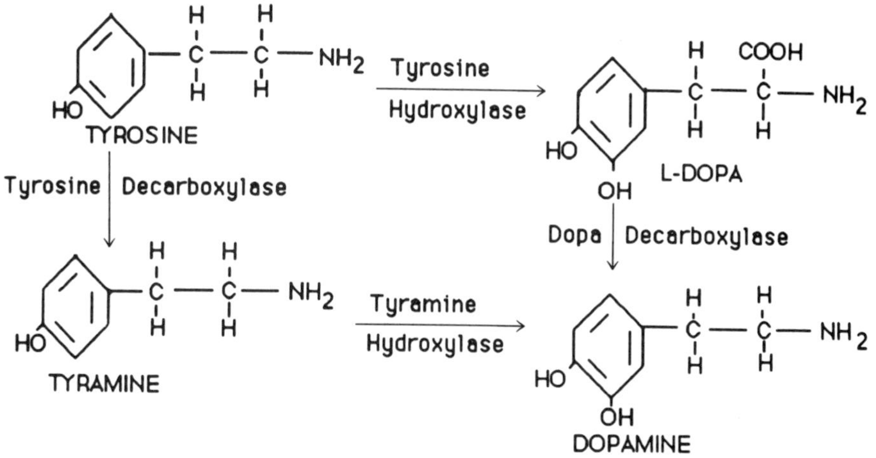

Figure 5-8. Synthetic pathway of dopamine—primary and alternate pathways.

located on the outer surface of the neuronal membrane and that "recognize" specific neurotransmitters in a highly selective way, much as a key fits into a lock.

The complexing of transmitter to receptor initiates a subsequent series of events that vary depending on the particular role that a specific type of receptor may perform. Postsynaptically, the initial message received by the receptor is then processed by a group of "second messengers" that work principally by activating enzymes. The best understood among these is the second messenger coupled with cyclic AMP, which appears to occur at both noradrenergic beta-receptors and at dopamine D_1 receptors. Within this system, the neurotransmitter-receptor interaction leads to a complexing of protein on the other side of the membrane, which then binds to adenylate cyclase and activates it, causing ATP to convert to cyclic AMP. Cyclic AMP then activates protein kinases, which in turn promote phosphorylation of key enzymes. Other second-messenger systems, associated with alpha$_1$-adrenergic receptors and M_1 muscarinic receptors, stimulate the breakdown of phospholipids, thereby increasing intracellular concentrations of phosphoinositides and diacylglycerol (DAG), which also in turn will lead to enzyme phosphorylation and activation. Other second-messenger systems, such as those mediated through D_2 receptors, are not yet known.

The Dopamine System

Dopamine, a catecholamine neurotransmitter, is the first product synthesized from tyrosine through the enzymatic activity of tyrosine hydroxylase. Its synthetic pathway and the subsequent ones of norepinephrine and epinephrine are shown in Figure 5-8.

There are three subsystems within the brain that use dopamine as their primary neurotransmitter. These all arise in the ventral tegmental area. One group, arising

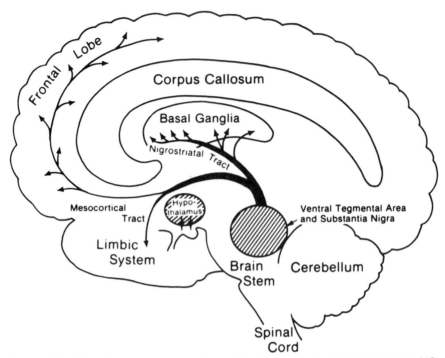

Figure 5-9. The dopamine system. Reprinted with permission from Andreasen NC: *The Broken Brain: The Biological Revolution in Psychiatry.* New York, Harper & Row, 1984, p 134. Copyright 1984 Nancy C. Andreasen.

in the substantia nigra, projects to the caudate and putamen and is referred to as the nigrostriatal pathway. Its terminations appear to be rich in both D_1 and D_2 receptors. A second major tract, called the mesocortical or mesolimbic (or mesocorticolimbic) projects to the prefrontal cortex and temporolimbic regions such as the amygdala and hippocampus. The concentration of D_2 receptors in these regions is minimal, whereas D_1 receptors predominate. The third component of the dopamine system originates in the arcuate nucleus of the hypothalamus and projects to the pituitary. The various dopamine subsystems are summarized in Figure 5-9.

As Figure 5-9 indicates, the dopamine system is fairly specifically localized in the human brain. Because its projections include only a limited part of the cortex and focus primarily on brain regions important to cognition and emotion, it is considered to be one of the most important neurotransmitter systems for the understanding of these functions, and potentially for the understanding of their disturbances in individuals suffering from psychosis. The efficacy of the neuroleptic drugs used to treat psychosis is highly correlated with their ability to block D_2 receptors (Figure 5-10). There is a modest but much weaker correlation with their

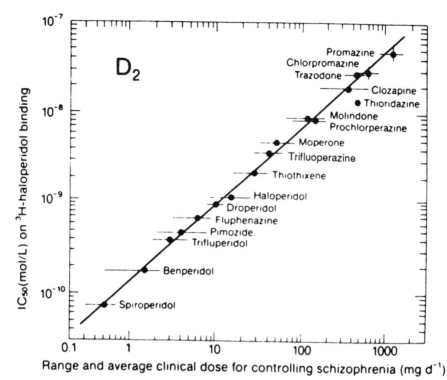

Figure 5-10. Correlation between drug potency and D_2 receptor blockade. Reprinted with permission from Seeman P: Dopamine receptors and the dopamine hypothesis of schizophrenia. Synapse 1:133–152, 1987.

ability to block D_1 receptors (Figure 5-11). Until the distribution of D_1 and D_2 receptors was more specifically mapped during recent years, it was assumed that the primary therapeutic effect of antipsychotic drugs occurred through D_2 blockade. This assumption is currently being reassessed, largely because of the rather sparse density of D_2 receptors in critical brain regions that mediate cognition and emotion, such as prefrontal cortex, amygdala, and hippocampus.

Understanding the projections of the dopamine system and the differential localization of D_1 and D_2 receptors clarifies some of the other actions of neuroleptic drugs. These drugs tend to have potent extrapyramidal effects, as a consequence of blocking dopamine receptors in the nigrostriatal pathway. Drugs that have a weak D_2 effect (of which clozapine is a recent example) are more likely to have fewer extrapyramidal side effects as a consequence of their weak D_2 blockade. If only we understood more specifically the brain regions from which the symptoms of psychosis arise, it would be possible to design a "rational pharmacology" that might target drugs to specific regions, based on what we know about the chemical anatomy of the brain. The rational pharmacology could capitalize both on the

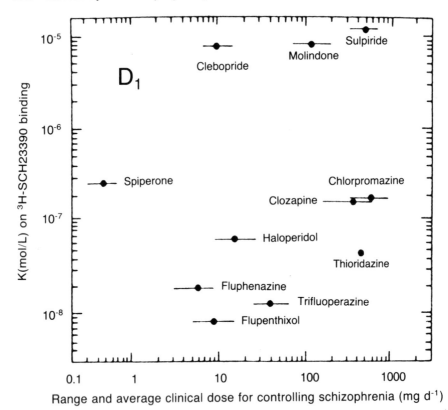

Figure 5-11. Correlation between neuroleptic potency and D_1 receptor blockade. Reprinted with permission from Seeman P: Dopamine receptors and the dopamine hypothesis of schizophrenia. Synapse 1:133–152, 1987.

distribution of D_1 and D_2 receptors and on the phenomena of co-localization, in that it is also known that only mesocorticolimbic projections have co-transmission with CCK.

The Norepinephrine System

The norepinephrine system arises in the locus coeruleus and sends projections diffusely throughout the entire brain (Figure 5-12). As Figure 5-12 illustrates, norepinephrine appears to exert effects on almost every brain region in the human brain, including the entire cortex, the hypothalamus, the cerebellum, and the brain stem. This distribution suggests that it may have a diffuse modulatory or regulatory effect within the CNS.

There is some evidence that norepinephrine may play a major role in mediating symptoms of major mental illnesses, especially mood disorders. Soon after they were developed, it was demonstrated that tricyclic antidepressants inhibit norepi-

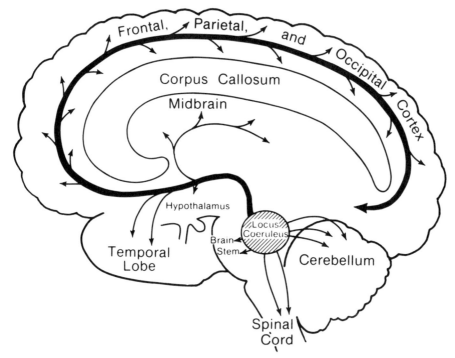

Figure 5-12. The norepinephrine system. Reprinted with permission from Andreasen NC: The Broken Brain: The Biological Revolution in Psychiatry. New York, Harper & Row, 1984, p 134. Copyright 1984 Nancy C. Andreasen.

nephrine reuptake, thereby enhancing the amount of norepinephrine available to stimulate postsynaptic receptors. Likewise, the MAO inhibitors also enhance noradrenergic transmission by inhibiting neurotransmitter breakdown. As described below, however, it is also clear that many antidepressants have mixed noradrenergic and serotonergic activities. Thus, the original "catecholamine hypothesis of affective illness," which suggested that depression was due to a functional deficit of norepinephrine at crucial nerve terminals whereas mania was due to a functional excess, is probably an oversimplification.

The Serotonin System

Serotonergic neurons have a distribution strikingly similar to norepinephrine neurons (Figure 5-13). Serotonergic neurons arise in the raphe nuclei, localized around the aqueduct in the midbrain. They project to a similar wide range of CNS regions, including the entire neocortex, the basal ganglia, temporolimbic regions, the hypothalamus, the cerebellum, and the brain stem. As is the case with the norepinephrine system, the serotonin system appears to be a general modulator.

A "serotonin hypothesis of depression" has also been proposed, largely because

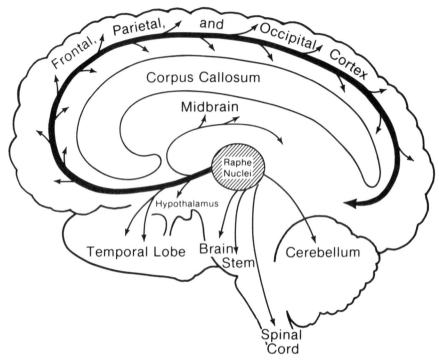

Figure 5-13. The serotonin system. Reprinted with permission from Andreasen NC: The Broken Brain: The Biological Revolution in Psychiatry. New York, Harper & Row, 1984, p 135. Copyright 1984 Nancy C. Andreasen.

antidepressant medications also facilitate serotonergic transmission by blocking reuptake. Some investigators postulate that serotonin may also play a role in psychosis, because one subtype of serotonin receptor, the 5-HT$_2$ receptor, has been found to be a receptor site for hallucinogens such as lysergic acid diethylamide (LSD).

The Acetylcholine System

Like dopamine, acetylcholine has a relatively more specific localization in the human brain (Figure 5-14). The cell bodies of a major group of cholinergic neurons are located in the nucleus basalis of Meynert, which lies in the ventral and medial regions of the globus pallidus. Neurons from the nucleus basalis of Meynert project throughout the cortex. The second group of acetylcholine projections originating in the diagonal band of Broca and the septal nucleus project to the hippocampus and cingulate gyrus. A third group of cholinergic neurons are local circuit neurons that enter main structures within the basal ganglia.

The acetylcholine system plays a major role in the encoding of memory, although the precise mechanisms are not understood. Patients with Alzheimer's disease show

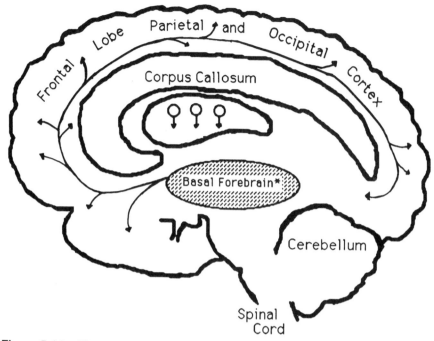

Figure 5-14. The acetylcholine system. *Includes the nucleus basalis of Meynert, the diagonal band of Broca, and the medial septal nucleus.

losses of acetylcholine projections both to the cortex and to the hippocampus, and blockade of muscarinic receptors produces impairment in memory. Dopamine and acetylcholine share heavy concentrations of activity within the basal ganglia, and the drugs used to block the extrapyramidal side effects of neuroleptics are cholinergic agonists, suggesting a possible reciprocal relationship between dopamine and acetylcholine in the modulation of motor activity and possibly of psychosis as well.

The GABA System

GABA is an amino acid neurotransmitter, as is glutamate. These two major amino acid neurotransmitters appear to serve complementary functions, with GABA playing an inhibitory role, whereas glutamate plays an excitatory role.

GABAergic neurons are a mix of local circuit and long-tract systems. Within the cerebral cortex and the limbic system, GABAergic neurons are predominantly local circuit. The cell bodies of GABAergic neurons in the caudate and putamen project to the globus pallidus and substantia nigra, making them relatively long tract. Long-tract GABAergic neurons also occur in the cerebellum.

The GABA system has substantial importance for the understanding of the neurochemistry of mental illness. Many of the anxiolytic drugs act as GABA agonists, thereby increasing the inhibitory tone within the CNS. Loss of the long-tract GABA neurons connecting the caudate to the globus pallidus releases the latter structure from inhibitory control, thereby permitting the globus pallidus to "run free" and produce the choreiform movements that characterize Huntington's chorea.

The Glutamate System

Glutamate, an excitatory amino acid neurotransmitter, is produced by pyramidal cells throughout the cerebral cortex and hippocampus. It has already been noted, for example, that the projections from the prefrontal cortex to the basal ganglia are glutaminergic.

It has been observed for many years that glutamate, in addition to being a neurotransmitter, is also potentially a neurotoxin if present in amounts that produce excessive neuronal excitation. Recently, this observation was coupled with observations about the psychological and biochemical effects of phencyclidine (PCP) to suggest a possible role for glutamate in either psychosis or neurodegenerative diseases such as Huntington's chorea. PCP blocks the effects of activating one subgroup of glutamate receptors, the N-methyl-D-aspartate (NMDA) receptors, probably by blocking the cation channel that the NMDA receptor activates. PCP intoxication produces a psychosis characterized by withdrawal, stupor, disorganized thinking and speech, and hallucinations. The possible relationship among PCP, its characteristic psychosis, and its effects on the glutamate system suggest that glutamate may play some role in producing (or protecting against) the symptoms of psychosis. Such diseases could be produced by excessive glutamatergic activity, which might produce neuronal degeneration through excessive excitation.

The Genetics of Mental Illness

It has been recognized for many years that mental illnesses tend to run in families. Evidence that disorders are familial is sometimes said to imply that they are "genetic" as well, but this is not necessarily the case. *Genetic* disorders are precisely that: coded in segments of DNA. The history of research in the familial aggregation of mental illnesses has been one of an increasing ability to determine more specifically the degree to which mental illnesses actually are genetic in the literal sense. The era of molecular biology and molecular genetics has arrived. This era has been supported by a long history of research in the familial aggregation of mental illnesses, which has established that the study of familial transmission is relevant to understanding the mechanisms of mental illness. The newer molecular approaches offer substantial additional insights.

Studies of Familial Aggregation

Studies of familial aggregation have offered the first line of evidence for the familial nature of major mental illnesses, as well as some indication that many mental illnesses may have a genetic component. The solid and increasingly methodologically rigorous studies of the prevalence of mental illnesses in families should not be minimized as we enter the era of molecular genetics; they have provided a major contribution. Such studies are usually divided into three broad groups: family studies, twin studies, and adoption studies. Each of these types of studies offers different perspectives on the genetics of disorders.

Family studies typically begin with the *proband method*. That is, an individual, or proband, is identified and used as the index case because he or she suffers from a particular disorder of interest, such as bipolar affective disorder or schizophrenia. Thereafter, all available first-degree relatives are typically evaluated. Early genetic studies used the *family history method*, which involves interviewing the proband and one or two additional family members about whether other members of the family have had any history of mental illness. This method is quick and simple, but less methodologically rigorous.

Gradually, the family history method has nearly been supplanted by the *family study method*, which involves directly interviewing all available first-degree relatives. The introduction of structured interviews and diagnostic criteria has presumably produced a steady increase in the accuracy of such family studies. In family studies, the prevalence of a specific disorder under investigation is also evaluated in some appropriately selected control group. For example, patients entering the hospital for hernia repair might represent the control group for the probands, whereas all their first-degree relatives would serve as the control group for the first-degree relatives of the mentally ill probands. If an increased rate of the specific mental illness under study is observed in the first-degree relatives of the mentally ill probands, then investigators conclude that a disorder is familial and possibly genetic.

Such studies do not exclude the possibility that the disorder is purely familial, however, and not due to a specifically genetic cause. Disorders could run in families because of learned behavior, role modeling, or predisposing social environments. For example, depression tends to run in families, and this could represent either genetic transmission or social learning; responding to stressful life events with a depressive coping style could easily be a learned adaptive mechanism passed on from parents to children through role modeling. Likewise, antisocial behavior also tends to run in families; although possibly genetic in origin, antisocial behavior could also be an adaptive response to social deprivation, nurtured by peer pressure from "gangs" that tend to cluster in impoverished inner cities.

As discussed in more detail in the various chapters on specific disorders (Section II of this volume), many major mental illnesses have been shown to be familial through family studies. Alzheimer's disease, schizophrenia, bipolar and unipolar mood disorders, anxiety disorders, and antisocial personality all tend to have increased rates in first-degree relatives of probands suffering from these various disorders. Thus, many major mental illnesses are highly familial. The test for the geneticist, however, is to determine whether they are also truly genetic.

Thus, investigators have turned to other methods in addition to family studies

Table 5-2.   Pairwise rates of schizophrenia, schizoid disorder, other mental disorders, and normality among sets of monozygotic twins: a summary of study results

Study	Number of pairs	Schizophrenia[a] (%)	Schizoid disorder[b] (%)	Other disorders[c] (%)	Normal (%)
Luxenburger 1928[d]	14	72	14		14
Rosanoff et al. 1934	41	61		7	32
Kallmann 1946	174	69	21	5	5
Slater and Crowie 1971	37	64		14	22
Kringlen 1967	45	38		29	33
Fischer 1973	21	48	5	5	43
Gottesman and Shields 1982	22	50	9	9	23

[a] Includes both confirmed and presumptive diagnoses.
[b] So diagnosed by the investigators.
[c] Includes as examples alcoholic, psychopath (Kallmann); psychopathic, suicide (Slater and Crowie); alcoholic, character neurosis (Kringlen).
[d] Includes only co-twins of certain schizophrenic patients.

to identify a more purely genetic component. Before techniques were available to look directly at DNA, the best methods were *twin studies* and *adoption studies*.

Twin studies.   These typically begin with ascertainment of a proband twin, who may be monozygotic or dizygotic, and who suffers from the disorder of interest. The co-twin is then evaluated to determine whether he or she also suffers from the illness (i.e., is concordant). The concordance rate on monozygotic twins can then be compared with that in dizygotic twins (using only same-sex twins among the dizygotic twins to help control for random cultural and genetic noise). The higher the rate of concordance in monozygotic twins as compared with dizygotic twins, the greater the degree of genetic influence.

The rationale behind twin studies is based on the fact that monozygotic twins have identical genetic material, whereas dizygotic twins theoretically share on average 50% of their genetic material in common (the percentage can actually run from 0 to 100%, but it should average out to 50% across large numbers of twin pairs). Thus, if a disorder were totally genetic and totally penetrant, the concordance rate in monozygotic twins would theoretically be 100%, whereas that in dizygotic twins would be 50%. In fact, actual rates for both groups are lower for most major mental illnesses that have been studied with the twin method. Table 5-2 shows the concordance rates for schizophrenia in the various twin studies that have been conducted to date.

Although powerful, twin studies do not provide a perfect method for looking at the genetics of major mental illnesses. Because twins are reared together, role modeling could again be an influential factor, particularly for milder disorders that have a potentially prominent "psychological" component, such as depression. This psychological component could theoretically be greater in monozygotic than in dizygotic twins, because monozygotic twins are often treated as "identical" by their parents and peers. The development of major mental illness in one's identical co-twin is clearly a serious psychological stressor that could be influential in the development of a disorder in the unaffected twin. If the unaffected twin is led to believe that he or she is indeed "identical" with the co-twin, he or she might develop a mental illness as part of a self-fulfilling prophecy. Alternatively, he or she might develop it out of sympathetic identification with a co-twin with whom he or she has been intimately nurtured for most of his or her life. Thus, environmental factors are not completely disentangled through the use of the twin method.

The twin method has been used less for the study of major mental illnesses because they are methodologically quite difficult. Nevertheless, twin studies have been completed for some disorders, including schizophrenia, affective disorder, and alcoholism. In general, the twin method has tended to support the familial nature and potentially the genetic aspect of most disorders to which it has been applied.

Adoption studies. These represent the most refined technique for disentangling environmental and genetic influences. In adoption studies, the population targeted for study is the adopted children of parents with a major mental illness, who were adopted at birth and reared by parents lacking the disorder. These children can be compared with a control group consisting of the adopted children of psychiatrically normal mothers. To whatever extent the rate of illness is higher in the adopted children of the mothers with the specific mental illness, that mental illness can be considered to be transmitted genetically rather than environmentally. In this model, learned behavior and role modeling of parents with illness have been excluded, because the child has been reared apart from the ill parent.

Like all paradigms, however, this one also has inherent limitations and problems. Accurate diagnosis in the father is sometimes difficult, often relying on case registers and historical information rather than direct interview. Of even more concern is the fact that information about the biological mother of the child may not be available, and the mother may not even be able to identify the specific biological father due to having multiple sex partners.

An additional problem with adoption studies (and of family studies in general) is the fact of assortative mating. *Assortative mating* refers to the tendency of individuals with a specific mental illness to mate with, or marry, a person who has a similar illness. This may occur because of a "like attracts like" phenomenon, or it may occur as a consequence of simple social convenience, because the partners often meet one another in mental hospitals and sometimes have few friends who are not mentally ill because of the social handicaps produced by some mental illnesses. Whatever the mechanism, assortative mating produces problems for family and genetic studies, because it gives the offspring a double genetic loading.

Adoption studies are the most difficult to complete, largely because of problems in obtaining access to appropriate samples. Some major adoption studies have been done in Scandinavian countries, which have excellent epidemiological registries. Adoption data are available for schizophrenia, affective disorder, and antisocial personality. In all cases, they add to the evidence for genetic factors in these disorders.

Genes Versus Environment in Major Mental Illnesses

As the above summary indicates, there is considerable evidence indicating that some mental illnesses are familial and that some may be genetic as well. Twin and family data provide particularly strong evidence in this regard, although family studies provide the weakest evidence for a purely genetic cause. Nevertheless, it seems unlikely that a familial propensity toward very serious illnesses such as Alzheimer's disease or schizophrenia could be explained purely on the basis of role modeling and learned behavior.

To understand the potentially complicated interactions between genes and environment, however, one must recognize that environmental factors are not necessarily psychological. Recent research with brain imaging techniques has suggested that other types of environmental factors, such as perinatal injuries, may have some influence on the development of severe mental disorder, particularly schizophrenia and affective disorders. Because these studies, using both computerized tomography and MRI, have shown that male patients have a significant increase in ventricular size compared with both female patients and normal control subjects, and because males are more vulnerable to perinatal injuries, these findings from neuroimaging suggest that physical environmental factors may also play a role in the development of major mental illnesses such as affective disorders or schizophrenia. These environmental factors could be perinatal, infectious, or traumatic, because male children appear to be more vulnerable to developing birth injuries, to having prenatal problems (i.e., a higher rate of spontaneous abortion), and possibly to developing infections as well. Because one common complication of difficult labor and delivery is periventricular hemorrhage, mechanisms of this type might explain the increased rate of ventricular size in male patients suffering from either schizophrenia or bipolar illness. The mechanism by which periventricular injury might predispose to the later development of schizophrenia or affective disorder is unclear; significant major subcortical structures such as the thalamus lie on the borders of the ventricles, and many major neurochemical tracts arising in the reticular core send white matter projections along the borders of the ventricles (e.g., the dopamine system arising in the ventral tegmental area, the norepinephrine system arising in the locus coeruleus).

Twin studies using neuroimaging have also been done in a cohort of individuals suffering from schizophrenia. The earliest twin study examined ventricular size in a group of monozygotic twins discordant for schizophrenia compared both with dizygotic twins and with normal monozygotic twins. In this study, conducted by Reveley et al., the ill monozygotic twins were found to have larger ventricular size than the well twins. (A summary of their data is shown in Table 5-3.) Further, the well monozygotic twins who had a schizophrenic co-twin also tended to have larger ventricular size than did monozygotic twin pairs who were both well.

Thus, these results appear to suggest a combined genetic and environmental interaction. Both twins from the ill cohort tended to have bigger ventricles that normal twins, suggesting a genetic contribution to ventricular size that might reflect an underlying predisposition to the illness. Because the ill twin also had bigger

Table 5-3. Ventricle-to-brain ratios (VBRs) in normal twins and in monozygotic twins discordant for schizophrenia

| Twin status | n | Age ± SE | VBR | | | |
			Overall (mean ± SE)	Mean intrapair difference	r	h² (%)
MZ normal	22	39 ± 3	4.2 ± 0.6	0.36	.98	98
DZ normal	16	38 ± 4	5.1 ± 0.6	1.90	.35	70
MZ schizophrenic	7	38 ± 3	8.6 ± 0.2			
MZ schizophrenic co-twins	7	38 ± 3	6.5 ± 0.2	2.16	.87	87

Note. MZ = monozygotic. DZ = dizygotic.
Source. Adapted from Reveley AM, Reveley MA, Clifford CA, et al: Cerebral ventricular size in twins discordant for schizophrenia. Lancet 1:540–541, 1982.

ventricles than the well co-twin, however, these findings also suggest that some type of environmental factor was necessary to "release" an underlying genetic diathesis that both twins shared. This release, presumably something such as a birth injury, is what caused the ill co-twin to develop the schizophrenia.

The findings of the Reveley group in England are now being replicated in a similar study conducted at the National Institute of Mental Health in the United States. In this study as well, the ill twin in a discordant monozygotic twin pair can consistently be identified on the basis of structural brain abnormalities seen with neuroimaging (in this instance MRI).

Thus, numerous information sources suggest that it may be difficult to find purely genetic models that will explain some major mental illnesses. In general, patterns of transmission within families do not appear to follow simple Mendelian patterns. The neuroimaging data suggest the importance of environmental factors, in this case biological environmental factors. Psychological factors, such as role modeling, certainly cannot be excluded and may also be highly relevant. Thus, in some cases, and perhaps in many, it may be necessary to use multifactorial models to explain the etiology of major mental illnesses.

Molecular Genetics

Molecular genetics provides an alternative approach to the descriptive studies discussed above. The techniques of molecular biology provide methods for looking directly at the genetic material itself and offer the hope of being able to identify the gene or genes that might produce an illness either by working in isolation or by interacting with environmental factors to cause the illness. Initially, pursuing the principles of parsimony, investigators are seeking a single major locus. Although at least some forms of major mental illness may be too complex to be explained on the basis of a single gene, this strategy is well worth pursuing, because the reward would be very great if a single locus were identified, even in a subset of families or individuals.

Methods of molecular genetics.   The techniques of molecular genetics depend on the fact that many genetic loci are polymorphic; that is, genes are not simply a continuous series of base sequences that provide coding information to produce proteins. Instead, the information coded by the base pairs is divided by "spacers" in the DNA that vary in length. The spacers themselves have no known function, and they are edited out when messenger RNA is produced to initiate protein synthesis. They exist, however, in the genomic DNA.

Genetic variation and transmission can be studied through the use of these restriction fragment length polymorphisms (RFLPs). RFLPs are small pieces of DNA (typically measured in kilobases and consisting of somewhere between 1,000 and 10,000 base pairs) that can be seen after the DNA is digested or cut with an enzyme known as a restriction endonuclease; a restriction endonuclease is a bacterial enzyme that recognizes a specific base sequence and digests or cuts it out specifically. Differences in the lengths of these restriction fragments are inherited in classic Mendelian patterns. Therefore, if a single gene producing a disease is embedded within an RFLP or itself represents an RFLP, its transmission can be mapped within families and the genetic pattern of transmission thereby identified. Thus, the term *restriction fragment length polymorphism* refers to the variation in fragment length (polymorphism) produced by the spacers occurring between coding information. They are referred to as restriction fragment length polymorphisms because they are identified through the use of the restriction enzymes that cut the DNA and permit the identification of these variable fragment lengths.

Typically, these measurements are made in the laboratory with Southern blotting techniques and various other methods. A basic understanding of the techniques of molecular biology and molecular genetics has become part of our scientific cultural heritage in the 1980s and 1990s. Various comprehensive and useful summaries of molecular biology are available; one of the best is the *Scientific American* publication *Recombinant DNA: A Short Course* (Watson et al. 1983).

To study the genetics of major mental illnesses such as bipolar disorder or schizophrenia, two different strategies are available. These are sometimes referred to as the *candidate gene approach* and the *reverse genetics approach.*

The candidate gene approach starts with the identification of some specific gene that might have pathophysiological relevance to the disorder of interest. During the past decade, molecular biologists have been actively engaged in cloning many genes. The cloned genes obviously have applications beyond those involved in the study of genetics, i.e., they can be used as an inexpensive method for synthetically manufacturing medically useful products such as hormones. Not all genes are polymorphic, but those that are can be used to study the genetic transmission of diseases. Examples of such polymorphic genes that can be used in the candidate gene approach include neuropeptide-Y, beta nerve growth factor, dopamine, and MAO. Candidate genes that might be relevant to mental illness include those that are involved in neurotransmission and hormonal regulation.

The strength of the candidate gene approach is that it directly permits investigators to decide whether the particular protein has any relevance to the production of a major mental illness. When families of sufficient size are studied and it is determined that the particular gene sorts with the individuals who suffer from the illness, then that particular protein has been identified as a causative mechanism. Likewise, if the study is negative, the protein has been excluded as a cause. To date, the candidate gene approach has been used only minimally, and no positive candidate gene studies have been reported for major mental illnesses.

The positive work reported to date has involved the second strategy, linkage studies using RFLPs. This approach is referred to as *reverse genetics* because the investigator does not begin with a specific gene in mind. Here, the unit of interest is the RFLP, which is used to map the genome. If evenly spaced polymorphisms are used to map the genome, then the entire body of human DNA can be mapped with only 150 polymorphisms.

Linkage studies with RFLPs must begin with large, informative families, involving multiple generations in which a substantial number of individuals suffer from the disorder of interest. Samples of their DNA can be collected through creating cell cultures of lymphocytes. Their genomes can then be scanned to determine whether a specific variation in restriction fragment length is linked to the presence of the specific disorder at some chromosomal location. Because of the size of the human genome, this process is relatively labor-intensive. Nevertheless, it has had a highly successful application in Huntington's chorea, where linkage was relatively quickly established on chromosome 4 through the study of a large Venezuelan pedigree. This led, 2 years later, to the development of a premorbid test for the disease. Nevertheless, illustrating the intransigent puzzles inherent in human biology, the gene itself has not yet been identified; we still do not know what the abnormal structural or regulatory protein is that produces Huntington's chorea. Thus, even with a clear, relatively simple, autosomal dominant disease for which the chromosomal locus has been identified, the final answer that we seek will not come easily.

Studying the genetics of major mental illnesses with RFLPs has presented much more complex problems, because in general RFLPs are not fully penetrant and not clearly due to single loci. At present, two major positive studies of affective disorder have been reported. The work of Egeland et al. (1987), with a large pedigree from the Old Order Amish, appeared to show autosomal dominant transmission with reduced penetrance and to establish linkage between bipolar illness and chromosome 11. Subsequent reanalysis of the pedigree, however, has reduced the significance of their finding. A study by Baron et al. (1987) showed close linkage between bipolar illness and the X chromosome marker for color blindness, confirming much earlier work indicating the possibility of X chromosome linkage in bipolar illness based on the "old-fashioned" methods of clinical testing for color blindness or red cell antigens. No linkage studies have been completed for unipolar disorder, and none are likely to appear quickly. A linkage for schizophrenia has been reported on chromosome 5, but several nonreplications of this finding have also been reported.

The results of these linkage studies illustrate some of the problems involved in applying molecular genetics to the study of mental illness, as well as the requirements for a good linkage study. One fundamental requirement, which is not easily obtained, is the availability of informative families. An informative family has large numbers of family members who are ill, and it also has the illness running through only one side of the family (i.e., only through the father or the mother of the proband). If the illness is contributed through both sides, it becomes much more difficult to determine linkage because the illnesses diagnosed may be genetically heterogeneous. Theoretically, the disorder that runs within a single family and derives from one side is considered to be homogeneous in the literal sense (i.e., deriving from the same gene).

Heterogeneity is a serious problem in linkage studies. If a disorder is relatively common and affects large numbers of the population, and if it is caused by several different genes, then substantial noise is added to the system because it becomes difficult or impossible to tell whether the clinical manifestations are linked to one gene or the other. Depression in particular is a very common disorder. Thus, for the study of mood disorder, a genetic isolate such as the Old Order Amish is an ideal sample because there has been very little marriage in or out, and the disorder is more likely to be homogeneous within a family. Such genetic isolates are, of course, difficult to find. Further, isolates have their own inherent problems for genetic research, because findings may not be generalizable. Nevertheless, if a gene is identified in an isolate and its metabolic pathway studied and found to be informative, this might yield useful information concerning the pathophysiology of more common forms of the disorder. This hope has informed the study of Huntington's chorea, for example, although it has not been realized.

The disorders within such informative families must be reliably and accurately diagnosed, and ideally, environmental phenocopies should be relatively rare. For this reason, severe disorders such as bipolar disorder or schizophrenia present much easier cases than do depression or anxiety. Both of the linkage studies of bipolar illness described above relied on bipolar individuals as their index cases, and both used standard structured interviews such as the Schedule for Affective Disorders and Schizophrenia (SADS). Nevertheless, both used a broad definition of bipolar illness, including as "cases" individuals who suffered from unipolar depression as well. This increases the number of affected patients for analysis, but with the potential risk of introducing noise and possible environmental phenocopies. This problem is substantially greater in the study of milder disorders such as depression, because the diagnostic boundaries are less clear and the potential for environmental phenocopies is much greater. Although bipolar disorder appears to be relatively homogeneous clinically, most investigators share a consensus that depression is probably heterogeneous, and a definitive method for identifying subtypes has not yet been developed.

Thus, evidence accumulated to date suggests that many major mental disorders are familial, and that some forms are genetic and probably even caused by a single major genetic locus. Once a genetic locus is identified through linkage studies using RFLPs, the next step is to focus within that restriction fragment and identify the DNA sequence that codes for the specific gene producing the disorder. As the case of Huntington's chorea indicates, this next step is not necessarily easy. Once the abnormal gene is found and its product identified, then the potential exists for either improved treatment, or perhaps ultimately for prevention. A second major advantage of identifying a locus using linkage studies is that it becomes possible to do genetic counseling and to identify those unaffected individuals susceptible to developing the disease who may transmit it to their children. The ethical implications are profound. Measured against what was known and what could be done 30 years ago, recent achievements in genetics have been substantial. Measured against what remains to be done both scientifically and morally, however, these achievements seem quite modest.

Bibliography

Andreasen NC: Brain imaging: applications in psychiatry. Science 239:1381–1388, 1988

Andreasen NC (ed): Brain Imaging: Applications in Psychiatry. Washington, DC, American Psychiatric Press, 1989

Baron M, Risch N, Hamburger R, et al: Genetic linkage between X-chromosome markers and bipolar affective illness. Nature 326:289–292, 1987

Björklund A, Hökfelt T, Swanson LW: Handbook of Chemical Neuroanatomy, Vol 5: Integrated Systems of the CNS, Part I. Amsterdam, Elsevier, 1987

Botstein D, White RL, Skolnick MH, et al: Construction of a genetic linkage map in man, using restriction fragment length polymorphisms. Am J Hum Genet 32:314–331, 1980

Cooper JR, Bloom FE, Roth RH: The Biochemical Basis of Neuropharmacology, 5th Edition. New York, Oxford University Press, 1986

Coyle JT: Neuroscience and psychiatry, in The American Psychiatric Press Textbook of Psychiatry. Edited by Talbott JA, Hales RE, Yudofsky SC. Washington, DC, American Psychiatric Press, 1988, pp 3–32

Creese I, Burt DR, Snyder SH: Dopamine receptor binding predicts clinical and pharmacological potencies of anti-schizophrenic drugs. Science 192:481–483, 1972

Doane BK, Livingston KF: The Limbic System: Functional Organization and Clinical Disorders. New York, Raven, 1986

Egeland JA, Gerhard DS, Pauls DL, et al: Bipolar affective disorders linked to DNA markers on chromosome 11. Nature 323:646–650, 1987

Emson PC: Chemical Neuroanatomy. New York, Raven, 1983

Fischer M: Genetic and environmental factors in schizophrenia: a study of schizophrenic twins and their families. Acta Psychiatr Scand [Suppl] 238:9–142, 1973

Fuster JM: The Prefrontal Cortex: Anatomy, Physiology, and Neuropsychology of the Frontal Lobe, 2nd Edition. New York, Raven, 1989

Gottesman II, Shields J: Schizophrenia: The Epigenetic Puzzle. New York, Cambridge University Press, 1982

Gusella JF, Wexler NS, Conneally PM, et al: A polymorphic DNA marker genetically linked to Huntington's disease. Nature 306:234–238, 1983

Heston LL: The genetics of schizophrenic and schizoid disease. Science 167:249–256, 1970

Isaacson RL: The Limbic System, 2nd Edition. New York, Plenum, 1982

Jones EG, Peters A: Cerebral Cortex, Vol 6: Further Aspect of Cortical Function, Including Hippocampus. New York, Plenum, 1987

Kallmann FJ: The genetic theory of schizophrenia: an analysis of 691 schizophrenic twin index families. Am J Psychiatry 103:309–322, 1946

Kandel ER, Schwartz JH: Principals of Neural Science, 2nd Edition. New York, Elsevier, 1985

Kelsoe JR, Ginns EI, Egeland JA, et al: Re-evaluation of the linkage relationship between chromosome 11p loci and the gene for bipolar affective disorder in the Old Order Amish. Nature 342:238–243, 1989

Kety SS, Rosenthal D, Wender PH, et al: Mental illness in the biological and adoptive families of adopted schizophrenics. Am J Psychiatry 128:302–306, 1971

Kringlen E: Heredity and Environment in the Functional Psychoses: An Epidemiological-Clinical Twin Study. Oslo, Universitetsforlaget, 1967

Luxenburger H: Vorlufiger bericht ber psychiatrische Serienuntersuchungen und Zwillinge. Zeitschrift fur die Gesamte Neurologie und Psychiatrie 116:1167–1171, 1928

Nauta WJH, Feirtag M: Fundamental Neuroanatomy. New York, WH Freeman, 1986

Rosanoff AJ, Handy LM, Plesset IR, et al: Etiology of so-called schizophrenic psychoses with special reference to their occurrence in twins. Am J Psychiatry 91:247–286, 1934

Seeman P, Lee T, Chau-Wong M, et al: Antipsychotic drug doses and neuroleptic-dopamine receptors. Nature 261:717–719, 1976

Slater E, Crowie V: The Genetics of Mental Disorders. London, Oxford University Press, 1971

Stuss DT, Benson DF: The Frontal Lobes. New York, Raven, 1986

Watson JD, Tooze J, Kurtz DT: Recombinant DNA: A Short Course. New York, WH Freeman, 1983

Self-assessment Questions

1. What is the standard anatomic definition of the prefrontal cortex? Describe the functions performed by the prefrontal cortex. Contrast the "euphoric syndrome" with the "apathetic syndrome." List several neuropsychological tests used to assess prefrontal function.

2. Describe the limbic system, listing the structures included in it, and describe the functions of the amygdala and hippocampus in relation to memory.

3. Discuss possible relationships between abnormalities in the frontal system, the memory system, and the language system in relation to the symptoms of psychosis.

4. Describe the location of cell bodies and projections for the dopamine system, the norepinephrine system, the serotonin system, and the acetylcholine system.

5. Describe the mechanisms by which abnormalities in GABA neurons may produce Huntington's chorea. Describe the functions of glutamate and its possible relationship to the symptoms of the psychosis, using PCP as a model.

6. Describe the relative strengths of family studies, twin studies, and adoption studies as methods for determining the familial nature of mental illnesses and the degree to which purely genetic factors play a causal role.

7. Discuss the possible interaction between genes and environmental factors in producing mental illness, using neuroimaging studies of schizophrenia as an example.

8. Describe the candidate gene approach versus the reverse genetics approach for studying molecular mechanisms of mental illness. Describe the two different positive linkage studies for bipolar illness and their implications for possible heterogeneity of major mental illnesses.

Section II

Psychiatric Disorders

Chapter 6
Organic Mental Disorders

When age has crushed the body with its might,
The limbs collapse with weakness and decay,
The judgment limps, and mind and speech give way.

Lucretius

The organic mental disorders encompass a variety of mental disturbances and syndromes, each initiated or maintained by a physical injury or insult, such as the effect of a drug or brain trauma. Organic disorders may mimic any of the major syndromes, so that the types of mental disturbances are as wide ranging as psychiatry itself. According to DSM-III-R, the essential feature of these disorders is a psychological or behavioral abnormality associated with transient or permanent brain dysfunction. To diagnose an organic mental disorder, the presence of a specific organic factor (or factors) must be demonstrated and judged to be etiologically related to the abnormality. The organic factor is demonstrated by the history, physical examination, or laboratory tests. In many cases, an organic factor may be inferred, but may not be possible to demonstrate unequivocally.

Organic disorders have been recognized for centuries. For example, in the 17th century, Morgagni, the great Italian anatomist, made correlations between the clinical picture of mental patients and postmortem changes in their brains. However, it was not until the late 19th century when the brain syndromes and their pathology were systematically investigated and described, mostly by the great neuropathologist-psychiatrists Alzheimer, Pick, Nissl, and Brodmann. Even Freud believed that most mental disorders would ultimately be found to have a neuroanatomical basis.

139

Table 6-1.   Organic mental disorders

Delirium
Dementia
Organic mood syndrome
Organic delusional syndrome
Amnestic syndrome
Organic hallucinosis
Organic anxiety syndrome
Organic personality syndrome
Organic mental syndrome not otherwise specified

In this chapter, we describe the two major organic mental syndromes, delirium and dementia, which are both characterized by global intellectual impairment, followed by a description of organic disorders that are associated with specific or isolated symptoms, such as dysphoric mood (Table 6-1).

Delirium

Delirium is a syndrome characterized by impaired attention, perceptual disturbances, and intellectual impairment. Delirium may develop over hours or days and may be alarming to observers, creating a sense of urgency. Indeed, because delirium is initiated and maintained by organic factors, it represents an emergency situation requiring immediate attention and careful evaluation.

Delirium is surprisingly common, especially among persons who are medically ill. Among medical patients at general hospitals, approximately 10–15% develop a delirium during their hospitalization, and delirium is particularly common among postsurgical and elderly patients (e.g., intensive care unit [ICU] psychosis). Delirium is also associated with high mortality—an estimated 40–50% of patients will die within 1 year.

Clinical Findings

The hallmark of delirium is the relatively rapid development of global cognitive impairment combined with disorientation and confusion. Although the presentation of delirium may differ among patients, several features are characteristic, including

1. Clouding of consciousness evidenced by either diminished or increased alertness
2. Attention deficit, so that the patient may be distractible and unable to focus his or her attention sufficiently
3. Perceptual disturbances so that misinterpretations are made of environmental stimuli (e.g., illusions and hallucinations, often visual)
4. Sleep-wake cycle disturbances characterized by a worsening of symptoms at night ("sundowning")
5. Disorientation to place, date, or person

Table 6-2.   DSM-III-R diagnostic criteria for delirium

A. Reduced ability to maintain attention to external stimuli and to appropriately shift attention to new external stimuli.

B. Disorganized thinking as indicated by rambling, irrelevant, or incoherent speech.

C. At least two of the following:

   1. Reduced level of consciousness
   2. Perceptual disturbances, such as misinterpretations, illusions, or hallucinations
   3. Disturbance of sleep-wake cycle with insomnia or daytime sleepiness
   4. Increased or decreased psychomotor activity
   5. Disorientation to time, place, or person
   6. Memory impairment

D. Clinical features develop over a short period of time (usually hours to days) and tend to fluctuate over the course of a day.

E. Either 1 or 2:

   1. Evidence from history, physical examination, or laboratory tests of a specific organic factor(s) judged to be etiologically related to the disturbance.
   2. In the absence of such evidence, an etiologic organic factor can be presumed if the disturbance cannot be accounted for by any nonorganic mental disorder.

6. Memory impairment, typically recent rather than remote memory
7. Incoherence, so that the patient may be unable to communicate intelligibly
8. Altered psychomotor activity, resulting in restlessness and agitation, or excessive somnolence

The diagnostic criteria for delirium are presented in Table 6-2. Characteristically, delirium fluctuates from day to day or hour to hour. At times the patient may appear normal but later in the day may be disoriented and hallucinating. The following case example illustrates delirium.

An 84-year-old retired police chief was brought to the emergency room by his family, who reported a 4- to 5-day history of lassitude, lower-extremity weakness, bladder incontinence, and intermittent confusion and memory impairment. They reported that the patient had fallen 4 weeks earlier and had sustained a scalp laceration requiring suturing. There was no history of alcohol use. When examined, the patient was cooperative but drowsy and easily distracted. Although oriented to person, he was disoriented to date and situation. Memory for recent events was poor, and he was unable to recall three objects either immediately or at 3 minutes. He could not name the current president, but remembered President Franklin Roosevelt. Interestingly, the patient was an acquaintance of one of the author's (D.W.B.) deceased grandfathers and was able to speak at length of this remote relationship.

A presumptive diagnosis of delirium was made, and a workup for organic causes was begun. Computerized tomography (CT) showed the presence of bilateral chronic subdural hematomas. The patient was transferred to the neurosurgery service where burr hole evacuation was performed. The delirium cleared, but the patient had a residual dementia and was eventually transferred to a long-term nursing facility.

Etiology

Delirium almost always occurs in persons with serious medical, surgical, or neurologic illness or in a drug intoxication or withdrawal state. In fact, the development of a delirium may precede other manifestations of an underlying physical disorder; therefore, the presence of an unexplained delirium should lead to an immediate search for an organic factor that may have initiated the disturbance. Because delirium is a syndrome, and not a disease, it is best seen as the final common pathway from many potential causes. Most causes of delirium lie outside the central nervous system (CNS) and include metabolic abnormalities, such as those caused by infection, febrile illness, hypoxia, hypoglycemia, drug withdrawal states, hepatic encephalopathy, or postoperative changes. Other causes lie within the CNS, such as brain abscesses, trauma, and postictal states. Although delirium may be influenced by the environment, the environment should never be considered the main cause of delirium, except in rare cases of total sensory deprivation.

Because the differential diagnosis of delirium is so broad, an evaluation must be thorough. The history and physical examination, however, will probably steer the clinician a particular way. A workup must include a complete physical examination in which attention is paid to focal neurologic signs, papilledema, and frontal lobe release signs (e.g., suck, snout, palmomental, and rooting reflexes), which are characteristic of global deficit states. Laboratory tests should include routine blood and urine studies (e.g., complete blood count [CBC], urinalysis), chest X ray, CT (or magnetic resonance imaging [MRI]), electrocardiogram (ECG), lumbar puncture (in selected patients), toxic screen, blood gases, and electroencephalogram (EEG). Although laboratory test results will vary depending on the underlying cause of the delirium, delirious patients are likely to have temperature elevations and abnormal EEGs that are diffusely slow.

The major problem in differential diagnosis is distinguishing delirium from a functional confusional state, such as may be found in a schizophrenic or manic patient. Typically, the delirious patient has a more acute presentation and is globally confused, and the hallucinations (often visual) tend to be fragmented and disorganized. The delirious patient is less likely to have a personal or family history of psychiatric illness. Be cautioned, however, that the presence of a preexisting psychiatric illness does not preclude the possibility of developing a delirium.

Clinical Management

First, it is essential that the underlying physical condition be corrected, if possible. Until the condition is corrected, measures must be taken to maintain the patient's health and safety, including constant observation, consistent nursing care, frequent reassurance, and repeated simple explanations. Restraints may be necessary, but can actually increase agitation in some patients. It is wise to minimize external stimulation, and experience has shown that delirious patients tend to do better in quiet, well-lighted rooms, because shadows or darkness may frighten them.

Medication should be used with caution because delirious patients are exquisitely sensitive to side effects. Unnecessary medication should be discontinued, including sedatives or hypnotics (e.g., benzodiazepines), which may have caused the delirium and can exacerbate sleep-wake cycle disturbances. For the highly agitated patient, low doses of a high-potency antipsychotic (e.g., haloperidol, thiothixene) may be helpful, but agents with significant anticholinergic properties (e.g., chlorproma-zine, thioridazine) should be avoided, as these can worsen or prolong the delirium. In fact, in surgical patients, plasma anticholinergic levels have been found to correlate with delirium. If sedation is absolutely necessary, low doses of short-acting benzodiazepines (e.g., oxazepam or lorazepam) may be helpful.

Recommendations for management of delirium

1. In the hospital, a quiet, restful setting that is well lighted is best for the confused patient.

2. Consistency of personnel is less likely to upset the delirious patient.

3. Reminders of day, date, time, place, and situation should be prominently displayed in the patient's room.

4. Medication for behavior management should be limited to those cases in which behavioral interventions have failed.

   - Only essential drugs should be prescribed and polypharmacy should be avoided.
   - Avoid sedative-hypnotics and anxiolytics.
   - Unmanageable behavior may also require low-dose neuroleptics, or alternatively, benzodiazepines with short half-lives (e.g., 0.5 mg lorazepam twice daily).

Dementia

Dementia is the global impairment of cognitive function, memory, and personality that occurs without a disturbance in consciousness or level of alertness (i.e., sensorium). The diagnostic criteria are listed in Table 6-3. The disability caused by dementia is severe enough to interfere with social or occupational functioning. Dementias are acquired, unlike mental retardation (which may be associated with these symptoms), which is congenital. The impairment created by dementia differentiates it from the mild memory change ("benign senescent forgetfulness") that occurs during normal aging. Remember that dementia is a clinical syndrome and not a diagnosis. Although the causes of dementia are many, its clinical presentations are remarkably similar. Most dementias are irreversible, but many can be controlled by therapeutic interventions, and a smaller number (up to 15%) may be reversed. A search for treatable causes is mandatory in the demented patient.

Dementia is, unhappily, quite common in the general population. About 5% of persons over age 65 years are severely demented, whereas 10% suffer mild dementia. At age 80 years, 20% or more suffer a severe dementia. Among elderly

Table 6-3. DSM-III-R criteria for dementia

A. Demonstrable evidence of impairment in short- and long-term memory.

B. At least one of the following:
   1. Impairment in abstract thinking
   2. Impaired judgment
   3. Other disturbances of higher cortical function, such as aphasia, apraxia, agnosia, and constructional difficulty
   4. Personality change

C. The disturbance in A and B significantly interferes with work or usual social activities or relationships with others.

D. Not occurring exclusively during the course of delirium.

E. Either 1 or 2:
   1. There is evidence from the history, physical examination, or laboratory tests of a specific organic factor(s) judged to be etiologically related to the disturbance.
   2. In the absence of such disturbance, an etiologic organic factor can be presumed if the disturbance cannot be accounted for by any nonorganic mental disorder.

Criteria for severity of dementia

Mild: Although work or social activities are significantly impaired, the capacity for independent living remains, with adequate personal hygiene and relatively intact judgment.

Moderate: Independent living is hazardous and some degree of supervision is necessary.

Severe: Activities of daily living are so impaired that continual supervision is required, e.g., patient is unable to maintain minimal personal hygiene, is largely incoherent or mute.

---

hospitalized patients and physically ill persons, the rates of dementia are higher still.

Clinical Findings

Dementia usually develops insidiously and is often easily overlooked and attributed to the normal process of aging. In its earliest stages, the only symptoms may be subtle changes in personality, a decrease in range of interests or apathy, and the development of labile or shallow emotions. Gradually, intellectual skills will be lost, noticed initially in work settings where high performance is required, and may be denied by the patient. These characteristics help to separate delirium from dementia and are highlighted in Table 6-4.

As the disorder advances, memory impairment becomes more pronounced, affecting immediate or recent memory preferentially; the changes in mood and personality become more exaggerated and social skills may be lost, whereas in earlier stages they may have helped to preserve the patient's image of health; psychotic symptoms may arise; judgment is impaired; and eventually language impairment, leading to perseveration, vagueness, or even aphasia, may develop. When the dementia is advanced, patients may be unable to perform basic tasks such as feeding themselves or caring for personal hygiene. Patients may forget names of friends

Table 6-4. Clinical features differentiating dementia from delirium

Dementia	Delirium
Chronic or insidious onset	Acute or rapid onset
Level of consciousness unimpaired early on	Level of consciousness clouded
Normal level of arousal	Agitation or stupor
Usually progressive and deteriorating	Often reversible
Common in nursing homes and psychiatric hospitals	Common on medical, surgical, and neurological wards

and be unable to recognize close relatives. Regression may include the development of infantile behavior, such as incontinence and extreme emotional lability. Finally, patients may become totally mute and unresponsive. At this stage, death usually occurs within months, although some patients may linger.

It is necessary to separate dementia from pseudodementia, an important condition that sometimes accompanies depressive illness. In this disturbance, the depressed patient appears to be demented. He or she is unable to remember correctly, cannot calculate well, and complains, often bitterly, of lost cognitive abilities and skills. Features that are helpful in differentiating dementia from pseudodementia are presented in Table 6-5. The importance of this distinction is obvious: the pseudodemented patient has a treatable illness, and is not truly demented. The "dementia" is an artifact of the depression.

Diagnosis

The best diagnostic test for dementia is a careful history, physical examination, and mental status examination. The Mini-Mental State Exam, a quick, at-the-bedside test, can be used to get a rough index of cognitive impairment. (This test is included in the Appendix.) Assessing orientation, memory, constructional abil-

Table 6-5. Clinical features differentiating pseudodementia from dementia

Pseudodementia	Dementia
Short duration	Long duration
Complaints of cognitive loss	Few complaints of cognitive loss
Complaints of cognitive dysfunction, usually detailed	Complaints of cognitive dysfunction, usually imprecise
Communications of distress	Often appear unconcerned
Memory gaps for specific periods or events	Memory gaps for specific periods unusual
Attention and concentration usually well preserved	Attention and concentration faulty
"Don't know" answer typical	Near-miss answers frequent
Little effort to perform simple tasks	Patients struggle to perform tasks
Patients highlight failures	Patients delight in trivial accomplishments
Early loss of social skills	Social skills often retained
Mood change pervasive	Affect shallow and labile
History of prior psychiatric illness common	History of previous psychiatric illness uncommon

ity, and ability to read, write, and calculate, the test can be administered in 5 minutes. Thirty points are possible: a score of less than 25 is suggestive of impairment, and a score of less than 20 usually indicates definite impairment.

Laboratory testing is an important part of the workup. All patients with new onset of dementia should have a CBC, serum electrolytes, serum glucose, blood urea nitrogen (BUN), serum creatinine, liver and thyroid function tests, sedimentation rate, vitamin B_{12} and folate levels, serologic tests for syphilis and human immunodeficiency virus (HIV), urinalysis, ECG, and chest X ray. Most of the readily reversible metabolic, endocrine, vitamin deficiency, and infectious states, whether causal or complicating, will be uncovered by these simple tests, when combined with the history and physical findings. Other tests are helpful in carefully chosen patients: CT (or MRI) of the brain is appropriate in the presence of a history suggestive of a mass, or focal neurologic signs, or a dementia that is very brief in duration; and EEGs are appropriate for patients with altered consciousness or suspected seizures. Undue weight should not be placed on isolated findings. In some situations, other tests may be useful, including cerebral blood flow, lumbar puncture, and arterial blood gases. In particular, cerebral blood flow as measured by single photon emission computer tomography (SPECT) can be useful in the differential diagnosis of Alzheimer's dementia, because these patients have a relatively characteristic decrease in posterior temporoparietal blood flow. Hospitalization should be considered if the history is unclear, if the patient is suicidal, if acute deterioration has occurred without apparent cause, or if the social situation precludes adequate observation. The organic workup is summarized in Table 6-6.

Neuropsychological testing can often be very useful in the evaluation of dementia. Testing may be done to obtain baseline data by which to measure change both before and after treatment. Testing can also be helpful in evaluating bright individuals suspected of early dementia and when other test results (i.e., imaging studies) are ambiguous. Neuropsychological testing may also help distinguish delirium from dementia and depression.

Irreversible Causes of Dementia

Alzheimer's disease is the most common cause of the degenerative dementias and accounts for 50–60% of all cases of dementia. It affects between 1 and 2 million Americans. In DSM-III-R, Alzheimer's disease is divided into senile and presenile forms; however, the natural history and pathology of cases arising before and after the senium are identical, so there is no clear basis for such a distinction.

Alzheimer's disease usually begins insidiously in patients in their 50s, 60s, or beyond and usually leads to death within 6–10 years of its onset. Estimates of the prevalence of Alzheimer's disease range from 5% at age 65 to 20% by age 90. Symptoms begin gradually and progressively worsen over many years, resulting in near collapse of intellectual functioning. Physical findings are generally absent or present only in later stages and may include hyperactive deep tendon reflexes, Babinski's sign, and frontal lobe release signs. Many patients develop illusions, hallucinations, and delusions, findings that have been associated with accelerated

Table 6-6. Evaluation for organic mental disorders

1. Complete history

2. Thorough physical examination, including neurological examination

3. Mental status examination

4. Laboratory studies

   - Complete blood count (CBC), with differential
     Serum electrolytes
     Serum glucose
     Blood urea nitrogen (BUN)
     Creatinine
     Liver function tests
     Serology for syphilis and HIV
     Thyroid function tests
     Serum vitamin B_{12}
     Folate
   - Urinalysis and urine drug screen
   - Electrocardiogram
   - Chest X ray
   - Brain computerized tomography or magnetic resonance imaging

5. Neuropsychological testing

6. Optional tests

   - Cerebral blood flow (i.e., single photon emission computer tomography [SPECT])
   - Lumbar puncture

cognitive deterioration. Cortical atrophy and enlarged cerebral ventricles are seen with CT or MRI. Although not diagnosable during life, at autopsy characteristic brain pathology will be found, including senile plaques (degenerating neurons tangled around an amyloid core), neurofibrillary tangles (helical filaments tangled within neurons), neuronal granulovacuolar degeneration of nerve cell bodies, and Hirano bodies (elongated red structures often found in the hippocampus). Recent research has implicated primary degeneration of cholinergic neurons in the nucleus basalis of Meynert as a possible cause of Alzheimer's disease. Age-related memory disturbance in animals and humans may be associated with a cholinergic dysfunction. In response to these findings, investigators have tried to increase choline levels in patients with Alzheimer's disease with orally administered lecithin or tetrahydroaminoacridine (THA). Although modest success has been reported, it is too early to tell whether these agents will have any role in treating Alzheimer's disease.

Risk factors for Alzheimer's disease include female gender, a history of head injury, Down's syndrome, and having a first-degree relative with the disorder. In fact, up to 45% of first-degree relatives are affected with the disorder by age 86 years. In the familial form of the disease, molecular genetics studies have found defects on chromosome 21 that may be responsible for the accumulation of amyloid in blood vessels and neurons.

Pick's disease accounts for about 5% of the irreversible dementias and is clinically indistinguishable from Alzheimer's disease, only being definitively diagnosed after death. At autopsy, the brain exhibits distinctive frontotemporal atrophy and ventricular dilatation. Microscopic examination discloses neuronal loss with gliosis and the presence of Pick's bodies in the neurons. Pick's bodies contain masses of cytoskeletal elements that bind polyclonal antibodies against neurotubules and a monoclonal antibody against neurofilaments. Risk factors for Pick's disease include male gender and having a first-degree relative with the disorder.

Huntington's chorea is a neuropsychiatric disorder with autosomal dominant inheritance. Its gene has been located on the short arm of chromosome 4. Psychiatric manifestations range from mild anxiety to hallucinations and delusions, which may precede the onset of choreiform movements. Dementia occurs in the terminal phase of the illness.

Other illnesses associated with the dementia syndrome include diseases of the basal ganglia (Parkinson's disease), of the cerebellum (cerebellar, spinocerebellar, and olivopontocerebellar degeneration), and of the motor neuron (amyotrophic lateral sclerosis).

Other causes of irreversible dementias include parkinsonism-dementia complex of Guam, Jakob-Creutzfeldt disease, herpes simplex encephalitis, and multiple sclerosis. Numerous hereditary metabolic diseases are associated with irreversible dementia including Wilson's disease (hepatolenticular degeneration), metachromatic leukodystrophy, the adrenoleukodystrophies, and the neuronal storage diseases (e.g., Tay-Sachs).

Clinical Management

There are currently no drugs available that reverse the cognitive loss in Alzheimer's or other degenerative dementias. Medications are primarily useful for symptomatic treatment of associated depression, psychosis, agitation, aggressive behavior, or sleep disorders. In some cases, antipsychotics are required to allow the patient to remain within his or her family or social situation. The physician must find the lowest effective dose, a difficult task because these patients may not be able to tolerate side effects and may develop rigidity, akinesia, or tremors at relatively low doses. For long-term management of behavior problems, other medications may be useful, including propranolol, lithium carbonate, or carbamazepine. Case reports suggest that trazodone and buspirone may also have a limited role in the management of disturbed behavior.

The behavioral goals of treatment should be maintenance of the patient's socialization and provision of support for the family. Reality orientation may be worthwhile; reminiscence group therapy may be useful in maintaining socialization in selected patients. Even severely affected patients can react to familiar social activities and music. Self-help groups for family members provide educational and psychological support. Day care centers may provide needed relief for caregivers. A useful manual is *The 36-Hour Day* (Mace and Rabins 1981).

Recommendations for management of dementia
---

1. Both at home and in care facilities, patients usually respond better to low-stimulus environments than to high-stimulus situations.

   - Demented patients have difficulty interpreting sensory input and easily become overwhelmed.

2. Consistency and routine are important for reducing confusion and agitation.

3. Families are often overwhelmed by caring for a cognitively impaired relative.

   - Recommend that family members attend support groups, available in most communities.
   - Provide appropriate reading material.

4. Families should be given psychological support if the dementia patient requires institutionalization, to lessen the guilt they almost inevitably feel.

5. No medication has proven value for reversing or slowing the dementing process. Nonetheless, accompanying depression generally responds to antidepressants, and acute agitation or psychosis may respond to low-dose antipsychotics.

   - Avoid low-potency antipsychotics because of their anticholinergic side effects.
   - For long-term behavior management, lithium carbonate, propranolol, carbamazepine, and other agents have been tried, but benefit is inconsistent.

Treatable Forms of Dementia

Vascular disorders. *Multi-infarct dementia* is the second most common cause of dementia, accounting for 10% of cases. Its differentiation from the degenerative dementias includes its history of rapid onset and a stepwise deterioration occurring in patients in their 50s or 60s. This deterioration may be accompanied by focal neurologic impairment. The dementia is generally caused by multiple thromboembolic episodes occurring in persons with atherosclerotic disease of major vessels or heart valves. Patients with this disease commonly have high blood pressure or diabetes. There is generally a history of several strokes in the past, many of these "silent." Atherosclerosis in major arteries may be surgically correctable, but as atherosclerosis occurs diffusely among smaller intracranial vessels, it is not amenable to any specific intervention. In most cases, however, hypertension can be controlled, and early treatment of asymptomatic patients can help prevent or arrest the development of a multi-infarct dementia. Patients who have had or are at risk for stroke may benefit from the administration of anticoagulants or aspirin, which may prevent thrombus formation.

Subdural hematoma may produce a dementia itself or may complicate and add to the effects of other forms of dementia. Subdural hematomas are caused by a disruption of the veins that bridge the brain parenchyma and the meninges and are usually attributable to trauma. Predisposing causes for subdural hematoma include age over 60 years, alcoholism, epilepsy, and renal dialysis. The disorder is treated by evacuation of the hematoma through a burr hole in the skull.

Normal pressure hydrocephalus. This disorder is caused by excessive accumulation of cerebrospinal fluid (CSF), which gradually dilates the ventricles of the brain in the presence of normal CSF pressure. The flow of CSF from the ventricles to its usual site of absorption becomes obstructed so that fluid collects within the ventricles, resulting in the characteristic syndrome of dementia, gait disturbance, and urinary incontinence. Normal pressure hydrocephalus is generally idiopathic or the result of cerebral trauma.

Infections. Any infection that involves the brain is capable of producing a dementing illness. Many cases of dementia are prevented by the effective treatment of meningitis and encephalitis, whether caused by bacteria, fungi, protozoa, or viruses. Chronic infectious processes, e.g., those caused by bacteria (Whipple's disease), protozoa (syphilis), or fungi (cryptococcus), may affect the brain in such a way that the process is reversible and can be arrested, at least to some degree. Agents responsible for conditions such as Jakob-Creutzfeldt disease and progressive multifocal leukoencephalopathy (slow viruses) are resistant to any kind of treatment. Postinfectious encephalomyelitis, such as that occurring after a viral exanthem, may produce enough damage to leave the patient demented.

Dementia has also been attributed to acquired immunodeficiency syndrome (AIDS). The dementia may be caused by direct HIV infection of the nervous system, from intracranial tumors and infections (e.g., toxoplasmosis, cryptococcus), or from the indirect effects of systemic disease (e.g., septicemia, hypoxia, electrolyte imbalance). Because dementia may occur in the early stages of HIV infection, evaluation for HIV seropositivity is indicated for persons at high risk for infection (e.g., male homosexuals, drug addicts) who develop intellectual, mood, or behavior changes. For a more complete discussion of the psychiatric aspects of AIDS, see Chapter 21.

Metabolic disorders. Chronic diseases of the thyroid, parathyroid, adrenal, and pituitary glands can cause reversible dementias and are usually easily identified. Pulmonary diseases can produce dementia from hypoxia or hypercapnia. Chronic or acute renal failure may each cause a reversible dementia, as can liver failure (i.e., hepatic encephalopathy). Dementia is common in diabetic patients, particularly from hypoglycemic or hyperosmolar coma.

Nutritional disorders. Thiamine deficiency may lead to Wernicke-Korsakoff syndrome and Korsakoff's psychosis, an amnestic disorder. Both disorders are discussed later in this chapter. There are different mechanisms by which pernicious anemia can produce dementia, not all reversible. Folate deficiency is potentially reversible if recognized early. Pellagra (niacin deficiency), a major problem in underdeveloped countries, shows a dramatic response to niacin, even when mental changes have been present for a long time.

Treatable causes of dementia are summarized in Table 6-7.

Table 6-7. Treatable causes of dementia

Vascular
   Multiple infarcts
   Subacute bacterial endocarditis
   Decreased cardiac output
   Myocardial infarction, heart failure
   Collagen vascular diseases (e.g., lupus, polyarteritis)

Metabolic and endocrine
   Hypothyroidism
   Hyperparathyroidism
   Pituitary insufficiency
   Repeated hypoglycemia
   Respiratory acidosis
   Uremia
   Hepatic encephalopathy
   Porphyria
   Wilson's disease

Nutrition
   Pernicious anemia
   Alcoholism and thiamine deficiency
   Pellagra

Toxicity
   Bromides
   Mercury
   Others

Infections
   General paresis
   Cryptococcal meningitis
   Encephalitis
   Sarcoid
   Postinfectious encephalomyelitis

Mass effect
   Lymphoma and leukemia (with or without pathologic change)
   Intracranial tumor (e.g., subfrontal meningioma)
   Subdural hematoma

Subclinical seizures

Demyelinating disease

Normal pressure hydrocephalus

Specific Organic Syndromes

DSM-III-R defines six specific organically induced syndromes, highlighting their prominent symptoms: organic mood syndrome, organic delusional syndrome, amnestic syndrome, organic hallucinosis, organic anxiety syndrome, and organic personality syndrome. Cognitive or intellectual impairment is usually not prominent in these disorders. A residual category [organic mental syndrome not otherwise specified] has been created for patients presenting with a mixture of symptoms suggesting more than one of the organic syndromes. A person with prominent mood disturbance and gross intellectual impairment, for example, may be appropriate for this category.

Organic Mood Syndrome

Organic mood syndrome is characterized by depression, mania, or mixed mania and depression. The mood disturbance, according to DSM-III-R, must be accompanied by at least two neurovegetative symptoms such as insomnia, weight loss, or psychomotor agitation. Depression is a more common organically induced symptom than mania, although the latter has been attributed to such causes as head trauma, physical illness, or medication (e.g., azidothymidine [AZT] in AIDS patients). Typical patients with organic mood syndrome tend to be older and less likely to have a family history of mood disturbance. We recently saw the following patient at our hospital.

> Renee, a 29-year-old woman, was transferred for evaluation of depression and suicidal ideations. Although Renee had a long history of seclusiveness and undue social anxiety, she was otherwise psychiatrically well until 4 months before admission when she developed a depressive syndrome. One year earlier, she had been diagnosed with multiple sclerosis on the basis of slurred speech, gait ataxia, and multiple sclerotic plaques visualized by MRI.
>
> At admission, Renee admitted to low mood, appetite loss, poor energy, and low self-esteem and had psychomotor retardation. Before admission, Renee had written a suicide note and had been found in her room with insecticide sprays that she had been planning to kill herself with.
>
> Renee was diagnosed as having an organic affective disorder and received eight bilateral electroconvulsive treatments after she failed to respond to antidepressants. Her mood normalized, but she remained odd and seclusive.

As many as one-third of patients who have suffered a cerebrovascular stroke will experience depression in the 6- to 12-month period after the event. Interestingly, left hemisphere strokes appear to result in more depression than right hemisphere or brain stem strokes. Within the left hemisphere, the closer the lesion to the frontal pole, the more likely it is to produce depression. It is possible that these depressions are due to direct structural and biochemical effects. These patients tend to respond to tricyclic antidepressants (e.g., nortriptyline).

Organic Delusional Syndrome

An organic delusional syndrome may also occur and typically is drug related. Ingestion of psychostimulants (e.g., cocaine or amphetamines) may cause a syndrome that may be indistinguishable from paranoid schizophrenia. It has been suggested that Adolf Hitler developed persecutory delusions and delusions of grandeur from psychostimulants, which he was known to abuse. Although an amphetamine psychosis is usually self-limited, in rare cases delusions may persist for months or years after chronic abuse of psychostimulants. Delusional syndromes have also been associated with traumatic, metabolic, infectious, and other causes. The psychosis associated with temporal lobe epilepsy is often chronic and may not develop until 15 years or more have elapsed after the onset of psychomotor seizures.

Amnestic Syndrome

The main feature of amnestic syndrome is inability to remember recent events. Patients with this disorder may be oriented and alert, but cannot remember what happened a few hours earlier. This disorder may be caused by trauma, tumor, infection, infarction, seizures, or drugs, but the most common cause is alcohol abuse (Korsakoff's syndrome).

This alcohol-induced amnesia is probably related to chronic thiamine deficiency. This syndrome may occur in association with Wernicke-Korsakoff syndrome, characterized by the triad of gait ataxia, nystagmus, and mental confusion. It requires emergency treatment with thiamine, but once reversed, patients may suffer a residual amnestic disorder (i.e., Korsakoff's syndrome). Korsakoff's syndrome may not improve despite abstinence from alcohol and maintenance on thiamine, but is reversible in up to 50% of patients. Autopsies of patients with this syndrome show hemorrhage and sclerosis of the hypothalamic mammillary bodies and nuclei of the thalamus and more diffuse lesions in the brain stem, the cerebellum, and the limbic system.

Organic Hallucinosis

Organic hallucinosis is characterized by organically induced hallucinations in an otherwise clear sensorium and may be caused by tumors, trauma, encephalitis, or temporal lobe epilepsy. Auditory hallucinations may occur in heavy alcohol abusers after a period of abstinence or drop in blood ethanol level (e.g., alcohol hallucinations). Tactile hallucinations are often found in drug intoxication states (e.g., "coke bugs").

Organic Anxiety Syndrome

Organic anxiety syndrome was introduced in DSM-III-R after it was recognized that many drugs and illnesses produce symptoms of anxiety or panic. Examples include hyperthyroidism and caffeinism.

Organic Personality Syndrome

Organic personality syndrome refers to behavior and attitudinal changes due to a known or presumed organic cause. Such changes may represent an exaggeration of premorbid personality characteristics. A remarkable example of organic personality disorder is that of Phineas Gage, whose case is discussed in Chapter 5. The case illustrates the *frontal lobe syndrome,* typically associated with impaired judgment, disinhibition, amotivation, and *Witzelsucht* (silly humor and punning), but no intellectual impairment. Before the injury that destroyed his frontal lobes, Gage was a sober, responsible family man, and afterward became a loud, obnoxious, and foul-mouthed man, and was unable to keep a job.

The diagnosis is often used to describe the personality profile of some patients with temporal lobe epilepsy. These patients are often described as being "viscous," which reflects their tendency to become fixated on philosophical concerns and talk endlessly, unaware that the listener may not share their enthusiasm. Patients may display hypergraphia, hyperreligiousity, and disturbed sexuality (e.g., hyper- or hyposexuality). Several historical figures appear to fit this description, including Dostoyevski and Rasputin. Aggressive behavior may also occur as an interictal phenomenon, but is rarely a manifestation of a seizure. Anticonvulsants, such as carbamazepine, have been used to treat these interictal changes in the belief that if the seizure disorder is better controlled, the personality changes will stabilize or reverse. Carbamazepine has also been used to reduce aggressive tendencies in these patients. Although case reports suggest benefit, controlled trials are still needed.

Bibliography

Barnes R, Veith R, Okimoto J, et al: Efficacy of antipsychotic medications in behaviorally disturbed dementia patients. Am J Psychiatry 139:1170–1174, 1982

Black DW: Subdural hematoma—a retrospective study of the 'great neurologic imitator.' Postgrad Med 78:107–114, 1985

Black DW, Warrack G, Winokur G: The Iowa Record-Linkage Study, II: excess mortality in organic mental disorders. Arch Gen Psychiatry 42:78–81, 1985

Caine ED, Shoulson I: Psychiatric syndromes in Huntington's disease. Am J Psychiatry 140:728–733, 1983

Clarfield AM: The reversible dementias: do they reverse? Ann Intern Med 109:476–486, 1988

Consensus Conference: Differential diagnosis of dementing diseases. JAMA 258:3411–3416, 1987

Davison K: Schizophrenia-like psychoses associated with organic cerebral disorders: a review. Psychiatr Dev 1:1–34, 1983

Drevets WC, Rubin EH: Psychotic symptoms and the longitudinal course of senile dementia of the Alzheimer type. Biol Psychiatry 25:35–48, 1989

Dubin WR, Weis KJ, Zeccardi JA: Organic brain syndrome—the psychiatric impostor. JAMA 249:60–62, 1983

Flor-Henry P: Psychosis and temporal lobe epilepsy. Epilepsia 10:363–369, 1969

Francis J, Martin D, Kapoor WN: A prospective study of delirium in hospitalized elderly. JAMA 263:1097–1101, 1990

Golinger RC, Peet T, Tune LE: Association of elevated plasma anticholinergic activity with delirium in surgical patients. Am J Psychiatry 144:1218–1220, 1987

Greendyke RM, Kanter DR, Schuster DB, et al: Propranolol treatment of assaultive patients with organic brain disease—double-blind cross over, placebo controlled study. J Nerv Ment Dis 174:290–294, 1986

Heston LL, White JA, Mastri AR: Pick's disease—clinical genetics and natural history. Arch Gen Psychiatry 44:409–411, 1987

Katzman R: Alzheimer's disease. N Engl J Med 314:964–973, 1986

Levine AM: Case report: buspirone and agitation in head injury. Brain Injury 2:165–167, 1988

Lipsey JR, Robinson RG, Pearlson GD, et al: Nortriptyline treatment of post-stroke depression: a double blind study. Lancet 1:297–300, 1984

Mace NL, Rabins PV: The 36-Hour Day. Baltimore, MD, Johns Hopkins University Press, 1981

Mayeux R, Stern Y, Williams JBW, et al: Clinical and biochemical features of depression in Parkinson's disease. Am J Psychiatry 143:756–759, 1986

McAllister TW: Overview: pseudodementia. Am J Psychiatry 140:528–533, 1983

Medalia A, Scheinberg IH: Psychopathology in patients with Wilson's disease. Am J Psychiatry 146:662–664, 1989

Meyer JS, Judd DW, Tawaklna T, et al: Improved cognition after control of risk factors for multi-infarct dementia. JAMA 256:2203–2209, 1986

Pinner C, Rich CL: Effects of trazodone on aggressive behavior in seven patients with organic mental disorders. Am J Psychiatry 145:1295–1296, 1988

Rabins PV, Folstein MF: Delirium and dementia: diagnostic criteria and fatality rates. Br J Psychiatry 140:149–153, 1982

Robinson RG, Kubose KL, Star LB, et al: Mood changes in stroke patients: relationship to lesion location. Compr Psychiatry 24:555–566, 1983

Simpson DM, Foster D: Improvement in organically disturbed behavior with trazodone treatment. J Clin Psychiatry 74:191–193, 1986

Summers WK, Majovski LV, Marsh GM, et al: Oral tetrahydroamino-acridine in the long-term treatment of senile dementia, Alzheimer type. N Engl J Med 315:1241–1245, 1986

Williams KH, Goldstein G: Cognitive and affective response to lithium in patients with organic brain syndrome. Am J Psychiatry 136:800–803, 1979

Zubenko GS, Huff FJ, Beyer J, et al: Familial risk of dementia associated with a biologic subtype of Alzheimer's disease. Arch Gen Psychiatry 45:889–893, 1988

Self-assessment Questions

1. What are the differences between delirium and dementia?
2. What does a workup for an organic mental disorder consist of?
3. Describe Alzheimer's disease. What are its histopathological findings?
4. What is the pathognomonic finding in Pick's disease?
5. What triad of symptoms cluster in normal pressure hydrocephalus?
6. List reversible and irreversible causes of dementia.
7. What is pseudodementia? What are its typical signs?
8. How are dementia patients clinically managed?
9. What are the six specific organic mental syndromes?
10. Describe the frontal lobe syndrome.

Chapter 7

Schizophrenia

The psychopathology of schizophrenia is one of the most intriguing since it permits a many sided insight into the workings of the diseased as well as the healthy psyche.

Eugen Bleuler

Schizophrenia is probably the most devastating illness that psychiatrists treat. An estimated 1% of the population suffers from schizophrenia, which claims its victims at a youthful age and prevents their full participation in society. Schizophrenia also creates an enormous economic burden, costing society over $73 billion annually in direct and indirect costs. Despite its emotional and economic costs, schizophrenia has yet to receive sufficient recognition as a major health concern or the necessary research support to investigate its causes, treatments, and prevention.

History

Schizophrenia and related disorders have been recognized in almost all cultures and described throughout much of recorded time. Modern history dates to Emil Kraepelin, who is credited with identifying schizophrenia. His original term for

This chapter is adapted with permission from Black DW, Yates WR, Andreasen NC: Schizophrenia, schizophreniform disorder, and delusional (paranoid) disorders, in The American Psychiatric Press Textbook of Psychiatry. Edited by Talbott JA, Hales RE, Yudofsky SC. Washington, DC, American Psychiatric Press, 1988, pp 357–402. Copyright 1988 American Psychiatric Press, Inc.

schizophrenia, *dementia praecox,* was based on his observations that these patients developed their illness at a relatively early age and were likely to have a chronic and deteriorating course. Kraepelin was also instrumental in separating dementia praecox from manic-depressive illness, which had its onset distributed throughout life and a more episodic course. Dementia praecox was eventually renamed *schizophrenia,* a term coined by Bleuler to emphasize the cognitive impairment that occurs, which he conceptualized as a "splitting" of the psychic processes.

Bleuler believed that certain symptoms were fundamental to the illness, including affective blunting, disturbance of association (i.e., peculiar and distorted thinking), autism, and indecisiveness (ambivalence). Other symptoms such as delusions and hallucinations were regarded by him to be accessory because they could occur in other disorders, including manic-depressive illness. Bleuler's ideas earned acceptance throughout the United States, and generations of psychiatrists were taught the importance of Bleulerian fundamental symptoms ("the four A's"). Unfortunately, because these psychologically based symptoms are imprecise, the conceptualization of schizophrenia in the United States became increasingly broad. Later, the ideas of German psychiatrist Kurt Schneider, who emphasized first-rank or specific psychotic symptoms, were introduced, helping to reshape the concept of schizophrenia into one of a relatively severe psychotic disorder, bringing it back to the original ideas of Kraepelin. DSM-III-R represents a convergence of various points of view, with its Kraepelinian emphasis on course, the emphasis of specific delusions and hallucinations thought important by Schneider, and acknowledgment of the importance of Bleulerian fundamental symptoms.

Definition

According to DSM-III-R, a diagnosis of schizophrenia requires 1) the presence of characteristic psychotic symptoms for at least a 1-week duration; 2) deterioration in social and occupational functioning and self-care; 3) the ruling out of a major mood syndrome, or if present, the mood syndrome is brief in duration relative to the duration of the schizophrenic disturbance; 4) continuous signs of the disturbance for at least 6 months; 5) ruling out of an organic mental disorder; and 6) if there is a history of autistic disorder, that prominent hallucinations and delusions are now present (see Table 7-1 for more detail on DSM-III-R criteria for schizophrenia).

If an illness otherwise meets the criteria, but has a duration of less than 6 months, it is termed *schizophreniform disorder.* If the duration is less than 4 weeks, it may be classified as either a *brief reactive psychosis,* if there is evidence of obvious stress and emotional turmoil, or a *psychotic disorder not otherwise specified,* which is a residual category for psychotic disturbances that do not meet criteria for specific disorders.

Clinical Findings

Clinical findings in schizophrenia are protean and can change over time. Because of the variety of its manifestations, it has been said that to know schizophrenia is to

Table 7-1. DSM-III-R criteria for schizophrenia

A. Presence of characteristic psychotic symptoms in the active phase: either (1), (2), or (3) for at least 1 week (unless symptoms are successfully treated):

   1. Two of the following:

      a. Delusions

      b. Prominent hallucinations (throughout the day for several days or several times a week for several weeks, each hallucinatory experience not being limited to a few brief moments)

      c. Incoherence or marked loosening of associations

      d. Catatonic behavior

      e. Flat or grossly inappropriate affect

   2. Bizarre delusions (i.e., involving a phenomenon that the person's culture would regard as totally implausible, e.g., thought broadcasting, being controlled by a dead person)

   3. Prominent hallucinations (as defined in 1b above) of a voice with content having no apparent relation to depression or elation, or a voice keeping up a running commentary on the person's behavior or thoughts or two or more voices conversing with each other

B. During the course of the disturbance, functioning in such areas as work, social relations, and self-care is markedly below the highest level achieved before onset of the disturbance (or, when the onset is in childhood or adolescence, failure to achieve expected level of social development).

C. Schizoaffective disorder and mood disorder with psychotic features have been ruled out; i.e., if a major depressive or manic syndrome has ever been present during an active phase of the disturbance, the total duration of all episodes of a mood syndrome has been brief relative to the total duration of the active and residual phases of the disturbance.

D. Continuous signs of the disturbance for at least 6 months. The 6-month period must include an active phase (of at least 1 week, or less if symptoms have been successfully treated) during which there were psychotic symptoms characteristic of schizophrenia (symptoms in A), with or without a prodromal or residual phase, as defined below.

Prodromal phase: A clear deterioration in functioning before the active phase of the disturbance that is not due to a disturbance in mood or to a psychoactive substance use disorder and that involves at least two of the symptoms listed below.

Residual phase: Following the active phase of the disturbance, persistence of at least two of the symptoms noted below, those not being due to a disturbance in mood or to a psychoactive substance use disorder.

Prodromal or residual symptoms:

1. Marked social isolation or withdrawal
2. Marked impairment in role functioning as wage earner, student, or homemaker
3. Marked peculiar behavior (e.g., collecting garbage, talking to self in public, hoarding food)
4. Marked impairment in personal hygiene and grooming
5. Blunted or inappropriate affect
6. Digressive, vague, overelaborate, or circumstantial speech, or poverty of speech, or poverty of content of speech
7. Odd beliefs or magical thinking, influencing behavior and inconsistent with cultural norms, e.g., superstitiousness, belief in clairvoyance, telepathy, "sixth sense," "others can feel my feelings," overvalued ideas, ideas of reference
8. Unusual perceptual experiences, e.g., recurrent illusions, sensing the presence of a force or person not actually present
9. Marked lack of initiative, interests, or energy

   Examples: Six months of prodromal symptoms with 1 week of symptoms from A; no prodromal symptoms with 6 months of symptoms from A; no prodromal symptoms with 1 week of symptoms from A and 6 months of residual symptoms.

(continues)

Table 7-1.   DSM-III-R criteria for schizophrenia—*Continued*

E. It cannot be established that an organic factor initiated and maintained the disturbance.

F. If there is a history of autistic disorder, the additional diagnosis of schizophrenia is made only if prominent delusions or hallucinations are also present.

Classification of course. The course of the disturbance is coded in the fifth digit:

1—Subchronic. The time from the beginning of the disturbance, when the person first began to show signs of the disturbance (including prodromal, active, and residual phases) more or less continuously, is less than 2 years, but at least 6 months.
2—Chronic. Same as above, but more than 2 years.
3—Subchronic with acute exacerbation. Reemergence of prominent psychotic symptoms in a person with a subchronic course who has been in the residual phase of the disturbance.
4—Chronic with acute exacerbation. Reemergence of prominent psychotic symptoms in a person with a chronic course who has been in the residual phase of the disturbance.
5—In remission. When a person with a history of schizophrenia is free of all signs of the disturbance (whether or not on medication), "in remission" should be coded. Differentiating schizophrenia in remission from no mental disorder requires consideration of overall level of functioning, length of time since the last episode of disturbance, total duration of the disturbance, and whether prophylactic treatment is being given.
0—Unspecified.

know psychiatry. There are no pathognomonic symptoms specific to schizophrenia, but *hallucinations* have always been considered its hallmark. The hallucinations are perceptions experienced without an external stimulus to the sense organs and with a quality similar to a true perception. Schizophrenic patients can have auditory, visual, tactile, gustatory, olfactory, or a combination of these hallucinations, although auditory hallucinations are the most frequent. The hallucinations are commonly experienced as noises, music, or, more typically, "voices." The voices may be mumbled or heard clearly and they may speak words, phrases, or sentences. Visual hallucinations may be simple or complex. Olfactory and gustatory hallucinations are often experienced together, especially as unpleasant tastes or odors. Tactile hallucinations may be experienced as sensations of being touched or pricked, electrical sensations, or sensation of insects crawling under the skin (formication).

Delusions involve disturbance in thought rather than perception. Delusions are firmly held beliefs that are untrue as well as contrary to a person's educational and cultural background. Delusions occurring in schizophrenic patients may have somatic, grandiose, religious, nihilistic, or persecutory themes (Table 7-2). The type and frequency of delusions tend to differ according to culture. For example, in the Soviet Union, a patient may have delusions of being watched by the KGB; in the United States, a patient might worry about being spied on by the FBI or CIA. Certain types of hallucinations and delusions were considered "first rank" by Schneider, including clearly audible voices commenting on a person's actions, or arguing with each other about a patient or repeating aloud the patient's thoughts. Schneiderian delusions include themes of thought broadcasting, thought withdrawal, thought insertion, or being controlled (passivity). These symptoms are likely to occur in schizophrenic patients, but may also occur in affective disorder or organic states.

Formal thought disorder (disorganized speech) is also common in schizophrenic

Table 7-2. Varied content in delusions

Delusions	Foci of preoccupation
Grandiose	Possessing wealth, great beauty, or having a special ability (e.g., extrasensory perception); having influential friends; being an important figure (e.g., Napoleon, Hitler)
Nihilistic	Belief that one is dead or dying; belief that one does not exist or that the world does not exist
Persecutory	Being persecuted by friends, neighbors, or spouses; being followed or monitored or spied on by the government (e.g., FBI, CIA) or other important organizations (e.g., the Catholic church)
Somatic	Belief that one's organs have stopped functioning (e.g., that the heart is no longer beating) or are rotting away; belief that the nose or other body part is terribly misshapen or disfigured
Sexual	Belief that one's sexual behavior is commonly known; that one is a prostitute, pedophile, or rapist; that masturbation has led to illness or insanity
Religious	Belief that one has sinned against God; that one has a special relationship to God, or some other deity; that one has a special religious mission; that one is the Devil or is condemned to burn in Hell

patients, but is not specific to the illness. Positive types of thought disorder include marked incoherence, derailment, tangentiality, or illogicality, whereas negative thought disorder includes poverty of speech and poverty of content of speech.

A common symptom in schizophrenia is *lack of insight*. Patients generally do not believe that they are ill or abnormal in any way. The hallucinations and delusions are real to them and not imagined. Poor insight is one of the most difficult symptoms to treat, and it may persist even when other symptoms (e.g., hallucinations, delusions) respond to treatment.

Many schizophrenic patients develop diminished volition, various motor disturbances, and changes in social behavior. Abnormal behaviors range from catatonic stupor to excitement. In *catatonic stupor*, the patient may be immobile, mute, and unresponsive, and yet fully conscious. In *catatonic excitement*, the patient may exhibit uncontrolled and aimless motor activity. Patients may assume bizarre or uncomfortable postures, such as squatting, and maintain them for long periods. Patients may exhibit a *stereotypy*, which is a repeated, but non-goal-directed movement, such as rocking. They may also display mannerisms that are normal goal-directed activities, but are either odd in appearance or out of context, such as grimacing. Other common symptoms are *echopraxia*—imitating the movements and gestures of another person, *automatic obedience*—carrying out simple commands in a robotlike fashion, and *negativism*—refusing to cooperate with simple requests for no apparent reason.

Deterioration of social behavior often occurs along with social withdrawal. Patients may neglect themselves and become messy or unkempt and wear dirty or inappropriate clothing. Patients may ignore their surroundings so that they become cluttered and untidy. Patients may develop other odd behaviors that break social conventions, such as masturbating in public, foraging through garbage bins, or shouting obscenities. Many of today's "street people" are schizophrenic.

Schizophrenic patients often develop a reduced intensity of emotional response that leaves them indifferent and apathetic. *Anhedonia,* or the inability to experience pleasure, is also common. Expression of affect may be inappropriate, such as giggling over a relative's death, and is especially common in the disorganized subtype of schizophrenia. A full-blown depression may develop in up to 60% of schizophrenic patients. Depression is often difficult to diagnose because of the large overlap of symptoms between schizophrenia and depression. Antipsychotics may also cause what may appear to be a depression, but is actually a drug-induced akinesia. According to DSM-III-R, in well-established schizophrenia, the depression is diagnosed as depressive disorder not otherwise specified.

The following case example illustrates many of the symptoms found in schizophrenia.

Jane, a 55-year-old woman, was admitted to the hospital for evaluation after her landlord became concerned by her agitation. A former schoolteacher, Jane had lived in a series of rooming houses and had held only temporary jobs in the past 10 years. She was socially isolated and interacted with others only at her church.

Jane was born with a cleft palate that was surgically corrected at age 4 years. She was teased unmercifully as a child due to her appearance, despite good cosmetic results from the surgery. She was shy and socially awkward and had few friends, but was an avid reader and model student. Jane had little interest in boys, never dated, and after graduating from high school, briefly joined a convent. She eventually obtained her teaching certificate after graduating from college and lived with her mother. She was briefly hospitalized at age 25 after developing the belief that her neighbors were harassing her. Over the next 20 years, her beliefs evolved into a complex delusional system. She believed that she was at the center of a government cabal to change her identity. The FBI, the judicial system, the Roman Catholic Church, hospital personnel, and, it seems, most of her neighbors were believed to be involved in the plot. Neighbors, she believed, were recruited to spy on her, harass her, and generally make her life miserable. She would often overhear them plotting to assault or rape her.

As a result of her beliefs, Jane changed her residence about every 6 months. Unfortunately, she discovered that wherever she went, her new neighbors were also part of the plot to harass her. Still, she continued working, but was gradually relegated to substitute teaching positions until these opportunities eventually dried up. A doctor had suggested that she obtain disability benefits from the government, but because she denied having any mental illness, she refused to apply. She would obtain any temporary position that she could and, at admission, had been working several weeks in telemarketing schemes.

At age 49, Jane was briefly hospitalized after pounding on her ceiling and walls with a broom and yelling, in an attempt to stop her neighbors from harassing her. Reasons for her present hospitalization were similar. Although her landlord had complained of her yelling and screaming, Jane reported that she was simply responding to the discomfort her landlord and neighbors had caused by "zapping" her with electronic beams in an effort to harass her. She believed that electromagnetic waves were being used to control her actions and thoughts and described a bizarre sensation of electricity moving around her body when the landlord was near.

At the hospital, Jane wore simple clothing, but was always neatly groomed and dressed. She cooperated well with her physicians, had no evidence of depressed mood, but was clearly upset about her hospitalization, which she felt was unnecessary and inappropriate. Her speech was markedly circumstantial, but she spoke in a clear, strong voice that one might expect after years of teaching. She cooperated with her treatment plans. After 1 month of antipsychotic therapy, she remained delusional, but was no longer as concerned about her perceived harassment. Due to Jane's poor insight and history of medication noncompliance, she was placed on an intramuscular antipsychotic before discharge.

Many clinicians have found it useful to describe typical schizophrenic symptoms as either positive or negative. *Positive symptoms* include hallucinations, delusions, marked positive formal thought disorder (manifested by marked incoherence, derailment, tangentiality, or illogicality), and bizarre or disorganized behavior. *Negative symptoms* include alogia (e.g., marked poverty of speech or poverty of content of speech), affective flattening, anhedonia-asociality (e.g., inability to experience pleasure, few social contacts), avolition-apathy (e.g., anergia, lack of persistence at work or school), and attentional impairment. The frequency of these common symptoms in 111 schizophrenic patients is presented in Table 7-3. The subdivision resembles Bleuler's original distinction between fundamental and accessory symptoms. One of the authors (N.C.A.) has developed the Scale for the Assessment of Positive Symptoms (SAPS) and the Scale for the Assessment of Negative Symptoms (SANS) to evaluate these symptoms. These scales are included in the Appendix.

Schizophrenic patients often develop physical symptoms as well. Up to 75% have neurologic soft signs, such as abnormalities in stereognosis, graphesthesia, balance, and proprioception. Ocular abnormalities including both the absence and avoidance of eye contact and staring for long periods occur. Decreased or rapid blink rates and bouts of rapid blinking may occur. Smooth pursuit eye movement is often abnormal in schizophrenic patients and in their relatives. Some patients display vegetative symptoms that may involve disturbances of sleep, sexual interest, and bodily function. There is evidence of a reduction in stage 4 sleep. Many schizophrenic patients have inactive sex drives, and some develop chronic constipation. These symptoms may be caused by antipsychotics, but they were commonly described before antipsychotics became available.

As a group, chronic schizophrenic patients have odd personalities before the onset of their illness. A study of 52 chronic schizophrenic patients found that 35% had a DSM-III personality disorder premorbidly; 44% of these personality disorders were schizoid and the rest a mix of avoidant, paranoid, histrionic, compulsive, or other personality disorders.

Kraepelin believed that most schizophrenic patients became more cognitively impaired with time. Schizophrenic patients tend to have lower premorbid IQs than siblings and peers of similar social class origins, but IQ does not characteristically decline premorbidly or after the onset of schizophrenia. It is likely that observed changes in IQ are related to a patient's symptoms, which may affect test performance.

Table 7-3. Frequency of symptoms in 111 schizophrenic patients

Symptom	%	Symptom	%
NEGATIVE SYMPTOMS		**POSITIVE SYMPTOMS**	
● **Affective flattening**		● **Hallucinations**	
Unchanging facial expression	96	Auditory	75
Decreased spontaneous movements	66	Voices commenting	58
Paucity of expressive gestures	81	Voices conversing	57
Poor eye contact	71	Somatic-tactile	20
Affective nonresponsivity	64	Olfactory	6
Inappropriate affect	63	Visual	49
Lack of vocal inflections	73		
		● **Delusions**	
● **Alogia**		Persecutory	81
Poverty of speech	53	Jealous	4
Poverty of content of speech	51	Guilt, sin	26
Blocking	23	Grandiose	39
Increased response latency	31	Religious	31
		Somatic	28
		Delusions of reference	49
● **Avolition-apathy**		Delusions of being controlled	46
Impaired grooming and hygiene	87	Delusions of mind reading	48
Lack of persistence at work or school	95	Thought broadcasting	23
Physical anergia	82	Thought insertion	31
		Thought withdrawal	27
● **Anhedonia-asociality**			
Few recreational interests/activities	95	● **Bizarre behavior**	
Little sexual interest/activity	69	Clothing, appearance	20
Impaired intimacy/closeness	84	Social, sexual behavior	33
Few relationships with friends/peers	96	Aggressive-agitated	27
		Repetitive-stereotyped	28
● **Attention**			
Social inattentiveness	78	● **Positive formal thought disorder**	
Inattentiveness during testing	64	Derailment	45
		Tangentiality	50
		Incoherence	23
		Illogicality	23
		Circumstantiality	35
		Pressure of speech	24
		Distractible speech	23
		Clanging	3

Source. Adapted from Andreasen NC: The diagnosis of schizophrenia. Schizophr Bull 13:9–22, 1987.

Subtypes of Schizophrenia

DSM-III-R recognizes five subtypes of schizophrenia: paranoid, disorganized, catatonic, undifferentiated, and residual (Table 7-4). Their usefulness is primarily descriptive, for their reliability and validity are not established. As symptoms may

Table 7-4. DSM-III-R subtypes of schizophrenia

Paranoid	Undifferentiated
Disorganized (hebephrenic)	Residual
Catatonic	

vary over time, a patient may seem to fit several of these subtypes during the course of the illness.

The *paranoid* subtype involves preoccupation with one or more systematized delusions or frequently auditory hallucinations related to a single theme in the absence of formal thought disorder, flat or inappropriate affect, or bizarre behavior. Paranoid patients tend to have an older age at onset and are likely to be married, have children, and be employed.

Disorganized (hebephrenic) schizophrenic patients exhibit incoherence, marked loosening of associations, or grossly disorganized behavior. They also display flat or grossly inappropriate affect. The onset of this subtype occurs at an early age, with the development of nonparanoid symptoms such as avolition, flat affect, deterioration of habits, and cognitive impairment. These patients often seem silly and childlike and occasionally grimace, giggle inappropriately, and appear self-absorbed, often staring at themselves in mirrors.

Catatonic schizophrenia is a subtype dominated by stupor or mutism, negativism, rigidity, purposeless excitement, and bizarre posturing. This subtype of schizophrenia is reported to be less common than in the past, possibly a benefit of the modern treatment era.

The *undifferentiated* subtype of schizophrenia is a residual category for patients meeting criteria for schizophrenia but not criteria for the paranoid, disorganized, or catatonic subtypes.

Residual schizophrenia, as described in DSM-III-R, is a diagnosis for patients who no longer have prominent psychotic symptoms, but who once met criteria for schizophrenia and have continuing evidence of illness such as blunted affect or eccentric behavior.

Epidemiology

The prevalence of schizophrenia has been estimated at between 0.5 and 1%. In the Epidemiologic Catchment Area study in the United States, however, a lifetime prevalence for schizophrenia was found to range from 1 to 1.9%. This study found a preponderance of schizophrenia in women and persons aged 18–44 years. If these recent data are correct, there are between 2.4 and 4.6 million persons in the United States with schizophrenia. Prevalence rates are similar among different countries, but pockets of high prevalence have been reported in areas of Yugoslavia, Sweden, and Ireland, among Canadian Catholics, and among the Tamils in southern India. Low prevalence rates have been reported among the American Old Order Amish, Aboriginal tribes in Taiwan, and natives in Ghana. Blacks in the United States have traditionally had higher rates of schizophrenia, but this finding may be due to racial bias.

People can develop schizophrenia at any age, but the mean age at the first psychotic episode is 21.4 years for men and 26.8 years for women. Of persons with schizophrenia, 9 of 10 men, but only 2 of 3 women develop the illness by age 30. Age at onset is probably under both genetic and environmental control, but it is unknown why women develop the illness later than men. Patients with schizophrenia tend not to marry and are less likely to have children than persons in the general population. These facts are probably due to the illness itself, which impairs motivation, creates social isolation, and is associated with low sex drive. Schizophrenic patients also tend to be concentrated in low social classes, a finding most likely due to the "downward" drift resulting from impaired social and occupational functioning.

Schizophrenic patients have high suicide rates, and about 10% of schizophrenic patients will eventually commit suicide. Risk factors for suicide in schizophrenic patients include male gender, age under 30 years, unemployment, chronic course, prior depression, past treatment for a depression, and recent hospital discharge. Risk of homicide and other violent crimes is probably the same for schizophrenic patients as for the general population, despite unfortunate media depictions of mental illness.

Etiology and Pathophysiology

Hypotheses about the etiology and pathophysiology of schizophrenia can be grouped into genetic, environmental, and neurobiological causes.

Genetics

Evidence for a genetic contribution to schizophrenia is based on family studies, twin studies, and studies of adoptees. Summaries of individual family studies have shown siblings of schizophrenic patients to have about a 10% chance of developing schizophrenia, whereas children who have one parent with schizophrenia have a 5–6% chance. The risk of family members developing schizophrenia increases markedly when two or more family members have the illness. The risk of developing schizophrenia is 17% for persons with one sibling and one parent with schizophrenia and 46% for the children of two schizophrenic parents. Twin studies have been remarkably consistent in demonstrating high concordance rates for monozygotic twins averaging 46%, compared to 14% concordance in dizygotic twins. Adoption studies show that risk for schizophrenia is greater in the biological relatives of index adoptees who had schizophrenia than in the biological relatives of mentally healthy control adoptees.

Studies are now underway to find the schizophrenia "gene" with molecular genetic techniques (see Chapter 5 for a description of these techniques). A preliminary report suggested that the gene may lie on chromosome 5, although this finding has not been replicated. Many experts believe that because schizophrenia is heterogeneous, its etiology must be multifactorial, so that single-gene transmission would, at best, explain only a small fraction of the total cases. Like mental retardation, multiple mechanisms may lead to a similar clinical picture (i.e., phenotype), so that no single cause for schizophrenia is likely to emerge. In fact, polygenic models of the inheritance of schizophrenia tend to appear more consistent with published family and twin data than single-gene models.

Environmental Influences

Environmental hypotheses are divided into familial and extrafamilial (or physical) causes. Early theorists believed that bad parenting could lead to schizophrenia. Fromm-Reichmann wrote of the "schizophrenogenic mother," and Bateson warned of the "double-bind" situation, in which schizophrenic patients were thought to be subjected to ambiguous or confusing messages by their parents. Although these theories have been abandoned, they have led to more sophisticated family research on "expressed emotion." In a family environment, frequent and intense expression of emotion by relatives may occur. Although expressed emotion does not cause schizophrenia, it can lead to worsening of symptoms (e.g., agitation, hallucinations).

Extrafamilial (or physical) causes have also been thought to predispose to the development of schizophrenia. Schizophrenic patients are more likely than non-schizophrenic control subjects to have a history of birth injury and perinatal complications, which could result in a subtle brain injury setting the stage for the development of schizophrenia. Several investigators have hypothesized that schizophrenia may be the result of viral illness and cite birth seasonality as evidence. More schizophrenic individuals are born in the winter than in any other season. This suggests that as fetuses or neonates, many schizophrenic individuals may have suffered central nervous system damage due to an infection.

Neurobiology

Schizophrenia is widely believed to have a neurobiological basis. The most popular pathophysiologic explanation for schizophrenia is the *dopamine hypothesis,* which suggests that the symptoms of schizophrenia are due primarily to hyperactivity in the dopamine system. Evidence supporting this hypothesis includes the effectiveness of the antipsychotic medications, which block postsynaptic dopamine receptors, and the exacerbation of the symptoms of schizophrenia by stimulant drugs, such as amphetamine, which enhance dopamine transmission. Direct support for this hypothesis has been provided by postmortem brain studies and positron-emission tomography (PET). Other neurotransmitter systems may be involved in the neurochemistry of schizophrenia, including norepinephrine, serotonin, and gamma-aminobutyric acid (GABA), but these systems have been much less actively studied.

Neuroanatomic studies, some of which are reviewed in Chapter 5, have confirmed the presence of structural brain abnormalities in schizophrenia including ventricular enlargement, sulcal enlargement, and cerebellar atrophy. These abnormalities have not been explained on the basis of treatment with medication, length of illness, or treatment with electroconvulsive therapy (ECT). Some studies suggest that ventricular enlargement correlates with poor premorbid functioning, poor response to treatment, and cognitive impairment. Regional blood-flow studies have suggested that schizophrenic patients have a relative hypofrontality, whereas PET studies have shown decreased glucose utilization in the frontal lobes. These studies suggest that schizophrenia may be a frontal or temporolimbic disease.

Course and Outcome

Schizophrenia begins with a *prodromal phase* that precedes the active phase of the illness, usually by about 1 year. This phase consists of the gradual development of social withdrawal, peculiar behavior, deterioration in personal hygiene and grooming, and strange ideation. The prodrome is followed by an *active phase* in which psychotic symptoms, such as hallucinations and delusions, predominate. This phase is florid and alarming to friends and relatives and may result in medical intervention. A *residual phase* follows and is similar to the prodromal phase, although affective flattening and role impairment may be worse. Psychotic symptoms may persist during this phase, but may not be as troublesome to the patient. The residual phase may be interrupted by repeated recurrences of the active phase, or "acute exacerbations." The frequency and timing of these exacerbations is unpredictable, although stressful situations may precede these relapses. Relapses may be preceded by changes in thought, feeling, and behavior noticed by the patient and family members. There is a tendency for the symptoms of schizophrenia to change over time. Early in their illness, patients may show a preponderance of positive symptoms, but over time they may develop more negative or defect symptoms.

Studies of outcome in schizophrenia are difficult to compare directly, but according to a review of six outcome studies, 13% of patients had a good outcome, 42% had an intermediate outcome, and 45% had a bad outcome. Good outcome was defined as no hospital readmission during follow-up and bad outcome as continuous hospitalization during follow-up, or moderate to severe intellectual or social impairment. In one of the best-known outcome studies, the "Iowa 500" (Tsuang et al. 1979), 200 schizophrenic patients hospitalized in the 1930s and 1940s were followed up in the 1970s. Twenty percent of patients were psychiatrically well at follow-up, but 45% remained incapacitated. Twenty-one percent were married or widowed, but 67% had never married; 35% were economically productive but 58% had never worked. In general, this and other studies demonstrate that schizophrenia is a devastating illness that affects every aspect of the patient's life.

It is difficult to predict outcome in individual patients based on these studies. However, predictors of good outcome include acute onset, short duration of illness, lack of prior psychiatric history, presence of affective symptoms or confusion, good premorbid adjustment, steady work history, marriage, and older age at onset. Poor prognostic features include insidious onset, long duration of symptoms, history of psychiatric problems, affective blunting, obsessive-compulsive symptoms, assaultiveness, premorbid personality disorder, poor work history, celibacy, and young age at onset. Prognostic features in schizophrenia are summarized in Table 7-5.

Interestingly, schizophrenic patients are more likely to experience a good outcome now than 100 years ago, either because the illness has changed or because neuroleptic medication and other treatments have altered the natural history of the illness. Another possibility is that our definitions of good outcome have changed. For example, "good outcome" now may include patients living in care facilities or nursing homes who have minimal symptoms, but clearly are not well. For reasons that are not well understood, cross-cultural studies have shown that patients in

Table 7-5. Features associated with good and poor outcome in schizophrenia

Feature	Good outcome	Poor outcome
Onset	Acute	Insidious
Duration	Short	Chronic
Psychiatric history	Absent	Present
Affective symptoms	Present	Absent
Sensorium	Clouded	Clear
Obsessions/compulsions	Absent	Present
Assaultiveness	Absent	Present
Premorbid functioning	Good	Poor
Marital history	Married	Never married
Psychosexual functioning	Good	Poor
Neurological functioning	Normal	Soft signs present
Structural brain abnormalities	None	Present
Social class	High	Low
Family history of schizophrenia	Negative	Positive

less-developed countries tend to have better outcomes than those in more-developed countries. It may be that the schizophrenic person is better accepted in less-developed societies, has fewer external demands, and is more likely to be taken care of by family members. Women, in general, tend to have a better outcome than men in their response to medication and in long-term course.

Differential Diagnosis

Diagnosis of schizophrenia should be thought of as a diagnosis of exclusion because the consequences of the diagnosis are severe and limit therapeutic options. There are no definitive tests for schizophrenia, so the diagnosis rests on historical and clinical information. It is important that a thorough physical examination and history rule out organic causes for schizophrenic symptoms (see Table 7-6 for differential diagnosis). Atypical presentations should be carefully investigated.

Psychotic symptoms are found in many other illnesses including substance abuse (e.g., hallucinogens, phencyclidine (PCP), amphetamines, cocaine, alcohol), intoxication due to commonly prescribed medications (e.g., corticosteroids, anticholinergics, L-dopa), infections, metabolic and endocrine disorders, tumors and mass lesions, and temporal lobe epilepsy of many years duration.

Routine laboratory tests may be helpful in ruling out organic etiologies. Testing may include a complete blood count (CBC), urinalysis, liver enzymes, serum creatinine, blood urea nitrogen (BUN), thyroid function tests, and serologic tests for evidence of an infection with syphilis or human immunodeficiency virus (HIV). Computerized tomography or magnetic resonance imaging may be useful in selected patients to rule out alternative diagnoses, or during the initial workup for new-onset cases.

The major differential diagnosis involves separating schizophrenia from mood disorder, delusional disorder, or personality disorder. The chief distinction from mood

Table 7-6.   Differential diagnosis of schizophrenia

Psychiatric illness	Medical illness
Major depression	Temporal lobe epilepsy
Schizoaffective disorder	Tumor, stroke, brain trauma
Brief reactive psychosis	Endocrine/metabolic disorders (e.g., porphyria)
Schizophreniform disorder	
Delusional disorder	Vitamin deficiency (e.g., B$_{12}$)
Induced psychotic disorder	Infectious (e.g., neurosyphilis)
Panic disorder	Autoimmune (e.g., systemic lupus erythematosus)
Depersonalization disorder	
Obsessive-compulsive disorder	Toxic (e.g., heavy metal poisoning)
Personality disorders (e.g., "eccentric" cluster)	**Drugs**
	Stimulants (e.g., amphetamine, cocaine)
	Hallucinogens (e.g., phencyclidine [PCP])
	Anticholinergics (e.g., belladonna alkaloids)
	Alcohol withdrawal
	Barbiturate withdrawal

disorder is that in schizophrenia a full depressive or manic syndrome is either absent, develops after the psychotic symptoms, or is brief in duration relative to the duration of psychotic symptoms. Unlike delusional disorder, schizophrenia is characterized by bizarre delusions, and hallucinations are common. Patients with personality disorders, particularly those disorders within the "eccentric cluster" (e.g., schizoid, schizotypal, or paranoid), may be characterized by indifference to social relationships and restricted affect, bizarre ideation, or odd speech, but are not psychotic.

Clinical Management

The mainstay of treatment for schizophrenia is antipsychotic medication. All antipsychotics, with minor exceptions, have proved to be superior to placebo in the treatment of schizophrenia, reportedly due to their action to block postsynaptic dopamine receptors. None is demonstrated to be superior to another, so the choice of drug depends on the patient and his or her illness. An exception may be clozapine, which is reportedly effective in up to 30% of patients refractory to other antipsychotics. However, its high cost and potential for causing agranulocytosis will limit it usefulness. Attempts to correlate plasma concentration of antipsychotics and their metabolites with therapeutic response have been generally unsuccessful, although improvement may correlate with haloperidol plasma levels between 5 and 15 ng/ml.

The acutely psychotic or agitated schizophrenic patient requires rapid control of symptoms. A daily dosage of antipsychotic of about 800 mg of chlorpromazine (or its equivalent) will produce improvement in many patients within several days or weeks; higher dosages may increase the likelihood of adverse side effects and lower dosages may be ineffective.

Highly agitated patients who are out of control may need immediate pharmacologic control. In these situations, doses of high-potency antipsychotics should be repeated every 30–60 minutes intramuscularly or orally up to the equivalent of 30–60 mg of haloperidol over 6 hours. This dosing scheme is called *rapid neuroleptization*. It is likely that its effectiveness in subduing patients results from sedation, not specific antipsychotic effect. If sedation is the desired effect, a more rational approach to these patients is sedation with benzodiazepines acutely, simultaneously starting them on antipsychotics, remembering that it may take weeks for antipsychotic actions to take hold.

Patients benefiting from short-term treatment with antipsychotics are candidates for long-term prophylactic treatment, which has as its goal the sustained control of psychotic symptoms. Due to the potential of these medications to produce tardive dyskinesia, a potentially irreversible movement disorder, continuing benefit must be clearly established. Maintenance for 1 year is appropriate after an initial psychotic episode, usually at doses in the range of one-third to one-half of the original dose. After two such episodes, patients will probably benefit from longer prophylaxis (up to 5 years). Thirty to fifty percent of patients on maintenance neuroleptics ultimately relapse, but 70% relapse without medication. Of course, many patients relapse due to their noncompliance with their medication regimens.

Clinicians should periodically reassess whether the patient requires continued maintenance treatment. Because many patients develop more defect (negative) symptoms over time, they may have less need for antipsychotic medication, which tends to work most effectively in controlling positive symptoms. Further information about antipsychotics and their rational use is found in Chapter 24.

ECT is rarely useful in treating schizophrenia, unless a catatonic syndrome is present or the patient has developed a severe depression. Psychosurgery has no role in the treatment of schizophrenia. Other physical treatments including insulin coma therapy and hemodialysis have been abandoned due to ineffectiveness.

Adjunctive psychotropic medications are occasionally useful in the schizophrenic patient, but their role has not been clearly defined. Many patients benefit from anxiolytics (e.g., benzodiazepines) if anxiety is prominent. Lithium carbonate may be useful to reduce impulsive and aggressive behaviors, hyperactivity, or excitation or to stabilize mood. Antidepressants have been used to treat depressed schizophrenic patients. Although early studies suggested that antidepressants were not helpful in treating depressed schizophrenic patients and could cause a worsening of thought disorder, these recommendations are now being revised. Other medications including propranolol, carbamazepine, and clonidine have been used experimentally, but have no current role in the treatment of schizophrenia.

Psychosocial approaches to treatment play an important role in the management of schizophrenic patients and, like somatic treatments, must be tailored to fit individual needs. The fit will depend on the patient, the phase of illness, and the living situation.

Although dynamically oriented approaches are rarely helpful, supportive therapy that is reality oriented and pragmatic is useful. The clinician should assist the patient

Table 7-7. Reasons to hospitalize the schizophrenic patient

1. When the illness is new, to rule out alternative diagnoses, and to stabilize the dose of antipsychotic medication.
2. For special medical procedures, such as electroconvulsive therapy.
3. When aggressive or assaultive behavior presents a danger to the patient or others.
4. When the patient becomes suicidal.
5. When the patient is unable to properly care for himself or herself (e.g., refuses to eat or take fluids).
6. When medication side effects become disabling or potentially life threatening (e.g., severe pseudoparkinsonism, severe tardive dyskinesia, neuroleptic malignant syndrome).

in developing new coping strategies, testing reality, resolving concrete problems, and identifying both stressors and prodromal symptoms of relapse.

A vexing problem facing patients, their family members, and clinicians is deciding when the patient should enter the hospital. Long-term institutionalization is now rare, and most patients, if hospitalized, stay briefly in special psychiatric hospitals, or in psychiatric units found in general hospitals. Stays tend to be short (e.g., weeks to months), and the patient is returned to the community. Reasons to hospitalize a schizophrenic patient include the patient being a danger to self or others or refusing to properly care for himself or herself (e.g., not eating or taking fluids) or need for special medical observation, tests, or treatments. The reasons are summarized in Table 7-7. In some cases, a court order will need to be obtained for hospitalization if the patient is a danger to self or others and refuses hospitalization.

In the hospital, an active milieu characterized by high levels of support, a practical problem-solving approach, and broad delegation of responsibility with clear lines of authority tends to be superior to a custodial milieu for schizophrenic patients. The milieu must not be overly stimulating, however. Token economies in which patients are provided a high degree of ward structure and are rewarded for desired behaviors seem to be effective in controlling behavior in the hospital; however, this improvement may not generalize to situations outside the hospital.

Group therapy may be threatening to some patients, and counterproductive in the paranoid patient, but can help to provide social skills training and provide a format to allow friendships to develop. Family therapy has proved to be important. Research has shown that a family environment characterized by harsh criticism and emotional overinvolvement tends to precede schizophrenic relapse. Families must be educated about the nature of schizophrenia and the need for long-term management based on realistic expectations. They should also be provided instruction on how to reduce "expressed emotion."

Some patients are unable to live at home or may be better off living apart from their families. Group residential treatment centers (halfway houses) may be appropriate for them. Many patients will be unable to work regularly, but a sheltered workshop may provide simple repetitive work that will allow the patient to maintain contact with the community, allow the development of interpersonal relationships, and provide additional income.

Recommendations for management of the schizophrenic patient

1. Treat psychotic symptoms aggressively with medication.
   - Remember that all antipsychotics are equally effective (except clozapine, which may be more effective), so choice of drug depends on patient tolerance and side effects.
   - Intramuscular medication is useful in uncooperative or poorly compliant patients.

2. Engage the patient in an empathic relationship.
   - This task may be particularly challenging, as many schizophrenic patients are unemotional, aloof, and withdrawn.
   - Be practical; help the patient with problems that matter to him or her, such as finding adequate housing.

3. Help the patient find a daily routine that he or she can manage to help improve socialization and reduce boredom.
   - Day hospital programs are available in many areas.
   - Sheltered workshops that provide simple, repetitive chores may be helpful.

4. Develop a close working relationship with local social services.
   - Patients tend to be poor and disabled; finding adequate housing and food takes the skills of a social worker.
   - Assist the patient in obtaining disability benefits.

5. Family therapy is important for the patient living at home, or one who still has close family ties.
   - As a result of illness, many patients will have broken their family ties.
   - Families desperately need education about schizophrenia and need to learn how to reduce their "expressed emotion."
   - Help family members find a support group through referral to a local chapter of the Alliance for the Mentally Ill (AMI).

Bibliography

Andreasen NC: The diagnosis of schizophrenia. Schizophr Bull 13:9–22, 1987

Andreasen NC, Olson S: Negative v. positive schizophrenia: definition and validation. Arch Gen Psychiatry 39:789–794, 1982

Andreasen NC, Ehrhardt JC, Swayze VW, et al: Magnetic resonance imaging of the brain in schizophrenia: the pathophysiological significance of structural abnormalities. Arch Gen Psychiatry 47:35–44, 1990

Baron M: Genetics of schizophrenia. Biol Psychiatry 21:1051–1066, 1986

Black DW: Mortality in schizophrenia—the Iowa Record-Linkage Study. Psychosomatics 29:55–60, 1988

Black DW, Boffeli TJ: Simple schizophrenia: past, present, and future. Am J Psychiatry 146:1267–1273, 1989

Breier A, Astrachan BM: Characterization of schizophrenic patients who commit suicide. Am J Psychiatry 141:206–209, 1984

Buchanan RW, Kirkpatrick B, Heinrichs DW, et al: Clinical correlates of the deficit syndrome of schizophrenia. Am J Psychiatry 147:290–294, 1990

Buchsbaum MS, DeLisi LE, Holcomb HH, et al: Anteroposterior gradients in cerebral glucose use in schizophrenia and affective disorders. Arch Gen Psychiatry 41:1159–1166, 1984

Carlson A: The current status of the dopamine hypothesis of schizophrenia. Neuropsychopharmacology 1:179–186, 1988

Casanova MF, Kleinman JE: The neuropathology of schizophrenia: a critical assessment of research methodologies. Biol Psychiatry 27:353–362, 1990

Cutting J: Outcome in schizophrenia: overview, in Contemporary Issues in Schizophrenia. Edited by Kerr TA, Snaith RP. Washington, DC, American Psychiatric Press, 1986, pp 433–440

Dubin WR, Waxman HM, Weiss KJ, et al: Rapid tranquilization: the efficacy of oral concentrate. J Clin Psychiatry 46:475–478, 1985

Falloon IRH, Boyd JL, McGill CW: Family Care for Schizophrenia: A Problem-Solving Approach to Mental Illness. New York, Guilford, 1984

Farde L, Wiesel FA, Stone-Elander S, et al: D_2-dopamine receptors in neuroleptic-naive schizophrenic patients: a positron emission tomography study with [^{11}C]raclopride. Arch Gen Psychiatry 47:213–219, 1990

Kane J, Honigfeld G, Singer J, et al: Clozapine for the treatment of resistant schizophrenia. Arch Gen Psychiatry 45:789–796, 1988

Machon RA, Mednick SA, Schulsinger F: The interaction of seasonality, place of birth, genetic risk and subsequent schizophrenia in a high risk sample. Br J Psychiatry 143:383–388, 1983

McGlashan TH: The Chestnut Lodge follow-up study, II: long-term outcome in schizophrenia and the affective disorders. Arch Gen Psychiatry 41:586–601, 1984

Pfohl B, Winokur G: The evolution of symptoms in institutionalized hebephrenic/catatonic schizophrenics. Br J Psychiatry 141:567–572, 1982

Reynolds GP: Beyond the dopamine hypothesis: the neurochemical pathology of schizophrenia. Br J Psychiatry 155:305–316, 1989

Sherrington R, Brynjolfsson J, Petursson H, et al: Localisation of a susceptibility locus for schizophrenia on chromosome 5. Nature 336:164–166, 1988

Torrey EF: Surviving Schizophrenia: A Family Manual. New York, Harper & Row, 1983

Tsuang MT, Woolson RF, Fleming JA: Long-term outcome of major psychoses, I: schizophrenia and affective disorder compared with psychiatrically symptom-free surgical conditions. Arch Gen Psychiatry 36:1295–1306, 1979

Weinberger DR, Bigelow LB, Kleinman JE, et al: Cerebral ventricle enlargement in chronic schizophrenia: an association with poor response to treatment. Arch Gen Psychiatry 37:11–13, 1980

Wong DF, Wagner HN, Tune LE, et al: Positron emission tomography reveals elevated D2 dopamine receptors in drug-naive schizophrenics. Science 234:1528–1563, 1986

Self-assessment Questions

1. What were Bleuler's "four A's"? What were his fundamental and accessory symptoms?
2. How is schizophrenia diagnosed? What is its differential diagnosis?
3. What are typical signs/symptoms of schizophrenia?
4. What are the subtypes of schizophrenia?
5. What is the prevalence and sex distribution of schizophrenia? What is its age at onset?
6. What recent developments have occurred in the study of the genetics of schizophrenia?
7. What evidence supports a neurobiological basis for schizophrenia?
8. What is the natural history of schizophrenia?
9. How is schizophrenia managed, both pharmacologically and psychosocially?
10. When should the schizophrenic patient be hospitalized?

Chapter 8

Delusional Disorder and Other Psychotic Disorders

In a sense, the paranoiac's behavior is justified; he perceives something that escapes the normal person; he sees clearer than one of normal intellectual capacity, but his knowledge becomes worthless when he imputes to others the state of affairs he thus recognizes.

Sigmund Freud

Although schizophrenia is clearly the most significant psychotic disorder, and mood disorder with psychotic features is the most common, several less well known psychotic disorders are seen by psychiatrists and are briefly reviewed in this chapter (Table 8-1). These disturbances include delusional disorder, schizoaffective disorder, schizophreniform disorder, brief reactive psychosis, induced psychotic disorder, and psychotic disorder not otherwise specified.

Delusional Disorders

Delusional disorders constitute a small but important group of disturbances characterized by the presence of well-systematized nonbizarre delusions accompanied by affect appropriate to the delusion, occurring in the presence of a relatively well-preserved personality.

175

Table 8-1.   Other psychotic disorders

Delusional disorder

- Erotomanic type
- Grandiose type
- Jealous type
- Persecutory type
- Somatic type
- Unspecified type

Schizoaffective disorder

Schizophreniform disorder

Brief reactive psychosis

Induced psychotic disorder

Psychotic disorder not otherwise specified

The former term for the disorder, *paranoid disorder,* was discarded because of the ambiguity inherent in the term *paranoid,* which is often construed to mean "persecutory." The delusions observed in delusional/paranoid disorders are not restricted to themes involving persecution or jealousy, but may include grandiose, erotomanic (i.e., delusions of being loved), and somatic delusions. The paranoid disorders have a long history, and the term itself is from the Greek *para nous* meaning "mind beside itself," a term originally used to describe insanity. The term was revived in the 19th century by German psychiatrists interested in disorders characterized by delusions of persecution and grandeur. Kraepelin separated paranoia from dementia praecox (schizophrenia) and used the term to describe persons with systematized delusions, an absence of hallucinations, and a prolonged course without recovery, but not leading to mental deterioration. Bleuler also believed that paranoia was separate from dementia praecox, but that hallucinations could occur in some patients.

Delusional disorder is estimated to have a prevalence in the community of between 24 and 30 per 100,000 and is rare in psychiatric hospitals. In one study, only 0.14% of hospitalized psychiatric patients admitted over a 55-year period had a delusional disorder. It is generally considered to be a disorder of middle to late adult life, and it affects more women than men. Most patients seen in hospitals are married at the time of the first admission, are often from low socioeconomic classes, and are often immigrants.

It is not known what causes delusional disorder, although genetic, environmental, and psychodynamic mechanisms have been used to explain its etiology. Family studies have generally concluded that delusional disorder is probably not related to either schizophrenia or affective disorders, but delusional disorder is so uncommon that it is difficult to demonstrate that it runs in families. However, paranoid personality has been found in relatives of delusional disorder probands.

Table 8-2. DSM-III-R diagnostic criteria for delusional disorder

A. Nonbizarre delusion(s) (i.e., involving situations that occur in real life, such as being followed, poisoned, infected, loved at a distance, having a disease, being deceived by one's spouse or lover) of at least 1 month duration.

B. Auditory or visual hallucinations, if present, are not prominent [as defined in schizophrenia, criterion A(1)(b)].

C. Apart from the delusion(s) or its ramifications, behavior is not obviously odd or bizarre.

D. If a major depressive or manic syndrome has been present during the delusional disturbance, the total duration of all episodes of the mood syndrome has been brief relative to the total duration of the delusional disturbance.

E. Has never met criterion A for schizophrenia, and it cannot be established that an organic factor initiated and maintained the disturbance.

It is possible that psychosocial stressors may lead to delusional disorder in some persons. For example, *migration psychosis,* generally persecutory in nature, has been described in persons migrating from one country to another (although it is possible that persons in whom paranoia is prone to develop may be more likely to emigrate than others). Prison psychosis has been described in which isolation in prison, especially solitary confinement, may lead to paranoia.

Psychodynamic formulations of paranoia derive from Freud's analysis of the Schreber case. Schreber, a distinguished jurist, developed a paranoid psychosis in midlife. Freud believed that his persecutory delusions stemmed from unconscious homosexual urges defended against by the ego-defense mechanisms of denial and projection. Although Freud's ideas are helpful in allowing us to understand delusional disorder in some patients, their use in treating patients has been disappointing.

Delusional disorder tends to run a chronic, unremitting course. Unlike patients with schizophrenia, patients with delusional disorder are generally self-supporting and remain employed. The disorder is diagnostically stable, and it is unlikely that these patients, if properly diagnosed, will develop schizophrenia.

The diagnosis of delusional disorder is appropriate when nonbizarre delusions are present, have lasted at least 1 month, and involve situations that occur in real life (Table 8-2). Behavior is generally not odd or bizarre apart from the delusion or its ramifications. In addition, in delusional disorder, there is an absence of the bizarre delusions that may occur in schizophrenia (i.e., impossible delusions, such as being controlled by Martians), an absence of grossly disorganized speech or behavior, an absence of prominent hallucinations, and an absence of a mood disorder or organic mental disorder. The core feature, however, is a well-systematized, encapsulated, nonbizarre delusion. The term *systematized* is used to indicate that the delusion and its ramifications fit into a complex, all-encompassing scheme that makes logical sense to the patient. The term *encapsulated* indicates that, apart from the delusion or its ramifications, the patient generally behaves in a normal way, or at least is not perceived as especially unusual.

Table 8-3. Varied themes in delusional disorder in 29 patients

Theme	%
Jealous	38
Persecutory	35
Litigious/legal	17
Sexual	17
Scientific (i.e., special knowledge)	3

Source. Adapted from Winokur G: Delusional disorder (paranoia). Compr Psychiatry 18:453–479, 1977.

Common themes in patients with delusional disorder are presented in Table 8-3. Sexual problems and depressive symptoms are frequent complications, and patients may show overtalkativeness or circumstantiality, especially when discussing their delusions. Associated features of delusional disorder may include anger, social isolation and seclusiveness, eccentric behavior, suspiciousness, hostility, and, rarely, violence. Many patients become litigious and end up as lawyers' clients rather than as psychiatrists' patients.

According to DSM-III-R, delusional disorder includes the following subtypes: *persecutory type*, in which there is a belief that one is being malevolently treated in some way; *erotomanic type* (de Clerambault's syndrome), in which there is a belief that a person, usually of higher status, is in love with the patient; *grandiose type*, in which there is a belief that one is of inflated worth, power, knowledge, or identity or has a special relation to a deity or famous person; *jealous type*, in which the delusion is that one's sexual partner is unfaithful; and *somatic type*, in which the delusion is that a person has some physical defect, disorder, or disease, such as acquired immunodeficiency syndrome (AIDS). There is a residual category (*unspecified type*) for patients who do not fit the previous categories, for example, those who have been ill less than 1 month. The following case example illustrates the erotomanic subtype.

Doug, a 33-year-old restaurant manager, was brought to the hospital under court order for evaluation and treatment. The accompanying papers alleged that he had harassed and threatened a young woman.

The patient had an uneventful childhood growing up in a small midwestern town. Although quiet and bookish, he had several friends while growing up. He excelled in school and graduated from college with honors. He later returned to school for a Master's degree.

After admission, the following story unfolded. Doug had had a four-and-a-half-year fantasy relationship with a comely shop clerk who had recently married. Doug had become convinced that the young woman was in love with him, although they had never met. He took as evidence of her affection glances and smiles that they had exchanged when they occasionally crossed paths in their small town. After becoming convinced of her love, he mailed a "sexual business letter" to her after learning her name and address. Love letters continued over the next few years, and Doug kept careful track of her whereabouts. There were no other formal communications, but the letters indicated his belief in her infatuation over him and his desire that she act on it. In one letter he wrote: "What do you think I am? A can of vegetables that can just sit on your shelf to open or throw away whenever it suits you?"

The young woman complained about these letters to the police, who warned Doug not to call or write her. This warning had little effect. Interestingly, Doug himself complained to the police about his imagined harassment by her. The woman and her husband finally sought a court order for Doug's hospitalization when the letters to her had developed a more threatening tone, and a restraining order had failed to keep him away from the shop where she worked. Doug had felt jilted by the woman's relationship and subsequent marriage and had suggested in recent letters that the three get together to "work things out."

At the hospital, Doug was noted to be neatly groomed, articulate, and indignant about his hospitalization. Although he was notably circumstantial in describing his fantasy relationship, he clearly had no evidence of a mood disorder, hallucinations, or bizarre delusions. He reported a history of a similar relationship 10 years earlier, consisting mostly of letters, which had ended when the girl had moved out of town. Although Doug was a loner with few friends and had never had a sexual relationship, he was highly functional in his position at work and was active in several community organizations.

Several variants of delusional disorder have been described, including *Capgras' syndrome*, in which a patient believes that a person closely related to him or her has been replaced by a double (this belief was the theme of the 1950s "B" horror movie, *Invasion of The Body Snatchers*), and the *Fregoli syndrome*, in which the patient identifies a familiar person in various other people he or she encounters. The patient may maintain that although there is no physical resemblance between the familiar persons and others, they are nonetheless psychologically identical.

A careful diagnostic evaluation is necessary to rule out other functional or organic illnesses that could have caused the delusions. The workup must include a physical examination to rule out alcoholism, drug-induced states, dementia, and infectious, metabolic, and endocrine disorders. Routine laboratory tests may be indicated depending on the results of the history and physical examination. Computerized tomography or magnetic resonance imaging may be useful in selected patients, especially when mass lesions are suspected.

The major differential diagnosis remains in separating delusional disorder from mood disorders with psychotic features, schizophrenia, and paranoid personality. The chief distinction from mood disorders is that in delusional disorder a depressive or manic syndrome is absent, developed after the psychotic symptoms, or was brief in duration in relation to the psychotic symptoms. Unlike schizophrenia, delusional disorders are characterized by nonbizarre delusions and generally either absence of hallucinations or hallucinations that are not prominent. Furthermore, patients with delusional disorders do not develop other schizophrenic symptoms such as incoherence or grossly disorganized behavior, and personality is generally preserved. Persons with paranoid personality are suspicious and hypervigilant, but are not delusional.

There are no systematic data comparing treatments in delusional disorder. None-theless, a combination of psychosocial and physical measures seems prudent. Most patients have little insight about their illness and refuse to acknowledge a problem, so that the initial obstacle is getting the patient to the physician. After establishing a therapeutic relationship, the physician may gently challenge the patient's beliefs by showing how they interfere with the patient's life. Tact and skill are necessary to persuade a patient to accept treatment, and the physician must neither condemn nor collude in the beliefs. The patient must be assured of the confidential nature of the patient-physician relationship. Insight-oriented psychotherapy and group therapy are not recommended because suspiciousness and hypersensitivity may lead to misinterpretation. However, psychosocial treatment recommendations are based on clinical impression, not on empirical evidence.

For reasons that are not understood, delusional disorder has a poor response to antipsychotic medication, although these medications probably should be tried. Delusions and anxiousness may be decreased, but rarely disappear completely. If a patient does respond to antipsychotics, depot forms may sometimes be useful in preventing noncompliance due to suspiciousness. Other medications including anxiolytics and antidepressants may be indicated for accompanying anxiety or depressive syndromes, respectively, but have not been systematically evaluated in patients with delusional disorder.

Recommendations for management of delusional disorder

1. Because the patient with delusional disorder is so suspicious, it may be very difficult to establish a therapeutic relationship.
   - Building a relationship will take time and patience.
   - The therapist must neither condemn nor collude in the delusional beliefs of the patient.
   - The patient must be assured of complete confidentiality.

2. Once rapport is established, gently challenge the delusional beliefs, and point out how they are interfering with the patient's functioning.
   - Tact and skill will be needed to convince the patient to accept treatment.

3. A patient with delusional disorder may be more accepting of medication if it is explained as treatment for the anxiety, dysphoria, and stress that the patient is invariably experiencing as a result of his or her delusions.

4. Treatment for the jealous subtype may include separation and divorce. Unfortunately, the delusional beliefs of infidelity may transfer to future lovers or spouses.

Schizoaffective Disorder

The term *schizoaffective* was first used in 1933 by Kasanin to describe a group of patients with concurrent schizophrenic and affective symptoms, a history of a precipitating stressor, acute onset, and a family history of mood disorder. Kasanin believed that these patients had a subtype of schizophrenia, even though they

Table 8-4. DSM-III-R diagnostic criteria for schizoaffective disorder

A. A disturbance during which, at some time, there is either a major depressive or a manic syndrome concurrent with symptoms that meet the A criterion of schizophrenia.

B. During an episode of the disturbance, there have been delusions or hallucinations for at least 2 weeks, but no prominent mood symptoms.

C. Schizophrenia has been ruled out, i.e., the duration of all episodes of a mood syndrome has not been brief relative to the total duration of the psychotic disturbance.

D. It cannot be established that an organic factor initiated and maintained the disturbance.

Specify: **bipolar type** (current or previous manic syndrome) or **depressive type** (no current or previous manic syndrome)

recovered from their symptoms. After his initial description, patients with this mix of symptoms tended to receive a variety of diagnoses, such as atypical schizophrenia, good-prognosis schizophrenia, cycloid psychosis, and reactive schizophrenia, because there was little agreement about definition or the relationship of these disorders to schizophrenia or mood disorders.

In the past decade, the concept of schizoaffective disorder has been better defined and has been subjected to more intensive study. In all likelihood, patients with schizoaffective disorders probably constitute two groups, i.e., patients with mood disorders and patients with schizophrenia. Schizoaffective disorder probably does not represent an independent psychosis.

Because of its relatively imprecise definition, it is impossible to know its distribution in the community, although its prevalence is probably less than 1%; it is more frequently diagnosed in women. It is a commonly used diagnosis in psychiatric hospitals and clinics, but is primarily a diagnosis of exclusion.

According to DSM-III-R, schizoaffective disorder is a disturbance during which, at some time, there is either a depressive or manic syndrome concurrent with psychotic symptoms characteristic of schizophrenia, such as bizarre delusions or catatonic behavior; during an episode of the disturbance, hallucinations or delusions have been present for 2 or more weeks without prominent mood symptoms. Further, organic factors have been ruled out as a cause. The criteria specify two subtypes: the *bipolar type*, if the patient has had a current or previous manic syndrome, or the *depressive type*, in which no manic syndromes have been present. These criteria, presented in Table 8-4, represent an advance over DSM-III, in which, unlike other diagnoses, no criteria were provided.

The differential diagnosis for schizoaffective disorder consists primarily of schizophrenia, mood disorders, and organic disorders. In schizophrenia, the duration of all episodes of mood syndrome are brief relative to the total duration of the psychotic disturbance, and, by definition, schizophrenia leads to poor functioning in areas such as work, social relations, and self-care. Mood disorders, commonly associated with psychotic symptoms, are generally not associated with episodes of psychosis in the absence of a depression or mania. Organic disorders may be associated with psychoses and mood syndromes, but it is usually clear from the history, physical examination, or laboratory tests that a specific organic factor has initiated and maintained the disturbance, such as treatment with corticosteroids.

Because schizoaffective disorder probably represents a heterogeneous group of patients, it is difficult to talk about etiology. Family studies have shown an increased prevalence of both schizophrenia and mood disorders in relatives of schizoaffective patients, but because most of the studies use different diagnostic criteria, it is hard to know what to make of their conclusions. In general, schizoaffective patients have higher rates of schizophrenia and lower rates of mood disorders in their families than patients with mood disorder, but higher rates of mood disorder and lower rates of schizophrenia than patients with schizophrenia. Most other etiologic indicators also suggest that schizoaffective disorder is a "mixed bag" consisting of schizophrenic patients with severe mood symptoms and mood disorder patients with severe psychoses. In these patients, the disorders may be clinically indistinguishable and, of course, etiologically heterogeneous.

The signs and symptoms of schizoaffective disorder include those seen in schizophrenia and the mood disorders. The symptoms may present together or in an alternating fashion, and psychotic symptoms may be mood congruent or mood incongruent. The course and prognosis of schizoaffective disorder is variable and represents a middle ground between outcome in schizophrenia and outcome in mood disorder. Some studies, however, suggest that schizoaffective disorder, bipolar type, has an outcome similar to that for bipolar disorder, and that schizoaffective disorder, depressed type, has a prognosis similar to that of schizophrenia. Poor prognosis is indicated by poor premorbid adjustment, insidious onset, lack of a precipitating factor, predominance of psychotic symptoms, early onset, unremitting course, and a family history of schizophrenia.

The treatment of schizoaffective disorder depends on the symptom cluster that is manifested. The principles that apply for treatment of these patients apply to all psychiatric patients. If the patient is suicidal, is a danger to self or others, or is unable to properly care for himself or herself, hospitalization is necessary. Lithium carbonate will be useful in treating a manic syndrome, and antipsychotics for treating psychosis. Lithium is also useful in the long-term prophylaxis of schizoaffective disorders, particularly the bipolar type. The depressed schizoaffective patient may benefit from treatment with antidepressants and antipsychotics concurrently. The schizoaffective bipolar patient who does not respond to lithium should have a trial of carbamazepine, and possibly a combination of the two agents. Patients not responding to medication often respond to electroconvulsive therapy.

Schizophreniform Disorder

The term *schizophreniform* was first used in 1939 by Langfeldt to describe psychoses that were acute and reactive and occurred in persons with normal personalities. Rather than listing it as a subtype of schizophrenia, DSM-III-R lists the disorder under psychotic disorders not elsewhere classified. The definition of schizophren-

Table 8-5. DSM-III-R diagnostic criteria for schizophreniform disorder

A. Meets criteria A and C of schizophrenia.

B. An episode of the disturbance (including prodromal, active, and residual phases) lasts less than 6 months. (When the diagnosis must be made without waiting for recovery, it should be qualified as "provisional.")

C. Does not meet the criteria for brief reactive psychosis, and it cannot be established that an organic factor initiated and maintained the disturbance.

Specify: **without good prognostic features** or **with good prognostic features,** i.e., with at least two of the following:

1. Onset of prominent psychotic symptoms within 4 weeks of first noticeable change in usual behavior or functioning
2. Confusion, disorientation, or perplexity at the height of the psychotic episode
3. Good premorbid social and occupational functioning
4. Absence of blunted or flat affect

iform disorder requires: 1) active psychotic symptoms, 2) that the symptoms are not due to an organic mental disorder, 3) that criteria for brief reactive psychosis are not met, and 4) that duration is less than 6 months (see Table 8-5 for the complete list of criteria).

The diagnosis changes to schizophrenia once the symptoms have extended past 6 months, even if the only symptoms remaining are residual ones. The diagnosis is to be considered provisional in patients who have not recovered, because many persons who meet criteria for schizophreniform disorder will eventually go on to meet criteria for schizophrenia. In the past, patients with schizophreniform disorder would have been referred to as having *acute schizophrenia.*

This relatively new diagnosis has little empirical support, and the few relevant studies have yielded conflicting data. For example, one study found schizophreniform and schizophrenic patients to have similar structural brain abnormalities, but another investigator concluded that at least a portion of schizophreniform patients have a mood disorder, based on family history, treatment response, and neuroendocrine testing.

One long-term follow-up study indicates that patients with schizophreniform disorder have a heterogeneous outcome. Outcome measures used in the study (e.g., living situation, marital status, psychiatric symptoms) show that schizophreniform patients were more similar in outcome to schizophrenic patients than to mood disorder patients. This finding implies that some patients with schizophreniform disorder actually have a mood disorder, and that the others, probably the majority, go on to develop schizophrenia. The study also found that the morbidity risk for mood disorder among first-degree relatives of schizophreniform patients was no different from that observed among relatives of schizophrenic patients, but was significantly lower than that observed among relatives of mood disorder patients. Clearly, the proper boundaries of this disorder remain in question. Its main use is to guard against premature diagnosis of schizophrenia.

Treatment of schizophreniform disorder has not been systematically evaluated, but the principles of its management are similar for that of an acute exacerbation of schizophrenia, which is described in Chapter 7.

Brief Reactive Psychosis

In a brief reactive psychosis, a patient develops psychotic symptoms and emotional turmoil in response to a severe emotional stressor. This diagnosis, along with posttraumatic stress disorder and adjustment disorders, constitutes one of the few diagnoses in DSM-III-R for which a specified causative factor is identified.

In the past, patients with these disorders would have been diagnosed as having reactive, hysterical, or psychogenic psychoses. The diagnosis does not imply a relationship with schizophrenia. This disorder is similar to what Scandinavian psychiatrists regard as *reactive psychoses*, which arise in persons with vulnerable constitutions who are subjected to stress.

This rarely used diagnosis has been poorly studied, so the prevalence and sex ratio of brief reactive psychoses are not known. The disorder is thought to occur more commonly in persons of low socioeconomic status and those with personality disorders, especially borderline and schizotypal disorders.

Signs and symptoms are similar to those seen in schizophrenia, including hallucinations, delusions, or grossly disorganized behavior. However, in brief reactive psychosis, emotional turmoil as evidenced by rapid shifts from one mood to another, or overwhelming perplexity, is required for the diagnosis. The disturbance, by definition, lasts a few hours to 1 month with a full return to premorbid functioning, and it is not due to a mood disorder with psychotic features (see Table 8-6).

The differential diagnosis of brief reactive psychosis includes schizophrenia, mood disorders, organic disorders, factitious disorder with psychological symptoms, and malingering. In schizophrenia, onset is usually insidious, and there is no precipitating event. In mood disorders, a full mood syndrome is present, although psychotic symptoms, emotional turmoil, and a precipitating event may be found. In organic disorders, there will be evidence from the history, laboratory tests, or physical examination of an organic factor, such as drug intoxication, that initiated and maintained the disturbance. In factitious disorder with psychological symptoms, there will be evidence of intentional production of the symptoms coupled with the need to assume a sick role that may bring secondary gain (i.e., more attention from family members). In malingering, the symptoms are voluntarily produced in response to an external motivation (i.e., escaping from military duties). In some patients, the differential diagnosis between brief reactive psychosis, factitious disorder, and malingering will be very difficult, and prolonged observation will be needed to help clarify the diagnosis.

As in any acute psychosis, hospitalization may be necessary for the safety of the patient. Because brief reactive psychoses are probably self-limiting disorders, no specific treatment is indicated, and the hospital milieu itself may be sufficient to help the patient recover. Antipsychotic or anxiolytic medications may be helpful early on, especially if the patient is highly agitated or experiencing great emotional

Table 8-6. DSM-III-R diagnostic criteria for brief reactive psychosis

A. Presence of at least one of the following symptoms indicating impaired reality testing (not culturally sanctioned):

   1. Incoherence or marked loosening of associations
   2. Delusions
   3. Hallucinations
   4. Catatonic or disorganized behavior

B. Emotional turmoil, i.e., rapid shifts from one intense affect to another, or overwhelming perplexity or confusion.

C. Appearance of the symptoms in A and B shortly after, and apparently in response to, one or more events that, singly or together, would be markedly stressful to almost anyone in similar circumstances in the person's culture.

D. Absence of the prodromal symptoms of schizophrenia, and failure to meet the criteria for schizotypal personality disorder before onset of the disturbance.

E. Duration of an episode of the disturbance from a few hours to 1 month, with eventual full return to premorbid level of functioning. (When the diagnosis must be made without waiting for the expected recovery, it should be qualified as "provisional.")

F. Not due to a psychotic mood disorder (i.e., no full mood syndrome is present), and it cannot be established that an organic factor initiated and maintained the disturbance.

turmoil. Once the patient is sufficiently recovered, the therapist can assist the patient by exploring the meaning of the psychotic reaction and of the triggering stressor itself. Supportive psychotherapy should help to restore morale and self-esteem.

Induced Psychotic Disorder

Induced psychotic disorder occurs when the delusional system of a patient (secondary case) develops in the context of a close relationship with another person (or persons) (primary case) who already has an established delusion. The delusion in the patient is similar to that found in the primary case. According to DSM-III-R, the second person did not have a psychotic disorder before the onset of an induced delusion or the prodromal symptoms of schizophrenia (Table 8-7).

The disorder was termed *shared paranoid disorder* in DSM-III to highlight the

Table 8-7. DSM-III-R diagnostic criteria for induced psychotic disorder

A. A delusion develops (in a second person) in the context of a close relationship with another person, or persons, with an already established delusion (the primary case).

B. The delusion in the second person is similar in content to that in the primary case.

C. Immediately before the onset of the induced delusion, the second person did not have a psychotic disorder or the prodromal symptoms of schizophrenia.

possibility that several persons may share a similar delusion. In the past, this disorder has also been called *folie à deux*. The disorder is apparently rare, and information is limited to case reports. The disorder was first described in the late 19th century and may affect persons in all socioeconomic classes. Most cases involve two members within the same family.

The proposed mechanism for the development of shared paranoid disorder is the presence of a dominant person with an established delusional system and a more submissive person who develops the induced psychotic disorder, thereby gaining the acceptance of the more dominant individual. Because it is rare, the natural history is unknown, but clinical lore suggests that separation may result in rapid improvement in the submissive person.

Psychotic Disorder Not Otherwise Specified

Psychotic disorder not otherwise specified, or atypical psychosis, is a residual category for persons with psychotic symptoms such as hallucinations, delusions, or grossly disorganized behavior who do not clearly fit into any of the other better-defined categories. For example, a person with persistent auditory hallucinations, but who is otherwise well adjusted, employed, and socially competent, would fit this category. The category should also be used to classify psychoses about which there is inadequate information to make a specific diagnosis.

Certain culture-bound syndromes may fit this category, including the interesting condition known as *koro*. Indigenous to China and other parts of the Far East, an individual with koro develops the belief that the genitals are retracting into the body. Typically, a man believes that his penis is retracting, whereas a woman may believe that her breasts are retracting. There is usually no history of psychopathology, and the disorder remits spontaneously, although folk remedies may be used. These remedies include having the relatives pull on the person's genitals to prevent them from retracting. Epidemics of koro have been documented to occur in remote parts of China.

Bibliography

Clayton PJ: Schizoaffective disorders. J Nerv Ment Dis 170:646–650, 1982

Coryell WH, Tsuang MT: Outcome after 40 years in DSM-III schizophreniform disorder. Arch Gen Psychiatry 43:324–328, 1986

Fogelson DL, Cohen BM, Pope HG: A study of DSM-III schizophreniform disorder. Arch Gen Psychiatry 39:1281–1285, 1982

Kasanin J: The acute schizoaffective psychoses. Am J Psychiatry 90:97–126, 1933

Kendler KS: The nosologic validity of paranoia (simple delusional disorder: a review). Arch Gen Psychiatry 37:699–707, 1980

Kendler KS: Demography of paranoid psychoses (delusional disorder). Arch Gen Psychiatry 39:890–902, 1982

Kendler KS, Masterson C, Davis K: Psychiatric illness in first degree relatives of patients with paranoid psychosis, schizophrenia, and medical illness. Br J Psychiatry 147:524–531, 1985

Kendler KS, Spitzer RL, Williams JBW: Psychotic disorders in DSM-III-R. Am J Psychiatry 146:953–962, 1989

Langfeldt G: Schizophreniform States. Copenhagen, E Munksgaard, 1939

Levitt JJ, Tsuang MT: The heterogeneity of schizoaffective disorder: implications for treatment. Am J Psychiatry 145:926–936, 1988

Maj M: Lithium prophylaxis in schizoaffective disorder—a prospective study. J Affective Disord 14:129–135, 1988

Munoz RA, Amado H, Hyatt S: Brief reactive psychosis. J Clin Psychiatry 48:324–327, 1987

Opjordsmoen S: Long-term course and outcome in delusional disorder. Acta Psychiatr Scand 78:556–586, 1988

Pope HG, Lipinski JF, Cohen BM: Schizoaffective disorder: an invalid diagnosis? A comparison of schizoaffective disorder, schizophrenia, and affective disorder. Am J Psychiatry 137:921–927, 1980

Sacks MH: Folie à deux. Compr Psychiatry 29:270–277, 1988

Targum SD: Neuroendocrine dysfunction in schizophreniform disorder—correlation with six month clinical outcome. Am J Psychiatry 140:309–313, 1983

Tseng WS, Kan-Ming M, Hsu J, et al: A sociocultural study of koro epidemics in Guangdong, China. Am J Psychiatry 145:1538–1543, 1988

Watt JAG: The relationship of paranoid states to schizophrenia. Am J Psychiatry 142:1456–1458, 1985

Weinberger DL, DeLisi LE, Perman GP, et al: Computed tomography in schizophreniform disorder and other acute psychiatric disorders. Arch Gen Psychiatry 39:778–783, 1982

Winokur G: Delusional disorder (paranoia). Compr Psychiatry 18:453–479, 1977

Winokur G: Familial psychopathology and delusional disorder. Compr Psychiatry 26:241–248, 1985

Self-assessment Questions

1. How does delusional disorder differ from schizophrenia?
2. What are systematized encapsulated delusions?
3. What are the subtypes of delusional disorder?
4. How does schizoaffective disorder differ diagnostically from both schizophrenia and psychotic mood disorders?
5. Why is schizoaffective disorder a controversial diagnosis?
6. What evidence is there to link schizophreniform disorder to either schizophrenia or the mood disorders?
7. What is the differential diagnosis of a brief reactive psychosis?
8. How is a brief reactive psychosis managed?
9. What is the commonly accepted treatment for the secondary case in induced psychotic disorder?
10. What is koro?

Chapter 9

Mood (Affective) Disorders

I see the lost are like this, and their curse
To be, as I am mine, their sweating selves. But worse.

Gerard Manley Hopkins

The mood disorders are characterized primarily by a disturbance in the emotions and feelings that we refer to as "mood." The disturbance may manifest itself as either elation or unhappiness, and the two clinical syndromes associated with these extremes are referred to as mania and depression. Most people suffering from mood disorder have some type of depression, but a few experience mood swings between the two "poles" of mood disorder and are therefore referred to as having bipolar mood disorder. Mood disorders are very common, and they usually respond well to treatment. Learning to diagnose and treat these disorders is as basic and fundamental a skill in medicine as the diagnosis and management of myocardial infarction or streptococcal pharyngitis.

History

The recognition that humans suffer from some recognizably abnormal syndrome characterized by a disorder in mood has been present for many millennia. Perhaps the oldest medical document available to us is from ancient Egypt, the Ebers papyrus, and it describes a medical condition characterized by severe despondency that is equivalent to modern concepts of depression. In the Old Testament, the "case" of Saul is described in the book of Samuel during the 8th century B.C. Saul,

King of Israel, develops periods of severe depression, guilt, and incapacity. Several different treatments are attempted, including placing a young woman in his bed and having the young shepherd David play soothing music for him. He responds to the music of David for a time and even accepts David as a member of the royal household. Later, however, he relapses again, becomes severely psychotic, and even attempts to kill David and his own son Jonathan.

Another term for this disorder, "melancholy," appears in Hippocratic writings of the 4th century; *melancholy* literally means "black bile," and it reflects the belief that this disorder was due to a chemical imbalance of the humors of the body. Clear explicit references to disorders of mood continue through classical times up to the present. St. Augustine, St. John of the Cross, Shakespeare's Hamlet, John Keats, William James, and Leo Tolstoy are only a few of the many notable examples who have described their personal struggles with periods of depression or despondency.

Affective disorders are thus historically among the oldest psychiatric syndromes that have been recognized. They are also extremely common and "psychologically understandable." We have all experienced mild periods of despondency after some personal loss or failure, and it is therefore very easy to identify with and sympathize with people who suffer from the more severe forms of the illness. As later portions of this chapter will indicate, effective treatments for affective illnesses have become available during the past few decades, making these among the most treatment-responsive disorders in psychiatry and in medicine generally. Working with patients with mood disorders tends, therefore, to be very gratifying.

An additional aspect of mood disorder that makes it quite intriguing is its possible association with giftedness or creativity. As early as the 4th century B.C., Aristotle commented that "those who have become eminent in philosophy, politics, poetry, and the arts have all had tendencies toward melancholia." People with mood disorders may, as a group, be somewhat more creative or gifted than the general population. For example, in a group of successful creative writers selected from the rotating faculty at The University of Iowa Writers' Workshop, the rate of affective illness was nearly three times greater than that of a socioeconomically and educationally equivalent control group. The list of notable writers who clearly have had affective illness is long, including Robert Lowell, Ernest Hemingway, Sylvia Plath, John Berryman, and Ann Sexton.

Many eminent philosophers, scientists, and politicians have had affective illness as well. Aristotle cites both Plato and Alexander the Great as examples. Oliver Cromwell, Martin Luther, and Abraham Lincoln are probably examples as well. It is a sad commentary on the stigma attached to mental illness in our society that American presidential candidates are screened for a history of psychiatric illness, and even the untrue attribution of such a history is considered to be an effective form of mudslinging. Many of our great leaders of the past would have been prevented from accomplishing their missions had a history of mood disorder been considered grounds for disqualification.

These disorders are variously referred to as either "affective" or "mood" disorders. DSM-III-R uses the term "mood disorders," but DSM-III and much of the clinical and research literature use the alternate term. Although more traditional and more widely used, the concept of an abnormality of affect as a unifying principle for these disorders is somewhat problematic on several grounds. The term "affect" is sometimes used to refer to the external expression of an internal state (i.e., mood); the distinction between mood and affect also sometimes turns on transient versus sustained states, with mood being more transient and affect being more sustained (mood is to weather as affect is to climate). According to this distinction, the abnormality in affective or mood disorders is more often one of mood. Further, as is clear from Chapter 7 on schizophrenia, patients with schizophrenia often have pronounced abnormalities in affect that are fundamental to the illness, and therefore, schizophrenia is in some respects an "affective disorder." Thus, although the terms "affective" and "mood" disorders tend to be used interchangeably to refer to both depression and mania, the term "mood disorder" is probably preferable. Linguistic conventions are hard to wipe out, however, and so the term "affective disorder" is likely to remain entrenched for some time.

Clinical Findings and Diagnostic Criteria

The mood disorders fall into two broad syndromes, depression and mania.

Major Depressive Episode

Because feelings of sadness and despondency are very much part of normal human experience, having diagnostic criteria to demarcate pathological sadness from normal responses to stress and injury is particularly important. The DSM-III-R criteria for an episode of major depression appear in Table 9-1. These criteria specify that the patient have at least five symptoms of depression (and one of them must be depressed mood or loss of interest or pleasure). These five symptoms are drawn from a list of nine included in criterion A. These characteristic symptoms define major depression, and they must be present for at least 2 weeks in order to rule out transient fluctuations in mood. The remaining three criteria serve to rule out other conditions, such as abnormalities in mood due to an "organic" factor (e.g., myxedema), bereavement, schizoaffective disorder, schizophreniform disorder, or other psychotic conditions.

Because major depression is perhaps the most common psychiatric illness that clinicians working in any branch of medicine are likely to encounter, it is probably worthwhile to commit the nine characteristic symptoms to memory. This can be done through the use of a simple mnemonic: "Depression Is Worth Seriously Memorizing Extremely Gruesome Criteria. Sorry." (DIWS MEGCS) The initials stand for: Depressed mood, Interest, Weight, Sleep, Motor activity, Energy, Guilt, Concentration, Suicide. In conducting clinical interviews with patients to determine whether the patient is depressed, the clinician will repeatedly find himself mentally running through this list of symptoms. Consequently, it is convenient to

Table 9-1. DSM-III-R diagnostic criteria for major depressive episode

A. At least five of the following symptoms have been present during the same 2-week period and represent a change from previous functioning; at least one of the two symptoms is either (1) depressed mood, or (2) loss of interest or pleasure. (Do not include symptoms that are clearly due to a physical condition, mood-incongruent delusions or hallucinations, incoherence, or marked loosening of associations.)

   1. Depressed mood (or can be irritable mood in children and adolescents) most of the day, nearly every day, as indicated either by subjective account or observation by others

   2. Markedly diminished interest or pleasure in all, or almost all, activities most of the day, nearly every day (as indicated either by subjective account or observation by others of apathy most of the time)

   3. Significant weight loss or weight gain when not dieting (e.g., more than 5% of body weight in a month), or decrease or increase in appetite nearly every day (in children, consider failure to make expected weight gains)

   4. Insomnia or hypersomnia nearly every day

   5. Psychomotor agitation or retardation nearly every day (observable by others, not merely subjective feelings of restlessness or being slowed down)

   6. Fatigue or loss of energy nearly every day

   7. Feelings of worthlessness or excessive or inappropriate guilt (which may be delusional) nearly every day (not merely self-reproach or guilt about being sick)

   8. Diminished ability to think or concentrate, or indecisiveness, nearly every day (either by subjective account or as observed by others)

   9. Recurrent thoughts of death (not just fear of dying), recurrent suicidal ideation without specific plan, or a suicide attempt or a specific plan for committing suicide

B. 1. It cannot be established that an organic factor initiated and maintained the disturbance.

   2. The disturbance is not a normal reaction to the death of a loved one (uncomplicated bereavement).

   Note: Morbid preoccupation with worthlessness, suicidal ideation, marked functional impairment or psychomotor retardation, or prolonged duration suggest bereavement complicated by major depression.

C. At no time during the disturbance have there been delusions or hallucinations for as long as 2 weeks in the absence of prominent mood symptoms (i.e., before the mood symptoms developed or after they have remitted).

D. Not superimposed on schizophrenia, schizophreniform disorder, delusional disorder, or psychotic disorder not otherwise specified.

have it stored in an accessible memory bank so that the evaluation can be done fluently and smoothly.

As DSM-III-R criteria imply, the basic abnormality in depression is an alteration in mood: a person who is depressed feels sad, despondent, "down in the dumps," or full of despair. Although the dysphoric mood is most frequently expressed as complaints of feeling sad, occasionally patients will complain of feeling tense or irritable, with only a small component of sadness, or of having lost their ability to feel pleasure or to experience interest in things they normally enjoy.

The depressive syndrome is frequently accompanied by a group of "vegetative" symptoms, such as decreased appetite or insomnia. The decreased appetite often leads to some weight loss, although occasionally depressed persons will force themselves to eat in spite of decreased appetite, or they may be urged and encouraged to eat by a parent or spouse so that the weight loss is minimal. Less frequently, depression expresses itself as a desire to eat excessively and is accompanied by weight gain.

Insomnia may be initial, middle, or terminal. *Initial insomnia* means that the patient has difficulty falling asleep, often tossing or turning for several hours before dozing off. *Middle insomnia* refers to awakening in the middle of the night, remaining awake for an hour or two, and finally falling asleep again. *Terminal insomnia* refers to awakening early in the morning and being unable to return to sleep. Patients with insomnia will often worry and ruminate during the time when they are lying awake. Patients who have terminal insomnia may have more severe depressive syndromes. Depressed patients may also complain of restless sleep, indicating that they have awakened so frequently throughout the night that they scarcely got any sleep at all. These various types of sleep disturbance have been well documented by electroencephalogram (EEG) research in sleep laboratories. Occasionally, the sleep difficulty may involve a need to sleep excessively: the patient may complain of feeling chronically tired and needing to spend 10–14 hours each day in bed.

Motor activity is often altered in depression. Patients may subjectively complain of feeling either slowed down or agitated, but objective evidence is required as well to ensure that the symptom is truly present. A patient with psychomotor retardation may sit quietly in a chair for hours without speaking to anyone, simply staring into space. When she gets up and moves about, she walks at a snail's pace, her speech is slow, and her replies are brief and laconic. If asked about her thinking, she may complain that it is markedly slowed down. On the other hand, the agitated patient is restless and seems extremely nervous. The agitated patient may complain more of irritability or tenseness than of depression. He is unable to sit in a chair and frequently paces about. He may wring his hands or perform some other stereotyped and repetitive nervous gesture such as drumming his fingers on a table, pulling on his hair or clothing, or playing with objects in his hands. His speech is usually somewhat rapid, and he may complain in a high-pitched and staccato whine about the various miseries from which he is suffering.

Depressed patients also complain frequently of fatiguing too easily, or having a marked decrease in their energy level. In a general medical setting, this may be one of the most common presenting complaints of depression, and the clinician will need to probe to determine whether the easy fatigability is due to a depressive syndrome.

Feelings of worthlessness and guilt are also very common in depression. The depressed person may lose confidence in herself so that she is fearful of going to work, taking examinations, or assuming responsibility for household tasks. She may avoid answering the phone or returning phone calls in order to avoid responsibilities or social relationships that she feels unable to handle. She may become completely hopeless and full of despair, believing that her situation can never be improved, or even that she does not deserve to feel better. The depressed person may feel quite guilty over actual or fantasized misdeeds that she has committed in the past. Usually the "misdeed" is seen as more terrible than it actually was, so that the person believes that she should be a social pariah because of a lie told as a child, or sent to prison for a long term because of a questionable deduction taken on an income tax return.

Complaints of difficulty in concentrating or thinking clearly are also common in depression. The depressed person feels that he functions less well at work, is unable to study, or (in severe cases) is even unable to perform simple cognitive tasks such as watching a football game on television or reading "escape fiction."

Depressed patients may think a great deal about death or suicide. This may be seen either as an escape from their suffering, or a deserved punishment for their various misdeeds. The suicidal patient often expresses the notion that "everyone would be better off without me." Suicide risk is high in depressed patients and should always be assessed carefully (see Chapter 20 for more detail on evaluation and management of the suicidal patient).

In addition to the nine core symptoms summarized in the diagnostic criteria, other symptoms may also occur in patients suffering from depression. *Diurnal variation,* another vegetative symptom, is a fluctuation in mood during the course of a 24-hour day; it may reflect some type of neuroendocrine abnormality in depression. Most typically, the patient states that his mood is worse in the morning, but that it improves as the day progresses, so that he feels best in the evening. Less frequently, this problem is reversed, with the patient stating that he feels best in the morning.

The patient's sex drive may decrease markedly, so that he or she has no interest in sex, or even begins to experience impotence and/or anorgasmia. The depressed patient may also complain of other physical symptoms such as constipation or dry mouth.

Occasionally patients experience *masked depression,* meaning that the full depressive syndrome is not immediately obvious, because the patient does not report a depressed mood. Nevertheless, decreased interest and substantial clustering of symptoms elicited by systematic inquiry does indicate that the patient is nevertheless depressed. This syndrome may be especially important in a primary-care setting. For example, an older person may come in complaining primarily of many physical symptoms that are troubling her so much that she is unable to concentrate, unable to work, and unable to sleep. She will deny that her mood is despondent or irritable, stating that she is indeed upset, but would feel fine if only the physical symptoms were corrected. These symptoms are often pain or gastrointestinal problems, such as piercing headache, burning pains in the rectum, or persistent heartburn. Although a careful medical workup reveals no physical abnormalities, the patient usually continues to insist on the depressive symptoms. When the "masked" depression clears, the clustering of physical complaints tends to disappear totally.

Patients who are severely depressed may experience psychotic symptoms such as delusions or hallucinations. These are usually consistent with the depressed mood; for example, the depressed person may hear the voice of the devil speaking to him and telling him that he has fallen so far from God's ways that his soul is forever lost and that he will be tormented in hell throughout eternity. He may begin to believe that the world is coming to an end and that he has seen various "signs" as indicators of its impending demise. He may develop the delusion that the FBI or police are following him and bugging his house or office in order to catch him in the various misdeeds that his excessive guilt makes him believe he has committed. He may think that he has a fatal disease that is consuming his body and making his internal organs rot away. Less frequently, the delusions will not be consistent with depressed mood. For example, the patient may report that he is being spied on because he is on the verge of developing some great invention that others are attempting to steal from him—a persecutory delusion that is not directly related to depressed mood.

The following case example is relatively typical of a major depressive syndrome.

Wilma was brought to the hospital at the request of her family, and of her husband in particular. She described herself as being despondent and demoralized because her husband was having an affair with a woman who had previously been his secretary, Lydia, but her husband adamantly denied this and indicated that this belief was a delusion due to his wife's depressed condition.

Wilma admitted to a depressed mood, plus a full constellation of depressive symptoms, including feelings of worthlessness, suicidal thoughts, hypersomnia, increased appetite and weight gain, decreased interest and enjoyment in activities she normally found pleasurable (such as following the many activities of her four teenage children), and decreased energy.

When interviewed alone, she indicated that she was absolutely convinced that her husband, a successful local insurance agent, was secretly involved with another woman. She attributed most of her depressive symptoms to this situation, which she believed had been going on for at least 6 months (as had her depression). She had no specific evidence to support the occurrence of the affair, but indicated that her husband had been away more in the evenings, had a marked decrease in sexual interests, and had talked frequently about Lydia's secretarial skills until Wilma became jealous and angry. Due to pressure from Wilma, her husband eventually urged Lydia to seek another position, but Wilma believed that her husband was continuing to see Lydia secretly. Both in the presence of his wife and when interviewed alone, Bill adamantly denied the affair. He indicated that he was a devout Catholic (as was Wilma) and that such behavior was strongly discordant with his religious beliefs, as well as risky to his community position. Bill indicated that his sexual interest had decreased because Wilma had become increasingly overweight and less attractive. Wilma had had one prior episode of depression that had been successfully treated with antidepressants approximately 5 years earlier.

A diagnosis of depression was therefore made again, and Wilma was placed on imipramine, with a dosage gradually increased to 150 mg per day. She showed some improvement on this, and both Bill and Wilma were also seen for marital counseling. Their relationship improved somewhat, but Wilma continued to be suspicious.

Wilma remained on antidepressants for the next 3 months and continued to see a psychotherapist at weekly intervals to learn techniques to decrease her chronic negative mind-set, her suspicious attitude toward her husband, and her tendency to use food as a way of raising her spirits.

After 3 months of psychotherapy, she came in one day with a new firmness of step and her eyes flashing with anger. While cleaning out the pockets of one of her husband's

Table 9-2. Frequency of typical symptoms in patients with depression

Symptom	%
Insomnia	100
Sadness of mood	100
Tearfulness	94
Poor concentration	91
Suicidal thoughts	82
Fatigue	76
Irritability	76
Psychomotor retardation	76
Anorexia	66
Diurnal variation	64
Hopelessness	51
Poor memory	35
Delusions	33
Suicide attempts	15
Auditory hallucinations	6

Source. Adapted from Winokur G, Clayton P, Reich T: Manic Depressive Illness. St. Louis, MO, CV Mosby, 1969.

suits in preparation for sending it to the cleaners, she found a love letter from Lydia. She did not confront Bill immediately, but instead followed him the next night when he indicated that he was going back to the office to get caught up on some dictation. Ten minutes after his departure, Wilma left, drove past Lydia's house, and found Bill's car parked in her garage. Thereafter, she confronted him, and he finally confessed to an affair that had been going on for nearly 2 years.

The direction of marital counseling changed sharply, and Bill was urged to seek individual psychotherapy himself. Wilma continued to require antidepressant medication for another 6 months, as she gradually came to terms with the fact of her husband's infidelity (which was actually more painful than having her suspicions discounted by both her husband and the medical community). Eventually, however, the couple was able to work through this situation, to remain married, and to establish a reasonably good relationship with one another.

The frequency of some of the common symptoms of depression is summarized in Table 9-2.

Manic Episode

The DSM-III-R criteria for a manic episode require the presence of an abnormally elevated, expansive, or irritable mood plus three from a list of seven characteristic symptoms. The criteria are similar to those used to define depression, but also have differences that reflect the greater severity of psychopathology that typically characterizes mania. Because a manic episode is an extreme event, no specific duration is required, although it is specified that the mood disturbance must be sufficiently severe to cause marked impairment, or to require hospitalization. As in the case of depression, the symptoms cannot be caused by an organic factor, schizoaffective disorder, schizophrenia, or other psychoses. The criteria for a manic episode appear in Table 9-3.

Table 9-3. DSM-III-R diagnostic criteria for manic episode

Note: A "manic syndrome" is defined as including criteria A, B, and C below. A "hypomanic syndrome" is defined as including criteria A and B, but not C, i.e., no marked impairment.

A. A distinct period of abnormally and persistent elevated, expansive, or irritable mood.

B. During the period of mood disturbance, at least three of the following symptoms have persisted (four if mood is only irritable) and have been present to a significant degree:
   1. Inflated self-esteem or grandiosity
   2. Decreased need for sleep, e.g., feels rested after only 3 hours of sleep
   3. More talkative than usual or pressure to keep talking
   4. Flight of ideas or subjective experience that thoughts are racing
   5. Distractibility, i.e., attention too easily drawn to unimportant or irrelevant external stimuli
   6. Increase in goal-directed activity (either socially, at work or school, or sexually) or psychomotor agitation
   7. Excessive involvement in pleasurable activities that have a high potential for painful consequences, e.g., the person engages in unrestrained buying sprees, sexual indiscretions, or foolish business investments

C. Mood disturbance sufficiently severe to cause marked impairment in occupational functioning or in usual social activities or relationships with others, or to necessitate hospitalization to prevent harm to self or others.

D. At no time during the disturbance have there been delusions or hallucinations for as long as 2 weeks in the absence of prominent mood symptoms (i.e., before the mood symptoms developed or after they have remitted).

E. Not superimposed on schizophrenia, schizophreniform disorder, delusional disorder, or psychotic disorder not otherwise specified.

F. It cannot be established that an organic factor initiated and maintained the disturbance.

Note: Somatic antidepressant treatment (e.g., drugs, ECT) that apparently precipitated a mood disturbance should not be considered an etiologic organic factor.

The manic patient's mood is typically cheerful, enthusiastic, and expansive. The cheerfulness often has an infectious quality, making interviewing an enjoyable and sometimes amusing experience. Sometimes, however, the patient's mood is simply irritable, particularly when thwarted, and such irritable manic patients can be quite difficult to manage. Because of their euphoria, manic patients usually have very little insight into their problems. In fact, they may deny that anything is wrong with them, and instead blame friends or family for attributing an abnormality to them that is in fact not present. Because manic disorder is characterized by other symptoms that are clearly pathological, such as poor judgment and extreme grandiosity, it is usually not difficult for the clinician to differentiate manic euphoria from a normal "good mood."

Manic patients typically "suffer" from inflated self-esteem and grandiosity, which may reach delusional proportions. Manic patients may believe that they have special abilities or powers, which clearly are outside the normal range for their educational background or intellectual achievement. They may develop plans to write books, cut records, lead religious movements, or undertake expansive business ventures. When the grandiosity reaches delusional proportions, patients may report that they are rock stars, famous athletes, politicians, or even religious figures such as the Messiah.

The euphoria and grandiosity are typically accompanied by increased energy, activity levels, and cognitive speed. Patients with mania usually require less sleep than usual, often getting by on only 2 or 3 hours per night. Unlike the patient with depression, the manic patient does not feel tired and does not complain about inability to sleep.

Manic patients tend to talk excessively and to manifest pressured speech. Thus, they answer questions at great length, continue to talk even when interrupted, and sometimes talk when no one is listening. Their speech is usually rapid, loud, and emphatic.

Underlying the pressured speech is probably a rapid flow of thought, sometimes referred to as "flight of ideas." This increased speed in cognitive functioning is inferred by listening to the patient's speech, which manifests derailment, incoherence, and distractibility. Manic patients tend to skip from one topic to another as they describe their experiences, ideas, or symptoms. Thus, positive formal thought disorder is quite common in mania.

Distractibility is observed both in their speech and in their social behavior. While speaking, they may shift their topic in response to some stimulus in the environment, and they manifest the same pattern of distractibility when trying to perform tasks or complete activities. Thus, the increased energy and cognitive productivity is usually not sufficiently well organized to produce the magnificent goals that are projected in the manic patient's grandiose plans.

Manic patients are often more physically active than usual as well. They may become more social and gregarious, going to bars, planning parties, or calling friends at all hours of the night. Interest in sex is often increased, leading the manic patient to exhaust his partner or to make inappropriate overtures to casual acquaintances or strangers. Patients with mania are usually physically restless and unable to sit still. The increased level of activity is often accompanied by poor judgment. Patients suffering from mania often overextend themselves in ways that lead them into serious trouble after the manic episode is over. They spend money excessively, commit themselves to projects that they are unable to complete, become involved in extramarital affairs, or engage in quarrels with business associates or family members who disagree with them or try to "slow them down."

As in the case of depression, the manic patient may manifest symptoms of psychosis. Indeed, psychotic symptoms are almost more the norm than the exception in mania. Approximately 50% of manic patients have psychotic symptoms, compared to only about 20% of patients suffering from depression. Psychotic symptoms may include either delusions or hallucinations and typically express themes consistent with the mood, such as delusions about special abilities or powers. Less commonly, the delusions may be mood incongruent and express themes that are not related to the euphoric and grandiose mood.

The following case example illustrates a relatively typical manic syndrome.

Charles was brought to the psychiatric emergency room by the local police, after he jumped from his seat in the middle of a performance of Les Miserables, ran on the stage, and began yelling that the injustices of the Reagan administration were as extensive and profound as those portrayed in the performance. He began conversing with Jean Valjean, urging him to leave the performance, to join the Democratic party, and to assist in the effort to place a Democrat in the American presidency. This speech was accompanied by an extensive speech on the injustice of "packing" the Supreme Court with a group of extreme conservatives.

In the emergency room, he indicated that he did not reside in Iowa City, but had come from Des Moines (100 miles away) to attend the performance and to consult with friends and colleagues at the law school. He described himself as a prominent lawyer, a graduate of Harvard Law School who had edited the Law Review, a close friend of the Kennedy family and other prominent Democrats, and a dedicated crusader against social injustice. He described the Reagan administration as a rerun of the industrial-totalitarian axis that had been created in Nazi Germany, complained about a conspiracy that he believed was under way to destroy the Democratic party either by persecution or assassination of key figures, and indicated that one of the purposes of his trip to Iowa City was to warn his colleagues at the law school about these dangerous circumstances.

His appearance was somewhat unkempt and disheveled, not consistent with his description of his prominent status. Although he was attired in an expensive-appearing pinstripe suit, his hair was uncombed, his eyes were red, and he was unshaven. He talked excitedly in a rapid manner, and his voice rose to a shout at times. His speech was disjointed and difficult to follow, as his topic changed from his own special importance and abilities to the various conspiracies that he thought were underway in the Reagan government. He described a complex internal structure in the Reagan administration that he believed would "lead to another Watergate," and he marshaled evidence to support this position by referring to special implications in programs that had recently run on television such as Dynasty or David Letterman. When admission to the hospital was proposed, he became physically agitated and tried to run away. He became physically combative at attempts to restrain him, asserting in a threatening manner that he was a former state wrestling champion who was also a finalist for the Olympic team in his weight class.

Because of his agitation, a decision was made to obtain an emergency holding order. His claims of special importance and abilities were discounted and attributed to his manic state. Later, as more history was obtained, it became evident that he was indeed a prominent attorney with many important national connections and also had been a star wrestler. The conspiracy against the Democratic party, although potentially bearing some credence, contained enough implausible elaborations to qualify as delusional thinking. Interviews with his family members also revealed that he had had one prior hospitalization for mania and had been treated for depression as an outpatient. He had been taking maintenance lithium, but had decided to discontinue it abruptly approximately 3 days before coming to Iowa City to attend the performance of Les Miserables. Within a day after discontinuing the lithium, he became increasingly euphoric, irritable, and grandiose. His wife had been reluctant to let him come alone, but he had insisted that he would be okay.

He was placed on a therapeutic dose of lithium and his symptoms cleared rapidly over the course of 4–5 days. He was able to leave the hospital and to return to work within 1 week. His second episode of mania helped him appreciate the importance of maintenance lithium, as his insight about his illness grew, and he has been able to prevent subsequent relapses and to function effectively.

Table 9-4 summarizes the frequency of some common symptoms of mania.

Classification and Subtypes

Controversy exists about the best way to define and classify the various disorders of mood. This controversy arises because the two major mood syndromes, but especially depression, seem to exist on a continuum of severity. Very mild periods of depression are probably normal, because most people experience them. Once an arbitrary dividing line is set to distinguish "mild normal blues" from "pathological blues," it is not clear whether the remainder of the depressive syndromes are a single disorder on a continuum of severity or whether they represent discrete disorders. Further, there is controversy whether bipolar disorder is simply a more severe form of depression, or whether it represents a different and discrete disorder. This controversy arises largely because family studies indicate that many relatives of bipolar patients suffer only from depression.

Table 9-4.   Frequency of typical symptoms in patients with mania

Symptom	%
Distractibility	100
Pressured speech	99
Euphoria	98
Lability	95
Flight of ideas	93
Insomnia	90
Grandiosity	86
Irritability	85
Hostility	83
Extravagance	69
Depression	68
Diurnal variation	67
Depression after mania	52
Delusions of any type	48
Increased alcohol consumption	42
Increased sexual intercourse	32
Auditory hallucinations	21
Increased sexual contacts (noncoital)	12
Promiscuity	11
Suicidal thoughts	7

Source. Adapted from Winokur G, Clayton P, Reich T: Manic Depressive Illness. St. Louis, MO, CV Mosby, 1969.

Table 9-5. DSM-III-R classification of mood disorders

Bipolar disorders	Depressive disorders
Bipolar disorder, manic	Major depression, single episode
Bipolar disorder, depressed	Major depression, recurrent
Bipolar disorder, mixed	Dysthymia
Cyclothymia	Depressive disorder not otherwise
Bipolar disorder not otherwise specified	specified

Bipolar and Unipolar Disorders

The DSM-III-R classification of mood disorders is summarized in Table 9-5. It represents the best compromise that can be achieved concerning subtypes of mood disorders based on existing evidence.

The mood disorders may be thought of as subdivided into two main groups: those that are more severe and those that are less severe. The severe mood disorders, which typically require somatic therapy and may require hospitalization, are major depressive disorder and bipolar disorder. This classification subdivides the two severe types of mood disorders into bipolar and "unipolar." The term *unipolar* is widely used by clinicians to refer to patients who have depression, but it is not included in DSM-III-R. Thus, patients are subdivided in DSM-III-R on a syndrome basis: those who have had an episode of mania are referred to as having bipolar disorder (even if they have not yet had a depression), whereas those who have had depression only are referred to as having major depressive disorder (i.e., are unipolar). Although patients who have had only mania without depression might logically be separated out as manic disorder or be considered to be unipolar, by convention such patients are referred to as bipolar, because nearly all patients who experience mania eventually develop depression.

This subdivision of severe forms of mood disorders into bipolar or major depressive (or bipolar or unipolar) is based on its predictive power. These two subforms of severe mood disorder typically have different familial patterns, require different treatments, and perhaps have a different pathophysiology and etiology.

The mood disorders are conditions that tend to recur, although some people who experience mood disorder have only a single episode and remain well for the rest of their lives. Because these disorders recur in many people, however, DSM-III-R provides a system so that patients can be characterized on a lifetime basis and described in terms of the current episode of illness that they are experiencing. Thus, for example, bipolar patients may be identified as bipolar, currently manic or bipolar, currently depressed. Some patients cycle rapidly within an episode and are referred to as "mixed." The mixed or rapidly cycling patient is one of the most difficult to manage.

The nature of the manic or depressive episode is further characterized in terms of its severity. This way of subdividing depression is summarized in Table 9-6. The subdivision for mania is identical.

The most severe form is psychotic mania or depression, which is characterized by florid psychotic symptoms such as delusions or hallucinations. Sometimes the

Table 9-6.   DSM-III-R types of major depressive episode

• **MILD:** Few, if any, symptoms in excess of those required to make the diagnosis, **and** symptoms result in only minor impairment in occupational functioning or in usual social activities or relationships with others.

• **MODERATE:** Symptoms or functional impairment between "mild" and "severe."

• **SEVERE, WITHOUT PSYCHOTIC FEATURES:** Several symptoms in excess of those required to make the diagnosis, **and** symptoms markedly interfere with occupational functioning or with usual social activities or relationships with others.

• **SEVERE, WITH PSYCHOTIC FEATURES:** Delusions or hallucinations. If possible, **specify** whether the psychotic features are mood congruent or mood incongruent.

Mood-congruent psychotic features: Delusions or hallucinations whose content is entirely consistent with the typical depressive themes of personal inadequacy, guilt, disease, nihilism, or deserved punishment.

Mood-incongruent psychotic features: Delusions or hallucinations whose content does not involve typical depressive themes of personal inadequacy, guilt, disease, death, nihilism, or deserved punishment. Included here are such symptoms as persecutory delusions (not directly related to depressive themes), thought insertion, thought broadcasting, and delusions of control.

psychotic symptoms are consistent with the patient's mood. For example, a depressed patient who feels guilty and despondent may suffer from elaborate religious delusions of sin and guilt, or may hear voices condemning him. A manic patient may develop grandiose delusions that he is a deity, a rock star, or an important political figure. Such delusions are characterized as *mood congruent,* and the subtype of mania or the subtype of manic or depressive episode is therefore classified as manic/psychotic/mood congruent, or depressed/psychotic/mood congruent. A very disturbed patient suffering from mania or depression may display psychotic features that are not congruent with her mood; for example, a manic patient may believe that she is being tormented by demons. *Mood incongruent* delusions or hallucinations are a relatively worse prognostic feature, and so this form of psychotic mood disorder is delineated as a separate category.

Melancholia and Seasonal Mood Disorder

Two additional subtypes of depression are recognized: melancholia and seasonal mood disorder. The criteria for melancholia appear in Table 9-7.

Melancholia is thought to identify a relatively severe form of depression that is more likely to respond to somatic therapy. The concept of melancholia is based on an older historic distinction between endogenous versus reactive depression, a distinction that was based both on presumed etiology and a characteristic clustering of symptoms. In the original definitions of *endogenous depression,* it had no precipitating factors (*endo-genous* = "grows from within"), whereas a *reactive depression* occurred in reaction to some stressful life event such as a divorce or loss of a job.

Table 9-7. DSM-III-R diagnostic criteria for melancholia

The presence of at least five of the following:

1. Loss of interest or pleasure in all, or almost all, activities
2. Lack of reactivity to usually pleasurable stimuli (does not feel much better, even temporarily, when something good happens)
3. Depression regularly worse in the morning
4. Early morning awakening (at least 2 hours before usual time of awakening)
5. Psychomotor retardation or agitation (not merely subjective complaints)
6. Significant anorexia or weight loss (e.g., more than 5% of body weight in a month)
7. No significant personality disturbance before first major depressive episode
8. One or more previous major depressive episodes followed by complete, or nearly complete, recovery
9. Previous good response to specific and adequate somatic antidepressant therapy, e.g., tricyclics, ECT, MAO inhibitors, lithium

The term *endogenous* has been abandoned, as has the requirement that there can be no precipitating events, because increasing evidence has suggested that severe depressions may be triggered by various physiological or psychological stressors.

As traditionally defined, endogenous depression has a characteristic set of symptoms, most of which are used to define melancholia in DSM-III-R. These include pervasive loss of interest or pleasure, inability to respond to pleasurable stimuli, diurnal variation, terminal insomnia, severe psychomotor retardation, and anorexia or weight loss. These symptoms are predominantly "vegetative," and sometimes this subtype of depression is referred to as vegetative. A substantial body of research has suggested that this clustering of symptoms predicts a good response to antidepressant medication or electroconvulsive therapy (ECT). Frequently, patients with this clustering of symptoms have a past history of somatic therapy with good response.

DSM-III-R specifies another possible type of affective disorder as well, *seasonal mood disorder*. The criteria for seasonal mood disorder are summarized in Table 9-8. Clinicians have recognized for many decades that some individuals have a characteristic onset of affective symptoms in relation to changes of season, with depression typically occurring more frequently during winter months, and remissions or changes from depression to mania during the spring. Because this seasonal pattern has important implications for prevention and treatment, a seasonal subtype has recently been specified.

Dysthymia and Cyclothymia

DSM-III-R also recognizes two somewhat milder forms of affective disorder, dysthymia and cyclothymia.

Dysthymia (sometimes referred to as *depressive neurosis*) is a chronic and persistent disturbance in mood that has been present for at least 2 years and is characterized by relatively typical depressive symptoms, such as anorexia, insomnia, decreased energy, low self-esteem, difficulty concentrating, and feelings of hopelessness. Be-

Table 9-8.   DSM-III-R diagnostic criteria for seasonal pattern

A. There has been a regular temporal relationship between the onset of an episode of bipolar disorder (including bipolar disorder not otherwise specified [NOS]) or recurrent major depression (including depressive disorder NOS) and a particular 60-day period of the year (e.g., regular appearance of depression between the beginning of October and the end of November).

   Note: Does not include cases in which there is an obvious effect of seasonally related psychosocial stressors, e.g., regularly being unemployed every winter.

B. Full remissions (or a change from depression to mania or hypomania) also occurred within a particular 60-day period of the year (e.g., depression disappears from mid-February to mid-April).

C. There have been at least three episodes of mood disturbance in three separate years that demonstrated the temporal seasonal relationship defined in A and B; at least two of the years were consecutive.

D. Seasonal episodes of mood disturbance, as described above, outnumbered any nonseasonal episodes of such disturbance that may have occurred by more than three to one.

cause dysthymia is a mild chronic disorder, only two of these symptoms are necessary for diagnosis, but they must have persisted more or less continuously for at least a 2-year period. Criteria for dysthymia appear in Table 9-9.

Patients with dysthymia are chronically unhappy and miserable. Some also develop the relatively more severe major depressive syndrome; when the major depressive episode clears, these patients subsequently return to their chronic state of dysthymia. The coexistence of these mild and severe forms of depression is referred to as *double depression.*

A second mild affective syndrome is *cyclothymia,* a condition in which the patient has mild swings between the two poles of depression and hypomania. While in the manic phase, the person appears to be high, but is not so high as to be socially or professionally incapacitated. During the depressed phase, the individual has some symptoms of depression, but these are not severe enough to meet criteria for a full major depressive episode (i.e., five symptoms persisting for 2 weeks). Thus, the individual with cyclothymia tends to swing from high to low with a chronic mild instability of mood. The criteria for cyclothymia appear in Table 9-10.

Other Subtypes Not Appearing in DSM-III-R

There are other important disorders that do not appear in DSM-III-R. Several other classification systems or subtypes of mood disorder are frequently discussed clinically and have been the subject of intensive research investigation. Although these do not appear in DSM-III-R, they are sufficiently widely accepted that the clinician should have at least some familiarity with them.

Bipolar II disorder is mentioned in DSM-III-R as an example of "bipolar disorder not otherwise specified," although it is not listed as a specific subtype. Bipolar II

Table 9-9. DSM-III-R diagnostic criteria for dysthymia

A. Depressed mood (or can be irritable mood in children and adolescents) for most of the day, more days than not, as indicated either by subjective account or observation by others, for at least 2 years (1 year for children and adolescents).

B. Presence, while depressed, of at least two of the following:
   1. Poor appetite or overeating
   2. Insomnia or hypersomnia
   3. Low energy or fatigue
   4. Low self-esteem
   5. Poor concentration or difficulty making decisions
   6. Feelings of hopelessness

C. During a 2-year period (1 year for children and adolescents) of the disturbance, never without the symptoms in A for more than 2 months at a time.

D. No evidence of an unequivocal major depressive episode during the first 2 years (1 year for children and adolescents) of the disturbance.

   Note: There may have been a previous major depressive episode, provided there was a full remission (no significant signs or symptoms for 6 months) before development of the dysthymia. In addition, after these 2 years (1 year in children and adolescents) of dysthymia, there may be superimposed episodes of major depression, in which case both diagnoses are given.

E. Has never had a manic episode or an unequivocal hypomanic episode.

F. Not superimposed on a chronic psychotic disorder, such as schizophrenia or delusional disorder.

G. It cannot be established that an organic factor initiated and maintained the disturbance, e.g., prolonged administration of an antihypertensive medication.

Specify primary or secondary type:

   Primary type: The mood disturbance is not related to a preexisting, chronic, nonmood, Axis I or Axis III disorder, e.g., anorexia nervosa, somatization disorder, a psychoactive substance dependence disorder, an anxiety disorder, or rheumatoid arthritis.
   Secondary type: The mood disturbance is apparently related to a preexisting, chronic, nonmood Axis I or Axis III disorder.

Specify early onset or late onset:

   Early onset: Onset of the disturbance before age 21.
   Late onset: Onset of the disturbance at age 21 or later.

---

disorder is characterized by relatively mild symptoms of mania that typically occur either before or after periods of depression, but also may occur independently. These mild manic episodes are not sufficiently severe to require hospitalization, although they may lead to personal, social, or work difficulties. During the mild bipolar phase, the patient is upbeat, shows signs of poor judgment, and has other indices of mania such as increased energy or insomnia, but does not meet full criteria for a manic episode. Bipolar II disorder appears to "breed true" within families, in that relatives of bipolar II patients themselves have higher rates of bipolar II disorder than either bipolar I (i.e., meets criteria for a full manic episode)

Table 9-10. DSM-III-R diagnostic criteria for cyclothymia

A. For at least 2 years (1 year for children and adolescents), presence of numerous hypomanic episodes (all of the criteria for a manic episode, except criterion C which indicates marked impairment) and numerous periods with depressed mood or loss of interest or pleasure that did not meet criterion A of major depressive episode.

B. During a 2-year period (1 year in children and adolescents) of the disturbance, never without hypomanic or depressive symptoms for more than 2 months at a time.

C. No clear evidence of a major depressive episode or manic episode during the first 2 years of the disturbance (or 1 year in children and adolescents).

Note: After this minimum period of cyclothymia, there may be superimposed manic or major depressive episodes, in which case the additional diagnosis of bipolar disorder or bipolar disorder not otherwise specified should be given.

D. Not superimposed on a chronic psychotic disorder, such as schizophrenia or delusional disorder.

E. It cannot be established that an organic factor initiated and maintained the disturbance, e.g., repeated intoxication from drugs or alcohol.

or unipolar major depression. Bipolar II patients also tend to have a high rate of comorbidity with other disorders, such as substance abuse.

Patients with depression are also sometimes subdivided into primary and secondary subtypes. *Primary depression* is depression occurring in a person who has never had any other psychiatric illness. *Secondary depression* occurs in a person who previously has had another psychiatric diagnosis, the most common being alcoholism, other substance abuse, panic disorder and other anxiety disorders, and antisocial personality.

This subclassification was originally introduced to facilitate research, because investigators seeking genetic patterns of transmission or neurochemical indicators of depression wished to study relatively "pure" examples of depression. Patients with secondary depression were thought to have a disorder more closely related to their antecedent diagnosis (e.g., alcoholism) than to the depressive disorders. Secondary depression is, however, clinically important in its own right. Studies have indicated rather consistently that patients with secondary depression tend to be more difficult to manage, in that they have more suicidal thoughts and suicide attempts, are less compliant with treatment, and tend to improve less with treatment and to have a higher relapse rate. No doubt some of this increased morbidity in secondary depression is related to the fact that patients have two illnesses, depression and some other disorder such as alcoholism, both of which have their own inherent morbidity.

A distinction between *neurotic depression* and *psychotic depression* is also sometimes made. This subdivision tends to be based primarily on severity. Although the term *neurotic* suggests that internal conflicts may either cause or characterize the disorder, many clinicians who refer to depression as "neurotic" mean only that it is relatively mild or relatively chronic; the DSM-III-R concept of dysthymia corresponds rather closely to this position. Sometimes the term *neurotic* is used predictively to refer to a depression that is not likely to respond to medication and is more appropriately treated with some form of psychotherapy. Likewise, some clinicians use the term *psychotic* as nosological shorthand to mean that a patient is more likely to need inpatient treatment and to respond to medication or ECT, is at higher risk for suicide, and has difficulty in maintaining an adequate level of functioning at work and at home.

Approximately 20% of patients with major depression are actually psychotic, in that they have delusions or hallucinations. Because the terms *neurotic* and *psychotic* have been used so imprecisely, DSM-III-R abandoned this approach as a way of subdividing depression into two large groups, although the basic concepts are still included at the extreme ends of the classification system (i.e., psychotic major depression and dysthymia).

Epidemiology

Because epidemiologic surveys of the prevalence or incidence of mood disorder have not used identical criteria to define mood disorders, the incidence and prevalence are uncertain. One study done in New Haven, Connecticut, which used diagnostic criteria closely equivalent to DSM-III-R, has indicated that approximately 4.3% of the population is suffering from depression at any given time. Investigators in Iceland have reported a current rate of 3.8%, whereas investigators in Denmark have reported 3.4%. Estimates of lifetime prevalence vary, but it seems likely that somewhere between 8 and 20% of the population will experience a significant depression at some time, depending on how narrowly or broadly "significant depression" is defined.

Depression is more common in women than in men; at present, the ratio in the United States is approximately 2:1. The age at onset for major depression appears to be getting steadily lower, a phenomenon referred to as the *cohort effect*; that is, a proportionately larger number of individuals in the "baby boom" generation have had episodes of major depression, in comparison with older individuals. In the baby boomers, the age at onset is reported as earlier than in older individuals.

Bipolar disorder is much less common than unipolar major depression. The lifetime prevalence for bipolar disorder is between 0.5 and 1%. Bipolar disorder is also more common in women than in men, with a ratio of approximately 3:2.

Data from the Epidemiologic Catchment Area study show that dysthymia has a lifetime prevalence of approximately 3% and is more common in women under age 65, unmarried persons, and persons with low income. There are no comparable figures for cyclothymia.

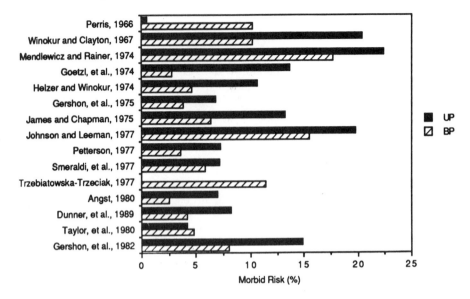

Figure 9-1. Morbid risk for bipolar (BP) and unipolar (UP) illness in first-degree relatives of bipolar probands.

Etiology and Pathophysiology

Many different ideas have been advanced to explain the pathophysiology and etiology of mood disorders. These explanations encompass the domains of genetics, social and environmental factors, and neurobiological factors.

Genetics

It has been recognized for many years that mood disorders tend to run in families. As discussed in Chapter 5, however, evidence that mood disorders tend to run in families does not necessarily indicate genetic transmission. Role modeling, learned behavior, social environmental factors such as economic deprivation, and physical environmental factors such as prenatal and perinatal birth complications may all provide nongenetic contributions to the development of a disorder, and these contributions could themselves be familial. (For example, before the advent of antibiotics, tuberculosis tended to run in families for environmental rather than genetic reasons.)

Studies of familial aggregation in mood disorders have provided empirical evidence that these disorders run in families. Data from family studies are summarized in Figures 9-1 and 9-2. Figure 9-1 summarizes data based on studies that used bipolar patients as the index cases. Figure 9-2 shows the rates of bipolar illness in the first-degree relatives of unipolar patients. Nearly all studies show significantly increased rates of mood disorder, and especially bipolar disorder, in the first-degree relatives of bipolar patients in comparison with normal control subjects. Unipolar patients

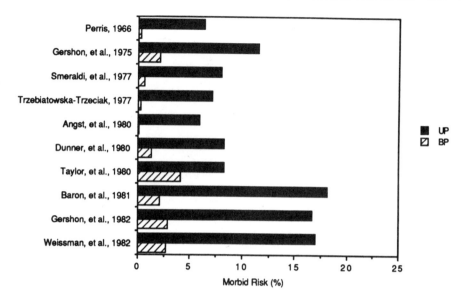

Figure 9-2. Morbid risk for bipolar (BP) and unipolar (UP) illness in first-degree relatives of unipolar probands.

tend to have much less bipolar illness among their first-degree relatives, but a high rate of unipolar illness. Control rates vary from study to study, but typically in the normal population are around 1% for bipolar disorder and between 5 and 15% for unipolar disorder; rates vary depending on the methods of definition.

As these figures indicate, the first-degree relatives of bipolar patients tend to have a higher rate of bipolar illness than the first-degree relatives of unipolar patients, although unipolar illness is also quite common in their first-degree relatives. On the other hand, the first-degree relatives of unipolar patients have lower rates of bipolar illness and higher rates of unipolar illness. Thus, not only are these disorders familial, but they also tend to "breed true." The fact that they do not breed *perfectly* true (i.e., bipolar illness *only* in the relatives of bipolar patients, and unipolar illness *only* in the relatives of unipolar patients) also suggests the possibility that these two forms of mood disorder may not be totally distinct from one another.

Twin and adoption studies have complemented these family studies and provided evidence to suggest that mood disorders are genetic in addition to familial. The twin studies are summarized in Table 9-11. The total number of available twin pairs is under 500; the overall monozygotic-to-dizygotic twin ratio in this entire sample is approximately 4:1 (65:14). Within individual studies, the monozygotic-to-dizygotic ratio ranges from a high of 75:0 to 57:23. These data are certainly sufficient to indicate that affective illness must have a strong genetic component. Adoption studies also support this conclusion.

Mood disorders were the first among the major mental illnesses to be studied with the techniques of molecular biology using the linkage method. Two types of

Table 9-11. Concordance rates for affective illness in monozygotic and dizygotic twins

Study	Monozygotic twins		Dizygotic twins	
	Concordant pairs/total pairs	Concordance (%)	Concordant pairs/total pairs	Concordance (%)
Luxenberger 1930	3/4	75.0	0/13	0.0
Rosanoff et al. 1935	16/23	69.6	11/67	16.4
Slater 1953	4/7	57.1	4/17	23.5
Kallmann 1954	25/27	92.6	13/55	23.6
Harvald and Hauge 1965	10/15	66.7	2/40	5.0
Allen et al. 1974	5/15	33.3	0/34	0.0
Bertelsen 1979	32/55	58.2	9/52	17.3
Totals	95/146	65.1	39/278	14.0

linkage have been reported. In a study of the Old Order Amish, linkage to the short arm of chromosome 11 was reported for bipolar disorder, a finding not supported by a subsequent reanalysis. In several other studies, X linkage has been reported for bipolar disorder. It is quite possible that several different genetic mechanisms could produce different forms of bipolar illness, so that a finding of linkage to different chromosomes is not unlikely.

It seems virtually certain that if a single gene exists for mood disorder, its penetrance is incomplete and is likely to be variable. The fact that monozygotic twins are not 100% concordant is just one piece of evidence that indicates a lack of full penetrance. Operationally, this means that individuals are carrying the gene, but not expressing it clinically, a fact that makes it difficult to identify a "case" and reduces the strength of the statistical analyses on which linkage studies depend.

Many other problems are likely to continue to plague the search for a "bipolar gene" or a "depression gene," including environmental phenocopies (especially a problem for depression), lack of clarity in the boundaries between unipolar and bipolar forms of mood disorder, clinical heterogeneity of the disorders, and probable genetic heterogeneity as well. Nevertheless, in spite of the difficulties involved, it seems certain that the efforts of molecular geneticists will produce valuable information that will prove useful in understanding the mechanisms that produce mood disorder.

Social and Environmental Factors

Early empirical research focused extensively on the question of whether stressful life events might be considered to "cause" mood disorders, particularly depression. The questions pursued in this research are supported by intuition and common sense, which suggest that misfortune is likely to produce sadness, particularly if the misfortunes are severe, multiple, or persistent, and if the individual experiencing them is vulnerable or predisposed either because of a genetic vulnerability or a variety of early life experiences rendering him more sensitive to stress, such as the loss of a parent early in life.

The results of this research are conflicting, with some studies suggesting that life events may indeed influence the development of mood disorders, whereas others have found no relationship. These conflicting results are difficult to interpret because many of the studies (both positive and negative) have methodological problems, due largely to the inherent difficulty of the topic being studied. Some of the early explanations of this question approached it from an "either/or" perspective; i.e., psychosocial stressors were conceived of as the *only* cause of depression, and the role of familial predisposition was not explored, or other studies tended to assume that depression could only be caused by biological factors and did not adequately examine the effects of psychosocial stressors.

A major confounder in many of these studies is the effect of depression itself on life events. Once an individual has developed an episode of depression or mania, the occurrence of the illness may produce many changes in psychosocial status, such as divorce, loss of job, or poor academic performance. The prior experience of a depressive episode may color future perceptions as well, making individuals who have had depression perceive relatively neutral life events in a more grim or pathological way. Thus, the only truly rigorous approach to examining the effects of the life events on depression is to assess their frequency *before* the onset of a first episode of depression. Because this approach would require large epidemiological samples, it has never been applied.

Perhaps the best approach to the psychosocial–life-event literature is to return to the intuitive and commonsense perspective with which this research endeavor began. That is, individuals who suffer losses are likely to feel sad or despondent, and a sufficient accumulation of losses may produce demoralization and depression. Indeed, the neuroendocrinologic research described below provides some support for this point of view. It seems distinctly possible that a series of stressful life events could induce a biological reaction, such an outpouring of cortisol that, once initiated, is difficult to stop and could initiate or exacerbate the presence of a true depressive syndrome that is both socially-psychologically and biologically based. One genetic factor that could be transmitted within families might be a tendency to be neurobiologically oversensitive to the effects of psychosocial stress.

The cohort effect for mood disorders, described above, also provides some evidence to suggest that psychosocial factors may have some influence on the development of mood disorders. This cohort effect was observed in a very large collaborative study of more than 1,000 patients suffering from mood disorder, their first-degree relatives, and a sample of normal control subjects. When the subjects in this study were divided into cohorts, based on their current age and their age at onset of depression (for those who had suffered an episode of major depression), it became clear that people in the younger age ranges were having a steadily earlier age at onset and an increased rate of mood disorder.

Various possible explanations for this cohort effect have been explored. It does not appear to be a consequence of better memory in younger individuals, involving a more recent approximation to the actual age at onset in these younger people. Because most of the people with an early onset of mood disorder are in the baby boom generation, it may reflect the impingement of various economic and social stresses on this cohort. The baby boomers have experienced more intensive competition in a variety of spheres than any generation in recent history. Because of the large number of individuals in this cohort, they have had to compete with one another for college admission and jobs in an economy that has declined substantially from that of their parents, due to pressures of recession and inflation. They have been through the "Age of Aquarius" and its subsequent abandonment, seen various cultural heroes assassinated, and participated in the tragedy of the Vietnam War. It is not precisely clear how these various economic and social stresses would produce a high rate of depression in this cohort, but the cohort effect is not consistent with any purely genetic explanation of depression, and it is one piece of evidence suggesting the continuing importance of social and environmental factors to the development of mood disorders.

Psychodynamic and other purely psychological explanations for mood disorders have also been proposed. Depression may be usefully conceptualized as "anger turned inward." Individuals vulnerable to depression may find it socially or ethically unacceptable to overtly express anger that they feel about unfairness or misfortunes that they have experienced; instead of ventilating and eliminating their anger, they instead turn it in against themselves, criticize and castigate themselves, and become depressed. Mania is sometimes conceptualized as a "defense against an underlying depression." According to this view, a person experiencing mania is in fact suffering from an underlying depression, but fights against it psychologically by increasing her energy and activity and artificially elevating her mood. Nevertheless, periods of depression tend to break through from time to time. This interpretation of mania is consistent with some well-observed clinical phenomena, such as the tendency of some manic patients to have bursts of depressive mood in the midst of a manic episode, as well as the tendency of many manic patients to experience depression immediately after a manic episode.

Neurobiology

Neurobiological studies of mood disorders have pursued three major areas of investigation: abnormalities in neurotransmission, abnormalities in neurophysiologic function (especially sleep), and abnormalities in neuroendocrine function.

Abnormalities in Neurotransmission

The catecholamine hypothesis of mood disorders has been widely investigated and is at least partially supported by evidence, although it is undoubtedly an oversimplification. This hypothesis postulates that depression is caused by a deficit of norepinephrine at crucial nerve terminals throughout the brain. It receives its greatest support from what is known about the mechanisms of action of antidepressant drugs.

Many antidepressants, such as imipramine, have been shown to increase the amount of norepinephrine functionally available at nerve terminals by inhibiting reuptake. Other medications that are also effective in treating depression, the monoamine oxidase (MAO) inhibitors, also increase the amounts of norepinephrine available to receptors by inhibiting breakdown of norepinephrine through MAO. Reserpine, known to deplete monoamines, tends to worsen depression. Finally, some studies (but not all) have demonstrated that patients with depression may have a decrease in 3-methoxy-4-hydroxyphenylglycol (MHPG), a major metabolite of brain norepinephrine. There is some suggestion that the finding of decreased MHPG is more prominent in bipolar patients suffering from depression than in unipolar and especially nonmelancholic patients.

Support also exists for serotonin abnormalities in depression. In this case, a functional deficit is also postulated. As for norepinephrine, the bulk of the evidence comes from the studies of the mechanism of drug action and from the study of serotonin metabolites in patients suffering from depression. Some antidepressant medications, particularly the newer ones such as fluoxetine, have potent and relatively specific effects on the serotonin system, further suggesting that dysregulation of serotonin may contribute to the development of depression. Patients suffering from severe depression have also been noted to have a decrease in the major serotonin metabolite, 5-hydroxyindoleacetic acid (5-HIAA) in their cerebrospinal fluid, and decreased numbers of $5\text{-}HT_2$ receptors have been observed in postmortem brains of individuals who have committed suicide.

Dysregulation in the acetylcholine system has also been proposed as another possible neurochemical mechanism for the symptoms of depression. Acetylcholine appears to have an interactive relationship with the monoamine neurotransmitters: increased tone in the monoamine system leads to a decrease in cholinergic tone, and conversely, increased cholinergic tone leads to a decrease in monoamine activity. Administration of cholinergic agonists tends to produce a variety of symptoms characteristic of depression, such as psychomotor slowing or the subjective experience of dysphoria.

Abnormalities in Neurophysiologic Function

Neurophysiologic abnormalities have also been extensively studied in mood disorder. The largest and most consistent body of data involves the use of sleep EEG. Studies have consistently demonstrated that patients suffering from depression have various EEG abnormalities during sleep, including decreased slow-wave sleep (i.e., "deep sleep"), a shortened time before the onset of rapid eye movement (REM) sleep (the period when dreams and nightmares occur), and longer periods of REM sleep, than do normal subjects. These three types of abnormality are referred to as decreased delta sleep, decreased REM latency, and increased REM density, respectively. All these abnormalities in sleep EEG are consistent with the subjective complaints of insomnia that depressed patients express. Depressed patients typically state that they do not sleep very deeply or very long; their decreased delta sleep indicates that they indeed do not sleep as deeply as normal, and the abnormalities in REM sleep are consistent with their complaints of light, fitful sleep.

Abnormalities in Neuroendocrine Function

Neuroendocrine abnormalities have also been extensively explored in patients suffering from depression. Early research in this area suggested that depressed patients had larger quantities of cortisol metabolites in their urine than did normal subjects, as well as higher blood levels of cortisol and abnormal diurnal variation in cortisol production. As the dexamethasone suppression test (DST) became available in internal medicine as a means for assessing patients suffering from Cushing's disease, this test was applied as well to psychiatric patients to explore the possibility of neuroendocrine dysregulation in depression and to attempt to determine the place on the hypothalamic-pituitary-adrenal (HPA) axis where this abnormality might occur.

It is now clear that somewhere between 30 and 70% of patients suffering from severe depression do not show normal suppression of cortisol secretion following the administration of dexamethasone. For a time, an abnormal DST was thought to provide a potential tool in the differential diagnosis of depression, because some psychiatric patients (e.g., schizophrenic patients) appeared rather consistently to have normal DSTs. As more evidence has become available, however, it has become clear that there are relatively high rates of DST nonsuppression in other psychiatric conditions such as anorexia nervosa, dementia, and substance abuse.

Although the DST is no longer widely used as a laboratory test, it is likely that abnormalities in neuroendocrine dysfunction in mood disorders may help illuminate their pathophysiologic mechanisms. Other aspects of the neuroendocrine system have been explored in addition to the HPA axis. Depressed patients have been shown to have a blunting of growth hormone output in response to insulin challenge and a blunted production of thyroid-stimulating hormone (TSH) in response to thyrotropin-releasing hormone (TRH). The abnormalities across various neuroendocrine target organs (e.g., adrenals, pancreas, thyroid) indicate that the abnormalities do not lie in these organs, and the patterns of abnormal response to challenge also suggest that the abnormality is not in the pituitary. More likely, the abnormality is at the level of the hypothalamus, a brain region regulated largely through monoamine neurotransmitters. The neuroendocrine data are consistent with a hypothesis of neurochemical dysregulation in the brain, and specifically a dysregulation within the catecholamine system.

Course and Outcome

Depressive Episode

A depressive episode may begin either suddenly or gradually. The duration of an untreated depressive episode may range from a few weeks to months or even years, although it is suspected that most depressive episodes clear spontaneously within approximately 6 months. Although the prognosis for any single depressive episode is quite good, particularly in view of the efficacy of the various antidepressant medications available, a substantial number of patients may experience a recurrence of depression at some time in their lives. Approximately 20% become chronically depressed.

Suicide is the most serious complication of depression. Approximately 15% of all hospitalized patients suffering from depression die by suicide. Several factors are suggestive of an increase in suicide risk: being divorced or living alone, history of alcohol or drug abuse, age over 40, history of a prior suicide attempt, and an expression of suicidal ideation (particularly when detailed plans have been formulated).

Risk of suicide should always be carefully evaluated in any patient suffering from depression, beginning with a direct inquiry as to whether the patient has considered taking his life. If the patient is considered to be at risk for suicide, he usually should be treated as an inpatient rather than as an outpatient, to minimize the risk. Suicide is discussed in more detail in Chapter 20.

Although suicide is the most important serious complication of depression, other social and personal complications may also occur. Decreased energy, poor concentration, and lack of interest may cause poor performance at school or work. Apathy and decreased sexual interest may lead to marital discord. Patients may attempt to treat depressive symptoms themselves with sedatives, alcohol, or stimulants, thereby initiating problems with drug and alcohol abuse.

Manic Episode

The onset of mania is frequently abrupt, although it may begin gradually over the course of a few weeks. The episodes usually last from a few days to months. They tend to be briefer and to have a more abrupt termination than depressive episodes. Although the prognosis for any particular episode is reasonably good, especially with the availability of effective treatments such as lithium and antipsychotics, the risk for recurrence is significant. Not uncommonly, an episode of mania is followed by an episode of depression. Some patients with bipolar disorder recover relatively fully, but a substantial subset continue to have chronic mild instability of mood, particularly recurrent episodes of mild depression.

The complications of mania are primarily social: marital discord, divorce, business difficulties, financial extravagance, and sexual indiscretions. Drug or alcohol abuse may occur during a manic episode. When mania is relatively severe, the patient may be almost completely incapacitated and require protection from the consequences of poor judgment or hyperactivity. In the past, this condition sometimes resulted in death from physical exhaustion. The excessive activity level continues to be a significant risk in patients with cardiac problems. A manic syndrome can switch rapidly to depression, with the risk for suicide being heightened when the patient becomes remorsefully aware of previous behavior. Patients rarely commit suicide while manic.

Differential Diagnosis

Depression

When evaluating depressed patients, the physician should always consider the possibility that the illness may result from some specific organic factor that induces a depressive syndrome, including sedatives, tranquilizers, antihypertensives, oral contraceptives, and glucocorticoids. Physical illnesses such as myxedema or systemic lupus erythematosus may also present with prominent depressive symptoms. If the depressive syndrome is judged to be largely the result of a specific organic agent or dysfunction that affects the central nervous system, the disorder is considered to be an organic mood disorder and is classified among the organic mental disorders. Treatment usually involves withdrawing or reducing the organic agent (i.e., medication) or treating the underlying physical illness.

A depressive episode in the elderly may be difficult to distinguish from the various dementias because both may be characterized by apathy, difficulty concentrating, and complaints of poor memory. If the features suggesting a depressive episode are at least as prominent as those suggesting a dementia, it is usually best to treat such patients for depressive symptoms, because a successful treatment will result in the disappearance of symptoms suggesting a possible dementia. Neuroimaging techniques such as single photon emission computer tomography (SPECT) and neuropsychological testing may also assist in the differential diagnosis. (See Chapter 4 for more detail on laboratory assessment and Chapter 6 for a discussion of pseudodementia.)

Dysphoric mood is a common symptom in schizophrenia. A depressive disorder can usually be distinguished from schizophrenia with several different clues. The dysphoric mood in schizophrenia is more typically apathetic or empty, whereas persons suffering from depression usually experience their mood as intensely painful. The onset of schizophrenia is usually more gradual, but patients suffering from schizophrenia also typically have a more severe deterioration in function than do patients suffering from depression. Patients with schizophrenia or major depression may suffer from psychotic symptoms, and thus, severe psychotic depression is often very difficult to distinguish from schizophrenia with acute onset. In this relatively difficult case, it is often best to treat the patient for depression and to observe the course of illness over time. If psychotic symptoms tend to persist after mood symptoms remit, then the diagnosis of schizophrenia or schizoaffective disorder is more likely.

People suffering from bereavement may have many depressive symptoms and experience them for a sufficient duration to meet criteria for a depressive episode. Nevertheless, such patients are not diagnosed as having depressive disorder, because the presence of the symptoms is considered to be a normal reaction. Further, the symptoms are usually self-limiting, clear spontaneously over time, have a different cause and prognosis than major depression, and usually do not respond to antidepressant medication. Consequently, such individuals are referred to as having *uncomplicated bereavement*.

Mania

Various medications (e.g., amphetamines or steroids) and various physical illnesses (e.g., Cushing's disease, frontal lobe tumor, or multiple sclerosis) may mimic the manic syndrome. As in the case of depression, an underlying organic cause for the symptoms should be carefully explored.

Among psychiatric conditions, the most important differential diagnosis is between mania and schizophrenia. Several features are useful in making this distinction. Personality and general functioning are usually satisfactory before and after an episode of manic disorder, even though mild disturbances in mood may occur. Although manic episodes may present with disorganized speech that is indistinguishable from the speech sometimes observed in schizophrenia, speech abnormalities in mania are always accompanied by a disturbance in mood and usually by overactivity and physical agitation. Although manic patients may experience delusions or hallucinations, these typically reflect the underlying disturbance in mood. (Mood-incongruent psychotic symptoms, of course, occur occasionally, making the differential diagnosis more difficult.)

It may be particularly difficult to distinguish an irritable and angry manic patient from an excited patient with paranoid schizophrenia, based on a simple cross-sectional evaluation. As in the case of a difficult differential diagnosis of depression, it is usually best to defer definitive diagnosis and to treat the patient as if manic, because mania carries a better prognosis.

Additional guidelines that make the diagnosis of manic episode more likely include a family history of affective disorder, good premorbid adjustment, and a previous episode of affective disorder from which there was complete or substantial recovery. On the other hand, if psychotic symptoms persist in the absence of an abnormality in mood, the diagnosis of schizophrenia or schizoaffective disorder is more likely.

Clinical Management

Good psychopharmacologic management is fundamental to the treatment of mood disorders. Both depression and mania usually respond remarkably well to the wide array of medications that are available. A more detailed discussion of antidepressant and antimanic medications and ECT appears in Chapter 24.

In the management of depression, the clinician's first decision must be whether the patient has a transient situational disturbance or a chronic personality problem (e.g., borderline personality) that mimics a major depressive episode (indicating that psychotherapy would be more effective), or whether he has a syndrome that is likely to respond to medications. DSM-III-R criteria are helpful in this regard, but not all patients who meet criteria will require medication. Some features suggestive of a good response to antidepressant medications include the presence of "vegetative" symptoms such as insomnia or weight loss, meeting criteria for melancholia, history of prior episodes of depression (particularly if they have responded well to antidepressants), severe incapacitating symptoms, relatively acute onset of symptoms, and a family history of mood disorder.

Various medications are available to treat depression: tricyclics, MAO inhibitors,

---

Recommendations for management of depressed patients

1. Establish a hopeful, optimistic tone at the initial interview.

   - Assess the severity of the depressive syndrome, remembering that there may be individual and cultural differences in the way depression is experienced and expressed.
   - Don't attempt extensive psychological probing when the patient is deeply depressed.
   - Determine suicide risk initially, and reassess frequently.

2. Treat severe to moderate depression aggressively with somatic therapy.

   - Severely depressed or suicidal patients may require hospitalization.
   - Severely depressed outpatients may need frequent (e.g., twice weekly) brief (e.g., 10- to 15-minute) contacts for support and medication management until their depression lifts.
   - Most patients will require at least 16–20 weeks of maintenance medication after an initial episode, and thereafter should be given a trial of decreasing or discontinuing the medication. If symptoms reemerge, medication should be reinstituted.

3. Determine whether psychosocial stressors are present that are contributing to the depressed mood, and counsel the patient on ways to cope with them.

4. Depressed patients tend to "get down" on themselves because they have been depressed; help patients learn to abandon negative or self-deprecating attitudes toward their depression through cognitive therapy or other psychotherapeutic techniques.

---

and several newer antidepressants. In addition, ECT may be used for severe depressions, particularly if the patient is suicidal, and lithium is often used as a maintenance medication to prevent relapse in patients with a history of recurrent depression.

Many antidepressants are currently available. These medications vary in their side effects and their pharmacologic mechanism of action. They may be thought of as existing on a continuum, ranging from those that are more sedating (e.g., amitriptyline, doxepin, nortriptyline) to those that are less sedating and that may even have psychostimulant effects (e.g., desipramine, fluoxetine). In general, the more sedating antidepressants tend to be anticholinergic, and the less sedating to be less anticholinergic. In addition, among the older classic antidepressants such as amitriptyline, those that are more sedating have more mixed effects on both norepinephrine and serotonin reuptake, whereas the less sedating antidepressants tend to affect the norepinephrine system more exclusively. Some of the newer antidepressants, such as trazodone and fluoxetine, appear to have their primary effect on the serotonin system.

Although the neuropharmacology of antidepressants is increasingly understood and may eventually lead to "rational" approaches to treating depression as our knowledge of specific neurochemical mechanisms in individual patients increases, at present the choice of an antidepressant medication is largely empirical. Thus, clinicians typically select an antidepressant based primarily on the patient's presenting complaints. Patients with insomnia or anorexia may do better with more sedating medications, perhaps largely because they will begin to sleep better almost immediately, whereas patients with lethargy and lower levels of tension and anxiety may prefer the less sedating medications such as imipramine or fluoxetine. Fluoxetine, in particular, has a specific tendency to produce insomnia and weight loss, making it a useful drug for those patients with "atypical" depressions characterized by hypersomnia and weight gain.

Most antidepressant medications have a relatively long half-life, as well as a relatively long latency for clinical response. The long half-life permits physicians to prescribe antidepressants in a single daily dose, which is usually taken at bedtime for the more sedating antidepressants, but may be taken in the morning for the less sedating.

Patients should be warned about the various side effects of antidepressants, which some patients often find particularly discomforting. It is helpful to explain to the patient that she may feel worse before she feels better, and that she should not expect to see any clear response for 2–4 weeks, although patients sometimes do feel a slight improvement of some symptoms shortly after beginning their medication regimen. This message offers some hope, but it also encourages patients to stick with the medication even if they find the side effects unpleasant. It is also helpful to convey the fact that most patients who present with depression do respond eventually to some type of antidepressant medication and obtain relief from their symptoms.

The specific dose of antidepressant varies depending on the antidepressant, the patient's body size and ability to tolerate side effects, and the severity of the depression. For most patients, it is best to begin with a moderate dose (e.g., 25–50 mg of amitriptyline at bedtime for the first few days) and then to titrate the dosage upward after the patient's ability to tolerate side effects has been assessed. This approach is particularly important in the management of outpatients, who may find it difficult to remain alert at work or while studying if the medications are extremely sedating. Treatment can be more aggressive in inpatients, because they are not attempting to maintain a work schedule, and potentially dangerous side effects on the cardiovascular system can be monitored closely.

Because some antidepressants (e.g., nortriptyline) appear to have a therapeutic window, blood levels may be useful in monitoring dosages. A more detailed description of this issue, and of the pharmacology of antidepressants, is provided in Chapter 24.

If patients do not respond to a specific antidepressant within 4–6 weeks, a clinical trial of another antidepressant or recourse to ECT may be appropriate. This decision will be guided by the clinical picture of the patient. If the syndrome is severe and worsening, then ECT may be chosen. If the patient shows more characterologic or atypical features, a MAO inhibitor may be tried. Most often, however, the clinician will choose to try at least one other antidepressant, often with a different pharmacologic profile (e.g., a different balance of effects on norepinephrine, serotonin, and acetylcholine) from the previous one to which the patient has not responded. Before trying a new medication, the clinician should also establish that the patient is indeed complying with the regimen prescribed by checking blood levels.

Patients who respond to a given antidepressant should usually be maintained on it for at least 16–20 months. Thereafter, the clinician may choose to attempt to discontinue the medication, while monitoring the patient closely. Because some antidepressants produce undesirable side effects such as weight gain, and because conservative prescription of medications is always a good clinical guideline, discontinuance should almost always be attempted in patients who do not have a history of recurrent depression. The medication should be discontinued gradually because many patients experience some mild withdrawal effects if tricyclics are discontinued abruptly. In particular, insomnia is a problem. Patients sometimes subjectively experience these withdrawal symptoms as a recurrence or relapse. Other symptoms that occur on abrupt withdrawal of antidepressants include increased tension and nervousness, nightmares, and gastrointestinal symptoms such as nausea or even vomiting.

Patients with recurrent depressions will often need long-term maintenance. The maintenance dosage can sometimes be reduced from the one originally required to achieve a therapeutic effect (e.g., from 200 to 100 mg of imipramine at bedtime). Some patients benefit from lithium augmentation of antidepressants to enhance therapeutic response. Lithium prophylaxis to prevent depressive relapse may be particularly useful for those patients who have had three or four previous episodes of depression. Maintenance lithium dosages may range from 600 to 1,200 mg per day, and blood levels are usually maintained in the 0.6–0.8 meq/L range.

MAO inhibitors may be used to treat patients who do not respond to tricyclic antidepressants, or who are unable to tolerate their side effects. These medications should be used with caution, because they have potentially more dangerous side effects and interactions than do the tricyclics. Nevertheless, for a subset of patients, MAO inhibitors may be useful. These patients tend to be those characterized by "atypical depression," with symptoms such as hypersomnia, increased appetite, and personality difficulties such as rejection sensitivity.

ECT is the treatment of choice for some patients suffering from severe depression. Methods for administering and monitoring ECT, as well as its side effects, are described in more detail in Chapter 24. In general, indications for ECT include very severe depression, high potential for suicide, cardiovascular disease (which may preclude use of antidepressants), and pregnancy. ECT is highly effective in producing a rapid remission of depressive symptoms. Response occurs relatively consistently in approximately 80% of patients. Patients will need maintenance antidepressant treatment after the course of ECT is completed.

Lithium carbonate is the first-line treatment for manic disorder. Mania usually is a severe syndrome that requires hospitalization, and consequently, aggressive treatment can be initiated in the closely supervised hospital environment. Patients are typically placed on a dose of 1,200–2,400 mg per day, with a goal of achieving serum blood levels between 0.9 and 1.4 meq/L. Blood levels are usually monitored at least twice weekly at first. If the patient is severely agitated and psychotic,

---

Recommendations for management of manic patients

1. Use somatic therapies aggressively to treat manic symptoms as rapidly as possible.

2. Follow the patient closely as the mania "breaks" to determine whether a subsequent depression is emerging; if this occurs, treat it with antidepressants as needed.

3. After an episode of mania, patients should be placed on maintenance lithium; typically they will continue to take lithium for a number of years, and perhaps for the remainder of their life, to prevent subsequent relapses.

4. Patients should be followed regularly even when they are stable, to ensure continued compliance with lithium prophylaxis and to monitor blood levels.

5. Manic episodes can have devastating personal, social, and economic consequences; patients will usually require (at a minimum) supportive psychotherapy to help them cope with these consequences and maintain their self-esteem.

6. Family members should be provided with psychological support, as needed, and with educational materials to help them understand the disorder, its symptoms, and its need for continued treatment.

7. Patients with bipolar illness are often appreciative of being told about the "good side" of their illness: its association with creativity and high achievement.

---

antipsychotics should be added to lithium almost immediately. Antipsychotic dosages are typically in the range of 300–1,000 chlorpromazine equivalents. As the psychotic symptoms or agitation clear, the antipsychotic medications can be rapidly discontinued. Manic patients will almost always require maintenance lithium.

Patients who do not respond to lithium or antipsychotics may be given a variety of alternative treatments. ECT is also highly effective for mania, and it is indicated as a treatment of choice in the subset of patients who cannot be given lithium or antipsychotics (e.g., patients who are pregnant or who have severe cardiovascular disease). The most effective alternative medication used to treat mania is carbamazepine. It has consistently proved effective in a subset of lithium nonresponders. Treatment of mania is more fully explored in Chapter 24.

Experiencing an episode of mood disorder is often a major blow to the patient's confidence and self-esteem. Consequently, most patients will require some supportive psychotherapy in addition to whatever medications are prescribed. During the acute episode, the clinician will typically let the depressive "wound" begin to heal, but as the patient recovers, the clinician may begin to review with the patient the various social and psychological factors that may be causing distress or that may have worsened as a consequence of depression. Work, school performance, and interpersonal relationships may all be impaired because of a mood disorder. It is important to help the patient assess these problems, to recognize that his illness rather than he himself is responsible, and to instill confidence that he can now begin to restore and repair whatever injuries have occurred as a consequence of his episode of mood disorder.

Some patients will respond well to this type of brief supportive psychotherapy used as an adjunct to medications. Others may require more intensive psychotherapy depending on their personality structure, social situation, disability induced by the mood disorder, and environmental supports. These psychotherapies may include psychodynamic psychotherapy, cognitive therapy, or behavior therapy. The various psychotherapies are described in more detail in Chapter 23.

Some patients may respond to psychotherapy alone. In particular, a patient with a brief, situation-based depression may respond well to crisis intervention. A person presenting with depressive symptoms who is attempting to cope with a stressful life event, such as separation or divorce, may have a relatively painful and persistent mood disorder for weeks to months, yet not require the use of medications. These patients may also benefit substantially from supportive and psychodynamic therapy. Patients with chronic mild depression (e.g., dysthymia) may also be more likely to benefit from a treatment regimen that emphasizes psychotherapy as its primary tool. In particular, these patients are likely to benefit from cognitive therapy, behavior therapy, and long-term psychodynamic therapy.

Bibliography

Allen MG, Cohen S, Pollin W, et al: Affective illness in veteran twins: a diagnostic review. Am J Psychiatry 131:1234–1239, 1974

Andreasen NC: Concepts, diagnosis and classification, in Handbook of Affective Disorders. Edited by Pakel ES. New York, Guilford, 1982, pp 24–44

Andreasen NC, Rice J, Endicott J, et al: Familial rates of affective disorder: a report from the National Institute of Mental Health Collaborative Study. Arch Gen Psychiatry 44:461–469, 1987

Angst J, Frey R, Lohmeyer B, et al: Bipolar manic-depressive psychoses: results of a genetic investigation. Hum Genet 55:237–254, 1980

Asberg M, Thoren P, Traskman L, et al: 'Serotonin depression'—a biochemical subgroup within the affective disorders? Science 191:478–480, 1976

Baron M: Linkage between an X-chromosome marker (deutan colorblindness) and bipolar affective illness. Arch Gen Psychiatry 24:721–727, 1977

Baron M, Risch N, Hamburger R, et al: Genetic linkage between an X-chromosome marker and bipolar affective illness. Nature 326:289–292, 1987

Baxter LR, Schwartz JM, Phelps ME, et al: Reduction of prefrontal cortex glucose metabolism common to three types of depression. Arch Gen Psychiatry 46:243–250, 1989

Bertelsen A: A Danish twin study of manic-depressive disorders, in Origin, Prevention and Treatment of Affective Disorders. Edited by Schou M, Stromgren E. London, Academic, 1979, pp 227–239

Black DW, Nasrallah A: Hallucinations and delusions in 1,715 patients with unipolar and bipolar affective disorders. Psychopathology 22:28–34, 1989

Black DW, Winokur G, Nasrallah A: Treatment and outcome in secondary depression: a naturalistic study of 1087 patients. J Clin Psychiatry 48:438–441, 1987

Cadoret RJ: Evidence of genetic inheritance of primary affective disorder in adoptees. Am J Psychiatry 135:463–466, 1978

Carney MWP, Roth M, Garside RF: The diagnosis of depressive syndromes and the prediction of ECT response. Br J Psychiatry 111:659–674, 1966

Carroll BJ: The dexamethasone suppression test for melancholia. Br J Psychiatry 140:292–304, 1982

Carroll B, Curtis CG, Mendels J: Neuroendocrine regulation in depression. Arch Gen Psychiatry 33:1039–1044, 1976

Clayton PJ, Halikas JA, Maurice WL: The depression of widowhood. Br J Psychiatry 120:71–77, 1972

Coppen AJ, Doogan DP: Serotonin and its place in the pathogenesis of depression. J Clin Psychiatry 49 (suppl 8):4–11, 1988

Davis JM, Koslow SH, Gibbons RD, et al: Cerebrospinal fluid and urinary biogenic amines in depressed patients and healthy controls. Arch Gen Psychiatry 45:705–717, 1988

Gershon ES, Bunney WE, Leckman JF, et al: The inheritance of affective disorders: a review of data and hypotheses. Behav Genet 6:227–261, 1976

Gillin JC, Byerley WA: Sleep: a neurobiological window on affective disorders. Trends in Neuroscience 8:537–542, 1985

Glassman AH: Idoleamines and affective disorders. Psychosom Med 31:107–114, 1969

Gold PW, Rubinow DR: Neuropeptide function in affective illness: corticotropin-releasing hormone and somatostatin as model systems, in Psychopharmacology: The Third Generation of Progress. Edited by Meltzer HY. New York, Raven, 1987, pp 617–627

Gold PW, Goodwin FK, Chrousos GP: Clinical and biochemical manifestation of depression: relation to the neurobiology of stress (Parts 1 & 2). N Engl J Med 319:348–353, 1988

Harvald B, Hauge M: Genetics and the epidemiology of chronic diseases (PHS Publication No 1163). Edited by Neal JV, Shaw W, Shull WJ. Washington, DC, DHEW, 1965, pp 61–76

Huston PE, Locher LM: Manic-depressive psychosis: course when treated and untreated with electric shock. Archives of Neurology and Psychiatry 50:37–48, 1948

Jimerson DC: Role of dopamine mechanisms in the affective disorders, in Psychopharmacology: The Third Generation of Progress. Edited by Meltzer HY. New York, Raven, 1987, pp 505–511

Kallmann FJ: Genetic principles in manic-depressive psychosis, in Depression: Proceedings of the American Psychopathologic Association. Edited by Zubin J, Hoch P. New York, Grune & Stratton, 1954, pp 1–24

Keller MB, Lavori PW, Rice J, et al: The persistent risk of chronicity and recurrent episodes of non-biopolar major depressive disorder: a prospective follow-up. Am J Psychiatry 143:24–28, 1986

Kendell RE: The Classification of Depressive Illnesses. London, Oxford University Press, 1968

Klein DF: Endogenomorphic depression: a conceptual and terminological revision. Arch Gen Psychiatry 34:447–454, 1974

Klerman GL, Lavori PW, Rice J, et al: Birth cohort trends in rates of major depressive disorder among relatives of patients with affective disorder. Arch Gen Psychiatry 42:689–693, 1985

Kraepelin E: Manic-Depressive Insanity and Paranoia. Edinburgh, E & S Livingstone, 1921

Krishnan KRR, Manepalli AN, Ritchie JC, et al: Growth hormone-releasing factor stimulation test in depression. Am J Psychiatry 145:90–92, 1988

Kupfer DJ, Thase ME: The use of the sleep laboratory in the diagnosis of affective disorders. Psychiatr Clin North Am 5:3–25, 1983

Luxenberger H: Psychiatrisch-neurologische Zwillings-pathologie. Zentralblatt fur Diagesamte Neurologie und Psychiatrie 14:56–57, 145–180, 1930

Meller W, Kathol RG, Jaeckle RS, et al: HPA axis abnormalities in depressed patients with normal response to the DST. Am J Psychiatry 145:318–324, 1988

Meltzer HY: Lithium mechanisms in bipolar illness and altered intracellular calcium functions. Biol Psychiatry 21:492–510, 1986

Meltzer HY, Lowy MT: The serotonin hypothesis of depression, in Psychopharmacology: The Third Generation of Progress. Edited by Meltzer HY. New York, Raven, 1987, pp 513–526

Mendlewicz J, Rainer JD: Adoption study supporting genetic transmission in manic-depressive illness. Nature 268:327–329, 1977

Nemeroff CB: The role of corticotropin-releasing factor in the pathogenesis of major depression. Pharmacopsychiatry 21:76–82, 1988

Nurnberger JI Jr, Gershon ES: Genetics of affective disorders, in Neurobiology of Mood Disorders. Edited by Post RM, Ballenger JC. Baltimore, MD, Williams & Wilkins, 1984, pp 76–101

Pakel ES (ed): Handbook of Affective Disorders. New York, Guilford, 1982

Post RM, Ballenger JC: Neurobiology of Mood Disorders. Baltimore, MD, Williams & Wilkins, 1984

Rosanoff AJ, Handy L, Plesset IR: The etiology of manic-depressive syndromes with special reference to their occurrence in twins. Am J Psychiatry 91:725–762, 1935

Schildkraut JJ: The catecholamine hypothesis of affective disorder: a review of supporting evidence. Am J Psychiatry 122:509–522, 1965

Schildkraut JJ, Orsulak PJ, LaBrie RA, et al: Toward a biochemical classification of depressive disorders, II: application of multivariate discriminant function analysis to data on urinary catecholamines and metabolites. Arch Gen Psychiatry 35:1436–1439, 1978

Schildkraut JJ, Orsulak PJ, Schatzburg AF, et al: Toward a biochemical classification of depressive disorders, I: differences in urinary excretion of MHPG and other catecholamine metabolites in clinically defined subtypes of depression. Arch Gen Psychiatry 35:1427–1433, 1978

Siever LJ, Davis KL: Overview: toward a dysregulation hypothesis of depression. Am J Psychiatry 142:1017–1031, 1985

Slater E: Psychotic and neurotic illness in twins (Medical Research Council Special Report Series No 278). London, Her Majesty's Stationery Office, 1953

Stahl SM: Regulation of neurotransmitter receptors by desipramine and other antidepressant drugs: the neurotransmitter receptor hypothesis of antidepressant action. J Clin Psychiatry 45:37–44, 1984

Weissman MM, Kidd KK, Prusoff BA: Variability in rates of affective disorders in relatives of depressed and normal probands. Arch Gen Psychiatry 39:1397–1403, 1982

Weissman MM, Leaf PJ, Bruce ML, et al: The epidemiology of dysthymia in five communities: rates, risks, comorbidity, and treatment. Am J Psychiatry 145:815–819, 1988

Whybrow PC, Akiskal HS, McKinney WT Jr: Mood Disorders: Toward a New Psychobiology. New York, Plenum, 1984

Winokur G, Clayton P, Reich T: Manic Depressive Illness. St. Louis, MO, CV Mosby, 1969

Winokur G, Black DW, Nasrallah A: Depressions secondary to other psychiatric disorders and medical illnesses. Am J Psychiatry 154:233–237, 1988

Self-assessment Questions

1. What are the nine symptoms used to define a major depressive episode in DSM-III-R?
2. What is the difference between mood-congruent and mood-incongruent delusions?
3. What are some symptoms that typically predict a good response to antidepressants?
4. What is the lifetime prevalence for bipolar disorder and for (unipolar) major depressive disorder?
5. Why have variable rates been reported for depression?
6. What is the "cohort effect"?
7. Review the evidence that suggests that mood disorders are familial and may be genetic.
8. Which neurotransmitter systems have been proposed to be dysfunctional in mood disorders?
9. What is the evidence indicating that neuroendocrine abnormalities occur in patients with mood disorders?
10. What is the difference between bereavement and a depressive episode?
11. Describe the first-line treatments for depression, as well as the various alternative treatments and their indications.
12. Describe the appropriate program of treatment for a manic episode. What alternative treatments are available?

Chapter 10
Anxiety Disorders

I stood stunned, my hair rose,
the voice stuck in my throat.

Virgil

Unlike depression, a syndrome recognized for centuries, the syndrome of anxiety has been recognized only in relatively recent times. Da Costa was first credited with describing anxiety as a disorder that he called "irritable heart" in the *American Journal of Medical Sciences* in 1871. Because chest pain, palpitations, and dizziness were the main symptoms of this syndrome, Da Costa thought the disorder was due to a functional cardiac disturbance characterized by hypersensitivity and sympathetic overreactivity. Physicians frequently diagnosed this syndrome in patients undergoing significant stress, such as during warfare. In fact, Da Costa first described this syndrome in a soldier who developed the disorder during the Civil War. Shortly thereafter, the condition was identified in many other settings, and it was variously referred to as "soldier's heart," the "effort syndrome," or "neurocirculatory asthenia."

While internists were emphasizing cardiovascular aspects of the anxiety syndrome, psychiatrists and neurologists became more concerned with its psychological aspects. Freud was responsible for recognizing anxiety as the core symptom in the syndrome and for introducing the term *anxiety neurosis.* Freud's conceptualization brought the patient's inner subjective feelings to the forefront, emphasizing the sense of fearfulness, terror, panic, and impending doom.

The relative relationship of physical and psychological symptoms of anxiety has remained a matter of debate. Early in the 20th century, psychologist William James

227

Table 10-1. Anxiety disorders

Panic disorder
  With agoraphobia
  Without agoraphobia
Agoraphobia
Social phobia
	Simple phobia
	Obsessive-compulsive disorder (see
	  Chapter 11)
	Generalized anxiety disorder
	Posttraumatic stress disorder

postulated that the psychological experience of anxiety is nothing more than an awareness of the physical symptoms of anxiety, thus implying that the physical experience is primary. Freud, on the other hand, believed that the psychological symptoms of anxiety were primary and led to the development of physical symptoms. Whichever is primary, the relationship is probably interactive once the symptoms have begun.

Because nervousness and fear are common human emotions that nearly everyone has experienced at one time or another, defining the boundaries of anxiety disorder is a matter of debate. It is important that physicians recognize the difference between pathological anxiety and anxiety as a normal or adaptive response. Feeling anxiety when being attacked by a grizzly bear is a normal and natural response and prepares the individual for the classic "flight or fight" response. Feeling anxiety before taking an examination or giving a talk is also normal and adaptive as long as the alertness or tension does not become excessive or handicapping. Even classic phobias, such as fear of heights, may reflect some primitive adaptive response. The potentially adaptive mechanism of anxiety or arousal, so useful in humans in coping with the stresses and threats of life, becomes a disorder only when anxiety becomes crippling or disabling.

Until 1980, panic disorder and generalized anxiety were classified together as *anxiety neurosis*, the term introduced by Freud. In DSM-III, anxiety neurosis was divided, as it had been discovered that panic disorder and generalized anxiety disorder were each associated with a different natural history, familial aggregation, and response to treatment. At the same time, a new diagnosis, posttraumatic stress disorder (PTSD), was introduced. In this chapter, we review panic disorders, agoraphobia, simple and social phobias, generalized anxiety disorder, and PTSD. Although obsessive-compulsive disorder (OCD) is classified as an anxiety disorder, there is considerable uncertainty about its true relationship to the other anxiety disorders. OCD is discussed in Chapter 11. The anxiety disorders are presented in Table 10-1.

Panic Disorder and Agoraphobia

Panic disorder consists of recurrent panic (or anxiety) attacks occurring at a frequency of four per month, or a single panic attack that is followed by at least 4 weeks of fear of having another attack. By definition, at some time during the disturbance, one or more panic attacks that occurred were unexpected and not

Table 10-2. DSM-III-R criteria for panic disorder

A. At some time during the disturbance, one or more panic attacks (discrete periods of intense fear or discomfort) have occurred that were 1) unexpected, i.e., did not occur immediately before or on exposure to a situation that almost always caused anxiety, and 2) not triggered by situations in which the person was the focus of others' attention.

B. Either four attacks, as defined in criterion A, have occurred within a 4-week period, or one or more attacks have been followed by a period of at least a month of persistent fear of having another attack.

C. At least four of the following symptoms developed during at least one of the attacks:
   1. Shortness of breath (dyspnea) or smothering sensations
   2. Dizziness, unsteady feelings, or faintness
   3. Palpitations or accelerated heart rate (tachycardia)
   4. Trembling or shaking
   5. Sweating
   6. Choking
   7. Nausea or abdominal distress
   8. Depersonalization or derealization
   9. Numbness or tingling sensations (paresthesias)
   10. Flushes (hot flashes) or chills
   11. Chest pain or discomfort
   12. Fear of dying
   13. Fear of going crazy or of doing something uncontrolled

   Note: Attacks involving four or more symptoms are panic attacks; attacks involving fewer than four symptoms are limited symptom attacks.

D. During at least some of the attacks, at least four of the C symptoms developed suddenly and increased in intensity within 10 minutes of the beginning of the first C symptom noticed in the attack.

E. It cannot be established that an organic factor initiated and maintained the disturbance, e.g., amphetamine or caffeine intoxications, hyperthyroidism.

Note: Mitral valve prolapse may be an associated condition, but does not preclude a diagnosis of panic disorder.

---

triggered by certain specific situations that might cause anxiety in normal persons, such as being robbed at gunpoint. Additionally, during the attacks, at least 4 of 13 characteristic symptoms have occurred, such as shortness of breath, dizziness, palpitations, or trembling or shaking. Diagnostic criteria for panic disorder are presented in Table 10-2.

Agoraphobia is a disabling complication of panic disorder characterized by phobic avoidance. The term *agoraphobia* derives from Greek, meaning "fear of the marketplace," and although many people with agoraphobia are uncomfortable in shops and markets, their true fear is to be separated from their source of security. The agoraphobic person may fear having a panic attack in a public place and embarrassing himself or herself, or having a panic attack and not being near a family physician or medical clinic. Agoraphobics tend to avoid crowded places, such as shops, restaurants, theaters, and church. Many have difficulty driving long distances (i.e., being away from help should a panic attack occur), crossing bridges, and

Table 10-3. Common situations that either provoked or relieved anxiety in 100 agoraphobics

Situations that provoke anxiety		Situations that relieve anxiety	
Situation	%	Situation	%
Standing in line at a store	96	Being accompanied by spouse	85
An appointment	91	Sitting near the door in church, etc.	76
Feeling trapped at hairdresser, etc.	89	Focusing thoughts on something else	63
Increasing distance from home	87	Taking the dog, baby carriage, etc., along	62
Particular places in neighborhood	66	Being accompanied by friend	60
Cloudy, depressing weather	56	Reassuring self	52
		Wearing sunglasses	36

Source. Adapted from Burns LE, Thorpe GL: The epidemiology of fears and phobias (with particular reference to the National Survey of Agoraphobics). J Int Med Res 5 (suppl 5):1–7, 1977.

driving through tunnels. Many insist on being accompanied to places they might otherwise avoid. Severe agoraphobia leads many patients to become housebound. Common situations that either provoke or relieve anxiety in people with agoraphobia are presented in Table 10-3.

Although they were originally conceptualized as separate disorders, evidence suggests that panic disorder and agoraphobia represent a single illness. Diagnostic criteria for agoraphobia are presented in Table 10-4.

The following case example illustrates both panic disorder and agoraphobia.

Susan, a 32-year-old housewife, presented to the outpatient clinic for evaluation of anxiety. She reported the onset of panic attacks at age 13, which she remembered as terrifying. She could still remember her first attack, which occurred during a history class. "I was just sitting in class when my heart began to beat wildly, my skin began to tingle, and I began feeling shaky. There was no need for me to feel nervous," she observed. For the next 19 years, attacks had been chronic and unrelenting, occurring up to 6–10 times daily. To Susan, the panic was devastating: "I grew up all those years feeling that I wasn't quite normal."

Soon after the onset of panic attacks, Susan developed phobic avoidance of crowded places, particularly disliking shopping centers, grocery stores, movie theaters, and restaurants. As a religious person, she attended church, but would sit in a pew near

Table 10-4. DSM-III-R criteria for agoraphobia without history of panic disorder

A. Agoraphobia: Fear of being in places or situations from which escape might be difficult (or embarrassing) or in which help might not be available in the event of suddenly developing a symptom(s) that could be incapacitating or extremely embarrassing. Examples include: dizziness or falling, depersonalization or derealization, loss of bowel or bladder control, vomiting, or cardiac distress. As a result of this fear, the person either restricts travel or needs a companion when away from home, or else endures agoraphobic situations despite intense anxiety. Common agoraphobic situations include being outside the home alone, being in a crowd or standing in line, being on a bridge, and traveling in a bus, train, or car.

B. Has never met the criteria for panic disorder.

an exit. Her agoraphobic symptoms waxed and waned over the years, and although she had never been housebound, at times she would insist on having her husband or a friend accompany her when she had to go shopping.

Susan had never sought treatment before and thought that no one could help her. She had gone to emergency rooms for evaluation, but had never been diagnosed with panic disorder. As Susan got older, she tried to ignore her feelings, believing that to admit them was a sign of weakness. She never told her husband of 15 years about her panic.

Susan was placed on an experimental medication (fluvoxamine, a novel antidepressant) and within 1 month was free of panic attacks and within 3 months no longer had agoraphobic symptoms. At a 6-month follow-up, she remained free of all anxiety-related symptoms. Susan reported feeling like a new person and felt much better about herself.

Epidemiology and Clinical Findings

According to the Epidemiologic Catchment Area study, 2–3% of women and 0.5–1.5% of men have panic disorder. The prevalence of agoraphobia is slightly higher. Panic disorder and agoraphobia each typically have an onset in the mid 20s, although age at onset may vary. Mean age at onset in panic disorder is 27 years, and 79% of panic disorder patients develop the disorder before age 30 years.

There are usually no precipitating stressors before the onset of panic disorder or agoraphobia. Many patients, however, will report that panic attacks came on after an illness or accident, the breakup of a relationship, postpartum, or after taking mind-altering drugs, such as LSD or marijuana.

The initial panic attack is generally alarming and may provoke a visit to a nearby emergency room where routine laboratory work including an electrocardiogram are inevitably found to be normal. The patient is usually told that the symptoms are due to "nerves."

If the panic attacks recur, the patient may be referred for an extensive medical workup. When no obvious physical cause for the anxiety is found, a psychiatrist is generally consulted. Typically, the psychiatrist's consultation is preceded by six or seven other evaluations, especially by cardiologists, neurologists, or gastroenterologists, depending on the target symptoms that the patient develops (see Table 10-5).

Attacks generally have a sudden onset, peak within minutes, and last 5–30 minutes. Although many patients claim that their attacks may last hours or even all day, it is likely that their continuing symptoms represent a recurrence of panic, or mild symptoms that persist after an attack. Common symptoms in panic disorder are presented in Table 10-6.

Etiology and Pathophysiology

Neurobiological models are currently the most popular ones used to explain the etiology of panic disorder. Possible biological disturbances underlying panic may

Table 10-5.   Specialists consulted depending on target symptoms of panic disorder

Specialist	Target symptoms
Pulmonologist	Shortness of breath; hyperventilation; smothering sensations
Dermatologist	Sweating; cold, clammy hands
Cardiologist	Palpitations; chest pain or discomfort
Neurologist	Tingling and numbness; imbalance; dizziness; derealization or depersonalization; tremulousness or jitteriness; lightheadedness
Otolaryngologist	Choking sensation; dry mouth
Gynecologist	Hot flashes; sweating
Gastroenterologist	Nausea; diarrhea; abdominal pain or discomfort (i.e., "butterflies")
Urologist	Frequent urination

include increased catecholamine levels in the central nervous system, an abnormality in the locus coeruleus (an area of the brain stem regulating alertness), carbon dioxide hypersensitivity, disturbances in lactate metabolism, and abnormalities of the gamma-aminobutyric acid (GABA) neurotransmitter system. Experimental data support each of these disturbances to some extent, but none explain all of the manifestations of panic disorder. Many of the competing theories are based on the ability of different substances to induce panic attacks, such as isoproterenol (a beta-antagonist), carbon dioxide, or sodium lactate. Recent theories highlight the role of GABA, which slows neurotransmission.

Genetic studies are compatible with biological models of panic disorder. Family studies have found a higher rate of panic disorder in relatives of probands with panic disorder than in relatives of normal subjects. For example, one study found a morbidity risk for panic disorder of 25% among first-degree relatives of patients with panic disorder compared to only 2% among normal control subjects. Early

Table 10-6.   Common symptoms reported by patients with panic disorder and agoraphobia

Symptoms	%	Symptoms	%
Fearfulness or worry	96	Restlessness	80
Nervousness	95	Trouble breathing	80
Palpitations	93	Easy fatigability	76
Muscle aching or tension	89	Trouble concentrating	76
Trembling or shaking	89	Irritability	74
Apprehension	83	Trouble sleeping	74
Dizziness or imbalance	82	Chest pain or discomfort	69
Fear of dying or going crazy	81	Numbness or tingling	65
Faintness/lightheadedness	80	Tendency to startle	57
Hot or cold sensations	80	Choking or smothering sensation	54

Source. Adapted from Noyes R, Clancy J, Garvey MJ, et al: Is agoraphobia a variant of panic disorder or a separate illness? Journal of Anxiety Disorders 1:3–13, 1987.

twin studies showed a higher concordance rate for anxiety disorder among monozygotic twins than dizygotic twins, a finding that indicates that genetic influences predominate over environmental influences. However, these early studies were flawed by including a mixed group of anxiety patients. Another study, however, found that anxiety disorders accompanied by panic attacks were five times more frequent in monozygotic than in dizygotic twins. There have been no adoption studies specifically of panic disorder.

Psychodynamic formulations of symptom formation have stressed the importance of *repression*, a common defense mechanism. Repression, Freud believed, is the mental mechanism that holds out of conscious reach all unacceptable sexual thoughts, impulses, or desires. When the psychic energy attached to these unacceptable elements becomes too strong to be held back by repression, they are brought into consciousness in a distorted way and are manifested by anxiety. Learning theorists, meanwhile, hold that anxiety is conditioned by the fear of certain environmental stimuli. For example, anxiety attacks are believed to be a conditioned response to a fearful situation; for example, a car accident might be paired with the experience of heart palpitations and anxiety. Long after the accident, palpitations alone, whether during vigorous exercise or minor emotional upset, become capable in themselves of provoking the conditioned response of an anxiety attack.

Course and Outcome

Different studies of panic disorder tend to describe different outcomes, due in part to the varied criteria used. In an early study, 173 patients were followed over 20 years. On follow-up, nearly 12% of the patients were well, 73% had symptoms, but no or mild disability, and 15% had moderate to severe symptoms. A 5-year follow-up of patients seen on a psychiatric consultation service found that 16% were well and 51% were mildly impaired. These studies suggest that over a long period, it is not unreasonable to expect that 50–70% of anxiety disorder patients will show some amount of improvement, although total remission is uncommon.

Panic disorder patients show increased risk for peptic ulcer and hypertension and higher mortality rates, higher suicide rates, and a larger number of deaths due to circulatory disease than expected.

The course of agoraphobia tends to parallel that of panic disorder, as the two are usually related. It tends to be chronic, but may wax and wane. If panic disorder is treated, the agoraphobia usually improves as well.

A potential complication of panic disorder is the development of alcohol abuse or dependence or use of other substances in an attempt at self-medication. This complication is important to keep in mind when evaluating patients with substance abuse, in order to look for the possibility that their illness began with spontaneous panic attacks or chronic anxiety.

Differential Diagnosis

In the evaluation of panic disorder, it is important to rule out other physical and psychiatric disorders that may mimic panic (see Table 10-7). The physical mani-

Table 10-7.   Differential diagnoses of anxiety

● **Medical illness**	● **Drugs**
Angina	Caffeine
Cardiac arrhythmias	Aminophylline and related compounds
Congestive heart failure	Sympathomimetic agents (e.g.,
Hypoglycemia	decongestants and diet pills)
Hypoxia	Monosodium glutamate
Pulmonary embolism	Psychostimulants and hallucinogens
Severe pain	Alcohol
Thyrotoxicosis	Withdrawal from benzodiazepines and
Carcinoid	other sedative-hypnotics
Pheochromocytoma	Thyroid hormones
Ménière's disease	Neuroleptic drugs

● **Psychiatric illness**

Schizophrenia
Mood disorders
Personality disorders
Adjustment disorder with anxious
  mood

festations of panic disorder are compatible with many physical disorders, for example, hyperthyroidism, hyperparathyroidism, pheochromocytoma, diseases of the vestibular nerve, hypoglycemia, and supraventricular tachycardia.

A relationship between mitral valve prolapse (MVP) and panic disorder has been proposed. MVP is usually a benign condition that occurs more frequently in panic disorder patients than in normal subjects, leading many clinicians to regard panic symptoms as a manifestation of MVP. However, studies have shown that panic disorder patients with or without MVP have a similar natural history, course of illness, and response to treatment. The presence of MVP does not preclude a diagnosis of panic disorder.

Other psychiatric disorders must also be ruled out, particularly depression. Patients with primary depression often have panic attacks and anxiety. Panic attacks may also occur in patients with generalized anxiety, schizophrenia, depersonalization disorder, somatoform disorder, and personality disorders.

Clinical Management

Panic disorder has traditionally been treated with a combination of individual psychotherapy and medication. Although results with psychodynamic psychotherapy have been disappointing, cognitive-behavior psychotherapy, recently applied to panic disorder, appears to have promise in helping patients to accept a more benign interpretation of their distressing symptoms.

Behavior treatment of panic attacks involves breathing exercises and relaxation training. Supportive psychotherapy is helpful in boosting the generally low morale of patients and improving their self-esteem. In addition, the therapist can help the patient to problem solve, recommend books and other reading materials about panic and agoraphobia, and encourage the patient to enter feared situations, such as shopping in a grocery store.

Antidepressants, including tricyclic antidepressants and monoamine oxidase (MAO) inhibitors, are important in the pharmacologic treatment of panic and agoraphobia. MAO inhibitors are generally reserved for patients who do not respond to tricyclics. Depressed mood is not a requirement for these drugs to be effective in blocking panic attacks. The benzodiazepine alprazolam has also proved useful in blocking panic attacks, but has a tendency to become habit forming.

Dosages of tricyclic antidepressants in the range from 150 to 300 mg daily are usually required. Dosages of alprazolam typically range from 2 to 6 mg daily. Once panic attacks have remitted, the patient should remain on medication for 6 months to 1 year to prevent early relapse. After this period, it is advisable to taper the dosage of medication. Although panic disorder tends to recur, up to two-thirds of patients will not relapse immediately after cessation of medication. Some patients will need to take medication chronically, however.

Beta-adrenergic blocking drugs, like propranolol, are reported to be useful in anxiety disorders, but they appear much less effective than antidepressants or alprazolam.

Panic disorder patients should be advised to eliminate caffeine from their diets because its anxiogenic effects tend to exacerbate the disorder.

Generalized Anxiety Disorder

Generalized anxiety disorder (GAD) is a relatively new disorder, having been first included in DSM-III in 1980. It is characterized by generalized, persistent anxiety without the specific symptoms that characterize either phobic disorders, panic disorder, or OCD (i.e., phobias, panic attacks, obsessions, and compulsions).

The diagnostic criteria require that generalized anxiety disorder not be diagnosed when the symptoms are due to another illness such as major depression or schizophrenia, or the generalized anxiety occurs in the context of a panic disorder, social phobia, or OCD. The anxiety or worry in GAD should not relate purely to having a panic attack, being embarrassed in public, being contaminated, or gaining weight, as in anorexia nervosa. The criteria also require that the individual have 6 of 18 symptoms from three categories including motor tension (e.g., trembling, muscle tension and restlessness, fatigue), autonomic hyperactivity (e.g., shortness of breath, palpitations, dizziness, hot flashes), or vigilance and scanning (e.g., feeling keyed up, exaggerated startle response, irritability). Furthermore, organic factors such as hyperthyroidism or caffeinism should be ruled out. The condition must exist for 6 months or longer. The complete criteria for GAD are listed in Table 10-8.

Epidemiology

Community surveys have shown that GAD is common, with a prevalence of up to 6.4% and a slight male preponderance. It tends to start in the early 20s, although

Table 10-8.   DSM-III-R criteria for generalized anxiety disorder

A. Unrealistic or excessive anxiety and worry (apprehensive expectation) about two or more life circumstances, e.g., worry about possible misfortune to one's child (who is in no danger) and worry about finances (for no good reason), for a period of 6 months or longer, during which the person has been bothered more days than not by these concerns. In children and adolescents, this may take the form of anxiety and worry about academic, athletic, and social performance.

B. If another Axis I disorder is present, the focus of the anxiety and worry in A is unrelated to it, e.g., the anxiety or worry is not about having a panic attack (as in panic disorder), being embarrassed in public (as in social phobia), being contaminated (as in obsessive-compulsive disorder), or gaining weight (as in anorexia nervosa).

C. The disturbance does not occur only during the course of a mood disorder or a psychotic disorder.

D. At least 6 of the following 18 symptoms are often present when anxious (do not include symptoms present only during panic attacks):

Motor tension
    1. Trembling, twitching, or feeling shaky
    2. Muscle tension, aches, or soreness
    3. Restlessness
    4. Easy fatigability

Autonomic hyperactivity
    5. Shortness of breath or smothering sensations
    6. Palpitations or accelerated heart rate (tachycardia)
    7. Sweating, or cold, clammy hands
    8. Dry mouth
    9. Dizziness or lightheadedness
   10. Nausea, diarrhea, or other abdominal distress
   11. Flushes (hot flashes) or chills
   12. Frequent urination
   13. Trouble swallowing or "lump in throat"

Vigilance and scanning
   14. Feeling keyed up or on edge
   15. Exaggerated startle response
   16. Difficulty concentrating or "mind going blank" because of anxiety
   17. Trouble falling or staying asleep
   18. Irritability

E. It cannot be established that an organic factor initiated and maintained the disturbance, e.g., hyperthyroidism, caffeine intoxication.

persons of any age may develop the disorder. Few patients with GAD seek treatment, and many see cardiologists or pulmonary specialists for specific symptoms. Because the disorder (as currently defined) is relatively new, the natural course and outcome are not known. Over 25% of patients with GAD, however, appear to develop panic disorder on follow-up, and the majority develop episodes of depression.

Etiology

The etiology of GAD is unknown, although studies show that it is familial and that approximately 25% of first-degree relatives are affected, female relatives more often than male relatives. Male relatives are likely to have alcoholism. One twin study reported a concordance rate of 50% in monozygotic twins and 15% in dizygotic twins. Several different neurotransmitter systems have been implicated in the disorder, including the noradrenergic, GABA, and serotonergic systems in the frontal lobe and limbic system, but at present, the cause of GAD is unknown.

Differential Diagnosis

The differential diagnosis of GAD is the same as for panic disorder and agoraphobia. It is particularly important to rule out organic conditions such as caffeine intoxication, stimulant abuse, alcohol withdrawal, and sedative-hypnotic withdrawal. The mental status examination and history should explore the diagnostic possibilities of panic disorder, simple phobias, social phobia, OCD, schizophrenia, and major depression.

Clinical Management

Behaviorally oriented psychotherapy (e.g., relaxation training) may be helpful in assisting the patient to recognize and control anxiety symptoms, especially if the condition is mild. The patient should be educated about the chronic nature of the disorder and the tendency of symptoms to wax and wane, often together with external stressors that the patient may be experiencing.

Minor tranquilizers are the medications of choice for GAD. Benzodiazepines should be prescribed in a maintenance dosage (e.g., diazepam 5 mg three times daily, or 5–10 mg at bedtime) for short periods (e.g., weeks or months) when the anxiety is particularly severe. Beta-adrenergic blockers, such as propranolol (e.g., in doses of 40–160 mg per day in divided doses) may be effective, but are not as well studied in GAD. Treatment with benzodiazepines should be time limited to prevent the complications of tolerance and dependence.

An alternative medication is buspirone, a nonbenzodiazepine anxiolytic, whose onset of action is relatively slow (i.e., weeks), but it has the advantage over benzodiazepines of having little abuse potential. Tricyclic antidepressants have also been used, particularly sedating ones such as doxepin or amitriptyline, and may also be effective. The antipsychotic trifluoperazine has been shown to be effective but should not be used due to its potential to cause tardive dyskinesia. In general, antipsychotics should only be used in psychotic patients.

Phobic Disorders

A phobia is an irrational fear of specific objects, places or situations, or activities. Although fear itself is to some degree adaptive, particularly for animals and primitive man, the fear in phobias is irrational, excessive, and disproportionate to any actual danger. Three categories of phobia are described in DSM-III-R, including *agoraphobia*, which has already been described, *social phobias*, in which there is fear of

Table 10-9. DSM-III-R criteria for social phobia

A. A persistent fear of one or more situations (the social phobia situations) in which the person is exposed to possible scrutiny by others and fears that he or she may do something or act in a way that will be humiliating or embarrassing. Examples include: being unable to continue talking while speaking in public, choking on food when eating in front of others, being unable to urinate in a public lavatory, hand-trembling when writing in the presence of others, and saying foolish things or not being able to answer questions in social situations.

B. If an Axis III or another Axis I disorder is present, the fear in A is unrelated to it, e.g., the fear is not of having a panic attack (panic disorder), stuttering or trembling (Parkinson's disease), or exhibiting abnormal eating behavior (anorexia nervosa or bulimia nervosa).

C. During some phase of the disturbance, exposure to the specific phobic stimulus (or stimuli) almost invariably provokes an immediate anxiety response.

D. The phobic situation(s) is avoided, or is endured with intense anxiety.

E. The avoidant behavior interferes with occupational functioning or with usual social activities or relationships with others, or there is marked distress about having fear.

F. The person recognizes that his or her fear is excessive or unreasonable.

G. If the person is under 18, the disturbance does not meet the criteria for avoidant disorder of childhood or adolescence.

Specify generalized type if the phobic situation includes most social situations, and also consider the additional diagnosis of avoidant personality disorder.

humiliation or embarrassment in public places, and *simple phobia,* a category that includes specific phobias, such as the irrational and intense fear of snakes.

Persons with social phobia tend to have multiple fears of situations where they may be observed by other people. They also commonly fear speaking in public, eating in public restaurants, writing in front of other persons, or using public restrooms.

Simple phobias are usually isolated and involve objects that conceivably may cause harm, such as snakes, heights, flying, or blood, but the person's reaction to them is excessive.

Diagnostic criteria for social and simple phobias are presented in Tables 10-9 and 10-10, respectively. Examples of common simple phobias are presented in Table 10-11.

Epidemiology

Phobias are common in the general population. Social phobias reportedly affect 3–5% of the population, but simple phobias may affect up to 25% of the population at some point during their lives. Simple phobias are more prevalent among women, but social phobias affect men and women equally. Simple phobias tend to have their onset in childhood, most starting before age 7 years. Social phobias begin

Table 10-10. DSM-III-R criteria for simple phobia

A. A persistent fear of a circumscribed stimulus (object or situation) other than fear of having a panic attack (as in panic disorder) or of humiliation or embarrassment in certain social situations (as in social phobia).

Note: Do not include fears that are part of panic disorder with agoraphobia or agoraphobia without history of panic disorder.

B. During some phase of the disturbance, exposure to the specific phobic stimulus (or stimuli) almost invariably provokes an immediate anxiety response.

C. The object or situation is avoided, or endured with intense anxiety.

D. The fear or the avoidant behavior significantly interferes with the person's normal routine or with usual social activities or relationships with others, or there is marked distress about having the fear.

E. The person recognizes that his or her fear is excessive or unreasonable.

F. The phobic stimulus is unrelated to the content of the obsessions of obsessive-compulsive disorder or the trauma of posttraumatic stress disorder.

during adolescence, the majority having their onset before age 25 years. Among simple phobias, the most commonly feared objects or situations include animals, storms, heights, illness, injury, and death.

Despite the frequency of phobias in the general population, few phobic patients receive treatment, probably because they perceive their phobia as trivial and are rarely limited by them. Fear of snakes, for example, will hardly keep a person from succeeding socially or occupationally, unless the person is employed as a zookeeper. Consequently, patients with phobias comprise only 2–3% of psychiatric outpatients.

Table 10-11. Common simple phobias

Phobia	Focus of fear	Phobia	Focus of fear
Acrophobia	Heights	Logophobia	Words
Ailurophobia	Cats	Nyctophobia	Night
Amathophobia	Dust	Odynephobia	Pain
Apeirophobia	Infinity	Ophidiophobia	Snakes
Arachnephobia	Spiders	Phonophobia	Loud noises
Claustrophobia	Closed spaces	Photophobia	Light
Cynophobia	Dogs	Poinephobia	Punishment
Entomophobia	Insects	Pyrophobia	Fire
Frigophobia	Cold weather	Theophobia	God
Gynophobia	Women	Topophobia	Stage fright
Homophobia	Homosexuals	Triskaidekaphobia	Number 13
Kakorrhaphiophobia	Failure	Xenophobia	Strangers
Keraunophobia	Thunder		

Etiology

Phobic disorders tend to run in families, although there are few reports that deal specifically with social or simple phobias because most reports lump all phobias together, including agoraphobia. Twin studies show a higher rate of concordance for anxiety and phobic disorders in monozygotic twins than in dizygotic twins, however.

Learning may play an important role in the etiology of phobias. Behaviorists have pointed out that many phobias tend to arise in association with traumatic events, such as developing a fear of heights after sustaining a fall. Learning theory appears to explain many, but not all, cases of phobia, and other explanations are likely. Psychoanalysts have long held that phobias result from unresolved conflicts in childhood and attribute phobias to the use of displacement and avoidance as defense mechanisms against castration anxiety.

Clinical Findings

People with social and simple phobias experience fear when exposed to specific phobic situations, manifest autonomic arousal, and develop avoidance. Initially, exposure leads to an unpleasant subjective state of anxiety. This state, in turn, leads to typical physiologic manifestations of anxiety, including rapid heart beat, shortness of breath, jitteriness, etc.

In the dreaded situation, the person with social phobia develops overwhelming anxiety and fears that others will recognize this anxiety. The phobic person soon learns to avoid these unpleasant objects or situations, learning to avoid public-speaking engagements, eating in public, riding in public, or using public toilets. The phobia may gradually lead to avoidance of social gatherings, meetings with superiors, and eventually just about any social encounter. The person with social phobia develops anticipatory anxiety when forced to enter phobic situations and will learn to avoid them if possible.

For the person with simple phobia, the degree of distress varies with the prevalence of the avoided situation. For example, a hospital employee who fears blood may be in constant fear because of the availability of blood at hospitals. Apart from contact with the feared stimulus, these people are usually free of symptoms. A case example of a person with simple phobia follows.

John, a 13-year-old boy, was brought to the clinic by his mother. She reported that John wouldn't wear shirts that had buttons on them and was worried that this peculiarity would cause problems for John when he was older. Already, his mother pointed out, not being able to wear "regular" collared shirts had kept John out of scouting troops and the school orchestra because of the uniforms he would have to wear. Doctors had told John's mother in the past that he would outgrow this fear. John clearly was uncomfortable and appeared embarrassed by his mother's recitation of the story but admitted that it was all true. John said that at about age 4 he developed a fear of buttons, but wasn't sure why. Since then, he had worn only V-necked shirts or sweaters, and had refused to wear collared shirts. In fact, John said, just thinking about such shirts bothered him, and he even avoided touching his brother's shirts hanging in the closet that they shared.

Ten years later, John had finished college and had enrolled in graduate school. He had overcome the phobia by himself at age 16 and was able to wear regular collared shirts, but still reported that he avoided wearing these shirts when possible.

Course and Outcome

Social phobias tend to develop slowly, without obvious precipitants, and to be chronic and fluctuating. Variable degrees of disability may occur depending on the nature and extent of the feared situation. Degree of disability also depends on the occupation and position of the phobic person. For example, a business executive required to meet with the public as part of his or her job would face much greater disability from a social phobia than would a lighthouse keeper.

Simple phobias tend to remit spontaneously with age. When simple phobias persist into adulthood, they often become chronic, but rarely cause disability.

Complications of phobic disorders include depression or substance abuse. The frequency with which depression occurs in social or simple phobias has not been adequately studied but is certainly common. Many persons with social phobias become dependent on alcohol or sedative drugs and will use them to reduce their anxiety in feared situations. Phobic symptoms may precede the onset of pathological drinking, suggesting that these disorders have a role in the development of alcohol dependence in some patients.

Differential Diagnosis

The differential diagnosis of phobic disorders includes the other anxiety disorders such as panic disorder, GAD, affective disorders, and OCD. Phobias may occur in the context of these disorders, but tend to appear after the onset of the primary disorder. The psychiatric differential for social phobia includes depression, schizophrenia, and avoidant personality disorder. The irrational fear that characterizes phobias must be separated from a schizophrenic delusion. The differentiation of a simple phobia from OCD is often difficult, but in the OCD patient, the phobia tends to be just one of many obsessional thoughts. Differentiation between avoidant personality and social phobia may be difficult, and in fact, there is great overlap between the two disorders. In general, the avoidant person has no specific fears of objects or situations, but has a general discomfort of social situations and requires continual reassurance.

Phobic symptoms are common in depression, and ones that arise in the context of a depressive episode are generally mood congruent (i.e., fear of failure) and generally disappear when the depression has been successfully treated.

Clinical Management

Mild cases of social phobia may respond to behavior psychotherapy alone, but many patients will need medication. Patients with social phobias have been treated with some success with tricyclic antidepressants, MAO inhibitors, and alprazolam. These patients tend to be sensitive to tricyclic side effects and may develop jitteriness, irritability, and insomnia on low doses of imipramine. Patients tend to relapse when the drugs are discontinued. Phenelzine, a MAO inhibitor, may be more effective than tricyclics for social phobias, but is associated with dietary restrictions that may limit its use.

Behavior psychotherapy is useful in the treatment of both social phobias and simple phobias. *Systematic desensitization* and *flooding* are the most widely used forms of exposure. In the former, patients learn to gradually reduce their anxiety associated with feared situations. In flooding, patients are instructed to enter situations or do things that are generally associated with anxiety until the anxiety associated with the exposure (e.g., eating in restaurants) subsides. It is unlikely that progress will occur unless patients are persuaded to confront feared situations. Behavior techniques are discussed further in Chapter 23.

Individual supportive psychotherapy is also useful, especially when combined with behavior therapy or medication to help restore moral and self-confidence. Cognitive techniques can be used to help modify dysfunctional thoughts about fear of failure, humiliation, or embarrassment. Marriage or family counseling may be indicated when disturbed marital or family situations are contributing to the symptoms.

Posttraumatic Stress Disorder

Posttraumatic stress disorder (PTSD) develops in persons who have experienced a physically or emotionally traumatic event that is outside the range of normal human experience, such as combat, physical assault, rape, or disasters such as home fires. Its three major elements include reexperiencing the trauma through dreams or recurrent and intrusive thoughts, emotional numbing such as feeling detached from others, and symptoms of autonomic arousal such as irritability and exaggerated startle response. The diagnostic criteria for PTSD are listed in Table 10-12.

The term *posttraumatic stress disorder* was introduced in DSM-III, although the concept of this disturbance has a long history. In the past, this syndrome was recognized in wartime as "shell shock" or "war neurosis," because it was seen most commonly in war situations. Many of its typical symptoms, however, such as intrusive thoughts and autonomic arousal, were also recognized in victims of other traumatic events, such as natural disasters, and in DSM-I, the disorder was diagnosed as "gross stress reaction," a diagnosis dropped from DSM-II.

Epidemiology and Clinical Findings

The prevalence of PTSD in the general population has been estimated to be 0.5% among men and 1.2% among women. Most men with the disorder have experienced combat. For women, the most frequent stressor is a physical assault or rape. PTSD can occur at any age, and children have been reported to develop it, such as after

Table 10-12. DSM-III-R criteria for posttraumatic stress disorder

A. The person has experienced an event that is outside the range of usual human experience and that would be markedly distressing to almost anyone, e.g., serious threat to one's life or physical integrity; serious threat or harm to one's children, spouse, or other close relatives and friends; sudden destruction of one's home or community; or seeing another person who has recently been, or is being, seriously injured or killed as the result of an accident or physical violence.

B. The traumatic event is persistently reexperienced in at least one of the following ways:

1. Recurrent and intrusive distressing recollections of the event (in young children, repetitive play in which themes or aspects of the trauma are expressed)
2. Recurrent distressing dreams of the event
3. Sudden acting or feeling as if the traumatic event were recurring (includes a sense of reliving the experience, illusions, hallucinations, and dissociative [flashback] episodes, even those that occur upon awakening or when intoxicated)
4. Intense psychological distress at exposure to events that symbolize or resemble an aspect of the traumatic event, including anniversaries of the trauma

C. Persistent avoidance of stimuli associated with the trauma or numbing of general responsiveness (not present before the trauma), as indicated by at least three of the following:

1. Efforts to avoid thoughts or feelings associated with the trauma
2. Efforts to avoid activities or situations that arouse recollections of the trauma
3. Inability to recall an important aspect of the trauma (psychogenic amnesia)
4. Markedly diminished interest in significant activities (in young children, loss of recently acquired developmental skills such as toilet training or language skills)
5. Feeling of detachment or estrangement from others
6. Restricted range of affect, e.g., unable to have loving feelings
7. Sense of a foreshortened future, e.g., does not expect to have a career, marriage, or children, or a long life

D. Persistent symptoms of increased arousal (not present before the trauma), as indicated by at least two of the following:

1. Difficulty falling or staying asleep
2. Irritability or outbursts of anger
3. Difficulty concentrating
4. Hypervigilance
5. Exaggerated startle response
6. Physiologic reactivity on exposure to events that symbolize or resemble an aspect of the traumatic event (e.g., a woman who was raped in an elevator breaks out in a sweat when entering any elevator)

E. Duration of the disturbance (symptoms in B, C, and D) of at least 1 month.

Specify delayed onset if the onset of symptoms was at least 6 months after the trauma.

the Chowchilla school bus kidnapping incident in 1976. The prevalence of PTSD among survivors of catastrophes varies, but in one well-studied tragedy, the Coconut Grove nightclub fire in the 1940s, 57% of patients followed for 1 year suffered an acute posttraumatic syndrome.

PTSD may begin within hours or days of the stressor, but may be delayed for months or years. The disorder can be acute, but has been reported to last in some cases for 30 or 40 years. Symptoms tend to fluctuate and worsen during periods of stress. Predictors of good outcome include rapid onset of symptoms, adequate premorbid functioning, strong social supports, and an absence of psychiatric or medical comorbidity.

Etiology

The major etiologic event leading to PTSD is the stressor. Because not all persons who experience a major stressor develop PTSD, other variables such as underlying personality and biological vulnerability are probably important. Stressors of all types may contribute to the development of PTSD, but must be severe enough to be outside the range of normal human experience. Business losses, marital conflicts, or the death of a loved one, for example, are not considered stressors that lead to PTSD. At least for war, certain experiences are highly linked to the development of PTSD, such as witnessing a friend being killed in action, witnessing atrocities, and especially, participating in atrocities.

Individual differences that can predispose to the development of PTSD include age, history of emotional disturbance, and social support. Eighty percent of young children who sustain a burn injury, for example, show symptoms of posttraumatic stress 1–2 years after the initial injury, but only 30% of adults who suffer this injury have symptoms after 1 year. Persons with prior history of psychiatric treatment have a greater likelihood of developing the syndrome, presumably because the previous illness reflects a greater sensitivity to stress, and persons with adequate social support are less likely to develop the disorder than persons with poor support. Certain biological abnormalities have been found in persons with PTSD, such as decreased rapid eye movement (REM) latency in stage 4 sleep, and may play a role in its development.

Complications

Complications of PTSD may include violence and aggression, alcohol and drug abuse, and poor impulse control. Although many war veterans have claimed that PTSD has led them to commit criminal offenses, a study has found that felonious behavior in combat veterans occurred only in veterans who had had similar behavior before their military service.

Differential Diagnosis

The differential diagnosis for PTSD includes major depression, adjustment disorder, panic disorder, GAD, OCD, depersonalization disorder, factitious disorder, and malingering. Occasionally, a physical injury may have occurred during the stressor so that an organic mental disorder must be considered as well. Many patients with PTSD meet criteria for another Axis I disorder (e.g., major depression, panic disorder), in which case both disorders should be diagnosed.

Clinical Management

There are few controlled studies of pharmacologic and psychotherapeutic strategies for the treatment of PTSD. However, many experts believe that supportive psychotherapy after the onset of symptoms will help promote an abreaction (i.e., psychological release) of the traumatic event. Hypnosis and intravenous amobarbital sodium (i.e., "Amytal" interview) have been used to facilitate this. Group and family therapy have been advocated, particularly in association with Vietnam veterans. Behavioral methods, including relaxation training and systematic desensitization, have also been used.

Patients with PTSD are reported to benefit from antidepressant medication, including tricyclics or MAO inhibitors, alprazolam, carbamazepine, and antipsychotics, but more study is required before specific recommendations can be made. These medications are probably best reserved for patients with specific psychiatric syndromes in addition to PTSD, for example, in treating major depression with antidepressants or psychotic symptoms with antipsychotics.

Recommendations for treatment of anxiety disorders

1. Mild cases of panic may respond to behavioral interventions, but many patients will need medication (e.g., tricyclic antidepressants [TCAs], monoamine oxidase [MAO] inhibitors, alprazolam).

2. The agoraphobic patient should be gently encouraged to get out and explore the world.

   - Progress will not occur unless the phobic patient confronts the feared places or situations.

3. Behavior techniques (i.e., exposure, flooding, desensitization) will help most persons with simple and social phobias.

   - Some people with social phobia respond well to medication (e.g., TCAs, MAO inhibitors, alprazolam).

4. Generalized anxiety may respond to simple behavior techniques (e.g., relaxation training), but many patients will need medication (e.g., benzodiazepines).

   - Be sure that the benzodiazepine is prescribed for a limited time only (e.g., weeks or months).

5. Posttraumatic stress disorder tends to be chronic, but many patients will benefit from the support available in group therapy.

   - Group therapy has become especially popular with Vietnam veterans, and most veterans organizations can offer help in finding a group.

Bibliography

Andreasen NC: Neuropsychiatric complications in burn patients. International Journal of Psychiatry and Medicine 5:161–171, 1974

Aronson TA: A naturalistic study of imipramine in panic disorder and agoraphobia. Am J Psychiatry 144:114–119, 1987

Ballenger JC, Burrows GD, DuPont RL, et al: Alprazolam in panic disorder and agoraphobia: results from a multicenter trial, I: efficacy in short-term treatment. Arch Gen Psychiatry 45:413–422, 1988

Barlow DH: Anxiety and Its Disorders—The Nature and Treatment of Anxiety and Panic. New York, Guilford, 1988

Barlow DH, DiNardo PA, Vermilyea BB, et al: Co-morbidity and depression among the anxiety disorders. J Nerv Ment Dis 174:63–72, 1986

Breslau N, Davis GC: Post-traumatic stress disorder: the etiologic specificity of war time stressors. Am J Psychiatry 144:578–583, 1987

Burns LE, Thorpe GL: The epidemiology of fears and phobias (with particular reference to the National Survey of Agoraphobics). J Int Med Res 5 (suppl 5):1–7, 1977

Davidson J, Kudler H, Smith R, et al: Treatment of post-traumatic stress disorder with amitriptyline and placebo. Arch Gen Psychiatry 47:259–266, 1990

Friedman MJ: Toward rational pharmacotherapy for post-traumatic stress disorder: an interim report. Am J Psychiatry 145:281–285, 1988

Fyer AJ, Mannuzza S, Gallops MS, et al: Familial transmission of simple phobias and fears: a preliminary report. Arch Gen Psychiatry 47:252–256, 1990

Gorman JM, Liebowitz MR, Fyer A, et al: A neuroanatomical hypothesis for panic disorder. Am J Psychiatry 146:148–161, 1989

Greist JH, Jefferson JW, Marks IM: Anxiety and Its Treatment—Help Is Available. Washington, DC, American Psychiatric Press, 1986

Heimberg RG, Barlow DH: Psychosocial treatments for social phobias. Psychosomatics 29:27–37, 1988

Helzer JE, Robins LE, McEvoy L: Post-traumatic stress disorder in the general population: findings of the Epidemiologic Catchment Area survey. N Engl J Med 317:1630–1634, 1987

Hoehn-Saric R: Neurotransmitters in anxiety. Arch Gen Psychiatry 39:735–742, 1982

Lee MA, Flegel P, Greden JF, et al: Anxiogenic effects of caffeine in panic and depressed patients. Am J Psychiatry 145:632–635, 1988

Liebowitz MR, Fyer J, Gorman JM: Social phobia: review of a neglected anxiety disorder. Arch Gen Psychiatry 42:729–736, 1985

Marks IM: Fears, Phobias, and Rituals: Panic, Anxieties, and Their Disorders. New York, Oxford University Press, 1987

Meibach RC, Dunner D, Wilson LG, et al: Comparative efficacy of propranolol, chlordiazepoxide, and placebo in the treatment of anxiety. J Clin Psychiatry 48:355–358, 1987

Noyes R, Clancy J, Hoenk PR, et al: The prognosis of anxiety neurosis. Arch Gen Psychiatry 37:173–178, 1980

Noyes R, Clarkson C, Crowe R, et al: A family study of generalized anxiety disorder. Am J Psychiatry 144:119–124, 1987

Noyes R, Clancy J, Garvey MJ, et al: Is agoraphobia a variant of panic disorder or a separate illness? Journal of Anxiety Disorders 1:3–13, 1987

Pittman RK, Orr SP, Forgue D: Psychophysiologic assessment of post-traumatic stress disorder imagery in Vietnam combat veterans. Arch Gen Psychiatry 44:970–975, 1987

Reich J, Yates W: A pilot study of treatment of social phobia with alprazolam. Am J Psychiatry 145:590–594, 1988

Ross RJ, Ball WA, Sullivan KA, et al: Sleep disturbance as the hallmark of post-traumatic stress disorder. Am J Psychiatry 146:697–707, 1989

Roy-Byrne P (ed): Anxiety: New Findings for the Clinician. Washington, DC, American Psychiatric Press, 1989

Shaw DM, Churchill CM, Noyes R, et al: Criminal behavior and post-traumatic stress disorder in Vietnam veterans. Compr Psychiatry 28:403–411, 1987

Solomon Z, Weisenberg M, Schwarzwald J, et al: Post-traumatic stress disorder among front line soldiers with combat stress reaction: the 1982 Israeli experience. Am J Psychiatry 144:448–454, 1987

Terr LC: Chowchilla revisited: the effects of psychic trauma four years after a school bus kidnapping. Am J Psychiatry 140:1543–1550, 1983

Torgerson S: Genetic factors in anxiety disorders. Arch Gen Psychiatry 40:1085–1089, 1983

Zitrin CM, Klein DF, Woerner MG, et al: Treatment of phobias, I: comparison of imipramine hydrochloride and placebo. Arch Gen Psychiatry 40:125–138, 1983

Self-assessment Questions

1. What is the relationship between panic disorder and agoraphobia?
2. What is the "irritable heart" syndrome?
3. What are the findings in genetic studies of panic disorder?
4. What is the differential diagnosis of panic disorder?
5. What is the pharmacologic treatment of panic disorder? generalized anxiety disorder? social phobia?
6. What are social and simple phobias? How do they differ?
7. What is the natural history of the different anxiety disorders?
8. When does posttraumatic disorder develop? What factors predispose to its development?
9. What behavior treatments are useful in the different anxiety disorders?
10. When is anxiety normal and when is it abnormal?

Chapter 11
Obsessive-Compulsive Disorder

He had another peculiarity—This was his anxious care to go out or in at a door or passage by a certain number of steps from a certain point . . .

Boswell's Life of Johnson

Johnson, whose behavior (i.e., repeating rituals) was so carefully observed by Boswell, probably had obsessive-compulsive disorder (OCD). Shakespeare, in describing the guilt-laden hand-washing rituals of Lady Macbeth, appears to have had some familiarity with the symptoms of the disorder. More recently, industrialist Howard Hughes developed crippling contamination obsessions in late adulthood that resulted in a fanatic preoccupation with germs and a bizarre life of filth and neglect.

Like most mental illnesses, OCD has been recognized for centuries. It was first described in 1838 by Esquirol, a French psychiatrist. Earlier, rituals were probably regarded as personal quirks, or worse, as evidence of possession by the devil. One wonders how many luckless victims of OCD were burned at the stake.

By the end of the 19th century, obsessions and compulsions were generally believed to be manifestations of depressive illness. Later, in part due to the influence of Freud, these symptoms were recognized as a syndrome, *obsessional neurosis,* believed to result from intrapsychic conflicts. This view remained prominent until recently when biologically oriented research supported the disease model of OCD, and behaviorally oriented clinicians began to reconceptualize OCD in terms of learning theory. In 1980, obsessional neurosis was renamed *obsessive-compulsive disorder,* reflecting these new etiologic concepts. Although the cause of OCD is

249

Table 11-1. DSM-III-R criteria for obsessive-compulsive disorder

A. Either obsessions or compulsions:

Obsessions: (1), (2), (3), and (4):

  1. Recurrent and persistent ideas, thoughts, impulses, or images that are experienced, at least initially, as intrusive and senseless, e.g., a parent's having repeated impulses to kill a loved child, a religious person's having recurrent blasphemous thoughts.
  2. The person attempts to ignore or suppress such thoughts or impulses or to neutralize them with some other thought or action.
  3. The person recognizes that the obsessions are the product of his or her own mind, not imposed from without (as in thought insertion).
  4. If another Axis I disorder is present, the content of the obsession is unrelated to it, e.g., the ideas, thoughts, impulses, or images are not about food in the presence of an eating disorder, about drugs in the presence of a psychoactive substance use disorder, or guilty thoughts in the presence of a major depression.

Compulsions: (1), (2), and (3):

  1. Repetitive, purposeful, and intentional behaviors that are performed in response to an obsession, or according to certain rules or in stereotyped fashion.
  2. The behavior is designed to neutralize or to prevent discomfort or some dreaded event or situation; however, either the activity is not connected in a realistic way with whatever it is designed to neutralize or prevent, or it is clearly excessive.
  3. The person recognizes that his or her behavior is excessive or unreasonable (this may not be true for young children; it may no longer be true for people whose obsessions have evolved into overvalued ideas).

B. The obsessions or compulsions cause marked distress, are time-consuming (take more than an hour a day), or significantly interfere with the person's normal routine, occupational functioning, or usual social activities or relationships with others.

still unknown, its study has been reinvigorated by new research methods and the development of effective treatments that have altered its formerly poor prognosis.

Definition

The essential features of OCD are obsessions or compulsions, or more commonly both. According to DSM-III-R (see Table 11-1), obsessions are recurrent or persistent ideas, thoughts, impulses, or images that are experienced as intrusive and senseless. Common obsessions include fears of harming other persons or of sinning against God. For example, a person may have an obsessional thought to kill a loved one, or a religious person may have blasphemous thoughts.

Compulsions, on the other hand, are repetitive, purposeful, and intentional behaviors performed in response to obsessions or according to certain rules, or in a stereotyped fashion. Common examples of compulsions include repetitive hand washing or checking rituals. Compulsive rituals are meant to neutralize or prevent discomfort or prevent a dreaded event or situation. The rituals are not necessarily connected logically to the event or situation. For example, a person might think that if he did not reread the directions on a box of detergent, harm would come to his child. The frequency of obsessions and compulsions in a series of patients

Table 11-2. Frequency of common obsessions and compulsions in 24 patients with obsessive-compulsive disorder

Obsessions	%	Compulsions	%
Aggression	79	Cleaning	71
Contamination	67	Checking	67
Symmetry	63	Counting	50
Sexual	25		
Hoarding	25		
Religious	17		
Somatic	17		

from Iowa is presented in Table 11-2, and the varied content in common obsessions is shown in Table 11-3.

To receive a diagnosis of OCD, the patient must not only have either obsessions or compulsions, but these symptoms must cause marked distress, be time-consuming (more than 1 hour daily), or significantly interfere with the person's routine, occupational functioning, or usual social activities and relationships. The definition for impairment is vague, but the intent is clear; not only must the person have the abnormal thoughts or behaviors, but they must affect him or her in a significant way. Many normal persons, especially children, have obsessional thoughts or repetitive behaviors, but they tend not to cause distress or interfere with living. In fact, ritualistic behavior adds structure to our lives. Most of us have daily routines that have probably changed little in years, (e.g., shaving and having coffee in the morning, lunch at noon, dinner at 6 P.M. and retiring at 11 P.M.), and many of

Table 11-3. Varied content in obsessions

Obsession	Foci of preoccupation
Aggression	Physical or verbal assault on self or others (includes suicidal and homicidal thoughts); accidents; mishaps; wars and natural disasters; death
Contamination	Excreta, human or otherwise; dirt; dust; semen; menstrual blood; other bodily excretions; germs; illness, especially venereal diseases; AIDS
Symmetry	Orderliness in arrangements of any kind, e.g., books on the shelf, shirts in the dresser, etc.
Sexual	Sexual advances toward self or others; incestuous impulses; genitalia of either sex; homosexuality; masturbation; competence in sexual performance, etc.
Hoarding	Collecting items of any kind, e.g., string, shopping bags, etc.; inability to throw things out
Religious	Existence of God; validity of religious stories, practices, or holidays; committing sinful acts
Somatic	Preoccupation with body parts, e.g., nose; concern with appearance; belief in having disease or illness, e.g., cancer

Source. Adapted from Akhtar S, Wig NN, Varma VK, et al: A phenomenological analysis of symptoms in obsessive-compulsive neurosis. Br J Psychiatry 127:342–348, 1975.

us double-check locks, avoid stepping on cracks, and say prayers before meals. Rituals also enhance the spiritual life of many (e.g., religious catechism). But these daily rituals are accepted, desirable, and easily adapted to changing circumstances. To the OCD patient, however, rituals are a distressing and unavoidable way of life; the rituals control the patient, not vice versa. A case example of OCD and its crippling effects follows.

Todd, a 24-year-old, was accompanied to the psychiatric outpatient clinic by his mother for evaluation of obsessions and compulsive rituals. According to Todd, compulsive rituals began in childhood, including touching objects a certain number of times and rereading prayers in church. These symptoms were not disabling, and his illness had only worsened 2 years before evaluation.

After graduating from college, he moved to a large midwestern city to work as an accountant for a major firm. Soon after moving there, he began to check the locks on his doors frequently and to check his automobile for signs of intruders. Eventually, he began to check other things around his apartment, such as appliances, water faucets, and electrical switches. He also developed extensive grooming and bathing rituals. Because of his time-consuming rituals, he was often late for work, and in fact, his work load became too much for him, and he was forced to quit his job. As an accountant, he would find himself adding columns of numbers over and over to make sure that he had "done it right." In addition to extensive rituals, Todd also had substantial obsessional thinking, such as having thoughts of losing control and assaulting someone, yelling embarrassing words in public, becoming contaminated, and possibly contracting AIDS. He also worried about the arrangement and symmetry of objects. Much of the time his rituals consisted of debating whether or not he needed to actually conduct a ritual and, in fact, mentally rehearsing them. Todd admitted that his rituals were irrational and excessive, but felt powerless to control them. Efforts to resist them merely made the rituals worse.

Todd moved back into his parents' home, but his rituals became more extensive and eventually took up his entire day. Rituals would begin on arising in the morning and continue until he retired at night. The rituals mostly involved bathing (he showered for half an hour and had to wash his body in a specific fashion), dressing in a certain way, and repeating rituals, such as walking in and out of the door a certain number of times.

Todd was a slender, unkempt young man who had a scraggly beard, long hair, and unclipped fingernails. His shoes were untied, and he wore several layers of clothing. Because of his fear of contamination, he had refused to shave and wore the same clothes every day.

Todd was treated with fluoxetine 80 mg daily and quickly improved. Within 2 months, his rituals were reduced to less than 1 hour per day and his grooming had improved. After 6 months, Todd still had minor rituals, but reported that he felt like his old self. He had obtained a job coaching track at a nearby high school.

Epidemiology

OCD has an average age at onset in the mid 20s; one-third of patients have developed OCD by age 15 and nearly three-quarters by age 30. Onset of the illness tends to be sudden, occurring over a period of 1 month, generally in the absence of any obvious stressor or precipitant. Although the onset is usually clear-cut, it may be gradual and insidious in some patients. On average, 7.5 years pass between onset of obsessions and compulsions and the initiation of treatment, although the delay may now be less due to the availability of effective treatments.

The prevalence of OCD traditionally has been felt to be as low as 0.05% in the general community and 1–4% in a clinic population. However, data from the Epidemiologic Catchment Area study suggest that as many as 2–3% of the general population meet criteria for OCD at some point during their lives.

Men and women appear to be affected equally by OCD, although there may be a slight female preponderance. Interestingly, one study showed that 75% of childhood-onset patients were male, suggesting that there may be more than one form of OCD. OCD patients have normal intelligence, despite early reports that suggested above-average intellect.

Etiology and Pathophysiology

OCD has been explained in genetic, psychodynamic, behavioral, and neurobiological terms. No explanation accounts for all of the richness of the disorder, and it is likely that a combination of these explanations will be found to account for the disturbance.

Family studies generally have shown a high prevalence of obsessive-compulsive symptoms among first-degree relatives of OCD patients, including up to 8% of parents and 7% of siblings. Some recent family studies have also linked OCD and Tourette's syndrome, and others have shown an increased prevalence of depression in relatives of OCD patients. Twin studies have generally found a higher concordance of OCD among monozygotic twins than among dizygotic twins, suggesting that there is an inherited predisposition to OCD. More careful studies on this subject are needed before any conclusions about the genetics of OCD can be made.

Dynamically oriented clinicians have long explained OCD as a fixation at the genital stage of development and regression to the earlier anal stage. This stage of development generally involves a preoccupation with anger, dirt, magical thinking, and ambivalence. Fixation at this stage is characterized by an overdeveloped super ego and various neurotic defense mechanisms, such as isolation, undoing, reaction formation, and displacement (see Chapter 23). Although many obsessions and compulsive behaviors appear laden with symbolic meaning, psychodynamic approaches are usually not helpful in treating this disorder.

Some experts use learning theory to explain the development of OCD. They believe that anxiety, at least initially, becomes paired to specific environmental events (i.e., classical conditioning), for example, to becoming dirty. The person then engages in compulsive rituals designed to decrease the anxiety (e.g., hand washing). When the rituals successfully reduce the anxiety, the compulsive behavior is believed more likely to occur in the future (i.e., operant conditioning). Although behavioral models of OCD have had little empirical support, behavior techniques are important in treating the disorder.

Neurobiological models have also been used to explain OCD. Evidence for a biological basis for the disorder includes associations with head trauma, epilepsy, Sydenham's chorea, and an epidemic of encephalitis after World War I. OCD has also been linked to birth trauma, abnormal electroencephalograms, abnormal auditory evoked potentials, growth delay, and abnormalities in neuropsychological testing. Additional support for a biological origin comes from animal studies in which bilateral hippocampal lesions or chronic amphetamine administration led to stereotypic behaviors that resemble compulsive rituals.

New imaging techniques have provided evidence of basal ganglia abnormalities. With positron-emission tomography (PET), two groups of investigators showed increased metabolic rates in the caudate nuclei and in the prefrontal cortex. With quantitative computerized tomography, another group of investigators showed that caudate volume was significantly less than that of control subjects. It has been hypothesized that basal ganglia dysfunction may lead to the complex motor programs involved in OCD, whereas the prefrontal hyperactivity may be related to the tendency to ruminate and plan excessively and to think in an overabstract way. As discussed in Chapter 5, the prefrontal cortex has important connections with the basal ganglia.

The most widely studied biochemical model has focused primarily on the neurotransmitter serotonin, which has been implicated as mediating a variety of behaviors including impulsivity, suicidality, aggression, and obsessive-compulsive symptoms. The antiobsessional effect of clomipramine, which is a potent serotonin reuptake blocker, supports a role for serotonin in OCD. Other medications, such as fluoxetine, fluvoxamine, and zimelidine, reported to be effective for this disorder are also relatively specific for blocking the reuptake of serotonin. A reduction of obsessions and compulsions has been correlated with a reduction of platelet serotonin and cerebrospinal fluid 5-hydroxyindoleacetic acid (5-HIAA) during clomipramine treatment. However, findings with other serotonin measures, such as platelet tritiated imipramine binding, have been inconclusive. Clearly, further study is needed, and it is unlikely that serotonin will account for all of the manifestations of OCD.

Relationship Between OCD and Obsessive-Compulsive Personality

OCD has long been associated with perfectionism, obstinacy, and orderliness consistent with the psychodynamic view that OCD results from regression to the anal stage of development. These traits are now linked to obsessive-compulsive personality.

Although a majority of OCD patients are reported to have premorbid obsessive-

Table 11-4.   Differential diagnosis of obsessive-compulsive disorder

Anorexia nervosa	Simple phobia
Autistic disorder	Social phobia
Major depression	Tourette's syndrome
Posttraumatic stress disorder	Trichotillomania
Schizophrenia	

compulsive traits, a one-to-one relationship between obsessive-compulsive personality and OCD does not exist. Persons with obsessive-compulsive traits do not necessarily develop OCD, although they often suffer from depression. Conversely, a significant number of OCD patients do not have premorbid obsessive-compulsive traits. A further discussion of obsessive-compulsive personality can be found in Chapter 16.

Course and Outcome

Summarizing available studies, a 1974 review found that 54–61% of OCD patients develop a chronic or progressive course, 24–33% a fluctuating course, and 11–14% a phasic course with periods of remission. However, these studies were conducted before effective treatments were available; therefore, future outcome studies may yield more favorable results.

Mild or atypical symptoms and a well-adjusted premorbid personality have been associated with a good prognosis; early onset and schizotypal personality have been associated with poor prognosis. Obsessive-compulsive symptoms are usually worsened by depressed mood. In fact, it is often depression that leads the OCD patient to seek help, not the obsessions or compulsions.

Recurrent episodes of major depression occur in a majority of patients with well-established (primary) OCD. Patients with OCD may be socially isolated and remain unmarried. Patients with milder disorders may, however, have near-normal or normal social relationships. Although suicidal thoughts are often prominent in obsessional thinking, the rate of suicide is not increased over expectations based on the general population.

Differential Diagnosis

The diagnosis of OCD rests on the history and the mental status examination, not laboratory or psychological tests. The disorder overlaps many other psychiatric syndromes (see Table 11-4) which must be ruled out, including schizophrenia.

Both OCD and schizophrenia tend to be chronic and to respond poorly to treatment. Severe obsessional thoughts often resemble delusional thinking. For example, a 38-year-old disabled truck driver treated in our clinic had extensive cleaning and checking rituals and felt compelled to describe the rituals in a loud voice as he was performing them—so loudly, in fact, that neighbors complained. Although the patient did not wish to do so, he firmly believed that harm would come to his family if he did not announce his rituals in this fashion. Although this patient realized that his ritualistic chanting was unreasonable, his actions indicated a belief to the contrary. However, whereas obsessions are unwanted, resisted, and recognized by the sufferer as having an internal origin, delusions are typically not resisted and are looked on as being of external origin.

OCD patients may at times develop hallucinations or delusions, but longitudinal studies show that they are not at increased risk for developing schizophrenia.

Many patients with well-established OCD have episodes of recurrent major depression (secondary depression). Likewise, patients with primary unipolar depression often develop obsessional thinking, usually consisting of morbid preoccupations and guilty ruminations. In these patients, the ruminations are ego-syntonic, appear rational, although exaggerated, and are seldom resisted. Whereas the depressed patient tends to focus on past events, the OCD patient focuses on the prevention of future events.

There is also a close association between OCD and phobic and anxiety disorders. Both OCD and anxiety disorder patients have avoidant behavior, show intense subjective and autonomic responses to certain objects or situations, and respond to behavioral interventions. Many persons with OCD are diagnosed as having simple phobias, such as a fear of germs. Alternatively, OCD patients may worry about public scrutiny and receive a diagnosis of social phobia.

Other disorders are also suggestive of OCD. Tourette's syndrome, characterized by vocal and motor tics, often coexists with OCD. Autistic disorder, a childhood disorder characterized by repetitive or stereotyped behaviors, may resemble OCD. Posttraumatic stress disorder is characterized by recurrent, intrusive ego-dystonic thoughts that may suggest obsessional thinking. Trichotillomania, or compulsive hair pulling, is classified as an impulse control disorder, but may, in fact, be related to OCD. Anorexia nervosa may also resemble OCD, as both involve ritualistic behavior, although in anorexia the behavior is desired and not resisted. Many anorexic patients also meet criteria for OCD.

Clinical Management

Historically, the treatment of OCD has been felt to be difficult and unsatisfactory. Recent developments in the treatment of OCD have changed this picture and have instilled a greater sense of optimism. The mainstays of treatment are pharmacotherapy and behavior therapy.

Behavior therapies, which tend to be more successful for ritualizers, emphasize exposure paired with response prevention. Briefly, a patient is exposed to a dreaded situation, event, or stimulus using a number of techniques (e.g., imaginal exposure, systematic desensitization, or flooding) and is then prevented from carrying out

---

Recommendations for management of obsessive-compulsive disorder (OCD)

1. Educate the patient about his or her illness

   - To reduce the patient's feelings of isolation, fear, and confusion
   - To reassure the worried patient that people with OCD rarely act on their frightening or violent obsessions
   - By pointing out the "up" side of OCD—that people with this disorder are usually conscientious, dependable, and likable
   - By recommending lay literature and suggesting that he or she join the OCD Foundation (New Haven, CT)

2. Establish an empathic relationship.

   - Do not tell patients to stop their rituals. They can't. That's why they are seeing you.
   - Explain that talking about the obsessions and compulsions will not make them worse.

3. Set limited goals with behavior therapy—don't tackle all rituals at once.

   - Find out what makes the rituals worse and what alleviates them.
   - Work on rituals one at a time and start with simple goals (e.g., reducing the amount of time spent in the shower from 40 to 35 minutes).

4. Use medication in moderate and severe cases.

   - Use clomipramine or fluoxetine and be patient. A full response may take months.

---

the compulsive behavior that usually results. For example, a compulsive washer may be asked to handle dirty objects (e.g., a used tissue) and then be prevented from hand washing. Thought-stopping techniques are also used to interrupt obsessional thoughts (e.g., the therapist may announce in a loud voice "Stop!" to interrupt the cycle of thinking). Proponents of behavior therapies state that up to 75% of patients who stick with the treatment respond, although it is unclear how extensive the improvement is. (See Chapter 23 for a more detailed description of behavior therapy.)

Pharmacotherapy has been growing in importance, primarily due to studies showing that one drug, clomipramine, has clear antiobsessional properties. Clomipramine, a tricyclic antidepressant that is relatively specific for serotonin reuptake blockade, is administered in dosages ranging from 150 to 300 mg daily. Nearly 60% of patients receiving clomipramine experience marked or moderate improvement, although side effects may limit its usefulness. Many patients develop sedation, orthostatic hypertension, and anticholinergic side effects (e.g., dry mouth, constipation, visual blurring, urinary hesitancy). Many patients develop a hyperstimulatory reaction characterized by agitation, jitteriness, and insomnia. (See Chapter 24 for a complete discussion of tricyclic antidepressants.) Clomipramine works well for both obsessions and compulsions irrespective of depressive symptoms, and a range of improvement is seen, including full remission. Treatment may be long-term, as patients tend to relapse when the drug is discontinued.

Other medications that appear to have antiobsessional properties are the anti-depressants fluoxetine and fluvoxamine (currently under investigation). With fluoxetine, OCD patients may need higher dosages than depressed patients and may take several months to respond. Other psychoactive medications have been the subject of case reports, but it is not clear that they have any role in the treatment of OCD.

Psychosurgery (stereotactic cingulotomy) has also been reported to benefit up to 80% of patients receiving the surgery, but a series of 36 patients did not show consistent improvement as a result of this treatment. Clearly, patients referred for psychosurgery should be refractory to less dramatic interventions.

Psychotherapy is an important adjunct to both behavior and pharmacologic treatments. Although psychodynamic formulations have not proved helpful in the treatment of this disorder, supportive psychotherapy is useful in guiding rehabilitative efforts by helping to restore morale, to provide hope, to help with problem solving, to encourage treatment compliance, and to encourage risk taking, such as helping in getting a patient to expose himself or herself to dreaded situations. Support groups for OCD patients are now available in many parts of the country and appear to be helpful.

Bibliography

Akhtar S, Wig NN, Varma VK, et al: A phenomenological analysis of symptoms in obsessive-compulsive neurosis. Br J Psychiatry 127:342–348, 1975

Ballantine HT, Bouckoms AJ, Thomas EK, et al: Treatment of psychiatric illness by stereotactic cingulotomy. Biol Psychiatry 22:887–897, 1987

Baxter LR, Phelps ME, Mazziotta JC, et al: Local cerebral glucose metabolism rates in obsessive-compulsive disorder. Arch Gen Psychiatry 44:211–218, 1987

Black A: The natural history of obsessional neurosis, in Obsessional States. Edited by Beach HR. London, Methuen Press, 1974, pp 1–23

Black DW, Noyes R: Comorbidity in obsessive-compulsive disorder, in Comorbidity in Anxiety and Mood Disorders. Edited by Maser JD, Cloninger CR. Washington, DC, American Psychiatric Press, 1990, pp 305–316

DeVeaugh-Geiss J, Landau P, Katz R: Treatment of obsessive-compulsive disorder with clomipramine. Psychiatric Annals 19:97–101, 1989

Goodwin DW, Guze SB, Robins E: Follow-up studies in obsessional neurosis. Arch Gen Psychiatry 20:182–187, 1969

Hamburger SD, Swedo S, Whitaker A, et al: Growth rate in adolescents with obsessive-compulsive disorder. Am J Psychiatry 146:652–655, 1989

Hollander E, Schiffman E, Cohen B, et al: Signs of central nervous system dysfunction in obsessive-compulsive disorder. Arch Gen Psychiatry 47:27–32, 1990

Jenike MA, Baer L, Minichiello WE: Obsessive-Compulsive Disorders. Littleton, MA, PSG Publishing, 1986

Jenike MA, Buttolph L, Baer L, et al: Open trial of fluoxetine in obsessive-compulsive disorder. Am J Psychiatry 146:909–911, 1989

Karno M, Golding JM, Sorenson SB, et al: The epidemiology of obsessive-compulsive disorder in five U.S. communities. Arch Gen Psychiatry 45:1094–1099, 1988

Luxenberg JS, Swedo SE, Flament MF, et al: Neurochemical abnormalities in obsessive-compulsive disorder detected with quantitative x-ray computed tomography. Am J Psychiatry 145:1089–1093, 1988

Marks IM: Review: obsessive-compulsive disorders, in Fears, Phobias, and Rituals: Panic, Anxiety, and Their Disorders. Edited by Marks IM. New York, Oxford University Press, 1987, pp 423–456

Pato MT, Zohar-Kadouch R, Zohar J, et al: Return of symptoms after discontinuation of clomipramine in patients with obsessive-compulsive disorder. Am J Psychiatry 145:1521–1525, 1988

Perse TL, Greist JH, Jefferson JW, et al: Fluvoxamine treatment of obsessive-compulsive disorder. Am J Psychiatry 144:1543–1548, 1987

Rapoport JL: The neurobiology of obsessive-compulsive disorder. JAMA 260:2888–2890, 1988

Rapoport JL: The Boy Who Couldn't Stop Washing. New York, EP Dutton, 1989

Zohar J, Insel TR, Zohar-Kadouch RC, et al: Serotonergic responsivity in obsessive-compulsive disorder. Arch Gen Psychiatry 45:167–172, 1988

Self-assessment Questions

1. How is OCD diagnosed?
2. What is the prevalence and sex distribution of OCD?
3. What defense mechanisms are thought to operate in OCD?
4. What evidence supports a neurobiological model for OCD?
5. What is the prognosis in OCD? What may change the prognosis of OCD in the future?
6. What is the differential diagnosis of OCD?
7. How are obsessions distinguished from delusions?
8. What are some of the behavior techniques used to treat OCD?
9. What is the purported mechanism of action of antiobsessional medications?
10. When is cingulotomy indicated?

Chapter 12
Somatoform and Related Disorders

So it is that a patient can confront his doctor with his symptoms, and put on him the whole onus of their cure.

Mayer-Gross, Slater, and Roth, Clinical Psychiatry

Somatoform disorders are characterized by physical complaints that occur in the absence of identifiable physical pathology. These conditions have been noted throughout recorded time and continue to baffle patients and practitioners. Typically, these common disorders are seen by primary-care physicians and other specialists, such as neurologists and cardiologists, rather than by psychiatrists. Patients with these disorders take up an inordinate amount of the clinician's time and energy. For example, in one study of somatizing patients seen in a primary-care practice, 28% of patient contacts involved emotional illness (not somatoform disorder per se), and these consultations took up 48% of the physician's time.

There are seven somatoform disorders (Table 12-1). They share the common feature of excessive concern with bodily symptoms that is not explainable on the basis of physical or laboratory evidence.

History

Although we now recognize several discrete somatoform disorders, their history has intertwined. Somatization disorder, formerly known as *hysteria*, was recognized

Portions of this chapter are adapted with permission from Black DW: Somatoform disorders. Prim Care 4:711–724, 1987. Copyright 1987 W.B. Saunders Company.

Table 12-1. DSM-III-R somatoform disorders

Somatization disorder	Body dysmorphic disorder
Conversion disorder	Undifferentiated somatoform disorder
Hypochondriasis	Somatoform disorder not otherwise specified
Somatoform pain disorder	

in the ancient world, when Greek physicians thought it resulted from a displaced uterus. Their treatment was to attract the "wandering uterus" back to its proper place by putting aromatic substances in the region of the vagina. Although Galen rejected this idea, the theory of uterine pathology persisted until Willis suggested that hysteria was caused by a disorder of the brain.

Hypochondriasis is derived from Greek, having the literal meaning "below the cartilage," referring to the area under the ribs housing various organs. The term has been used since the 17th century to associate changes in mental state with changes in the organs of the hypochondriac patient, which, it was believed, led to a preoccupation with bodily symptoms. In the 17th century, Sydenham suggested a close relationship between hysteria and hypochondriasis, and over the next two centuries, clinicians viewed hypochondriasis as the masculine version of hysteria, which occurred mostly in females.

In the 19th century, Charcot, a French neurologist working at the Salpêtrière, became interested in the bizarre and baffling manifestations of hysteria. He believed that strange emotions could produce hysterical symptoms in predisposed individuals. Hysteria later became Freud's central concern in the early years of psychoanalysis, his interest having developed while working in Paris with Charcot, who was treating hysteria with hypnosis. Psychoanalysts became very interested in hysteria, which they viewed as an illness designed to work out unconscious conflicts. In their seminal book on hysteria, Freud and his associate Breuer argued that hysterics suffer from the memories of emotionally charged ideas that had been stored in the unconscious, which they cannot easily consciously recall, but which continue to trouble them. Conversion, an ego-defense mechanism, was believed to convert psychic energy into bodily symptoms leading to hysteria. Thus, conversion was believed to give rise to both primary gain (i.e., the anxiety arising from a psychological conflict is kept from the patient's conscious mind) and secondary gain (i.e., support and sympathy from family and friends).

Gradually the term *hysterical* was used to mean any demanding patient whose symptoms were unexplained. So many different meanings developed from the term *hysteria* that a neutral term, *Briquet's syndrome*, was proposed for the disorder. In 1859, Paul Briquet, a French physician, had described hysteria as a polysymptomatic disorder. His concepts have been refined over the past 40 years, and diagnostic criteria (i.e., "Briquet's checklist"), developed in 1962, were later modified for inclusion in DSM-III and DSM-III-R as somatization disorder.

Although hysteria and hypochondriasis had been thought similar, use of the term *hypochondriasis* became restricted to less clearly delineated complaints of pain and discomfort. A hypochondriac, it was believed, was morbidly preoccupied with bodily function, unlike the hysteric, who exhibited "la belle indifference," or a strange lack of concern with the symptoms. Freud furthered the distinction between the two disorders by classifying hypochondriasis as a true neurosis, which implied that common everyday disturbances (e.g., sexual frustration) played a role in its etiology, whereas hysteria was conceptualized as a psychoneurosis (e.g., determined by early life experiences).

The concept of hypochondriasis continued to vacillate. In the early 20th century, it was argued that hypochondriasis was a valid disorder. This view was later challenged because patients with hypochondriacal symptoms were felt to often have other primary disorders, such as depression. Although the term has been little used and was, in fact, excluded from DSM-I, it was restored in DSM-II and subsequent editions. Its validity as a primary disorder has still not been adequately determined.

Somatization Disorder

Somatization disorder is a malady beginning early in life, affecting mostly women, and is characterized by recurrent and multiple bodily symptoms affecting most of the organ systems. The physical complaints, often dramatically described, are unexplained and typically include pain, anxiety- and mood-related symptoms, gastrointestinal disturbance, and psychosexual symptoms. To fulfill the criteria for the diagnosis of somatization disorder, patients must have at least 13 of 35 unexplained symptoms (see Table 12-2). For the clinician to count a symptom, the patient must report that it caused him or her to take a medicine other than aspirin, to alter his or her life pattern, or to see a physician; in the physician's judgment the symptom cannot be adequately explained by a physical disorder or an injury, nor can it be attributed to the side effects of medication, drugs, or alcohol or result from a panic (anxiety) attack.

In making the diagnosis, it is useful to have old medical charts available and to interview the patient on more than one occasion. Because of their many symptoms, patients may not recall old ones and may not have sufficient time to report new symptoms in one sitting. The frequency of common symptoms in somatization disorder are summarized in Table 12-3, and complaints from a typical patient are presented in Table 12-4.

Although a simple count of symptoms appears arbitrary, several studies have shown that this approach identifies a homogeneous group of patients who have a predictable course and outcome. The diagnosis is highly reliable and stable over time. The following case example illustrates the variety of symptoms found in somatization disorder and their stability over time.

A 26-year-old housewife presented for medical evaluation with a chief complaint of weakness and malaise with duration of 1 year. Other symptoms were soon unraveled: burning pain in her eyes, muscular aches and pains in her lower back, headaches, a stiff neck, abdominal pain "on both sides and below the navel," and vomiting "glassy white stuff—as if I were poisoned." Nine months earlier, she had been hospitalized

Table 12-2. DSM-III-R criteria for somatization disorder

A. Many physical complaints or a belief that one has been sickly, beginning before the age of 30 and persisting for several years.

B. At least 13 symptoms from the list below. To count a symptom as significant, the following criteria must be met:

    1. No organic pathology or pathophysiologic mechanism (e.g., a physical disorder or the effects of injury, medication, drugs, or alcohol) to account for the symptom or, when there is related organic pathology, the complaint or resulting social or occupational impairment is grossly in excess of what would be expected from the physical findings

    2. Has not occurred only during a panic attack

    3. Has caused the person to take medicine (other than over-the-counter pain medication), see a doctor, or alter life-style

Symptom list

Gastrointestinal symptoms:

    1. **Vomiting (other than during pregnancy)**
    2. Abdominal pain (other than when menstruating)
    3. Nausea (other than motion sickness)
    4. Bloating (gassy)
    5. Diarrhea
    6. Intolerance of (gets sick from) several different foods

Pain symptoms:

    7. **Pain in extremities**
    8. Back pain
    9. Joint pain
  10. Pain during urination
  11. Other pain (excluding headaches)

Cardiopulmonary symptoms:

  12. **Shortness of breath when not exerting oneself**
  13. Palpitations
  14. Chest pain
  15. Dizziness

Conversion or pseudoneurologic symptoms:

  16. **Amnesia**
  17. **Difficulty swallowing**
  18. Loss of voice
  19. Deafness
  20. Double vision
  21. Blurred vision
  22. Blindness
  23. Fainting or loss of consciousness
  24. Seizure or convulsion
  25. Trouble walking
  26. Paralysis or muscle weakness
  27. Urinary retention or difficulty urinating

Sexual symptoms for the major part of the person's life after opportunities for sexual activity:

  28. **Burning sensation in sexual organ or rectum (other than during intercourse)**
  29. Sexual indifference
  30. Pain during intercourse
  31. Impotence

Female reproductive symptoms judged by the person to occur more frequently or severely than in most women:

  32. **Painful menstruation**
  33. Irregular menstrual periods
  34. Excessive menstrual bleeding
  35. Vomiting throughout pregnancy

Note: The seven items in boldface may be used to screen for the disorder. The presence of two or more of these items suggests a high likelihood of the disorder.

Table 12-3.   Common symptoms in somatization disorder

Symptom	%	Symptom	%
Nervousness	92	Sexual indifference	44
Back pain	88	Dysuria	44
Weakness	84	Aphonia	44
Joint pain	84	Other bodily pains	36
Dizziness	84	Vomiting	32
Extremity pain	84	Anesthesia	32
Fatigue	84	Thoughts of suicide	28
Abdominal pain	80	Burning pains in rectum, vagina, mouth	28
Nausea	80	Lump in throat	28
Headache	80	Felt life was hopeless	28
Dyspnea	72	Weight loss	28
Trouble doing anything because felt bad	72	Anorgasmia	24
Chest pain	72	Diarrhea	20
Abdominal bloating	68	Vomiting all 9 months of pregnancy	20
Constipation	64	Blindness	20
Anxiety attacks	64	Fits of convulsions	20
Depressed feeling	64	Fluctuations in weight	16
Visual blurring	64	Unconsciousness	16
Anorexia	60	Paralysis	12
Palpitations	60	Visual hallucinations	12
Fainting	56	Attempted suicide	12
Dyspareunia	52	Amnesia	8
Menstrual irregularity	48	Urinary retention	8
Food intolerances	48	Dysmenorrhea (prepregnancy only)	8
Excessive menstrual bleeding	48	Dysmenorrhea (premarital only)	4
Dysmenorrhea (other)	48	Deafness	4
Phobias	48		

Source.   Adapted from Perley MJ, Guze SB: Hysteria—the stability and usefulness of clinical criteria. N Engl J Med 266:421–426, 1962.

for evaluation of the abdominal pain and had had a barium enema examination and an upper gastrointestinal X-ray series, both negative.

Six months before her clinic visit, she had developed blurry vision and a sharp shooting pain in her rectum with walking and had noted passing blood and mucus in her stools. Sigmoidoscopic examinations were unremarkable, but she was nevertheless diagnosed as having "mild ulcerative colitis" and was treated with Azulfidine (sulfasalazine). Another barium enema examination was negative. Five months before her clinic visit, she noted "wasting" of her hands and reported needing a larger glove size for the right hand on which she had noticed a pulsating vessel and whitish nodules for the first time.

Other medical complaints developed, including joint pains, malaise, blotching and red spots on her skin in response to sun exposure, and swelling of her right ankle, both knees, elbows, wrists, and shoulders. She began to notice multiple bruises, which were slow to heal. Three months before her clinic visit, a physician diagnosed rheumatoid arthritis despite a normal sedimentation rate and administered injections of cortisone and adrenocorticotropic hormone (ACTH), which did not help.

At her clinic visit, she identified other symptoms, including a burning pain in her pelvis, hands, and feet, heavy vaginal bleeding passing "clots as large as a fist," abdominal bloating, malodorous stools with "bits of sudsy mucus," urinary urgency, cough incontinence, tingling and burning in hands and feet, and a belief that her

Table 12-4.   Complaints from a typical somatization disorder patient

Organ system	Complaint
Neuropsychiatric	"The two hemispheres of my brain aren't working properly." "I couldn't name familiar objects around the house when asked." "I was hospitalized with tingling and numbness all over and the doctors didn't know why."
Cardiopulmonary	"I had extreme dizziness after climbing stairs." "It hurts to breathe." "My heart was racing and pounding and thumping . . . I thought I was going to die."
Gastrointestinal	"For 10 years I was treated for nervous stomach, spastic colon, and gallbladder and nothing the doctor did seemed to help." "I got a violent cramp after eating an apple and felt terrible the next day." "The gas was awful—I thought I was going to explode."
Genitourinary	"I'm not interested in sex, but I pretend to be to satisfy my husband's needs." "I've had red patches on my labia and I was told to use boric acid." "I had difficulty with bladder control and was examined for a tipped bladder, but nothing was found." "I had nerves cut going into my uterus because of severe cramps."
Musculoskeletal	"I have learned to live with weakness and tiredness all the time." "I thought I pulled a back muscle, but my chiropractor says it's a disc problem."
Sensory	"My vision is blurry. It's like seeing through a fog, but the doctor said glasses wouldn't help." "I suddenly lost my hearing. It came back, but now I have whistling noises, like an echo."
Metabolic/endocrine	"I began teaching half days because I couldn't tolerate the cold." "I was losing hair faster than my husband was."

bowel movements "just don't look right." She also disclosed a 10-year history of recurrent tonsillitis and quinsy during her childhood.

She was next seen at the same medicine clinic 21 years later after referral by her primary-care physician for evaluation of multiple somatic complaints. Her symptoms were remarkably similar to those reported earlier, including muscle weakness, fatigue, and lack of energy. She complained of a right-sided tremor that caused her to spill food, migratory aches and pains, and feeling cold in her extremities and reported heavy menstrual flow: "I used 48 sanitary pads in a single day." She also noted feeling sick; having abdominal bloating, flatulence, frequent nausea and vomiting, and constipation; her skin becoming darker; and her scalp hair falling out.

A protracted medical workup followed, including thyroid function studies, a thyroid uptake scan, rheumatoid factor, antinuclear antibody (ANA) titer, electromyography, and consultations from neurology, ophthalmology, and gynecology. She reported to the neurologist a history of convulsions 10 years earlier, which she believed left her with a residual tremor. Several years after developing convulsions, she had experienced episodes of weakness, headache, and nausea and vomiting that would wax and wane over the next 2 years. She reported having been concerned with her face sagging, which had alerted a previous neurologist to consider the diagnosis of myasthenia gravis. The ophthalmologist obtained a history of double vision and having had six changes in her eyeglass prescription during the past year because of deteriorating vision. She confirmed a history of heavy and painful bleeding to the gynecologist and also a history of five dilation and curettage procedures during the previous 10 years. She also complained of a yellowish discharge during the last 4 days of her menstrual cycle that had an "odor of semen."

Six years later, at age 53, she was admitted to a psychiatric hospital. She had had a total hysterectomy and oophorectomy in the interim, but apart from menstrual-related symptoms continued to have the same unrelenting physical complaints. Again, a protracted medical workup was negative.

This woman's remarkable history of illness spanning 27 years leaves little doubt that she had an unrecognized somatization disorder. Her complaints were consistent over the years and had resulted in multiple evaluations and procedures. Despite the multiplicity of complaints, many quite alarming, the patient remained fit and physically healthy.

The Epidemiologic Catchment Area study showed an estimated lifetime prevalence of somatization disorder in the general population of approximately 0.4%. Somatization disorder is more common in rural areas and among the less educated, and many female patients report a history of abuse or molestation as children. It is doubtful that more than a few patients experience marked improvement or permanent remission on follow-up.

Unfortunately, somatization disorder often leads to repeated surgeries, drug abuse, marital instability, depression, and suicide attempts. Most somatization disorder patients also have personality disorders (e.g., antisocial, borderline, histrionic). Although there is no one-to-one relationship between somatization disorder (hysteria) and histrionic personality, between one-half and two-thirds of somatization disorder patients meet criteria for histrionic personality.

Somatization disorder is familial, and it is found in about 20% of the first-degree female relatives of patients with the disorder. Family studies also indicate a significant association between somatization disorder and antisocial personality. First-degree male relatives of patients with somatization disorder show high rates of both antisocial personality and alcoholism. These findings have led to the observation that depending on the sex of the individual, underlying genetic or environmental factors may lead to different but overlapping clinical manifestations.

The differential diagnosis includes other psychiatric syndromes such as panic disorder, major depression, and schizophrenia. The panic disorder patient typically has a variety of physical symptoms, but these symptoms occur almost exclusively during discrete panic attacks. The depressed patient may have physical complaints, but these complaints are usually overshadowed by dysphoria and prominent vegetative symptoms of depression (e.g., appetite loss, lack of energy, insomnia). Schizophrenic patients often have physical complaints, but are typically delusional (e.g., "my spine is a set of twirling plates"). Although somatic complaints are common to these disorders, the syndromes are sufficiently different that diagnosis should not be difficult.

Table 12-5.   DSM-III-R criteria for conversion disorder

A. A loss of, or alteration in, physical functioning suggesting a physical disorder.

B. Psychological factors are judged to be etiologically related to the symptom because of a temporal relationship between a psychosocial stressor that is apparently related to a psychological conflict or need and initiation or exacerbation of the symptom.

C. The individual is not conscious of intentionally producing the symptom.

D. The symptom is not a culturally sanctioned response pattern and cannot, after appropriate investigation, be explained by a known physical disorder.

E. The symptom is not limited to pain or a disturbance in sexual functioning.

Specify: **single episode** or **recurrent**

Conversion Disorder

According to DSM-III-R, conversion disorder is defined as loss of or alteration in functioning suggesting a physical disorder; therefore, pain is not included in the definition. Further, the physician has determined that the symptom is not under voluntary control and the symptom cannot, after appropriate investigation, be explained by a known physical disorder or pathophysiologic mechanism. DSM-III-R also requires that psychological factors be judged etiologically involved with the conversion symptom as evidenced by a close, temporal relationship between an environmental stimulus and the initiation or exacerbation of the symptom; that the symptom is not consciously or intentionally produced; and that the symptom is not a culturally sanctioned response pattern. The complete criteria are listed in Table 12-5.

Common conversion symptoms include paralysis, abnormal movements, inability to speak (aphonia), blindness, and deafness. Conversion symptoms usually conform to the patient's concept of disease rather than typical physiological patterns. For example, anesthesia may follow a stocking-and-glove pattern, and not a dermatomal distribution. Symptoms may occur in isolation, but generally occur within the context of a primary illness (e.g., major depression, somatization disorder, schizophrenia). When a conversion disorder occurs along with another disorder, both diagnoses are made.

An estimated 20–25% of patients admitted to general medical services have had conversion symptoms at some time during their life. In a survey of consecutive psychiatric consultations in a general hospital, 5% were for conversion symptoms. Conversion symptoms are more common in women, patients from rural areas, and persons having low socioeconomic status.

Psychodynamic, biological, cultural, and behavioral mechanisms have been used to explain conversion symptoms. According to psychodynamic interpretations, patients with certain developmental predispositions respond to particular types of stress with conversion symptoms. The stress causes anxiety by awakening intrapsychic conflicts, usually over sexuality, aggression, or dependence issues. The high frequency of conversion symptoms in patients with a history of head injury and other organic brain conditions, however, argues for a biological etiology. The predisposition of various ethnic and social (generally non-European) groups to respond to emotional stress with particular conversions illustrates the sociocultural contributions to etiology. Models have also been developed to explain symptoms as a learned behavioral excess or deficit that follows a particular event or psychological state and is reinforced by a particular event or set of conditions.

The diagnosis of conversion disorder is established by excluding organic disease and demonstrating the presence of psychological factors involved in the symptom formation. This distinction between functional and organic symptoms is not difficult when a patient's physical symptoms are inconsistent with physical findings and the psychological stress is unmistakable. However, the diagnosis should be made with caution, for up to 30% of patients diagnosed with conversion disorder are later found to have an organic illness that in retrospect accounts for the symptom. Further, there is a high incidence of concomitant organic illness in patients with conversion symptoms. In a controlled study of hospitalized psychiatric patients diagnosed with conversion hysteria in Australia and Great Britain, 63.5% of patients but only 5.5% of control subjects had coexisting or antecedent organic brain disorders.

There are many useful clues that the clinician can use to help establish a diagnosis of conversion. Studies of patients with conversion symptoms indicate a high prevalence of comorbidity (33–50%) with major depression, somatization disorder, schizophrenia, or a personality disorder. Thus, an unexplained symptom in a patient with serious preexisting psychopathology or a prior history of conversion symptoms is more likely to be functional than organic. Many patients with conversion symptoms are believed to be modeling symptoms based on a prior illness, or on the symptoms of an illness suffered by an important figure in the patient's life (e.g., a figure from childhood).

Other psychological criteria formerly thought to be helpful in distinguishing conversion symptoms from organic disorders have not been confirmed by research, including emotional stress before the onset of symptoms, a history of disturbed sexuality, sibling position, primary gain, secondary gain, histrionic personality, and "la belle indifference." Indeed, most patients with conversion symptoms do not have any specific personality type. Further, most patients with conversion symptoms do not show "la belle indifference," but instead are deeply interested in their symptoms.

Favorable prognosis is generally associated with acute onset, definite precipitation by a stressful event, good premorbid health, and the absence of organic illness or major psychopathology. Among favorable prognostic studies, in one, 83% of inpatients and outpatients were well or improved in 4–6 years of follow-up; in another, an immediate favorable response to treatment in 100% of psychiatric outpatients with only 20% having relapses at the end of a 1-year follow-up was found. Other studies have had less optimistic findings. One study from Britain noted that of 85 patients, 4 committed suicide, and of 60 patients still alive, 82% had an organic

Table 12-6.   DSM-III-R criteria for hypochondriasis

A. Preoccupation with the fear of having, or the belief that one has, a serious disease, based on the person's interpretation of physical signs or sensations as evidence of physical illness.

B. Appropriate physical evaluation does not support the diagnosis of any physical disorder that can account for the physical signs or sensations or the person's unwarranted interpretation of them, **and** the symptoms in A are not just symptoms of panic attacks.

C. The fear of having, or belief that one has, a disease persists despite medical reassurance.

D. Duration of the disturbance is at least 6 months.

E. The belief in A is not of delusional intensity, as in delusional disorder, somatic type (i.e., the person can acknowledge the possibility that his or her fear of having, or belief that he or she has, a serious disease is unfounded).

disorder, schizophrenia, a mood disorder, or severely disabling conversion symptoms. Because conversion disorder rarely occurs as an isolated event and usually occurs in the context of another disorder, it is likely that the outcome reflects the natural history of the primary disorder, such as major depression, somatization disorder, or schizophrenia.

Hypochondriasis

Hypochondriasis is defined in DSM-III-R as an unrealistic interpretation of physical signs or sensations as abnormal, leading to the preoccupation with or fear of having a serious illness. This preoccupation occurs in the absence of a demonstrable physical disorder that could account for the symptoms, and in the absence of another mental disorder such as schizophrenia, major depression, or somatization disorder, and has a duration of 6 months or more. See Table 12-6 for the complete set of criteria.

Hypochondriacal patients display an abnormal concern with their health and tend to amplify normal physiologic sensations and misinterpret them as indicators of disease. These patients often fear a particular disease (e.g., cancer or AIDS) and cannot be reassured despite careful and repeated examinations. The following case example illustrates hypochondriasis.

Mabel, an 80-year-old retired school teacher, was admitted for evaluation of an 8-month preoccupation with having colon cancer. The patient had a history of single-vessel coronary artery disease and diabetes mellitus controlled by oral hypoglycemic agents, but was otherwise well. There was no history of mental illness. On admission, she reported her concern about having colon cancer, like her two brothers. As evidence of possible cancer, she reported having mild diffuse abdominal pain and cited an abnormal barium enema examination that she had had a year earlier. (The examination revealed diverticulosis.)

Because of her concern about having cancer, she had seen 11 physicians, but each in turn had been unable to reassure her that she did not have cancer.

Despite her complaint, Mabel denied depressed mood, displayed a full affect, and appeared to enjoy life. She reported sleeping less than usual, but attributed this to her abdominal discomfort.

At the hospital, Mabel was pleasant and cooperative, but chose not to socialize with other patients, whom she characterized as "crazy." She continued to be preoccupied with the possibility that she had cancer despite our reassurance. A benzodiazepine was prescribed for her sleep disturbance.

Despite the popularity of the term *hypochondriasis* and the frequency with which physicians see patients with functional symptoms, not much is known about the disorder. Unlike somatization disorder, which starts early in life and affects mostly women, hypochondriasis may begin at any age, but peaks in the middle years, and is equally common in men and women. There usually is no precipitating stressor. The prevalence of hypochondriasis in the general population is unknown, but bodily symptoms commonly occur in 60–80% of healthy individuals in any given week, and intermittent worry about illness occurs in about 10–20% of normal persons and in about 45% of psychiatric outpatients. Although most patients can be reassured by physicians that their symptoms are benign, about 9% will doubt the physician's reassurance.

Like the patient with somatization disorder, hypochondriacal patients, too, may have complaints involving most organ systems, doctor-shop, receive many evaluations and unnecessary surgery, and become addicted to drugs as a result of their ongoing physical complaints. The distinction between hypochondriasis and somatization disorder rests on age at onset and the number of symptoms that a patient reports.

Like conversion symptoms, hypochondriacal symptoms may occur in the course of schizophrenia or mood disorders, both of which need to be ruled out. Clinical remission appears unlikely, and a waxing and waning course is typical.

Somatoform Pain Disorder

Pain is the major symptom in a somatoform pain disorder, which lasts at least 6 months (see Table 12-7 for complete criteria). Some investigators believe that somatoform pain disorder is a conversion symptom, but this belief is debatable.

Table 12-7. DSM-III-R criteria for somatoform pain disorder

A. Preoccupation with pain for at least 6 months.

B. Either (1) or (2):

1. Appropriate evaluation uncovers no organic pathology or pathophysiologic mechanism (e.g., a physical disorder or the effects of injury) to account for the pain.
2. When there is related organic pathology, the complaint of pain or resulting social or occupational impairment is grossly in excess of what would be expected from the physical findings.

Among patients with somatoform pain disorder, pain is often related to environmental stress, such as the breakup of a relationship, and generally occurs in the absence of identifiable organic disease or is grossly out of proportion to that expected from the physical pathology. A case example follows.

> Nancy, a 34-year-old school teacher, developed disabling lower back pain coincidental to a work-related lawsuit in which she alleged unfair treatment by her co-workers. She attributed the back pain to a trivial fall 6 months earlier in which she had twisted her ankle; extensive neurologic and orthopedic workups had failed to document any physiologic abnormality. She became preoccupied by her back pain, had to quit working, and joined a support group for chronic pain sufferers.

Patients with somatoform pain disorder are commonly seen by internists and general practitioners, mostly because of the physical nature of their complaints, which are often accompanied by a denial of psychiatric symptoms such as depressed mood.

These disorders have been explained by psychoanalysts as a defect in ego functioning underlying the experience and expression of feelings. Psychologically stressful events are believed to be translated into somatic symptoms, rather than allowing the individual to develop and elaborate appropriate emotions. The inability to express emotion is called *alexithymia* and is believed to characterize the mechanisms of other neurotic symptoms (e.g., somatization, anxiety, dissociation, conversion).

Unexplained pain often occurs in the course of other psychiatric disorders, such as schizophrenia, somatization disorder, or major depression. In one case series, 60% of depressed patients reported subjective complaints of pain. Conversely, depression is a frequent accompaniment of chronic pain, although most pain patients do not have fulminant vegetative symptoms of depression. Therefore, the clinician must take care to search for a major depression when chronic pain is present. According to DSM-III-R, both disorders may be diagnosed together.

Other Somatoform Disorders

There are three residual categories reserved in DSM-III-R for patients who do not clearly manifest the characteristics of the four major somatoform disorders: body dysmorphic disorder, undifferentiated somatoform disorder, and somatoform disorder not otherwise specified.

A patient with *body dysmorphic disorder* is usually preoccupied with a specific organ or body part rather than having diffuse complaints involving multiple organ systems; this condition is often termed *dysmorphophobia*. A patient may believe that he or she is suffering from a serious disease on the basis of a minor local lesion such as a freckle on a nose. Patients who focus on perceived defects in their facial appearance often seek plastic surgery. This condition needs to be differentiated from *monohypochondriacal paranoia* (delusional disorder, somatic type) in which a patient has a delusional belief that a body part, such as the nose, is grossly deformed or distorted. In body dysmorphic disorder, the patient will not be delusional and is willing to acknowledge the possibility that the perceived defect is trivial. Monohypochondriacal paranoia has been reported to respond to the antipsychotic pimozide.

The diagnosis of *undifferentiated somatoform disorder* is reserved for patients with multiple functional complaints lasting at least 6 months but who do not meet criteria for another somatoform disorder. The category *somatoform disorder not otherwise specified* is a residual category for patients with somatoform symptoms who do not meet the criteria for any specific somatoform disorder or adjustment disorder with physical complaints. Because these three residual categories are relatively new, information about their frequency and course are not available.

Clinical Management of the Somatoform Disorders

Despite the development of effective treatments for patients with schizophrenic, mood, or anxiety disorders, the fundamental management of patients with somatoform disorders has not changed substantially in the past 25 years. However, physicians are now more aware of these disorders and recognize that simple measures can have a profound impact on the care and treatment of patients who suffer from these disorders.

Recommendations for the treatment of somatization disorder, hypochondriasis, and somatoform pain disorder are similar. There is general agreement on treatment approaches among experienced clinicians. These recommended approaches are not based on controlled clinical trials, but on everyday experience. First, it is essential that the physician follow the Hippocratic oath and "do no harm." Polysymptomatic disorders often lead to repeated evaluations, surgeries, and medication that may have little or no relevance to the underlying disorder. Because symptoms may be exaggerated or misidentified (e.g., minor spotting during the menses may be reported as "gushing"), physicians may overreact and pursue the diagnostic equivalent of a "wild goose chase." Therefore, it is essential that physicians who encounter patients with multiple unexplained symptoms make a proper diagnosis. Nonpsychiatric physicians may find a psychiatric consultation to be extremely helpful in pinpointing the diagnosis, and in helping to formulate treatment plans. A proper diagnosis and treatment plan will help to place the patient's symptoms in context so that unnecessary evaluations and surgeries will be avoided.

Second, the physician needs to establish a long-term empathic relationship with the patient and, hopefully, will become the patient's primary and only physician. These patients have a tendency to doctor-shop, which only leads to more evaluations, greater expense, and the possibility of iatrogenic complications.

Third, it is important to see the patient at regular intervals so that he or she will not need to acquire new symptoms to see a physician. The purpose of the visit is to listen attentively and to respond to historical data without inquiring in detail about the physical symptoms reported. By avoiding placing the focus on symptoms, the physician is able to convey the message that physical complaints are not the most important or interesting thing about the patient. It is advisable to set specific appointments at brief intervals.

Fourth, it is important to minimize the use of psychotropic agents and prescription analgesics. Somatoform disorder patients often request medications, but there is usually little indication for them. Whether medication is ever justified, particularly as these patients are at risk for substance abuse, is debatable. There are no data to show that medication is beneficial in treating either somatization disorder or hypochondriasis; therefore, medication is not indicated unless another psychiatric syndrome develops that may be amenable to treatment, such as major depression.

Depression is common in somatoform disorder patients, but there is little empirical data about the effectiveness of antidepressants in these patients. In general, secondary depressions do not respond well to antidepressant medication, so physicians should not have unrealistically high expectations for the treatment. There is some evidence to suggest that chronic pain, including idiopathic pain, may be relieved by antidepressants, but this association has not been subjected to careful study. Occasionally, somatoform disorder patients will develop an anxiety syndrome, such as generalized anxiety disorder, and benefit from the short-term use of a benzodiazepine (e.g., diazepam or alprazolam). Because of their potential for abuse, benzodiazepine use should be sharply limited and closely monitored. Ground rules need to be established from the outset so that the patient will be aware that anxiolytic therapy is considered a temporary measure only.

Finally, it is important to realize that the lives of patients with these disorders revolve around their symptoms, and that they are highly resistant to referral for psychiatric treatment. Thus, the most important therapeutic approach available to the primary physician is a sound, long-term doctor-patient relationship.

These five simple measures have been demonstrated to lower health care costs in patients with somatization disorder. A group of patients receiving a psychiatric consultation with recommendations for conservative care experienced a 53% drop in health care costs, mostly due to fewer hospitalizations. There was no change in the patients' health status or satisfaction with their health care. Health care costs of control subjects did not change.

Recommendations for management of the somatoform disorders

1. Schedule the patient for brief, but frequent, visits.
   - As the patient improves, the time between visits can be extended.

2. Establish an empathic relationship to reduce the patient's tendency to doctor-shop.
   - Try to be the patient's only physician.

3. Focus on psychosocial problems, not the physical symptoms.
   - Don't try to talk patients out of their symptoms or tell them it is "all in their head." To the patient, the symptom is real and distressing.

4. Minimize the use of psychotropic drugs.
   - No medication has proven value in somatoform disorders.
   - These patients may tend to become dependent on drugs easily, particularly sedative-hypnotics.

5. Minimize medical evaluations to reduce expense as well as iatrogenic complications.
   - Simple (i.e., conservative) management is proven to reduce costs.

Systematic treatment of conversion symptoms has not been well established, but reassurance and suggestion are usually appropriate, along with efforts to resolve any stressful situation that may have provoked the reaction. The spontaneous remission rate for individual conversion symptoms is high, so that even without intervention, most patients will improve and will not suffer adverse complications from the disorder. A method using behavior modification has been described in which the patient is placed at complete bed rest with the use of a bed pan and is informed that use of ward facilities will parallel improvement. As the patient improves, the time out of bed is gradually increased, and eventually, full privileges are restored. Nearly all patients (84%), who had various conversion symptoms ranging from blindness to bilateral wrist drop, experienced full remission. By allowing the patient to "save face," this method may have the advantage of keeping secondary gain (e.g., escaping from noxious activities, obtaining desired attention from family, friends, and others) to a minimum and reducing the opportunity for acting out.

In treating the conversion disorder patient, hospital staff should remain supportive and demonstrate concern, while encouraging self-help. It may be explained to the patient that the disorder is caused by psychological factors. It is rarely helpful to confront patients about their symptoms or make them feel ashamed of them.

Some investigators believe that hypnosis or intravenous amobarbital sodium may help the patient to relive the events that provoked the conversion symptoms and to abreact (or express) accompanying emotions. Psychodynamically oriented clinicians have recommended insight-oriented psychotherapy, focusing on childhood sexual behavior and other problems that they believe central to the etiology of conversion. These techniques, however, have not proved to be any more effective than conservative approaches.

Related Disorders

There are several conditions related to the somatoform disorders in which physical illnesses are mimicked. In DSM-III-R, factitious disorders and malingering are categorized separately from somatoform disorders. Another common clinical syndrome, compensation neurosis, does not appear in DSM-III-R, but because of its clinical importance will be briefly discussed.

Factitious Disorders

According to DSM-III-R, factitious disorders result in the intentional production or feigning of physical or psychological symptoms. In these disturbances, there is presumably a psychological need to assume the sick role, as evidenced by the lack of external incentives for the behavior, such as economic gain, better care, or improved physical well-being. The disorder is not diagnosed in the presence of another severe Axis I disorder, such as schizophrenia. The criteria are listed in Table 12-8.

Table 12-8. DSM-III-R criteria for factitious disorders

With physical symptoms:

A. Intentional production or feigning of physical (but not psychological) symptoms.

B. A psychological need to assume the sick role, as evidenced by the absence of external incentives for the behavior, such as economic gain, better care, or physical well-being.

C. Occurrence not exclusively during the course of another Axis I disorder, such as schizophrenia.

With psychological symptoms:

A. Intentional production or feigning of psychological (but not physical) symptoms.

B. A psychological need to assume the sick role, as evidenced by the absence of external incentives for the behavior, such as economic gain, better care, or physical well-being.

C. Occurrence not exclusively during the course of another Axis I disorder, such as schizophrenia.

Patients with factitious disorders knowingly fake physical or emotional illnesses for reasons that are presumably unconscious. Many persons with the disorder appear to make hospitalization a way of life and have been called "hospital hoboes," or "peregrinating problem patients." The term *Munchausen syndrome* has also been applied to this condition to describe the patient who moves from hospital to hospital simulating various illnesses. *Munchausen* comes from the fictitious peregrinations of the 19th century Baron von Munchausen, who was known for his tall tales and fanciful exaggeration. Cases have even been noted of Munchausen syndrome by proxy: a parent repeatedly induces illness or simulates illness in his or her child, so that the child is repeatedly hospitalized.

The incidence of factitious disorder is unknown, because many cases probably go undetected. However, in one study involving fever of unknown origin, up to 10% of the fevers were diagnosed as factitious. Factitious symptoms can occur in almost any organ system, and the various symptoms produced are limited only by the imagination of the patient.

Patients with factitious disorders will generally use one of three strategies: 1) reporting symptoms suggesting an illness, although not having them; 2) producing false evidence of an illness, such as a factitious fever by applying friction to a thermometer to raise the temperature; or 3) intentionally producing symptoms of illness, for example, by injecting feces into a knee joint, or taking warfarin orally to induce a bleeding disorder. Common methods for producing a factitious disorder are presented in Table 12-9.

Although most cases of factitious disorder involve the simulation of physical illness, patients sometimes feign mental illness. This form of factitious disorder is apparently less common, and its diagnosis can be extremely difficult, due in part to the lack of objective physical or laboratory abnormalities in mental illness. Patients may report depression, delusions, or auditory hallucinations, or they may

Table 12-9. Methods used to produce factitious disorders in 41 patients

Method	%
Injection or insertion of contaminated substance	29
Surreptitious use of medications	24
Exacerbation of wounds	17
Thermometer manipulation	10
Urinary tract manipulation	7
Falsification of medical history	7
Self-induced bruises or deformities	2
Phlebotomy	2

Source. Adapted from Reich P, Gottfried LA: Factitious disorders in a teaching hospital. Ann Intern Med 99:240–247, 1983.

behave in a bizarre manner, all in an attempt to simulate mental illness. In a follow-up of nine patients with factitious psychosis, patients remained emotionally disturbed and had poor social functioning. All patients had severe personality disorders.

Studies suggest that factitious disorder is a chronic condition that starts early in adulthood, in persons who may have had prior experience with hospitalization or severe illness, either of themselves or someone close to them, such as a parent. The disorder causes severe impairment of social and occupational functioning, because these patients spend a great deal of time in the hospital. Factitious disorders have been associated with severe personality disorders, such as borderline or antisocial personality. In one study, the majority of patients had worked in medically related occupations, including medicine, nursing, and medical technology. Most had various abnormal personality traits, but none was diagnosed as having a major mental disorder (i.e., Axis I disorder). Ninety-three percent were women.

It is believed that patients with factitious disorder consciously produce the signs or symptoms of physical illness to obtain medical care. Although the patients are aware of their role in producing signs and symptoms of illness, they are typically unaware of their motivation for having done so. Only psychological inference may give us clues as to what these motivations are. Some investigators believe that these patients may have had a personal history of deprivation coupled with absent or inattentive parents, but found love and caring from health care providers. Therefore, by producing genuine illness, the patient may re-create the nurturing atmosphere experienced earlier. However, not all patients with factitious disorders have a background of deprivation, so these theories can only apply to a minority of patients.

The differentiation of factitious disorder from somatoform disorders and malingering, based on presumed psychological mechanisms, is presented in Table 12-10.

Diagnosis of factitious illnesses requires almost as much inventiveness as is displayed by the patient in producing symptoms. Clues to the diagnosis will include a long and involved medical history that does not correspond to the patient's apparent health and vigor, a clinical presentation that too closely resembles text-

Table 12-10.   Differentiating between somatoform disorders, factitious disorders, and malingering

Disorder	Mechanism of illness production	Motivation for illness production
Somatization disorder	Unconscious	Unconscious
Conversion disorder	Unconscious	Unconscious
Hypochondriasis	Unconscious	Unconscious
Somatoform pain disorder	Unconscious	Unconscious
Factitious disorder	Conscious	Unconscious
Malingering	Conscious	Conscious

Source.   Adapted from Eisendrath SJ: Factitious illness: a clarification. Psychosomatics 25:110–117, 1984.

book descriptions, a sophisticated medical vocabulary, demands for specific medications or treatments, and a history of excessive surgeries. When factitious disorder is suspected, previous hospital charts should be gathered and prior clinicians spoken to. In one case reported in the literature, the authors were able to document at least 15 different hospitalizations in a 2-year period before admission and learned that the medical evaluations had led to repeated cardiac catheterizations and angiograms and had also resulted in the complication of the loss of a limb. In this particular patient, clues to the diagnosis included the manner in which the patient presented his story, absence of family or friends at the hospital, presence of multiple surgical scars, and an absence of distress despite complaints of crushing retrosternal pain.

Treatment of patients with factitious disorder is difficult and frustrating. The first task in treatment is identifying the illness as factitious, so that additional, and potentially harmful, procedures are avoided. Because most of these patients are hospitalized on medical and surgical wards, a psychiatric consultation should be sought. The psychiatrist can assist with the diagnosis and help to educate the physicians and nurses about the nature of factitious disorders. Once sufficient evidence has been gathered to support the diagnosis, the patient should be confronted, preferably in a nonthreatening manner by the attending physician and the psychiatrist. In a follow-up of 42 patients, 33 patients were confronted; none signed out of the hospital or became suicidal, and although only 13 patients acknowledged causing their disorders, most improved after the confrontation and 4 became asymptomatic. It is difficult to know how extensive the improvement was or how long it may have lasted, however. The authors reported that their lawyers had advised that room searches could be justified legally and ethically in their pursuit of a diagnosis, just as a search would be justified in the case of the patient who was thought to be suicidal. In both situations, the condition could be life threatening.

Malingering

DSM-III-R classifies malingering with the V-code conditions, which are not attributable to mental illness, but which are a focus of attention or treatment.

Malingering is defined as the intentional production of false or grossly exaggerated physical or psychological symptoms, motivated by external incentives, such as avoiding military conscription or duty, avoiding work, obtaining financial compensation, evading criminal prosecution, obtaining drugs, or securing better living conditions.

Unlike factitious disorder, where symptoms are produced for presumably unconscious reasons, malingering is produced intentionally for reasons that are generally apparent to the malingerer. Although the prevalence of malingering is not known, it is believed that most malingerers are men who have obvious reasons to feign illness, such as prisoners, factory workers, or persons in other unpleasant settings where illness may provide a temporary escape from harsh responsibilities.

Malingering should be strongly suspected if any combination of the following is noted: medicolegal context of presentation (e.g., the person is being referred by his or her attorney for examination), marked discrepancy with the person's claimed disability and objective findings; the patient's lack of cooperation during the diagnostic evaluation and in complying with the treatment regimen; or the presence of antisocial personality disorder. The patient suspected of malingering should be thoroughly evaluated because most symptoms that patients report will be vague and unverifiable.

There is controversy about the correct approach to the malingerer. Some investigators feel that the malingerer should be confronted after sufficient evidence has been collected to confirm the diagnosis, whereas others feel that confrontations will simply disrupt the doctor-patient relationship and make the patient even more vigilant to possible detection. Clinicians who take the second position feel that it is best to approach the patient as though the symptoms are real, and symptoms can then be given up in response to treatment without the patient losing face.

Compensation Neurosis

Compensation or accident neurosis consists of psychologically motivated physical or mental symptoms occurring in situations in which the patient is the subject of an unsettled claim for compensation. Material incentive seems to increase or prolong the symptoms, which, according to clinical lore, improve when a single final payment is negotiated (the "greenback poultice"). Thus, as long as a claim continues, or if compensation depends on regular review of the continued disability, symptoms are believed likely to persist.

In these situations, it is almost impossible to decide to what extent the patient is producing the symptoms consciously or experiencing the result of an intrapsychic process. In most cases, bodily symptoms occur without demonstrable organic pathology, such as chronic low back pain.

In a follow-up study of 35 claimants with accident neurosis, few claimants had recovered, and the recovery that took place was unrelated to the time of compensation. Overprotection by relatives appeared to be the most important factor in prolonging the symptoms.

Bibliography

Bash IY, Alpert M: The determination of malingering. Ann NY Acad Sci 347:86–99, 1980

Coryell W, Norten SG: Briquet's syndrome (somatization disorder) and primary depression: comparison of background and outcome. Compr Psychiatry 22:249–256, 1981

Dickes RA: Brief therapy of conversion reactions: an in-hospital technique. Am J Psychiatry 131:584–586, 1974

Dworkin SF, Von Korff M, LeResch EL: Multiple pains and psychiatric disturbance: an epidemiologic investigation. Arch Gen Psychiatry 47:239–244, 1990

Eisendrath SJ: Factitious illness: a clarification. Psychosomatics 25:110–117, 1984

Katon W, Ries RK, Kleinman A: The prevalence of somatization in primary care. Compr Psychiatry 25:208–214, 1984

Kellner R: Hypochondriasis and somatization. JAMA 258:2718–2722, 1987

Kenyon FF: Hypochondriacal states. Br J Psychiatry 129:1–14, 1976

Lilienfeld SO, VanValkenberg C, Larntz K, et al: The relationship of histrionic personality disorder to antisocial personality and somatization disorders. Am J Psychiatry 143:718–722, 1986

Morrison J: Childhood sexual histories of women with somatization disorder. Am J Psychiatry 146:239–241, 1989

Murphy GE: The clinical management of hysteria. JAMA 247:2559–2564, 1982

Perley MJ, Guze SB: Hysteria—the stability and usefulness of clinical criteria. N Engl J Med 266:421–426, 1962

Pope HG, Jonas JM, Jones B: Factitious psychosis: phenomenology, family history, and long-term outcome of nine patients. Am J Psychiatry 139:1480–1483, 1982

Quill TE: Somatization disorder—one of medicine's blind spots. JAMA 254:3075–3079, 1985

Reich P, Gottfried LA: Factitious disorders in a teaching hospital. Ann Intern Med 99:240–247, 1983

Rosenblatt RM, Reich J, Dehring D: Tricyclic antidepressants in the treatment of depression and chronic pain-analysis of the supporting evidence. Anesth Analg 63:1025–1032, 1984

Shah KA, Forman MB, Freedman HS: Munchausen's syndrome and cardiac catheterization—a case of a pernicious interaction. JAMA 248:3008–3009, 1982

Slater ETO, Glithero E: A follow-up of patients diagnosed as suffering from "hysteria." J Psychosom Res 9:9–13, 1965

Smith GR, Monson RA, Ray DC: Psychiatric consultation in somatization disorder. N Engl J Med 314:1407–1413, 1986

Swartz M, Blazer D, George L, et al: Somatization disorder in a community population. Am J Psychiatry 143:1403–1408, 1986

Tarsh MJ, Roysten C: A follow-up study of accident neurosis. Br J Psychiatry 146:18–25, 1985

Self-assessment Questions

1. What is the origin of the terms *hysteria* and *hypochondriasis*?
2. How is somatization disorder diagnosed?
3. What do family studies of somatization disorder show?
4. Explain conversion as an ego-defense mechanism.
5. What are the risk factors for conversion disorder?
6. What is the natural history of the different somatoform disorders?
7. How does somatization disorder differ from hypochondriasis?
8. How are the somatoform disorders managed?
9. How do the somatoform disorders, factitious disorders, and malingering differ?
10. Explain compensation neurosis.

Chapter 13
Dissociative Disorders

*In a bright, unfamiliar voice that sparkled, the woman said,
"Hi, there, Doc!"*

Three Faces of Eve, *1957*

The history of dissociation parallels that of hysteria and hypnosis. Charcot at the Salpêtrière in Paris had recognized somnambulism, fugue, and multiple personality as manifestations of "la grande hysterie." Janet, Charcot's disciple, believed that dissociation of mental processes was the basis of all hysterical phenomena. According to Janet, dissociation is a defect of mental integration in which one or more groups of mental processes have become separated from consciousness and function independently. Freud, who also visited Charcot at the Salpêtrière, identified among the hysterical disorders those due to dissociation, which included altered states of consciousness, such as somnambulism, fugue, and multiple personality, and those due to conversion, which encompass sensory and motor phenomena, such as hysterical paraplegia and anesthesia. This distinction has proved useful and, in fact, is used in DSM-III-R, the former comprising the dissociative disorders, and the latter the somatoform disorders.

In the 20th century, interest in the dissociative disorders, particularly multiple personality, has waxed and waned. In the early part of the century, the syndrome of multiple personality fell into disrepute as many psychiatrists came to believe that it was caused by hypnosis, and that they were being duped by patients. However, cases continued to accumulate in the literature, and in the last decade, interest in the disorder has been revived. Hollywood and the popular press have never lost interest in dissociative disorders, especially amnestic states and multiple

283

Table 13-1.   Dissociative disorders

- Amnestic states

    Psychogenic amnesia
    Psychogenic fugue

- Multiple personality disorder

- Depersonalization disorder

- Dissociative disorder not otherwise specified

personality. These disorders have continued to fascinate the public for over 50 years as the subjects of movies and books.

According to DSM-III-R, dissociative disorders are characterized by a disturbance or alteration in the normally integrative functions of identity, memory, and consciousness. The disturbance may have a sudden or gradual onset, and its course may be transient or chronic. These disorders range from manifesting additional personalities, to developing disturbances in memory, to developing a feeling that one's own reality is lost.

These disorders tend to present in colorful ways. Their dramatic quality and their presumed rarity have probably contributed to the skepticism among many mental health professionals about their validity, particularly multiple personality. Recent reports suggest that these disorders may be more common than once thought.

The dissociative disorders include the amnestic states, multiple personality disorder, and depersonalization disorder. A residual category exists for dissociative disorders that do not meet the criteria for a specific disorder (Table 13-1).

Amnestic States

Memory loss from psychological causes is called *psychogenic amnesia* (Table 13-2). The disorder is defined as a single episode of sudden inability to recall important information, a loss too extensive to be explained by ordinary forgetfulness. The prevalence of psychogenic amnesia is unknown, but it has been reported to occur after severe physical or psychosocial stressors (e.g., natural disasters, war). In a study of combat veterans, 5–20% were amnestic for their combat experiences, and 5–14% of all military psychiatric casualties have amnestic syndromes.

Typically, perplexity, confusion, and disorientation occur initially, followed by

Table 13-2.   DSM-III-R criteria for psychogenic amnesia

A. The predominant disturbance is an episode of sudden inability to recall important personal information that is too extensive to be explained by ordinary forgetfulness.

B. The disturbance is not due to multiple personality disorder or to an organic mental disorder (e.g., blackouts during alcohol intoxication).

Table 13-3.   DSM-III-R criteria for psychogenic fugue

A. The predominant disturbance is sudden, unexpected travel away from home or one's customary place of work, with inability to recall one's past.

B. Assumption of a new identity (partial or complete).

C. The disturbance is not due to multiple personality disorder or to an organic mental disorder (e.g., partial complex seizures in temporal lobe epilepsy).

an awareness that the subject does not recall significant personal information, or even his or her own identity. The duration of amnesia may range from minutes to days, or in some cases even longer. In one series, 79% of amnestic episodes lasted less than a week.

Although the cause of amnesia is unknown, Freud explained it as the result of the repression of unacceptable thoughts and wishes that would otherwise cause distress. An alternative explanation is that amnesia is an innate ability to enter altered states in response to stressful stimuli.

Psychogenic amnesia typically has a sudden onset and rapid and spontaneous recovery, although gradual onset and recoveries are occasionally found. Recurrences may occur, particularly if the precipitating stressors remain or return.

Because recovery is spontaneous, it is doubtful that specific interventions are necessary. Hypnosis and intravenous amobarbital sodium ("Amytal") interviews have been used successfully in some patients to help in recovering memories. (See Chapter 24 for details about the technique.) Once the memory is recovered, some experts believe that it is useful to assist the patient in developing an understanding of his or her motivation behind the memory loss.

Psychogenic fugue is characterized by amnesia with inability to recall one's past and the assumption of a new identity, which may be partial or complete (Table 13-3). The fugue usually involves sudden, unexpected travel away from home or from one's customary place of work and by definition is not due to multiple personality or an organic mental disorder, such as one due to temporal lobe epilepsy.

Psychogenic fugue, like psychogenic amnesia, has been reported to occur in the context of severe psychological stress, including war and civilian and natural disasters. In some persons, personal rejections, losses, or financial pressures may precede the fugue, which is typically brief, lasting hours to days with a minimal amount of travel. A fugue can last for months and develop into a complicated pattern of travel and identity formation. Recovery of past memories and the resumption of the former identity usually occur abruptly, often over hours, but may take much longer. Hypnosis and/or intravenous amobarbital sodium ("Amytal") interviews have been reported to be helpful in assisting patients to recover missing memories.

A case example of a woman who suffered a fugue state follows.

Carrie, a 31-year-old attorney from a small midwestern town, was reported to the police as missing for 4 days, under mysterious circumstances. Normally dedicated and dependable, Carrie was known to have finished her day at work, had exercised at a health spa, and then failed to return home to her husband. Her car was later found abandoned in town. A search was mounted, and it was assumed that she had been abducted, or even murdered, especially after a headless corpse had turned up. Candlelight vigils were held, psychics were consulted, and friends blanketed the community with posters offering rewards for help in locating Carrie.

One month after her disappearance, Carrie called her father from Las Vegas, where she said she had been the entire time. She claimed to have suffered amnesia, had been admitted to a mental hospital, and was regaining her memory with the help of a psychologist. There was no history of mental illness, although she had been described by friends as a "free spirit."

Carrie stated that after jogging on the night of her disappearance, she had been physically assaulted, which prompted the amnesia, and she had been unable to recall her past. An assailant had forced her toward an alley, and an altercation ensued. Carrie said that during the struggle she was "struck in the head" and knocked unconscious. "When I came to, I was dazed, confused, and disoriented." Afterward, she had obtained transportation to Las Vegas and assumed a new name. Her condition soon became known to the police, who helped her receive medical care and treatment.

Carrie quickly recovered her memory and her identity. She returned home and resumed her legal practice.

The differential diagnosis of amnesia includes various organic disorders that can cause memory impairment, such as a brain tumor, closed head trauma, or a dementing illness. A complete workup should include a physical examination, mental status examination, toxicologic studies, electroencephalogram, and other measures when indicated. (The complete "organic workup" is listed in Table 6-6.) The chief differential will be among the different dissociative disorders, organic mental disorders, and malingering. If the amnesia develops into a period characterized by separate identity and experiences, psychogenic fugue and multiple personality must be considered.

In general, organic disorders are unlikely to have sudden onset and termination related to psychological stressors. Furthermore, memory impairments in many organic conditions are more severe for recent than for remote events, resolve slowly if at all, and are rarely followed by full return of memory. Additionally, disturbances in attention, disorientation, or a labile affect are characteristic of many organic disorders, but are unlikely in psychogenic amnesia. Memory loss from alcohol intoxication ("blackouts") is distinguished by the failure of full short-term recall and evidence of heavy substance abuse. Malingering involves the simulation of inability to recall one's past or representing oneself as having amnesia for behaviors that are alleged to be out of character (e.g., claiming amnesia for a crime). Careful observation in a hospital setting will be helpful in making the diagnosis.

Multiple Personality Disorder

Multiple personality disorder (MPD) is characterized by the development of two or more distinct personalities or personality states (Table 13-4). A *personality* is defined as a relatively enduring pattern of thinking and behavior exhibited in a

Table 13-4. DSM-III-R criteria for multiple personality disorder

A. The existence within the person of two or more distinct personalities or personality states (each with its own relatively enduring pattern of perceiving, relating to, and thinking about the environment and self).

B. At least two of these personalities or personality states recurrently take full control of the person's behavior.

wide range of social and personal contexts, but a *personality state* is not as well developed. In some patients with MPD, there may be at least two fully developed personalities, whereas in other patients there may be only one distinct personality and one or more personality states. According to DSM-III-R, at least two of these personalities or personality states must recurrently take full control of the person's behavior for the diagnosis to be made.

Although MPD has been described for centuries, most lay conceptions are based on media depictions, such as Eve and Sybil. The prevalence of MPD is not currently known, but is reportedly rare. A recent report from an inpatient unit and an outpatient clinic, however, suggests that it may be more common than originally thought.

Between 75 and 90% of patients with MPD are female, and the disorder is believed to have its onset in childhood, usually before age 9 years. MPD has been described as occurring in multiple generations and in siblings within families. MPD apparently runs a chronic course.

It is not known what causes MPD, although severe abuse during early childhood has been implicated. A current etiologic model holds that MPD is the result of self-induced hypnosis, in which individuals overwhelmed with abuse, psychological mistreatment, or neglect develop different personalities to deal with different aspects of trauma. In this sense, MPD may represent a form of posttraumatic stress disorder.

According to one large case series, the average number of personalities in the MPD patient is 7, although approximately one-half of the patients had more than 10 personalities. Over the course of the patient's life, however, different personalities may vary in the percentage of the time that they control a person's behavior.

The transition from one personality to another usually occurs suddenly, although it may be gradual. The switches are thought to be brought on by psychosocial stressors, conflict among the personalities, or intrapsychic conflicts. The personalities may or may not be aware of each other.

Common symptoms reported by patients with MPD and characteristic of their alternate personalities are presented in Table 13-5.

A case example of a patient with MPD seen in our hospital follows.

Cindy, a 24-year-old, was transferred from a hospital in another state to facilitate arrangements for placement in the community. At the other hospital, Cindy had been diagnosed as having a multiple personality disorder, although in the past she had received diagnoses of chronic schizophrenia, borderline personality disorder, schizoaffective disorder, and bipolar affective disorder.

Table 13-5.   Common symptoms in multiple personality disorder (MPD) and characteristics of alternate personalities in 50 patients

MPD symptoms	%	Alternate personality characteristics	%
Markedly different moods	94	Amnestic personalities	100
Exhibiting an alternate personality	84	Personalities with proper names (e.g.,	
Different accents	68	Nick, Sally)	98
Inability to remember angry outbursts	58	Angry alternate personality	80
Inner conversations	58	Depressed alternate personality	74
Different handwriting	34	Personalities of different ages	66
Different dress or makeup	32	Suicidal alternate personality	62
Unfamiliar people know them well	18	Protector alternate personality	30
Amnesia for a previously learned subject	14	Self-abusive alternate personality	30
Discovery of unfamiliar possessions	14	Opposite-sex alternate personality	26
Different handedness	14	Personalities with non-proper names	
		(e.g., "observer," "teacher")	24
		Unnamed alternate personality	18

Source.   Adapted from Coons PM, Bohman ES, Milstein V: Multiple personality disorder: a clinical investigation of 50 cases. J Nerv Ment Dis 176:519–527, 1988.

Cindy had been well until 3 years before admission when she developed "voices." She also developed other symptoms, including multiple somatic complaints, periods of amnesia, and self-abusive behaviors. Her family and friends noticed abrupt changes in her personality and mood and thought that Cindy had become a pathological liar because she would do or say things that she would later deny. She became chronically ill, was in and out of hospitals, and was puzzling to her doctors. She had trials of antipsychotics, antidepressants, lithium carbonate, and anxiolytics with little or no benefit. Cindy continued to get worse.

Cindy was a friendly, diminutive young woman and was clean and neatly groomed. There was no evidence of a formal thought disorder, but Cindy carefully described the "voices" that she had heard for many years. She reported that these "voices" were from nine separate personalities that, with the help of a therapist, she had learned about during her prior hospitalization.

The personalities ranged in age from 2 to 48 years, and two of the personalities were masculine. Her problem, she said, was her inability to control the switches among the personalities, which made her feel out of control. Cindy reported that she had been sexually abused by her father as a child and was made to perform unspeakable acts. She also reported visual hallucinations consisting of visions of her father coming at her with a knife. Although we were not able to confirm the history of sexual abuse, it was not unlikely based on what we had learned of her father.

Cindy cooperated well with the ward routine and looked forward to placement in the community. The nurses recorded several episodes of acting out, which occurred when Cindy switched to one of her troublesome personalities. The nurses noted that at these times, her voice would change in inflection and tone. Cindy would become childlike and appear bewildered. Cindy told us that her alternate personality Joy, an 8-year-old, was responsible for acting-out behaviors. Arrangements were made for individual psychotherapy, and the patient was discharged to the community.

Patients with MPD often have multiple physical complaints and may fulfill criteria for somatization disorder; headaches are particularly common. Patients often report time lapses ("losing time"), hearing voices (usually experienced as originating

Table 13-6. DSM-III-R criteria for depersonalization disorder

A. Persistent or recurrent experiences of depersonalization as indicated by either (1) or (2):
   1. An experience of feeling detached from, and as if one is an outside observer of, one's mental processes or body
   2. An experience of feeling like an automaton or as if in a dream

B. During the depersonalization experience, reality testing remains intact.

C. The depersonalization is sufficiently severe and persistent to cause marked distress.

D. The depersonalization experience is the predominant disturbance and is not a symptom of another disorder, such as schizophrenia, panic disorder, or agoraphobia without history of panic disorder but with limited symptom attacks of depersonalization, or temporal lobe epilepsy.

---

from within the head), and being told of behaviors for which the patient has no memory. Their symptoms and level of function may fluctuate, and multiple prior diagnoses are common.

These patients usually meet criteria for other disorders, including somatization disorder, borderline personality, and major depression. The differentiation from borderline personality is particularly difficult because the two disorders coexist in proportions ranging up to 70%, and many symptoms overlap, including mood instability, identity disturbance, and self-abusive behaviors. Many patients report hallucinations and delusional-like phenomena and may carry a prior diagnosis of schizophrenia or mood disorder with psychotic features, both of which need to be ruled out.

Many experts believe that long-term therapy is of value in helping patients to integrate their personalities, although there is little objective evidence to support this recommendation. Individual psychotherapy, often facilitated with hypnosis and/or intravenous amobarbital sodium, has also been used. In one follow-up study, motivated patients in treatment with therapists who had experience with MPD achieved integration and remission of symptoms.

No medication has proved beneficial in MPD. Antidepressants may be effective for coexisting depression, although their role in these patients has not been systematically evaluated. Some clinicians claim that different personalities require different medications. Although this belief may have some theoretical value, it runs counter to known pathophysiologic mechanisms of the major disorders. As with any patient, polypharmacy should be avoided.

Depersonalization Disorder

Depersonalization disorder is characterized by periods in which persons may have a strong and unpleasant sense of their own unreality, which may be associated with a sense that the environment is also unreal (Table 13-6). This experience often makes patients feel mechanical and separated from their thoughts, emotions, or identity.

Although the prevalence of depersonalization disorder is unknown, it is apparently common in mild form, and many normal persons have transiently experienced this phenomenon. Thus, it is only diagnosed when it is severe and persistent and causes marked subjective distress.

The disorder typically begins in adolescence or early adult life, and rarely begins after the age of 40 years. The cause of depersonalization is unknown, but Freud postulated that depersonalization, as an ego-defense mechanism, allowed a person to deny one's unacceptable feelings by denying one's experience of self.

Depersonalization disorder generally runs a chronic course with remissions and exacerbations. Exacerbations often follow psychological stress, such as the breakup of a relationship. Episodes of depersonalization usually come on suddenly and may last for minutes, hours, or days, and then gradually abate.

No treatment has proven value for this disorder, but benzodiazepines (e.g., diazepam, alprazolam) may be of help in managing the accompanying anxiety. Hypnotherapy has been reported to help some patients in learning to control episodes of depersonalization.

It is important to rule out other disorders that may be associated with depersonalization, such as schizophrenia, major depression, phobias, panic disorder, obsessive-compulsive disorder, drug abuse, sleep deprivation, partial complex seizures, and migraine.

Recommendations for treatment of dissociative disorders

1. Be sure that organic causes of amnesia or dissociation are completely ruled out.

2. Be patient and supportive. In most cases of amnesia, return of memory is rapid and complete.

3. The amobarbital sodium ("Amytal") interview may be helpful both diagnostically and therapeutically.

   - In many patients, the interview will help the patient to recover missing memories.
   - The interview can be helpful diagnostically in separating functional from organic causes of amnesia, because the functional patient may experience a return of memory, and the organic patient will tend to become more confused.

4. Multiple personality disorder (MPD) patients are especially vexing, and therapy may be long-term. You may wish to refer the patient to a therapist who has experience with these patients.

   - It may be useful to help patients gradually learn about the number and nature of their personalities.
   - A goal with MPD patients should be to help them learn how to control their switches and accept responsibility for their actions.

5. Medications have no proven value in the dissociative disorders.

Bibliography

Bliss EL: Multiple Personality, Allied Disorders, and Hypnosis. New York, Oxford University Press, 1986

Brauer R, Harrow M, Tecker GJ: Depersonalization phenomena in psychiatric patients. Br J Psychiatry 117:509–515, 1970

Coons PM, Bohman ES, Milstein V: Multiple personality disorder: a clinical investigation of 50 cases. J Nerv Ment Dis 176:519–527, 1988

Fahy TA: The diagnosis of multiple personality disorder: a critical review. Br J Psychiatry 153:597–600, 1988

Horevitz RP, Braun BG: Are multiple personalities borderline? Psychiatr Clin North Am 7:69–88, 1984

Kluft RP: An update on multiple personality disorder. Hosp Community Psychiatry 38:363–373, 1987

Meller YL: Depersonalization—symptoms, meaning, therapy. Acta Psychiatr Scand 66:451–458, 1982

Putnam FW, Guroff JJ: A clinical phenomenology of multiple personality disorder: review of 100 recent cases. J Clin Psychiatry 47:285–293, 1986

Schenk L, Bear D: Multiple personality and related dissociative phenomena in patients with temporal lobe epilepsy. Am J Psychiatry 138:1311–1315, 1981

Schreiber FR: Sybil. Chicago, IL, Henry Regnery, 1973

Thigpen CH, Cleckley HM: The Three Faces of Eve. New York, McGraw-Hill, 1957

Self-assessment Questions

1. What is dissociation?
2. How does psychogenic amnesia differ from psychogenic fugue?
3. What is the differential diagnosis of the dissociative disorders?
4. What is a current popular etiologic theory of multiple personality disorder?
5. What is depersonalization? How common is it?

Chapter 14

Alcoholism

At such gruesome moments, I would solace myself with thoughts of the wondrous gifts of alcohol, the manna that mankind so seldom appreciates.

W.C. Fields

People in virtually all cultures have consumed alcoholic beverages for medicinal purposes, religious ceremony, and recreation. It is likely that from the days when cave dwellers first drank beverages from fermented juices and grains, alcohol also has led to trouble. Drunkenness was condemned in the Old Testament and in later years was thought to represent Satan's influence. Despite these associations, production of all types of liquors, wine, and beer has flourished over the centuries, and, apart from failed attempts at controlling alcohol production and distribution, such as during Prohibition in the United States, attempts at control have largely been unsuccessful. Islamic countries specifically prohibit the use of alcohol for religious reasons, not for reasons of health.

A change has slowly taken place in how American society perceives the alcoholic person. Starting with ideas presented by the American physician Benjamin Rush and the British physician Thomas Trotter, the disease concept of alcoholism was planted. By the turn of the century, institutions had opened for the treatment of alcoholism, and societies and journals devoted to the study of alcoholism were established.

The disease concept waned during Prohibition, but revived after World War II, due in part to the influence of Jellinek's *Disease Concept of Alcoholism*, published in 1960, and the number of returning veterans with alcohol-related problems. The

Table 14-1. DSM-III-R criteria for psychoactive substance abuse

A. A maladaptive pattern of psychoactive substance use indicated by at least one of the following:

1. Continued use despite knowledge of having a persistent or recurrent social, occupational, psychological, or physical problem that is caused or exacerbated by use of the psychoactive substance
2. Recurrent use in situations in which use is physically hazardous (e.g., driving while intoxicated)

B. Some symptoms of the disturbance have persisted for at least 1 month, or have occurred repeatedly over a longer period of time.

C. Never met the criteria for psychoactive substance dependence for this substance.

debate on whether alcoholism is a disease is unending, although the position that it is has been endorsed by the American Medical Association and American Psychiatric Association.

The value of the disease model has been to encourage problem drinkers to seek help in a humane, nonjudgmental way. The drawback is that it tends to excuse drinkers from responsibility for an essentially voluntary behavior: no one forces the alcoholic person to drink.

Definition

According to DSM-III-R, all substance use disorders follow the same set of criteria, including alcohol abuse and dependence (Tables 14-1 and 14-2). The definition of dependence requires that the person exhibit at least three of nine behaviors and that some symptoms of the disturbance have persisted for at least 1 month or have occurred repeatedly over a longer period of time. The criteria focus on drinking behavior, impairment caused by drinking, and the development of tolerance or withdrawal symptoms. Further, severity of psychoactive substance dependence is rated as 1) mild, if there are few, if any, symptoms in excess of those required to make the diagnosis and there is only minimal impairment; 2) moderate; or 3) severe, if many symptoms in excess of those required to make the diagnosis are present and symptoms markedly interfere with functioning.

The definition for psychoactive substance abuse requires a maladaptive pattern of substance use and duration of longer than 1 month, but also that the person has never met criteria for psychoactive substance dependence. The concept of a general drug-dependence syndrome, introduced in DSM-III-R, has been endorsed by the World Health Organization.

Epidemiology

About two-thirds of American adults drink alcoholic beverages occasionally, and 12% are "heavy drinkers"—that is, persons who drink almost every day and become

Table 14-2. DSM-III-R criteria for psychoactive substance dependence

A. At least three of the following:

1. Substance often taken in larger amounts or over a longer period than the person intended
2. Persistent desire or one or more unsuccessful efforts to cut down or control substance use
3. A great deal of time spent in activities necessary to get the substance (e.g., theft), taking the substance (e.g., chain smoking), or recovering from its effects
4. Frequent intoxication or withdrawal symptoms when expected to fulfill major role obligations at work, school, or home (e.g., does not go to work because hung over, goes to school or work "high," intoxicated while taking care of his or her children), or when substance use is physically hazardous (e.g., drives when intoxicated)
5. Important social, occupational, or recreational activities given up or reduced because of substance use
6. Continued substance use despite knowledge of having a persistent or recurrent social, psychological, or physical problem that is caused or exacerbated by the use of the substance (e.g., keeps using heroin despite family arguments about it, cocaine-induced depression, or having an ulcer made worse by drinking)
7. Marked tolerance: need for markedly increased amounts of the substance (i.e., at least a 50% increase) in order to achieve intoxication or desired effect, or markedly diminished effect with continued use of the same amount

Note: The following items may not apply to cannabis, hallucinogens, or phencyclidine (PCP):

8. Characteristic withdrawal symptoms (see specific withdrawal syndromes under psychoactive substance–induced organic mental disorders)
9. Substance often taken to relieve or avoid withdrawal symptoms

B. Some symptoms of the disturbance have persisted for at least 1 month, or have occurred repeatedly over a longer period of time.

intoxicated several times a month. Drinkers tend to be young, relatively prosperous, well educated, and urban. According to the Epidemiologic Catchment Area study, the lifetime prevalence for alcohol dependence is almost 14%. In hospitals, however, the prevalence is far greater. Between 25 and 50% of medical/surgical patients in general hospitals are alcoholic, and an estimated 50–60% of psychiatric inpatients in some settings have coexisting alcoholism or other substance abuse. Alcoholism is the third leading cause of death in the United States.

There are about four alcoholic men to each alcoholic woman, and the typical age at onset is between 16 and 30 years. Onset in men is earlier than in women, although alcoholism in women progresses more rapidly.

Alcoholism rates tend to be very high in certain countries, including the Soviet Union, France, Ireland, and Korea, and very low in other countries, including China and the Islamic countries. Certain professions are prone to alcoholism, including waiters, bartenders, longshoremen, and musicians. Other groups that are predisposed to alcoholism include patients with antisocial personality, anxiety and mood disorders, and homosexuality.

Based on epidemiologic distinctions, a simple classification for alcoholism has been developed. The Type I alcoholic patient is characterized by early onset; personality characteristics of impulsivity, distractibility, and recklessness; antisocial personality; a family history positive for alcoholism; being male; and poor treatment response. Nearly 25% of alcoholic patients meet this description.

The Type II alcoholic patient is characterized by an adult onset, a gradually increasing consumption, personality characteristics of guilt, worry, dependency, and introversion, a lack of or modest family history of drinking, equal prevalence in males and females, and a better response to treatment than Type I alcoholism. About 75% of all alcoholic patients meet the Type II description.

Clinical Findings

There is no general picture that applies to the alcoholic person. Patterns of drinking and symptoms are diverse. In its earliest stages, alcoholism may be hard to identify. Symptoms may be minimal, and the patient will probably deny drinking excessively. Family members and co-workers are the most likely candidates to identify early symptoms in the alcoholic person, which may include an insidious change in work habits or productivity, lateness or unexplained absences, or minor personality disturbances, such as irritability or moodiness. As alcoholism advances, minor physical changes may occur, such as acne rosacea, the large red nose that develops in some alcoholic patients; palmar erythema, the red palms associated with higher estrogen levels circulating in the blood of alcoholic patients; or painless enlargement of the liver consistent with fatty infiltration, the earliest form of liver involvement in alcoholism. Other symptoms may include cigarette-burned fingers, an increased number of minor respiratory or other infections, blackouts, minor accidents and bruises, complaints by others about the drinker's driving skills, and perhaps an arrest or accident due to drunk driving.

As alcoholism advances, there may be increasing signs of liver disease, such as jaundice or ascites. Additional physical changes may occur, including testicular atrophy, gynecomastia, and the development of Dupuytren's contractures. At this stage, jobs may be lost, marriages forfeited, and families estranged due to the toll that alcohol takes. The following case example illustrates many of the clinical symptoms and findings of alcoholism and represents an example of the Type II alcoholic patient.

> John, a 63-year-old attorney, was brought to an alcohol rehabilitation unit by his wife and son. When he arrived, he smelled of alcohol and had a boozy appearance and slurred speech. In a loud, belligerent manner, he said that he wouldn't stay and attempted to leave. His wife intervened and told him that she would divorce him if he didn't stay and get help. He stayed.
>
> John had a 20-year history of excessive drinking. He had started drinking when in the Army during World War II and enjoyed drinking with his friends, mostly on social occasions. He had grown up in a house where alcohol had been prohibited for religious reasons. After the war, he married, attended law school, and established a successful career as a trial attorney. Although he always enjoyed a single beer or martini after work, the drinking never led anywhere.
>
> Then, in his mid-40s, his alcohol consumption began to increase, at first imper-

ceptibly, and then noticeably. John would drink several beers or cocktails in the evening and usually fall asleep afterward. He and his wife began to fight, mostly about his drinking, which he denied was a problem. He was occasionally belligerent with his four children, whom he generally ignored. He preferred to drink his beer and watch television.

A series of personal crises followed. John had an affair with a divorced woman, separated from his wife, was eventually divorced, and remarried. He had a falling out with his law partners, left the firm, and withdrew from his longtime friends. His drinking took a more serious turn. Although he was still able to practice law, his caseload dried up as lawyers in the small town became increasingly aware of his impairment. He began to drink in the morning (to calm his nerves, he said), took advantage of the three-martini lunch, and drank in the evening, usually passing out in a chair. He continued to deny his alcoholism, even when confronted by his new wife and his four children. He pointed out that he was still able to work and was not a "skid row" bum.

His doctor also became concerned. John had become overweight and hypertensive and had developed the stigmata of alcoholism: spider angiomas, acne rosacea, palmar erythema, and testicular atrophy. The progression of the alcoholism was so gradual that by the time of hospital admission no one could remember what John was truly like. All that people remembered was his boozy appearance, his occasional belligerence, and his social withdrawal.

The inpatient program consisted of individual, group, and family therapy sessions after a period of alcohol withdrawal, which was uneventful. By the end of his 30-day stay, John was noted by his family to be happier, optimistic, more talkative, and motivated. He had new ideas for improving his law practice and looked forward to the future. At 3-year follow-up, he had remained sober, had developed a satisfying relationship with his wife and children, and had a growing law practice.

Complications

Complications of alcoholism, summarized in Table 14-3, are medical, emotional, and social. Medical problems can range from benign fatty infiltration of the liver to death from an alcohol overdose. Almost all organ systems can be affected by heavy use of alcohol, the gastrointestinal tract perhaps suffering most. Minor problems include gastritis and diarrhea. Peptic ulcers may develop or be worsened by the direct toxic effect that alcohol has on the mucosa. Fatty infiltration of the liver occurs in almost all alcoholic patients, and Laennec's cirrhosis occurs in 10% of heavy drinkers. Pancreatitis may develop and lead to impaired glucose control and impaired digestion, or frank diabetes mellitus. Other complications include cardiomyopathy, thrombocytopenia, anemia, and myopathy.

The central and peripheral nervous systems may be damaged by both the direct and indirect effects of alcohol. Peripheral neuropathy commonly occurs in a stocking-and-glove distribution, probably from alcohol-induced vitamin B deficiency. Other nervous system effects include cerebellar damage leading to dysarthria and ataxia, and the Wernicke-Korsakoff syndrome, which is due to thiamine deficiency.

Table 14-3. Medical and psychosocial hazards associated with alcoholism

• **Drug interactions**
• **Gastrointestinal**
  Esophageal bleeding
  Mallory-Weiss tear
  Gastritis
  Intestinal malabsorption
• **Pancreatitis**
• **Liver disease**
  Fatty infiltration
  Alcoholic hepatitis
  Cirrhosis
• **Nutritional deficiency**
  Malnutrition
  Vitamin B deficiency
• **Neuropsychiatric**
  Wernicke-Korsakoff syndrome
  Cortical atrophy/ventricular dilatation
  Alcohol-induced dementia
  Peripheral neuropathy
  Myopathy
  Depression
  Suicide
• **Endocrine system**
  Testicular atrophy
  Increased estrogen levels
	• **Alcohol withdrawal syndromes**
	  "The shakes"
	  Withdrawal seizures ("Rum fits")
	  Alcohol hallucinosis
	  Alcohol withdrawal delirium ("delirium tremens")
	• **Infectious disease**
	  Pneumonia
	  Tuberculosis
	• **Cardiovascular**
	  Cardiomyopathy
	  Hypertension
	• **Cancer**
	  Oral cavity
	  Esophagus
	  Large intestine/rectum
	  Liver
	  Pancreas
	• **Birth defects**
	  Fetal alcohol syndrome
	• **Psychosocial**
	  Accidents
	  Crime
	  Spouse and child abuse
	  Job loss
	  Divorce, separation
	  Legal entanglements

The Wernicke stage of this syndrome consists of the triad of nystagmus, ataxia, and mental confusion, which readily reverses with an injection of thiamine. The Wernicke stage may lead to Korsakoff's syndrome, which involves an anterograde amnesia. This amnesia is characterized by the presence of *confabulation*, which occurs when patients invent stories to fill in memory gaps. The syndrome is associated with necrotic lesions of the mammillary bodies, thalamus, and other brain stem areas. Korsakoff's syndrome is not always permanent and may be reversible in up to one-third of patients. A mild dementia may occur, due to either vitamin deficiency or the direct effect of alcohol, although the exact cause is controversial. Alcoholism has also been found to enlarge the cerebral ventricles and widen cortical sulci, effects that are partly reversible. Neuropsychological testing of alcoholic patients shows intellectual deficits, primarily in conceptual shifting. Many of these cognitive deficits are reversible, particularly as the period of sobriety gets longer.

A *fetal alcohol syndrome* has been described. Abnormalities associated with alcohol teratogenicity include a characteristic facial appearance (i.e., small head circumference and/or flattening of the facial features), low IQ, behavior problems, and minor malformations. This syndrome occurs with a frequency between 1 and 2 per 100,000 live births. Women should probably be instructed to avoid alcohol altogether during pregnancy.

Traumatic injuries are common to the alcoholic person. Alcohol contributes to over one-half of all deaths due to motor vehicle accidents occurring annually.

Minor household injuries are frequent, as the alcoholic person may stumble and fall, sustaining bruises, fractures, and lacerations. The highly publicized deaths of actors William Holden and Natalie Wood testify to the lethal nature of these accidents. Subdural hematomas occur in many elderly alcoholic persons who fall, hitting their heads and tearing the bridging veins within the skull.

Cancer rates of the mouth, tongue, larynx, esophagus, stomach, liver, and pancreas are increased in alcoholism. The exact role of alcohol in many cancers is confounded by the effects of smoking and tobacco use. Alcohol interferes with male sexual function (i.e., can cause impotence) and fertility through direct effects on testosterone levels and testicular atrophy. Increased levels of female hormones (e.g., estrogen) can lead to the development of breast enlargement and a female pubic hair pattern in the alcoholic man.

Psychiatric complications include acute intoxication, alcohol withdrawal disorders (i.e., "the shakes"), amnestic syndromes such as Korsakoff's syndrome, and dementia. Secondary depression commonly occurs in up to 60% of patients with well-established (primary) alcoholism. In fact, alcohol itself can lead to depression from its direct effects on the brain. The depression may lead to risk for suicide, which occurs in 2–4% of alcoholic persons, although suicide in alcoholic persons may occur in the absence of depression. Alcoholic persons at risk for suicide include those with a history of interpersonal loss within the past year.

Other problems associated with alcoholism are largely social and occupational. Alcoholic persons have high rates of separation and divorce, frequent job problems, including absenteeism and job loss, and legal entanglements from their public intoxication, drunk driving, and bar fights. Alcoholism is also associated with increased risk for abuse of or dependence on other substances.

Etiology

Although its cause is unknown, genetic, behavioral, neurobiological, and psychodynamic mechanisms have been used to explain alcoholism. Family studies of alcoholism have consistently shown high rates of the disorder among first-degree relatives of alcoholic persons. In fact, about 25% of fathers and brothers of alcoholic persons themselves have alcoholism.

Alcoholism has also been associated with depression, criminal behavior, and antisocial personality in the families of alcoholic persons. Typically, depression occurs in the female relatives and alcoholism or antisocial personality in male relatives of alcoholic persons.

Twin studies have shown that monozygotic twins have a higher concordance rate for alcoholism than dizygotic twins. Adoption studies have shown that the biological relatives of alcoholic probands are significantly more likely to become alcoholic than the relatives of control adoptees. Males and females exhibit different patterns of genetic transmission. Male alcoholism is likely to be familial, whereas female alcoholism is sporadic.

Social and environmental factors are also important to the genesis of alcoholism.

Among adult adoptees, alcoholism is not only related to biological background of the proband, but to the environment in which the proband was reared as well.

Neurobiological theories of alcoholism are compatible with genetic theories; a stress-diathesis model hypothesizes that an environmental stressor will lead to alcoholism in persons who have inherited a vulnerability to alcoholism. Various explanations have been used to describe what the vulnerability might be: that alcohol leads to increased activity of endorphins (or morphine-like substances), creating an increase in preference for alcohol; that alcohol may, at least initially, increase relaxation in susceptible individuals, such as sons with alcoholic parents, as evidenced by slow-wave alpha activity on electroencephalogram; that sons with alcoholic parents may be particularly prone to high tolerance in early stages of alcoholism; and that unpleasant physiologic reactions, such as the *oriental flush*, might protect certain ethnic groups from alcoholism.

Behaviorists suggest that learning may play a role in alcoholism. Children tend to follow their parents' drinking patterns. Boys are encouraged to drink more than girls. Learning processes may contribute to the development of alcohol dependence through the repeated experience with withdrawal symptoms, in that relief of withdrawal symptoms by alcohol may reinforce further drinking.

Psychodynamically oriented clinicians suggest that overindulgent mothering and overprotection encourages infantile oral demands that may lead to adult alcoholism. Marital conflict in such parents or paternal attitudes that are alternately severe and overindulgent lead to inconsistency. Bewildered, the child evolves into a passive-dependent adult who turns to alcohol as a release from painful internalized emotions. Thus, the dynamically oriented physician would argue that the alcoholic patient may have been psychologically traumatized early in life and his or her personality fixated in the oral stage of development, characterized by overindulgence, a need for instant gratification, and selfishness. No characteristic personality pattern (except antisocial personality) or family constellation has been consistently identified in alcoholism research, however.

Course and Outcome

Alcoholism is associated with various outcomes. Investigators in a 1983 review of 10 major follow-up studies concluded that despite methodological differences, results were remarkably similar in indicating that 2–3% of alcoholic patients become abstinent each year, and 1% return to asymptomatic or "controlled" drinking. These findings were found true for both treated and untreated alcoholic samples, supporting the hypothesis that for some persons, alcoholism is self-limiting. In the 10 studies, 46–87% of the subjects remained alcoholic at follow-up, 8–39% had achieved abstinence, and 0–33% were asymptomatic drinkers.

Diagnosis

The diagnosis of alcoholism can usually be made on the basis of a careful history and mental status examination. However, because alcoholic persons are notorious for denying their illness and grossly underestimate the extent of their drinking, it is usually necessary to gather information from family members or other informants when alcoholism is suspected. Blood alcohol levels are often useful. A level of 150 mg/dl in a nonintoxicated person is strong evidence for alcoholism. Further, blood alcohol levels can be roughly correlated to level of intoxication:

0–100 mg/dl	A sense of well-being, sedation, and tranquility
100–150 mg/dl	Incoordination and irritability
150–250 mg/dl	Slurred speech and ataxia
>250 mg/dl	Passing out or unconsciousnes

Other laboratory measures may be useful, but none are diagnostic. Mean corpuscular volume (MCV) is increased in up to 95% of alcoholic patients. Alcoholic patients may develop increased high-density-lipoprotein (HDL) cholesterol, increased lactate dehydrogenase (LDH), decreased low-density-lipoprotein (LDL) cholesterol, decreased blood urea nitrogen (BUN), decreased red blood cell volume, and increased uric acid. Thirty percent of alcoholic patients will have evidence of a rib or vertebral fracture on chest X ray (versus 1% of control subjects). Liver enzymes are often abnormal. Gamma-glutamyltransferase (GGT) may be increased in 75% of alcoholic patients and is often the earliest laboratory sign of alcoholism. Transaminases (serum glutamic-oxaloacetic transaminase [SGOT] and serum glutamic pyruvic transaminase [SGPT]) are also increased. Mathematical models have been developed that combine the results of many different laboratory tests, allowing high sensitivity and specificity in the identification of alcoholism. However, these methods are generally useful for research only.

Clinical Management

Alcohol-induced organic disorders often require medical intervention. Intoxication, which rarely requires more than simple supportive measures, such as decreasing external stimuli and removing the source of alcohol, is the most common disorder requiring treatment. In cases of excessive intake of alcohol, in which respiratory compromise is present or likely, intensive care may be required.

Treatment of alcohol withdrawal depends on the syndrome exhibited (Table 14-4). These syndromes are usually precipitated by the abrupt withdrawal from alcohol, but may be seen in alcoholic patients who simply reduce their usual intake.

Uncomplicated alcohol withdrawal ("the shakes") (Table 14-5) begins 12–18 hours after the cessation of drinking and peaks between 24 and 48 hours. Untreated, the "shakes" subside within 5–7 days, but may linger. Minor withdrawal is characterized

Table 14-4.   Alcohol withdrawal syndromes

Minor withdrawal ("the shakes")
Alcoholic seizures ("rum fits")
Alcoholic hallucinosis
Alcoholic withdrawal delirium ("delirium tremens")

by tremors, nausea and vomiting, and signs of autonomic hyperactivity such as increased heart rate and blood pressure.

Alcoholic seizures ("rum fits") occur 7–38 hours after cessation of drinking and peak between 24 and 48 hours. These seizures consist of a burst of between one and six generalized seizures, but rarely lead to status epilepticus. Alcoholic seizures occur primarily in chronic, long-term alcoholic patients, and will precede delirium tremens in 30% of cases.

Alcohol hallucinosis (Table 14-6), characterized by vivid, unpleasant auditory hallucinations, has an onset within 48 hours of cessation of drinking and may last 1 week or more. In rare cases, the hallucinations may become chronic. These hallucinations occur in the presence of a clear sensorium.

The most dramatic withdrawal syndrome is *alcohol withdrawal delirium* ("delirium tremens") (Table 14-7). Delirium tremens occurs in a minority (5% of hospitalized alcoholic patients) of alcoholic patients, but in one-third of those who have had alcoholic seizures. Symptoms include the development of delirium (confusion and disorientation, perceptual disturbances, sleep-cycle disturbance, agitation), mild fever, and autonomic hyperarousal. The withdrawal delirium may begin 2–3 days after drinking stops, or after a significant reduction of intake, and symptoms peak on days 4 and 5 after drinking stops. On average, the syndrome typically lasts 3 days, but can persist for weeks. In the past, mortality rates of up to 15% were reported, although with good supportive care, deaths should now be rare. The following case example illustrates alcohol withdrawal delirium.

Dave, a 34-year-old unemployed veteran, had a 10-year history of chronic alcoholism, including a history of delirium tremens, alcoholic blackouts, and rum fits. He was also

Table 14-5.   DSM-III-R criteria for uncomplicated alcohol withdrawal

A. Cessation of prolonged (several days or longer) heavy ingestion of alcohol or reduction in the amount of alcohol ingested, followed within several hours by coarse tremor of hands, tongue, or eyelids, and at least one of the following:

  1. Nausea or vomiting
  2. Malaise or weakness
  3. Autonomic hyperactivity, e.g., tachycardia, sweating, elevated blood pressure
  4. Anxiety
  5. Depressed mood or irritability
  6. Transient hallucinations or illusions
  7. Headache
  8. Insomnia

B. Not due to any physical or other mental disorder, such as alcohol withdrawal delirium.

Table 14-6.   DSM-III-R criteria for alcohol hallucinosis

A. Organic hallucinosis with vivid and persistent hallucinations (auditory or visual) developing shortly (usually within 48 hours) after cessation of or reduction in heavy ingestion of alcohol in a person who apparently has alcohol dependence.

B. No delirium as in alcohol withdrawal delirium.

C. Not due to any physical or other mental disorder.

well known at the hospital for his unpleasant and critical attitude. He had been admitted multiple times for alcohol withdrawal and rehabilitation services, which seemed to have little impact on his drinking.

Dave came to the hospital requesting treatment for alcohol withdrawal. He stated that he had been drinking heavily since his last inpatient stay 3 months earlier, particularly during the week before seeking help. He had been drinking at least a quart of distilled liquor daily, and probably more. He was tremulous, hypertensive, and diaphoretic. A tapering chlordiazepoxide (Librium) protocol was instituted, but the next morning, Dave insisted on leaving the hospital against medical advice. He stated that he had more important things to do than letting the doctors "fool with him." During the evening before leaving the hospital, he had been mildly intrusive and had wandered around looking into other person's rooms, much to the annoyance of the nurses. They were happy to see him discharged.

Dave was brought back to the hospital the following day by the police, after he had been found wandering around town acting strangely. At the hospital, he was noticeably paranoid about people plotting against him, but also appeared to be confused. Although he knew where he was, he was unable to give the date or the year. By the next morning, Dave was floridly delirious and agitated. He was loud, aggressive, and disoriented to place, date, and situation. In addition, he was febrile, had very high diastolic blood pressure, and was diaphoretic. Because of his belligerence and physical restlessness, he was placed in seclusion, and restraints were required. Over the next 2 days, he was given nearly 1,200 mg of chlordiazepoxide, which was still not enough to quiet him. He remained loud and agitated. Intravenous hydration was required because of his poor oral intake. The nurses noted that on 1 of the 2 days he played an imaginary game of chess with imaginary playmates. He seemed to be in a world of his own, having a variety of hallucinatory experiences.

On the third day, Dave awakened fully oriented, was no longer hallucinating, but was mildly suspicious. Over the next few days, he returned to his normal baseline behavior and was eventually discharged to the community.

The management of alcohol withdrawal consists of 1) supportive measures, 2)

Table 14-7.   DSM-III-R criteria for alcohol withdrawal delirium

A. Delirium developing after cessation of heavy alcohol ingestion or a reduction in the amount of alcohol ingested (usually within 1 week).

B. Marked autonomic hyperactivity, e.g., tachycardia, sweating.

C. Not due to any physical or other mental disorder.

Table 14-8. Management of alcohol withdrawal syndromes

1. Chlordiazepoxide protocol
   - 50 mg q 4 hours × 24 hours, then
   - 50 mg q 6 hours × 24 hours, then
   - 25 mg q 4 hours × 24 hours, then
   - 25 mg q 6 hours × 24 hours, then discontinue

   The protocol should be started if three of seven parameters are met: systolic blood pressure >160, diastolic blood pressure >100, pulse >110, temperature >38.3°C, nausea, vomiting, tremors. The dose should be held if any of the following signs are present: nystagmus, sedation, ataxia, slurred speech, or the patient is asleep.

2. Thiamine: 50–100 mg po or im × 1; folic acid: 1 mg po daily

3. Phenytoin: 100 mg tid × 5 days, in patients with a history of withdrawal seizures

4. Haloperidol: 2–5 mg bid for patients with alcoholic hallucinosis

5. For delirium tremens,
   - Supplement chlordiazepoxide protocol as necessary (i.e., 50–100 mg q 2–4 hours) for agitation
   - Seclusion and restraints as necessary
   - Adequate hydration and nutrition

nutritional supplementation, 3) benzodiazepines, and 4) anticonvulsants in selected patients. Minor withdrawal can usually be treated on an outpatient basis, particularly in patients who have a history of uncomplicated withdrawal and a physician who is familiar with them. Management may include 25–50 mg of chlordiazepoxide four times daily decreased by one-fifth daily over the next 5 days, combined with daily visits to the physician to assess symptoms.

Inpatient treatment is best for patients with medical or psychiatric comorbidity, poor ability to follow instructions, poor social support, or a history of severe withdrawal symptoms. Nutritional supplementation should include oral thiamine and folic acid plus multivitamins and an adequate diet. Intramuscular thiamine may be administered if oral intake is not possible and should be given before any situation in which glucose loading is required, because glucose can deplete thiamine stores.

Chlordiazepoxide may be administered in doses starting at 50 mg orally six times daily on the first day. A specific protocol is recommended in Table 14-8. Chlordiazepoxide and other benzodiazepines are preferred for withdrawal because of their safety and cross-tolerance with alcohol. However, chlordiazepoxide is most often recommended because of its long half-life and low cost. Other benzodiazepines probably work as well. In patients with substantial liver damage, or the elderly, intermediate or short-acting benzodiazepines such as lorazepam or oxazepam may be best to use, due to their lack of metabolites and advantage of renal excretion.

Patients with a history of alcohol withdrawal seizures should receive low doses of phenytoin (100 mg orally three times daily for 5 days). Although this dosage produces low blood levels, it has been shown to reduce the risk of seizures. Diazepam may be used to interrupt the seizures should status epilepticus occur. Other agents have been used for treating withdrawal, including carbamazepine, clonidine, and propranolol, but their role in the treatment of withdrawal is not yet clear.

The delirious patient will require additional care that may include seclusion and restraints. The daily chlordiazepoxide may be supplemented as needed to control agitation; intravenous administration may be necessary. Intravenous hydration may also be necessary, although most alcoholic patients are overhydrated, not dehydrated, as is commonly believed.

Alcohol hallucinosis may be treated with antipsychotic medication. A small dose of haloperidol (2–5 mg orally twice daily) may be beneficial in relieving the potentially frightening auditory hallucinations. The medications are usually discontinued when the hallucinations cease.

Rehabilitation

Once alcohol detoxification has been accomplished, efforts at rehabilitation can be made. Rehabilitation has two goals: 1) that the patient remain sober, and 2) that coexisting disorders are identified and treated. In fact, perhaps two-thirds of alcoholic patients have additional psychiatric diagnoses including depression or anxiety disorders that may require specific treatment. Because alcoholism can itself cause depression, and most depressions lift with sobriety, antidepressants should be prescribed only to abstinent alcoholic patients who remain depressed after 2–4 weeks of sobriety.

Physicians should diagnose alcohol abuse or dependence when present. Patients should be told that they have a significant alcohol problem and that treatment is recommended. Although a diagnosis may not produce change, in some patients it may be the single most important step toward precipitating change.

Alcoholic patients should be encouraged to attend Alcoholics Anonymous (AA), a worldwide self-help group for recovering alcoholic persons. The meetings provide members with acceptance, understanding, forgiveness, and confrontation. With a program of 12 steps, new members are asked to admit their problems, give up a sense of personal control over the disease, make personal amends, and help others to achieve sobriety.

For the hospitalized alcoholic patient, a team approach is used. Group therapy is used to enable patients to see their own problems mirrored in others and to learn better coping skills. Family therapy is often important, as the family system that has been altered to accommodate the patient's drinking may often reinforce it. The issue of codependency is now popular, i.e., the notion that the alcoholic person's drinking is maintained (or enabled) by spouses, family members, or close friends. In family therapy, such issues can be addressed. Inpatient programs also provide education about the harmful effects of alcohol on the mind and the body.

Disulfiram (Antabuse) may be a helpful adjunct in maintaining abstinence in some patients. Disulfiram inhibits aldehyde dehydrogenase, an enzyme necessary for the metabolism of alcohol. Inhibiting this enzyme leads to the accumulation of acetaldehyde if alcohol is consumed. Acetaldehyde is toxic and leads to unpleasant symptoms, such as nausea, vomiting, palpitations, and hypotension. In rare cases, the effects may be fatal; therefore, disulfiram should not be prescribed in a cavalier manner. The typical dosage is 250 mg once daily. Interestingly, the deterrent effect of disulfiram appears to be psychological and is not dose dependent.

Chemical aversive conditioning has been used in the past. This has involved various aversive chemicals used to either induce vomiting (emetine, apomorphine) or apnea (succinylcholine) or electrical stimulation to produce pain. Although treatment effectiveness has been found to equal or exceed other modalities, the relatively greater risks of medical complications from these methods and their unpleasantness limit their usefulness.

Lithium carbonate has been used experimentally to treat alcoholism for more than 10 years. Lithium appears to enhance abstinence and to antagonize the effects of alcohol intoxication, effects independent from its effect on mood. However, further study is needed to learn which alcoholic patients are most likely to benefit from lithium therapy.

It is difficult to determine the effectiveness of inpatient programs to treat alcoholism. Although many outcome studies show benefits, the studies are not comparable in terms of patient population or treatment interventions used. Outcome literature shows that the predictors for a good outcome include having a stable marriage and home life, having a stable job, suffering less psychopathology (especially antisocial personality), and having a family history negative for alcoholism. Length of the inpatient program does not appear to be an important factor. In fact, patients sent involuntarily to rehabilitation programs appear to benefit as much as the voluntary patient. Nearly half of treated alcoholic patients will relapse, most commonly during the first 6 months after hospital discharge.

Recommendations for management of alcoholism

1. The alcoholic person needs acceptance, not blame.

2. Although it is tempting to refuse treatment to the chronic alcoholic person, based on his or her history of failure, it is always possible that the next rehabilitation may work. Don't give up!

3. Treatment of withdrawal syndromes should take place in an inpatient setting if the patient has a history of severe "shakes," hallucinosis, seizures, or delirium tremens. Other patients (the majority) can be handled as outpatients.
   - Chlordiazepoxide is standard treatment, but other benzodiazepines (e.g., lorazepam) work just as well.

4. Be sure to manage the patient's other emotional problems as well (e.g., panic disorder, depression), because untreated they may lead to a resumption of drinking.

5. Be sure to include the family in the treatment process.
   - Alcoholism affects every member of the family, and unresolved issues may lead to relapse.
   - Family members should be encouraged to attend Al-Anon, a support group for relatives of alcoholic persons.

Bibliography

Cadoret RJ, O'Gorman TW, Troughton E, et al: Alcoholism and antisocial personality—interrelationships, genetic and environmental factors. Arch Gen Psychiatry 42:162–167, 1985

Clancy J, Vanderhuth E, Campbell P: Evaluation of an aversive technique as a treatment for alcoholism-controlled trial with succinylcholine-induced apnea. J Stud Alcohol 28:476–485, 1967

Cloninger CR: Neurogenic adaptive mechanisms in alcoholism. Science 236:410–416, 1987

Eckardt MJ, Harford TC, Kaelber CT, et al: Health hazards associated with alcohol consumption. JAMA 246:648–666, 1981

Fawcett J, Clark DC, Aagesen CA, et al: A double-blind, placebo controlled trial of lithium carbonate therapy for alcoholism. Arch Gen Psychiatry 44:248–258, 1986

Frances RJ, Bucke S, Alexopoulous GS: Outcome study of familial and non-familial alcoholism. Am J Psychiatry 141:1469–1471, 1984

Fuller RK, Branchey L, Brightwell DR, et al: Disulfiram treatment of alcoholism—a Veterans Administration cooperative study. JAMA 256:1449–1455, 1986

Goodwin DW: Alcoholism and genetics. Arch Gen Psychiatry 42:171–174, 1985

Grant I, Adams KM, Reed R: Aging, abstinence, and medical risk factors in the prediction of neuropsychologic deficit among long-term alcoholics. Arch Gen Psychiatry 41:710–718, 1984

Helzer JE, Pryzbeck TR: The co-occurrence of alcoholism with other psychiatric disorders in the general population and its impact on treatment. J Stud Alcohol 49:219–224, 1988

Helzer JE, Robins LN, Taylor JR, et al: The extent of long-term moderate drinking among alcoholics discharged from medical and psychiatric treatment facilities. N Engl J Med 312:1678–1682, 1985

Helzer JE, Canino GJ, Yeh EK, et al: Alcoholism—North America and Asia: a comparison of population surveys with the Diagnostic Interview Schedule. Arch Gen Psychiatry 47:313–319, 1990

Holden C: Is alcoholism treatment effective? Science 236:20–22, 1987

Irwin M, Schuckit M, Smith TL: Clinical importance of age at onset in Type I and Type II primary alcoholics. Arch Gen Psychiatry 47:320–324, 1990

Jellinek EM: The Disease Concept of Alcoholism. New Haven, CT, College and University Press, 1960

Judd LL, Huy LY: Lithium antagonizes ethanol intoxication in alcoholics. Am J Psychiatry 141:1517–1521, 1984

Malcolm R, Ballenger JC, Sturgis ET, et al: Double-blind controlled trial comparing carbamazepine to oxazepam treatment of alcohol withdrawal. Am J Psychiatry 146:617–621, 1989

Pickins RW, Hatsukami DK, Spicer JW, et al: Relapse by alcohol abusers. Alcoholism 9:244–247, 1985

Stein LI, Newton JR, Bowman RS: Duration of hospitalization for alcoholism. Arch Gen Psychiatry 32:247–252, 1975

Streissguth AP, Clarren SK, Jones KL: Natural history of the fetal alcohol syndrome: a 10 year follow up of 11 patients. Lancet 2:85–91, 1985

Self-assessment Questions

1. Who originated the disease concept of alcoholism?
2. How is alcohol dependence diagnosed?
3. How do Type I and Type II alcoholic patients differ?
4. What are the clinical findings in alcoholism's earliest stage? middle stage? late stage?
5. List the medical complications of alcoholism.
6. What are the purported psychodynamic causes of alcoholism?
7. What laboratory abnormalities are associated with alcoholism?
8. What are the major withdrawal syndromes, and how are they treated?
9. Discuss the role of disulfiram in the treatment of alcoholism.
10. What are the predictors for good outcome for alcohol rehabilitation efforts?

Chapter 15

Psychoactive Substance Use Disorders

O true apothecary!
Thy drugs are quick.

William Shakespeare, Romeo and Juliet

Psychoactive substances are compounds that can alter one's state of mind. Alcohol, the most important psychoactive substance, is discussed in Chapter 14. Some agents have been around since antiquity, although some new ones are the products of modern organic chemistry techniques. A literal cornucopia of psychoactive substances are available in the United States, and these drugs have been subject to both appropriate and inappropriate use.

The problems resulting from substance abuse appear more extensive today than before, probably due to the increased availability and number of agents that are subject to experimentation and use. Drug problems cut across all social and economic boundaries. All age-groups have been affected, particularly adolescents and young adults. Due to the near-epidemic nature of illicit drug use and growing public concern, the government has acted to increase funding for research in the area of drug abuse, presidential commissions have been appointed, and since 1989, a drug "czar" has been in place to coordinate drug containment efforts.

In this chapter, we review the major categories of psychoactive substance use disorders and their corresponding substance-induced organic mental disorders. The major categories include sedative-hypnotic substance use disorders, opioid substance use disorders, central nervous system (CNS) stimulants and their associated dis-

Table 15-1. Categories of drug use disorders

● **Sedatives, hypnotics, and anxiolytics** Barbiturates Nonbarbiturates (e.g., meprobamate) Benzodiazepines	● **Stimulants** Amphetamines Methylphenidate Cocaine
● **Opiates** Heroin Meperidine Codeine Hydromorphone (Dilaudid)	● **Hallucinogens** ● **Arylcyclohexylamines** Phencyclidine ● **Cannabis** ● **Inhalants**

orders, the disorders of hallucinogen and arylcyclohexylamine use, cannabis (e.g., marijuana) use disorders, and disorders of inhalant use (Table 15-1).

Definition

As pointed out in Chapter 14, DSM-III-R introduced generic criteria for psychoactive substance abuse and dependence, a concept endorsed by the World Health Organization. The definition of *psychoactive substance dependence* includes at least three significant behaviors out of a nine-item list that includes psychosocial problems that indicate a serious degree of involvement with the drug. Severity criteria are included to indicate whether the dependence is mild, moderate, severe, in partial remission, or in full remission.

Psychoactive substance abuse tends to be a residual category for those who continue to abuse substances, despite problems caused by the use, but fail to meet criteria for dependence. The different criteria are geared toward separating individuals whose use of psychoactive substances is *hazardous* from those whose use is merely *harmful.* Clearly, overlap exists between abuse and dependence, and the disorders are probably better thought of as lying along a continuum, because either the abuse of or dependence on any psychoactive substance can result in similar types of problems.

Additionally, DSM-III-R identifies specific drug-induced organic mental disorders (e.g., sedative, hypnotic, or anxiolytic withdrawal, delirium, opioid withdrawal) that relate to the acute or chronic effects that psychoactive substances have on the CNS.

Epidemiology

Psychoactive substance use is widespread in the United States. It is probably impossible to know its true extent, because drug abusers may not readily cooperate with surveys, and much use is recreational and not necessarily accompanied by abuse or dependence. The Epidemiologic Catchment Area study in the early 1980s found that the combined category of drug abuse/dependence had a lifetime prevalence ranging from 5.5 to 5.8% in three urban centers. Among the respondents, drug abuse/dependence was more common in young persons, especially among those aged 18–24 years, men, blacks, and persons in urban settings. These statistics do not reveal the true extent of illicit drug use, however. For example, marijuana has been used by over one-quarter of Americans and is *regularly* smoked by about 20 million persons. Cocaine achieved great popularity in the 1980s, particularly among "yuppies" (i.e., young urban professionals), and nearly one-quarter of young Americans have used it, including nearly 7% of high school seniors. Patterns of use change, however, reflecting the fluctuating popularity of drugs, their availability, and their cost. Cocaine, for example, is now widely available and less expensive than in the past. A freebased derivative of cocaine, "crack," is even cheaper, and its use has become epidemic in inner cities and elsewhere. Opiates and barbiturates peaked in popularity long ago, and the estimated number of heroin addicts has remained stable for some time.

Among the bothersome trends in psychoactive substance abuse is the use of multiple agents. In fact, the use of one substance greatly increases the chance of that person using another. Some compounds are deliberately combined to produce a desired effect, e.g., cocaine and heroin. The extent of combined drug use is only now becoming apparent. In DSM-III-R, such use is classified as *polysubstance dependence*, i.e., when three or more compounds have been repeatedly used, but no single agent has predominated.

Etiology

Understanding psychoactive substance use involves a knowledge of the user, his or her environment, and the drug itself. None of these variables works in isolation, and it is probably the interaction of the three that leads to drug use disorders.

Dependence on various substances (e.g., tobacco, opium, alcohol) has been shown to be familial, so it is likely that many users have a constitutional vulnerability to drug use. In fact, adoption studies of drug abusers suggest that the disorders may be genetic as well.

Although no one personality pattern has been found to predict drug abuse, the frequency of personality disorders among drug abusers is very high. Certain personality characteristics appear to predispose persons to illicit drug use, including antisocial and borderline traits. Narcissistic traits have been identified as a possible risk factor in cocaine abusers. Other psychological characteristics also seen in drug abusers include hostility, low frustration tolerance, inflexibility, and low self-esteem. Although these traits may have led to the drug abuse, it is also just as likely that they may have resulted from the drug use.

Other physical and psychiatric conditions have been linked with drug abuse, including chronic pain, anxiety disorders, and depression. It is not hard to see how these disturbances could lead to substance abuse. Several longitudinal studies have shown that many traits precede and predict the use of psychoactive substances. Some predictive factors can be identified long before drug use begins, such as aggressiveness and rebelliousness manifested in childhood.

Other characteristics of the user may be important in predisposing to abuse, including the existence of opiate receptors in several brain regions, such as the limbic system. Opioid drugs interact directly with these brain receptors. Likewise, benzodiazepine receptors have been identified in the brain, and may play a role in sedative, hypnotic, or anxiolytic abuse. Knowledge of these neurotransmitter systems helps us to understand why drug abusers can become increasingly reliant on drugs while progressively ignoring other means to enjoy life (e.g., food, work, sex, family, friends).

The pharmacologic properties of the drug itself may contribute to abuse. Some compounds (e.g., opiates, sedatives, hypnotics, and anxiolytics) can produce rapid relief of anxiety. Stimulants generally relieve boredom and fatigue and provide a sensation of energy and increased mental alertness. Hallucinogens provide a temporary escape from reality. These properties all contribute to their abuse. Substances that do not provide such pleasurable sensations (e.g., phenothiazines) are rarely abused.

In general, drugs with rapid onset and briefer action (e.g., heroin, cocaine) are the preferred substances of abuse. Methods of administration that enhance the rapidity of onset are often exploited to provide added "kick," for example, sniffing, smoking, and intravenous use.

Tolerance and withdrawal phenomena also contribute to abuse, because users quickly learn that higher doses of some substances are needed to get the same effect, and that the drug itself can be used to prevent uncomfortable withdrawal symptoms.

Societal and family values also influence the use of illicit drugs. For example, if parents smoke, drink alcoholic beverages, or use psychoactive substances, their offspring are more prone to use illicit drugs, perhaps through modeling. Persons whose friends use drugs are more likely to use them too, which suggests the influence of one friend on another. A person may simply seek out as friends, however, those who share similar values and interests, hence leading to drug abuse. Susceptibility to the influence of friends has been associated with lack of a close relationship to parents, a large amount of time spent away from home, and increased reliance on peers as opposed to parents.

Drug laws can also have an effect. Antidrug laws have been tried for centuries (e.g., restricting alcohol, tobacco, and opium). Their success has been mixed, but laws have tended to be more successful in totalitarian (e.g., China, Soviet Union) than in democratic (e.g., Western Europe, United States) regimes. In some countries, drug use is proscribed for religious reasons (e.g., Islamic countries) and their use has severe consequences. Needless to say, drug abuse in these countries is uncommon.

The following case example illustrates many of the problems that beset substance abusers and some of the factors that lead to the abuse.

Laura was referred to the hospital for drug rehabilitation. The 21-year-old Native American worked as a nursing assistant in a care center in a small midwestern town.

Laura was adopted at an early age into a middle-class family and had several adopted brothers and sisters. Her adoptive parents made sure she was adequately clothed and fed, but provided little emotional nurturing or stability. As a child, she was sexually abused by one of her adoptive brothers and forced to have intercourse with him on a regular basis for several years. At age 12, she became pregnant, carried the baby to term, and gave it up for adoption.

Laura reported an extensive history of antisocial and delinquent behaviors and admitted to using a variety of psychoactive substances including marijuana, alcohol, amphetamines, cocaine, and, most recently, crack. To pay for her drug use, she had become a drug dealer at age 14 and later moved on to prostitution. Laura reported that she started smoking marijuana and drinking alcoholic beverages at about age 12 and had used the two substances on a regular basis since then. Several years later, she started to use amphetamines, and later added cocaine and crack. She also admitted to having tried an assortment of other drugs including PCP, LSD, and heroin.

In the 6 months before her hospitalization, she had graduated from snorting cocaine to injecting it intravenously, sometimes in combination with heroin. She told us that she enjoyed the "orgasmic" feeling that she received from the injections and had actually lost interest in sexual activity with her boyfriend as a result. The two would use drugs together, and she admitted that she used unclean needles despite her knowledge of their potential danger for transmitting human immunodeficiency virus (HIV). Her boyfriend, as described by Laura, was an unsavory character who was a drug dealer, had an extensive prison record, and worked as her pimp.

Laura had had prior psychiatric hospitalizations for depression and had had several for drug detoxification, one occurring after a suicide attempt. She had never remained in the hospital very long and usually left against medical advice.

Although Laura had been referred to our hospital under a court order for evaluation of substance abuse, she told us that despite her heavy use of drugs, she did not plan to give them up. Despite her resistance, she was referred to a drug rehabilitation center.

Sedative, Hypnotic, and Anxiolytic Substance Use Disorders

Sedatives, hypnotics, and anxiolytics have been used to provide sedation, induce sleep, relieve anxiety, prevent seizures (as muscle relaxants), and induce general anesthesia. All sedatives, hypnotics, and anxiolytics are cross-tolerant with one another and with alcohol. They are also all capable of producing physical and psychological dependence and withdrawal syndromes. Classes of these compounds include the barbiturates, nonbarbiturate sedative-hypnotics, and the benzodiazepines.

The history of sedative-hypnotics dates to 1903, when barbital, the first barbiturate, was introduced. Later, nonbarbiturate sedative-hypnotics (e.g., meprobamate) were synthesized. Benzodiazepines first became available in the 1960s. Because of their wide margin of safety, benzodiazepines have largely displaced barbiturates and nonbarbiturate sedative-hypnotics from the market. Whereas barbiturates are potentially fatal in overdose, the benzodiazepines produce almost no respiratory depression, and the ratio of lethal-to-effective dosage is extraordinarily high. Although the barbiturates and nonbarbiturate sedative-hypnotics are effective in providing both sedation and hypnosis (e.g., sleep induction), they are rarely used today. The main indication for phenobarbital now is as an anticonvulsant. Methaqualone, a nonbarbiturate sedative-hypnotic, no longer has any accepted medical use and is not manufactured in the United States, although it is readily available on the black market. The benzodiazepines are among the most widely prescribed medications in the United States, and about 15% of the general population is prescribed a benzodiazepine in any given year. Fortunately, studies have confirmed that most prescriptions for benzodiazepines are appropriate, and only a small minority of patients abuse the drugs. Further information about the rational use of sedatives, hypnotics, and anxiolytics is found in Chapter 24.

Sedative, hypnotic, or anxiolytic abuse involves a maladaptive pattern of use for 1 month or longer, whereas dependence requires the presence of at least three independent indications of inappropriate use, or problems directly attributable to the substance lasting 1 month or longer.

There may be two distinct groups of sedative, hypnotic, and anxiolytic abusers. The first group includes men and women in their teens or 20s who obtain the drugs illegally and use them for recreational purposes. Similar to the Type I alcoholic, this group is likely to have coexisting psychopathology, such as antisocial personality. The other group consists of middle-aged women who obtain the drug from their physician for complaints of nervousness and become physically dependent. Although in the past it was believed that there might be an "addictive personality" that is more prone to abusing these agents, no consistent personality profile has emerged.

Sedative, hypnotic, and anxiolytic dependence may eventually lead to physical and social problems, occupational difficulties (e.g., job loss), and problems with relationships. Dependent persons sometimes turn to crime to obtain their drug.

Not much is known about the natural history of sedative, hypnotic, or anxiolytic dependence, but like alcoholism, it is likely that the course is chronic and relapsing.

Sedative, hypnotic, or anxiolytic use is associated with intoxication, withdrawal, and withdrawal delirium. These syndromes vary little from drug to drug, although the withdrawal phenomena may be worse with the shorter-acting drugs and more prolonged with the longer-acting ones. The syndromes are similar to those seen with alcoholism, which is not surprising since they are cross-tolerant.

The symptoms of sedative, hypnotic, and anxiolytic intoxication are dose related. The intoxicated patient may show lethargy, impaired mental functioning, poor memory, irritability, self-neglect, and emotional disinhibition. As intoxication advances, slurred speech, ataxia, and impaired coordination develop. With higher doses, death may occur due to respiratory depression (although this complication does not occur with the benzodiazepines). The criteria for sedative, hypnotic, or anxiolytic intoxication are found in Table 15-2.

Withdrawal from barbiturates can be dangerous, unlike the withdrawal from other sedatives, hypnotics, and anxiolytics, which is merely uncomfortable. Withdrawal symptoms can occur when the substance is abruptly withdrawn, or from a

Table 15-2. DSM-III-R criteria for sedative, hypnotic, or anxiolytic intoxication

A. Recent use of a sedative, hypnotic, or anxiolytic.

B. Maladaptive behavior changes, e.g., disinhibition of sexual or aggressive impulses, mood lability, impaired judgment, impaired social or occupational functioning.

C. At least one of the following signs:
1. Slurred speech
2. Incoordination
3. Unsteady gait
4. Impairment in attention or memory

D. Not due to any physical or other mental disorder.

Note: When the differential diagnosis must be made without a clear-cut history or toxicologic analysis of body fluids, it may be qualified as "provisional."

reduction in dose. Symptoms of the barbiturate withdrawal syndrome are presented in Table 15-3. During the first 24 hours of withdrawal, the patient becomes anxious, restless, and apprehensive. Coarse tremors develop, and deep tendon reflexes become hyperactive. Weakness, nausea and vomiting, orthostatic hypotension, sweating, and other signs of autonomic hyperarousal occur. On the 2nd or 3rd day of withdrawal, grand mal seizures can occur. The seizures generally consist of a single convulsion or a burst of several convulsions, although status epilepticus rarely develops. A withdrawal delirium, associated with confusion, disorientation, and visual and somatic hallucinations, sometimes develops at this stage. Withdrawal symptoms in patients using longer-acting substances (e.g., phenobarbital, diazepam) tend to come on later and last longer than the symptoms from short-acting agents (e.g., amobarbital, lorazepam). The DSM-III-R criteria for sedative, hypnotic, or anxiolytic withdrawal are listed in Table 15-4.

Patients addicted to sedatives, hypnotics, or anxiolytics should be withdrawn from the drugs in the hospital, due to the severity of the withdrawal symptoms. Before initiating a tapering withdrawal schedule, a tolerance test should be administered using either pentobarbital or diazepam (see Table 15-5). The test should be administered to a patient who is not intoxicated. Once the level of tolerance has been established, the patient is withdrawn using phenobarbital or diazepam.

Table 15-3. Barbiturate withdrawal syndrome

Severity	Symptoms	Onset	Duration
Minor	Postural hypotension; nausea, vomiting, anorexia; tremors; sleeplessness; agitation/anxiety	12–24 hours	up to 14 days
Moderate	Status epilepticus; seizures; myoclonic jerking	2–3 days	up to 8 days
Dangerous	Death; hyperpyrexia; delirium tremens; hallucinosis	3–4 days	up to 14 days

Table 15-4. DSM-III-R criteria for uncomplicated sedative, hypnotic, or anxiolytic withdrawal

A. Cessation of prolonged (several weeks or more) moderate or heavy use of a sedative, hypnotic, or anxiolytic, or reduction in the amount of substance used, followed by at least three of the following:

   1. Nausea or vomiting
   2. Malaise or weakness
   3. Autonomic hyperactivity, e.g., tachycardia, sweating
   4. Anxiety or irritability
   5. Orthostatic hypotension
   6. Coarse tremor of hands, tongue, and eyelids
   7. Marked insomnia
   8. Grand mal seizures

B. Not due to any physical or other mental disorder, such as sedative, hypnotic, or anxiolytic withdrawal delirium.

Note: When the differential diagnosis must be made without a clear-cut history or toxicologic analysis of body fluids, it may be qualified as "provisional."

The initial dose is determined by substituting 30 mg of phenobarbital for every 100 mg of pentobarbital administered during the tolerance test. During withdrawal, the daily requirement of phenobarbital is decreased by 30 mg. The daily requirement of diazepam is decreased by 10 mg from an initial level equal to the intoxicating dose. On this schedule, the patient will be somewhat uncomfortable. If signs of withdrawal worsen or the patient becomes somnolent or intoxicated, the schedule may need to be adjusted. Some patients will present at the hospital already experiencing withdrawal symptoms, in which case pentobarbital or diazepam should be administered in sufficient doses to make the patient comfortable before the withdrawal procedure is initiated.

Although few patients who obtain legitimate prescriptions for sedatives, hypnotics, and anxiolytics abuse them, certain general rules should apply to all patients.

Table 15-5. Pentobarbital/diazepam tolerance test

1. Pentobarbital 200 mg (or diazepam 20 mg) is administered orally. Evaluate in 2 hours.

   • No tolerance—the patient is asleep but arousable
   • Tolerance 400–500 mg of pentobarbital (or 40–50 mg of diazepam)—the patient is grossly ataxic, has a coarse tremor or lateral nystagmus
   • Tolerance 600 mg of pentobarbital (or 60 mg of diazepam)—the patient is mildly ataxic
   • Tolerance 800 mg of pentobarbital (or 80 mg of diazepam)—the patient has slight nystagmus
   • Tolerance 1,000 mg of pentobarbital (or 100 mg of diazepam)—the patient is asymptomatic

2. If the patient remains asymptomatic, an additional oral dose of pentobarbital 200 mg (or diazepam 20 mg) is given.

   • Failure to become symptomatic at this dose suggests a daily tolerance of >1,600 mg of pentobarbital (or 160 mg of diazepam).

These medications should be targeted to specific symptoms or syndromes (e.g., generalized anxiety disorder) and their use limited if at all possible (e.g., weeks or months only). It is uncommon for patients, for example, to require chronic administration of benzodiazepines. In addition, the drug should be prescribed in the minimum necessary dosage to control the patient's symptoms, and prescriptions should generally be nonrefillable. Because of the proven safety and efficacy of benzodiazepines, there is no reason to prescribe the more dangerous barbiturates, except for their use as anticonvulsants, or the nonbarbiturate sedative-hypnotics.

Opioid Substance Use Disorders

The opiates include morphine, heroin, hydromorphone (Dilaudid), codeine, and meperidine. Meperidine is a synthetic opiate pharmacologically similar to morphine. The opiates are commonly used for pain control, and heroin is the only one of these substances not available in the United States for medical use. It is difficult to know how widespread opiate abuse is, but there are probably one-half million opiate addicts in the United States, a number that has been relatively stable over the years, despite growing public concern and increased efforts at rehabilitation.

Opiate abuse is more common in urban settings, males, and blacks. Addiction is also more common among physicians and other health care professionals, probably due to their easy access to the opiates. Many opiate addicts have other psychiatric disorders as well, particularly the other substance use disorders, antisocial and borderline personality disorders, and mood disorders.

The natural history of opiate addiction probably varies depending on the setting, suggesting that circumstances of exposure and availability are important factors in maintaining use. In a 12-year follow-up of opiate addicts treated by a U.S. government-operated treatment center, 98% had returned to the use of opiates within 12 months of release. A follow-up study in London found a relapse rate of 53% within 6 months. However, in a study of Vietnam veterans who had used opiates in Vietnam, fewer than 2% continued to use the substances after returning home. These discrepant findings suggest that there may be more than one type of user.

Opiates may lead to both abuse and dependence, like other psychoactive drugs. It is likely that opiate addiction leads to more crime than other compounds, due to their relatively high cost. Opiate addiction is associated with high fatality rates, because inadvertent fatal overdoses, deaths from accidents, and suicide are common in abusers. Opiate addicts are also at high risk for developing medical problems due to their poor nutrition and use of dirty needles for injecting the substance (e.g., heroin). Among the medical problems that plague opiate addicts are serum hepatitis, HIV infection, pneumonia, and cellulitis. Although it is not clear whether addicts grow out of their habit over the years, the death rate is high so that there are relatively few older abusers.

Opiate users tend to avoid physicians, and it is likely that when the patient is brought to medical attention it will be for reasons of opiate intoxication or with-

Table 15-6.   DSM-III-R criteria for opiate intoxication

A. Recent use of an opiate.

B. Maladaptive behavior changes, e.g., initial euphoria followed by apathy, dysphoria, psychomotor retardation, impaired judgment, impaired social or occupational functioning.

C. Pupillary constriction (or pupillary dilation due to anoxia from severe overdose) and at least one of the following signs:

1. Drowsiness
2. Slurred speech
3. Impairment in attention or memory

D. Not due to any physical or other mental disorder.

Note: When the differential diagnosis must be made without a clear-cut history, testing with an opioid antagonist, or toxicologic analysis of body fluids, it may be qualified as "provisional."

---

drawal phenomena. Due to the likelihood of comorbid medical problems (e.g., cellulitis) and poor physical condition, the opiate abuser needs a thorough medical evaluation.

Most heroin or morphine addicts take opiates intravenously, which produces flushing and an orgasmic sensation in the abdomen. This sensation is followed by euphoria and a sense of well-being. Drowsiness and inactivity, psychomotor retardation, and impaired concentration then develop. Physical signs that occur after a heroin addict "shoots up" (which may occur three or more times a day) include pupillary constriction, slurred speech, respiratory depression, hypotension, hypothermia, and bradycardia. Constipation, nausea, and vomiting are also common. Skin ulcers may develop at injection sites. DSM-III-R criteria for opiate intoxication are presented in Table 15-6.

Eventually, tolerance develops to most of the opiate effects, including the euphoria. Sexual interest diminishes, and in women, menstruation may cease. Daily use of opiates over days to weeks, depending on dosage and drug potency, will produce opiate withdrawal symptoms starting approximately 10 hours after the last dose with short-acting opiates (e.g., morphine, heroin) or a longer period of time for longer-acting substances (e.g., meperidine). Mild withdrawal symptoms include lacrimation, rhinorrhea, sweating, yawning, piloerection, hypertension, and tachycardia. More severe symptoms include hot and cold flashes, muscle and joint pain, nausea, vomiting, and abdominal cramps. Seizures may occur during meperidine withdrawal. All of these withdrawal symptoms have been seen in babies born to addicted mothers. In addition to the physical symptoms, psychological symptoms include severe anxiety and restlessness, irritability, insomnia, and decreased appetite. Patients may be extremely demanding and manipulative. The DSM-III-R criteria for opiate withdrawal are found in Table 15-7.

Patients addicted to opiates should be gradually withdrawn using methadone. First, tolerance to opiates must be established. When the patient develops initial symptoms of withdrawal, a dose of 10–20 mg of methadone is administered orally

Table 15-7.   DSM-III-R criteria for opiate withdrawal

A. Cessation of prolonged (several weeks or more) moderate or heavy use of an opiate, or reduction in the amount of opiate used (or administration of an opioid antagonist after a brief period of use), followed by at least three of the following:
1. Craving for an opiate
2. Nausea or vomiting
3. Muscle aches
4. Lacrimation or rhinorrhea
5. Pupillary dilation, piloerection, or sweating
6. Diarrhea
7. Yawning
8. Fever
9. Insomnia

B. Not due to any physical or other mental disorder.

Note: When the differential diagnosis must be made without a clear-cut history or toxicologic analysis of body fluids, it may be qualified as "provisional."

every 2–4 hours until withdrawal symptoms are suppressed. A heroin addict may require between 20 and 40 mg of methadone initially. Once the patient is stabilized, the methadone should be given on a once-daily or twice-daily schedule as the total daily amount is reduced by 10–20% of the stabilization dose daily. Most withdrawals from short-acting substances such as heroin or morphine take 7–10 days, and withdrawal from longer-acting substances such as methadone should proceed more slowly (e.g., over 2–3 weeks).

An alternative method for withdrawing patients from opiates is the use of clonidine, which provides good suppression of the autonomic signs of withdrawal. Patients do better with an abrupt switch to clonidine when the methadone dosage is first stabilized at 20 mg or less daily. The abrupt switch to clonidine may be started along with gradual low-dose naltrexone, an opioid antagonist. When clonidine is given in doses starting at 0.1–0.3 mg three times daily (which may be increased to 0.2–0.7 mg three times daily over an 8- to 14-day period), the use of clonidine for withdrawal may actually be safer and more effective than methadone withdrawal. Clonidine is not currently approved by the Food and Drug Administration for opiate withdrawal, however.

It is not uncommon to find patients tolerant to different substances, for example, both a sedative, hypnotic, or anxiolytic and an opiate. In these situations, it is safest to stabilize the patient on a dose of methadone, and to withdraw the sedative, hypnotic, or anxiolytic first, because sedative, hypnotic, or anxiolytic withdrawal is potentially the more dangerous syndrome.

Methadone maintenance treatment continues to be a major alternative in managing opiate addicts. In this approach, methadone, a long-acting opiate, is administered orally once daily. Because of its long half-life (between 22 and 56 hours in methadone-maintained subjects) and its wide distribution in the body, the drug creates few subjective effects or withdrawal symptoms. The rationale of methadone maintenance is that by switching addicts to methadone, their "drug hunger" is alleviated so that they are less preoccupied with drug-seeking behavior. For the most part, this treatment approach has been successful. The majority of patients in these well-regulated programs show significant decreases in opiate and nonopiate use, criminal activity, and depressive symptoms. They also show increases in gainful employment. Programs now espouse the view that methadone is a transitional treatment that leads to total abstinence. Methadone programs also emphasize ongoing individual and group psychotherapy to help keep the addict in the program, and to assist them in coping with day-to-day problems without resorting to drugs.

Central Nervous System Stimulant Use Disorders

CNS stimulants include dextroamphetamine, methylphenidate, methamphetamine, phenmetrazine, and cocaine. The action of these agents is to elevate mood, increase energy and alertness, decrease appetite, and slightly improve task performance. These drugs also cause autonomic hyperarousal, leading to tachycardia, elevated blood pressure, and pupillary dilation. Amphetamines were first used in the 1930s and have been prescribed for many conditions over the years, including depression, obesity, narcolepsy, and childhood attention-deficit disorder. Their rational use in the treatment of attention-deficit hyperactivity disorder is discussed in Chapter 24.

The abuse potential of stimulants was recognized relatively early, and illicit use of the drugs has become widespread. Because of their overuse in the 1970s (e.g., as diet pills), changes in the regulation of their legitimate distribution were made in an attempt to stem the tide of abuse. Unfortunately, many of these compounds are easy to synthesize, and although their legal use has declined, their illegal use continues to grow. One of the newest drugs to hit the black market, "ice," is a crystallized form of the easily synthesized methamphetamine.

Cocaine is included with these drugs because it has similar stimulant effects, although it differs structurally from the amphetamines. Derived from the coca plant, which is indigenous to certain countries in South America, cocaine has legitimate medical use as a local anesthetic. Because of its pleasurable stimulant effects, cocaine has always had a following in the United States. In fact, it was used in the late 19th century in various elixirs and tonics, including the original Coca-Cola formulation. Early researchers, including Sigmund Freud, became advocates of its use, but increasingly, cocaine became associated with sudden death, emotional and domestic problems, and addiction and was finally declared an illegal narcotic in the Harrison Act of 1914. Cocaine has continued to be very popular as a recreational drug, although until recently it was restricted to affluent groups because of its high cost. A low-cost derivative, "crack," became available for smoking in the 1980s.

The clinical syndromes produced by the CNS stimulants include those of abuse and dependence, intoxication, delirium, delusional disorder, and withdrawal. Amphetamine and cocaine intoxication are quite similar and are diagnosed on the basis of their recent use, maladaptive behavior (e.g., grandiosity, hypervigilance),

Table 15-8. DSM-III-R criteria for amphetamine or similarly acting sympathomimetic intoxication

A. Recent use of amphetamines or a similarly acting sympathomimetic.

B. Maladaptive behavior changes, e.g., fighting, grandiosity, hypervigilance, psychomotor agitation, impaired judgment, impaired social or occupational functioning.

C. At least two of the following signs within 1 hour of use:
1. Tachycardia
2. Pupillary dilation
3. Elevated blood pressure
4. Perspiration or chills
5. Nausea or vomiting

D. Not due to any physical or other mental disorder.

Note: When the differential diagnosis must be made without a clear-cut history or toxicologic analysis of body fluids, it may be qualified as "provisional."

and signs of autonomic hyperarousal (e.g., tachycardia or pupillary dilation). The DSM-III-R criteria for amphetamine intoxication are presented in Table 15-8.

Cocaine intoxication tends to cause tactile hallucinations (e.g., "coke bugs"), unlike the other stimulants. Psychological symptoms may include euphoria, disinhibition, an enhanced sense of mastery, sexual arousal, and improved self-esteem. Depending on how it is administered (e.g., intranasally, intravenously), users may also report a "rush" (i.e., rapid onset of euphoria). By smoking a purified cocaine base that has been "freed" from its salts and cutting agents by a chemical process (i.e., "freebasing"), users report an even more rapid, but short-lived, high. Common psychological and physical symptoms seen in 32 freebase cocaine abusers are presented in Table 15-9.

Table 15-9. Common psychological and physical symptoms in 32 freebase cocaine abusers

Psychological symptoms	%	Physical symptoms	%
Paranoia	63	Blurred vision	34
Visual hallucinations	50	Coughing	34
Craving	47	Muscle aches	34
Asocial behavior	41	Dry skin	28
Impaired concentration	38	Tremors	28
Irritability	31	Weight loss	25
Bad dreams	31	Chest pains	22
Hyperexcitability	28	Episodic unconsciousness	16
Violence	28	Difficult urination	16
Auditory hallucinations	25	Respiratory problems	9
Lethargy	25	Edema	9
Depression	25	Seizures	3
Business problems	25	Insomnia	3

Source. Adapted from Verebey K, Gold MS: From coca leaves to crack: the effects of dose and routes of administration in abuse liability. Psychiatric Annals 18:513–520, 1988.

Table 15-10.   DSM-III-R criteria for amphetamine or similarly acting sympathomimetic withdrawal

A. Cessation of prolonged (several days or longer) heavy use of amphetamine or a similarly acting sympathomimetic, or reduction in the amount of substance used, followed by dysphoric mood (e.g., depression, irritability, anxiety) and at least one of the following, persisting more than 24 hours after cessation of substance use:

　　1. Fatigue
　　2. Insomnia or hypersomnia
　　3. Psychomotor agitation

B. Not due to any physical or other mental disorder, such as amphetamine or similarly acting sympathomimetic delusional disorder.

Note: When the differential diagnosis must be made without a clear-cut history or toxicologic analysis of body fluids, it may be qualified as "provisional."

Stimulant intoxication can lead to fighting, agitation, impaired judgment, and transient psychosis. The psychosis may resemble paranoid schizophrenia with persecutory delusions, but usually subsides days or weeks after the drug use stops. In rare cases, the psychosis may last longer, but a diagnosis of schizophrenia should only be considered when it is clear that there is no continuing source of the drug. Antipsychotics have been used to treat the symptoms of stimulant-induced psychosis, although they may not be needed, because the psychosis is short-lived once the offending drugs have been stopped. Occasional patients who use stimulants develop a delirium, usually shortly after taking the drug, which disappears as the blood level drops. In some patients, binge-crash cycles may develop with psychostimulant abuse.

Cocaine has also been associated with serious medical complications such as acute myocardial infarction due to coronary artery constriction and anoxic brain damage due to cocaine-induced seizures.

No specific amphetamine withdrawal syndrome has been identified, although many users report fatigue and depression, nightmares, headache, profuse sweating, muscle cramps, and hunger from discontinuation of the drug. When this "crash" extends past 24 hours after the last use of the substance, DSM-III-R classifies these symptoms as amphetamine or similarly acting sympathomimetic withdrawal (Table 15-10). Withdrawal symptoms usually peak within 2–4 days. Depression may occur, peaking between 48 and 72 hours after the last dose of amphetamine. Separate criteria are presented in DSM-III-R for cocaine withdrawal, but are not included in this chapter because they are so similar to those of amphetamine withdrawal.

Amphetamine intoxication and amphetamine delusional disorder are generally self-limiting; therefore, no specific treatment is required. Antipsychotics may be prescribed for the psychosis, particularly if the person is agitated or dangerous. Elimination of the drug may be accelerated by acidifying the urine with ammonium chloride. A withdrawal depression that persists more than 2 weeks can be treated with tricyclic antidepressants, although their use in these cases has not been systematically evaluated. Desipramine, a tricyclic antidepressant, is now being advocated for use in cocaine withdrawal; it is reported to be helpful in reducing the craving for cocaine that many addicts experience on withdrawal. Similarly, flupentixol, an antipsychotic not available in the United States, is said to produce similar benefits for the "crack" cocaine user. Although these approaches to treating cocaine withdrawal show promise, their routine use in these patients is premature.

Hallucinogen Use Disorders

Hallucinogens are agents that induce psychotic-like experiences, such as hallucinations, perceptual disturbances, and feelings of unreality. Some persons believe that hallucinogens will bring one closer to God, or even expand one's mind. The drugs became very popular in the late 1960s and early 1970s when psychedelic substances were romanticized and self-styled drug gurus (e.g., Timothy Leary) advocated their use. Their use continues, although they are probably not as popular now.

Hallucinogens are a diverse group of compounds, most synthetic, and two (i.e., peyote and mescaline) are of botanical origin. Newer drugs, such as 3,4-methylenedioxymethamphetamine (MDMA) appear to cause less disorientation and perceptual distortion than older hallucinogens such as lysergic acid diethylamide (LSD) and have been popularized as mood drugs.

Hallucinogens are sympathomimetics and can cause tachycardia, hypertension, sweating, blurry vision, pupillary dilation, and tremors. They affect multiple neurotransmitter systems, including dopamine, serotonin, acetylcholine, and gamma-aminobutyric acid (GABA). Tolerance can develop to some hallucinogens (e.g., LSD). These compounds are probably not physically addicting, but many persons have become psychologically dependent on them.

Although the different hallucinogens differ in quality and duration of subjective effects, LSD can be taken as a prototype. The drug is short acting and rapidly absorbed. Onset occurs within an hour of ingestion, and the effects last 8–12 hours. In addition to autonomic hyperarousal, the drug causes various psychological reactions including profound alterations in perception (e.g., colors may be experienced as brighter and more intense; colors may be heard or sounds seen), and senses appear heightened. Emotions may become intense and labile. Religious feelings, introspection, and philosophical insight are reported to occur. In fact, these properties led psychiatrists to experiment with LSD and other hallucinogens for therapeutic purposes, such as for facilitating therapeutic communication, improving insight, and increasing self-esteem. DSM-III-R has termed this reaction a *hallucinogen hallucinosis*. See Table 15-11 for the complete list of criteria for this disorder.

Although many effects of hallucinogens are reported as pleasant, "bad trips" can occur when patients develop marked anxiety or paranoia. Another common undesirable effect is the *flashback*, a brief reoccurrence of a drug-induced experience that occurs in situations unrelated to taking the drug. Flashbacks may consist of visual distortion, geometric hallucinations, and misperceptions. This symptom leads to a DSM-III-R diagnosis of *posthallucinogen perception disorder* if the flashbacks

Table 15-11. DSM-III-R criteria for hallucinogen hallucinosis

A. Recent use of a hallucinogen.

B. Maladaptive behavior changes, e.g., marked anxiety or depression, ideas of reference, fear of losing one's mind, paranoid ideation, impaired judgment, impaired social or occupational functioning.

C. Perceptual changes occurring in a state of full wakefulness and alertness, e.g., subjective intensification of perceptions, depersonalization, derealization, illusions, hallucinations, synesthesias.

D. At least two of the following signs:
    1. Pupillary dilation
    2. Tachycardia
    3. Sweating
    4. Palpitations
    5. Blurring of vision
    6. Tremors
    7. Incoordination

E. Not due to any physical or other mental disorder.

Note: When the differential diagnosis must be made without a clear-cut history or toxicologic analysis of body fluids, it may be qualified as "provisional."

cause marked distress (see Table 15-12 for the criteria). Usually the disorder is self-limiting, but may become chronic in some persons.

Chronic psychosis has been reported in a minority of hallucinogen users, and it was once thought that these drugs could induce schizophrenia. Although these agents may possibly precipitate psychotic episodes in vulnerable persons, it is likely that users who develop schizophrenia would have developed the illness regardless of their hallucinogen use.

Arylcyclohexylamine Use Disorders

Phencyclidine (PCP) has also become a significant drug of abuse since the late 1960s and may be taken in a variety of ways (e.g., orally, intravenously, or in-

Table 15-12. DSM-III-R criteria for posthallucinogen perception disorder

A. The reexperiencing, following cessation of use of a hallucinogen, of one or more of the perceptual symptoms that were experienced while intoxicated with the hallucinogen, e.g., geometric hallucinations, false perceptions of movement in the peripheral visual fields, flashes of color, intensified colors, trails of images from moving objects, positive afterimages, halos around objects, macropsia, and micropsia.

B. The disturbance in A causes marked distress.

C. Other causes of the symptoms, such as anatomic lesions and infections of the brain, delirium, dementia, sensory (visual) epilepsies, schizophrenia, entoptic imagery, and hypnopompic hallucinations, have been ruled out.

Table 15-13.   DSM-III-R criteria for phencyclidine (PCP) or similarly acting arylcyclohexylamine intoxication

A. Recent use of phencyclidine or a similarly acting arylcyclohexylamine.

B. Maladaptive behavior changes, e.g., belligerence, assaultiveness, impulsiveness, unpredictability, psychomotor agitation, impaired judgment, impaired social or occupational functioning.

C. Within an hour (less when smoked, insufflated ["snorted"], or used intravenously), at least two of the following signs:

   1. Vertical or horizontal nystagmus
   2. Increased blood pressure or heart rate
   3. Numbness or diminished responsiveness to pain
   4. Ataxia
   5. Dysarthria
   6. Muscle rigidity
   7. Seizures
   8. Hyperacusis

D. Not due to any physical or other mental disorder, e.g., phencyclidine or similarly acting arylcyclohexylamine delirium.

Note: When the differential diagnosis must be made without a clear-cut history or toxicologic analysis of body fluids, it may be qualified as "provisional."

---

tranasally). Common street terms for the drug include angel dust and crystal. PCP was originally developed as an anesthetic agent for animals, and although it affects several neurotransmitter systems, its mechanism of action is still unknown. The drug may produce intoxication, delirium, and delusional and mood disorders and has been known to cause flashbacks.

Because of variation in dosages available on the streets, effects of PCP can vary widely. It is easy to manufacture and relatively cheap and, as a result, is often used to adulterate other illicit compounds. Onset of action may occur in as few as 5 minutes and generally peaks in 30 minutes. Users report feelings of euphoria, warmth, tingling, and derealization. With moderate doses, bizarre behavior may develop, accompanied by a blank stare, myoclonic jerks, confusion, and disorientation. With higher doses, users can become comatose and have convulsions. Death may occur due to respiratory depression. Unlike hallucinogens that dilate pupils, users of PCP have normal or small pupils. Chronic psychotic episodes have been reported to follow its use, and unlike the hallucinogens, PCP apparently can lead to long-term neuropsychological damage. The DSM-III-R criteria for PCP intoxication are found in Table 15-13.

Adverse reactions to PCP may require treatment. Diazepam has been used in reducing agitation, but severe behavior disturbances may require short-term antipsychotic use, preferably haloperidol, due to its relative absence of anticholinergic side effects. Phentolamine or other antihypertensive agents may be needed to reduce elevated blood pressure. Ammonium chloride can be used to acidify the urine to promote the drug's elimination.

Table 15-14.   DSM-III-R criteria for cannabis intoxication

A. Recent use of cannabis.

B. Maladaptive behavior changes, e.g., euphoria, anxiety, suspicious or paranoid ideation, sensation of slowed time, impaired judgment, social withdrawal.

C. At least two of the following signs developing within 2 hours of cannabis use:

1. Conjunctival injection
2. Increased appetite
3. Dry mouth
4. Tachycardia

D. Not due to any physical or other mental disorder.

Note: When the differential diagnosis must be made without a clear-cut history or toxicologic analysis of body fluids, it may be qualified as "provisional."

Cannabis

The active ingredient in marijuana is believed to be delta-9-tetrahydrocannabinol (THC). Marijuana, or *Cannabis sativa*, is a hemp plant that has been used for centuries for medicinal purposes. The plant itself contains various amounts of THC; plants used today tend to have a much higher THC content than was available in the past. Although marijuana has long been used for recreational purposes, it became popular among the drug subculture in the 1960s and 1970s and is probably less popular today. Nonetheless, of the illicit psychoactive compounds, marijuana is still probably the most widely used.

The substance is generally smoked in a cigarette (i.e., a joint), leading to intoxication in 10–30 minutes. THC and its metabolites are highly lipid soluble and accumulate in fat cells, having a half-life of approximately 50 hours. Intoxication may last 2–4 hours depending on the dose, although behavior changes may continue for many hours. Oral ingestion (usually from adding to baked goods) produces a slower onset of intoxication and more powerful effects.

Psychological effects of marijuana include euphoria, drowsiness, and a feeling of calm. Users also report feeling that time has slowed, develop increased appetite and thirst, feel that their senses are heightened, and report improved self-confidence. Physical symptoms include conjunctivitis (red eyes), a strong odor, pupillary dilation, tachycardia, dry mouth ("cotton mouth"), and coughing fits. Many effects reported by marijuana users are similar to those reported by LSD users, for example, the development of perceptual distortions, sensitivity to sound, and a feeling of oneness with the environment. Unwanted effects include anxiety and paranoia (e.g., suspiciousness, hyperalertness), impaired attention, and decreased motor coordination. Marijuana rarely causes severe reactions. The DSM-III-R criteria for cannabis intoxication are found in Table 15-14.

Marijuana users often report a morning hangover that can interfere with functioning. Marijuana has been shown to impair the transfer of material from immediate to long-term memory, and electroencephalogram studies show both a decrease and an increase in alpha rhythm patterns. Chronic use has been associated with an amotivational syndrome characterized by lack of persistence at schoolwork or any task that requires a prolonged attention period. Users may seem apathetic or inert and become unproductive; in fact, these symptoms resemble the apathy and amotivation seen in schizophrenia (e.g., Bleuler's fundamental symptoms). Many users develop cannabis abuse or dependence and develop the social, psychological, and medical problems attributable to marijuana. Often it is difficult to isolate the effects of marijuana because many of its regular users also take other drugs.

Adverse effects of marijuana usually do not require professional help. Occasionally, anxiolytics (e.g., diazepam) are needed to calm the highly anxious user. Because there is no characteristic withdrawal syndrome, detoxification is unnecessary.

Inhalants

Inhalants are a group of chemicals that produce psychoactive vapors. Popular inhalants include airplane glue, paint thinner, nail-polish remover, gasoline, and many other substances in aerosol cans including hair spray and room deodorizers. The active substances in the inhalants include toluene, acetone, benzene, and other organic hydrocarbons. Methods of inhalation may vary, but commonly, the substance is sprayed into a plastic bag and inhaled.

The use of volatile solvents is widespread, and it is estimated that 1 in 10 persons under age 17 years has experimented with them. Because they are widely available and cheap, inhalants are mostly used by young persons who may have trouble gaining access to other psychoactive substances.

Inhalants act as CNS depressants and produce an intoxication that is similar to alcohol but of shorter duration. Effects may last from 5 to 45 minutes after cessation of sniffing and include excitation, disinhibition, and a sense of euphoria. Less desirable symptoms include dizziness, slurred speech, and ataxia. Inhalants may also cause symptoms of an acute delirium (e.g., impaired concentration, disorientation). Hallucinations and delusions have been reported with their use. Other effects include loss of appetite, lateral nystagmus, hypoactive reflexes, and double vision. At higher doses, patients may become stuporous or comatose.

Most users of inhalants are male. Hispanics and Native Americans seem to be overrepresented in their use. Although experimentation with inhalants is extremely common, regular use is found primarily among lower socioeconomic groups, children of alcoholic parents, and children from abusive or disruptive homes.

No withdrawal syndrome from inhalants has been identified. Because inhalants often contain high concentrations of heavy metals, permanent neuromuscular and brain damage has occurred, and serious risk of irreversible damage to the kidneys, liver, and other organs from benzene and other hydrocarbons is possible.

Clinical Management of the Psychoactive Substance User

Although specific treatment approaches will differ depending on the primary agent of abuse, the pattern of abuse, and the personal characteristics of the abuser, there are general guidelines that apply to all psychoactive substance abusers. These guidelines are similar to those applied to the alcoholic patient and are summarized in Chapter 14.

Treatment can be thought of as having two phases—an acute phase and a chronic phase. In the acute phase, detoxification is the major goal. This goal may be difficult to achieve in some patients, for example, those with potentially serious withdrawal syndromes (e.g., from barbiturates or opiates), and easier in others (e.g., marijuana abusers) where there is no specific withdrawal syndrome. Hospitalization will be necessary for safe detoxification in some patients so that tolerance can be determined and a slow taper of medication monitored under medical supervision. Others, like the alcoholic patient, may be able to stop their drug use after having a physician make a diagnosis and explain its significance to the patient. In any event, the circumstances of detoxification should be determined by the patient and physician working together. Clearly, many drug addicts have serious medical conditions that the physician will also need to address during this phase of treatment. For example, a heroin addict may have an antecubital cellulitis and be seropositive for HIV; a cocaine addict may have an eroded nasal septum from sniffing the drug that has become secondarily infected.

Psychiatric comorbidity is also important to assess during this phase of treatment. Many, if not most, psychoactive substance abusers have additional psychiatric diagnoses that can have a profound impact on their treatment outcome. Abuse of other substances is the most common comorbidity, followed by mood disorders and personality disorders. Comorbidity always complicates treatment efforts and reduces the likelihood of success. Examples include the amphetamine abuser who develops a suicidal depression during withdrawal, and the heroin addict with an antisocial personality whose use seems, in part, to be motivated by membership in a street gang that celebrates drug use.

The second phase of treatment consists of efforts to rehabilitate the patient and to prevent future use of psychoactive substances. The success of this phase is almost completely dependent on the motivation of the patient, because there is no way to truly assess or enforce compliance (except, of course, by frequent and random drug screening tests and threats of punishment for noncompliance). Except in the military, in certain professions (e.g., pilots), and in totalitarian societies, such strict enforcement is neither possible nor desirable.

Multimodel approaches to the patient are needed for rehabilitation. Individual psychotherapy may be important in helping the patient to learn about motivation for using drugs, and in learning alternative methods of handling stressors. Group approaches, especially in the hospital, are useful in confronting patients with the seriousness of their problem and its significant effects on their life. Peer groups seem unequaled in their ability to achieve confrontation. Behavioral or cognitive approaches may be needed to help the patient to reverse habits that lead or exacerbate drug use, or to help the patient to correct cognitive distortions (e.g., "If I don't use drugs, I won't be popular with my friends."). Social skills training may be needed for some patients, to help them break a cycle of getting in with the "wrong crowd" and learn to meet and be accepted by more appropriate peers.

Family therapy and marital counseling will be a necessary adjunct in other patients; for example, the teenager whose inhalant use has led to considerable disruption of his family life, and the young man whose marriage is falling apart due to his cocaine addiction.

Medical approaches for the rehabilitation or maintenance phase of treatment are important for some patients. Methadone maintenance in opiate addicts has been popular for years and seems to have an established role in the treatment of at least some opiate addicts. Methadone maintenance provides a carefully monitored substitute addiction that allows the patient to function in the community. Patients with comorbid psychiatric disorders may, of course, benefit from ongoing somatic treatment for anxiety, depression, or psychosis. It is probably wise to avoid the use of benzodiazepines in these patients due to their abuse potential. The use of desipramine or flupentixol in cocaine abusers, discussed earlier in the chapter, can only be considered experimental.

Self-help groups have become an integral part of a comprehensive treatment approach to drug use disorders. Alcoholics Anonymous (AA) has led the way for the creation of sister groups, such as Cocaine Anonymous (CA), Narcotics Anonymous (NA), and Drugs Anonymous (DA). These groups are organized along the same lines as AA, following a 12-step program to provide an atmosphere in which recovering addicts can share their experiences. These programs are now available in many parts of the United States.

Recommendations for management of psychoactive substance use

1. Do not let your personal beliefs and attitudes about drug abuse interfere with your care of the addict.

   - Patients need consistent yet firm handling.
   - Neither condemn the addict, nor condone his or her behavior.

2. Be sure to consider both medical and psychiatric comorbidity. Many addicts have potentially serious medical problems that require treatment, significant addictions to other substances, mood disorder, or personality disorders.

3. Be prepared for relapses during the rehabilitation phase of treatment. Relapse is almost inevitable, but does not represent failure of the treatment program. Be there to help the patient get "back on the wagon."

4. Support groups can be very helpful to the patient, and referral to community-based organizations is essential.

Bibliography

Busto U, Sellers EM, Naranjo CA, et al: Withdrawal reaction after long-term therapeutic use of benzodiazepines. N Engl J Med 315:854–859, 1986

Cadoret RJ, Troughton E, O'Gorman TW, et al: An adoption study of genetic and environmental factors in drug abuse. Arch Gen Psychiatry 43:1131–1136, 1986

Charney DS, Henninger GR, Kleber HD: A combined use of clonidine and naltrexone as a rapid, safe, and effective treatment of abrupt withdrawal from methadone. Am J Psychiatry 143:831–837, 1986

Council on Scientific Affairs: Marijuana—its health hazards and therapeutic potentials. JAMA 246:1823–1827, 1981

Council on Scientific Affairs: Methaqualone—abuse limits its usefulness. JAMA 250:3052, 1983

Cregler LL, Mark H: Medical complications of cocaine abuse. N Engl J Med 315:1495–1500, 1986

Dinwiddie SH, Zorumski CF, Rubin EH: Psychiatric correlates of chronic solvent abuse. J Clin Psychiatry 48:334–337, 1987

Gawin FH, Kleber HD: Cocaine abuse treatment. Arch Gen Psychiatry 41:903–909, 1984

Gawin FH, Kleber HD, Byck R, et al: Desipramine facilitation of initial cocaine abstinence. Arch Gen Psychiatry 46:117–121, 1989

Gawin FH, Allen D, Humblestone B: Outpatient treatment of "crack" cocaine smoking with flupenthixol decanoate. Arch Gen Psychiatry 46:322–325, 1989

Gossop M, Johns A, Green L: Opiate withdrawal: inpatient versus outpatient programmes and preferred versus random assignment. Br Med J 293:103–104, 1986

Gossop M, Green L, Phillips G, et al: What happens to opiate addicts immediately after treatment: a prospective follow-up study. Br Med J 294:1377–1380, 1987

Halikas JA, Weller RA, Morse CL, et al: Regular marijuana use and its effect on psychosocial variables: a longitudinal study. Compr Psychiatry 24:229–235, 1983

Khantzian EJ, McKenna GJ: Acute toxic and withdrawal reactions associated with drug use and abuse. Ann Intern Med 90:361–372, 1979

Kozel NJ, Adams EH: Epidemiology of drug abuse: an overview. Science 234:970–974, 1986

Millman RB: Drug abuse and drug dependence, in Psychiatry Update: American Psychiatric Association Annual Review, Vol 5. Edited by Frances AJ, Hales RE. Washington, DC, American Psychiatric Press, 1986, pp 120–232

Nicholi AM: The non-therapeutic use of psychoactive drugs—a modern epidemic. N Engl J Med 308:925–933, 1983

O'Brien CP, Woody GE, McLellan AT: Psychiatric disorders in opioid dependent patients. J Clin Psychiatry 45:9–13, 1984

Vaillant GE: A 12-year follow-up of New York narcotic addicts. Arch Gen Psychiatry 15:599–609, 1966

Vardy M, Kay S: LSD psychosis or LSD induced schizophrenia? Arch Gen Psychiatry 40:877–883, 1983

Verebey K, Gold MS: From coca leaves to crack: the effects of dose and routes of administration in abuse liability. Psychiatric Annals 18:513–520, 1988

Woody GE, McLellan AT, Luborsky L, et al: A 12-month follow-up of psychotherapy for opiate dependence. Am J Psychiatry 144:590–596, 1987

Yates WR, Fulton AI, Gabel J, et al: Personality risk factors for cocaine abuse. Am J Public Health 79:891–892, 1989

Self-assessment Questions

1. How widespread is psychoactive substance abuse/dependence, and what are its risk factors?
2. Who appear to be the two types of sedative, hypnotic, or anxiolytic abusers?
3. Describe the withdrawal syndrome from sedatives, hypnotics, or anxiolytics.
4. Why are barbiturates especially dangerous?
5. Describe the pentobarbital/diazepam tolerance test.
6. Describe the opiate withdrawal syndrome and how it differs from sedative, hypnotic, or anxiolytic withdrawal.
7. What are the pharmacokinetics of cocaine?
8. Does LSD use lead to schizophrenia?
9. What are the symptoms of PCP intoxication?
10. What is the "amotivational" syndrome in association with marijuana?
11. Why are the inhalants dangerous substances of abuse?

Chapter 16
Personality Disorders

All is caprice, they love without measure those whom they will soon hate without reason.

Thomas Sydenham, 1682

Maladaptive character traits have been part of man's makeup since the dawn of time; their recognition as a mental illness termed *personality disorder* is relatively recent. The ancient Greeks, for example, observed and classified many of the mental illnesses that are recognized today, including mania, paranoia, and melancholia. They did not recognize personality disorders, however, but elaborated a system of four temperaments—sanguine, choleric, melancholic, and phlegmatic—to describe variations of personality type. The ancients felt that these temperaments were the embodiments of the four elements: earth, air, fire, and water. These four temperaments continued to be recognized through the 19th century. Kraepelin in fact characterized the personalities often found in manic-depressive patients or their relatives as depressive, hypomanic, or irritable, terms that corresponded to the Greek temperaments melancholia, sanguine, and choleric. These terms are still useful descriptively.

In the early 19th century, descriptive psychiatrists working in Europe and the United States described abnormal personality traits. The French psychiatrist Pinel described *manie sans delire* and used this term to describe patients who are prone to unexplained outbursts of rage and violence but who were not insane. This group of patients probably included many who would now be regarded as having antisocial personality. Prichard, an English physician, suggested the term *moral insanity* to describe persons who violated social norms, but were neither intellectually impaired

Table 16-1. DSM-III-R personality disorders

Cluster A (the "eccentric" disorders)	Cluster C (the "anxious" disorders)
• Paranoid • Schizoid • Schizotypal	• Avoidant • Dependent • Obsessive-Compulsive • Passive-Aggressive
Cluster B (the "dramatic" disorders)	
• Antisocial • Borderline • Histrionic • Narcissistic	

nor psychotic. The concept of moral insanity has persisted, and the closest equivalent currently is antisocial personality disorder. Later, Freud and other leaders of the psychoanalytic movement attempted to describe character along the lines of psychosexual development (e.g., oral, anal, phallic, and genital). These stages of development are discussed later in the chapter.

More recently, attempts have been made to describe the various personality types important to clinicians. In DSM-III and DSM-III-R, for example, 11 personality types are described. These manuals use a "polythetic" schema, in which a combination of four or five of eight or nine items can trigger the corresponding diagnosis. An advantage of polythetic schemata is their greater coverage, which occurs at the expense of diminished specificity. For example, a person may receive a diagnosis of borderline personality, even in the absence of impulsivity, undue anger, or unstable interpersonal relationships, as long as five other items are present.

Although the polythetic approach offers more rigorously defined subtypes than were available before, they are not perfect. Normal personality variants and the way these shade into more dysfunctional types are left out. Additionally, few persons with personality disorders show exclusively the traits of the diagnosed personality disorder and usually manifest traits belonging to several of the defined personality types. As a result, many clinicians believe that a dimensional approach to the diagnosis of personality disorder is preferable, in which scales are used to measure different qualities, such as narcissism.

Most clinicians probably think along both dimensional and categorical lines simultaneously. For example, in describing patients, a patient may be diagnosed as having an obsessive-compulsive personality with avoidant and narcissistic features, meaning that the person satisfies the diagnosis for obsessive-compulsive personality disorder but has features consistent with both avoidant and narcissistic personality disorders.

According to DSM-III-R, there are 11 distinct personality disorders, in addition to a residual category (personality disorder not otherwise specified) for those with mixed or atypical traits that do not fit into the better-defined categories. Further, the 11 disorders are grouped into three separate personality "clusters" according to their clinical similarity. These clusters include the eccentric disorders (Cluster A), the dramatic disorders (Cluster B), and the anxious disorders (Cluster C) (Table 16-1).

Definition

Personality disorders are coded on Axis II in an attempt to separate them from the major mental disorders (Axis I). Theoretically, a person may have both Axis I and Axis II disorders, with some exceptions. For example, personality disorders are not diagnosed in persons with chronic psychotic disorders (e.g., schizophrenia) that are so devastating to the personality that the concept of personality disorder becomes meaningless for them. In fact, many persons with personality disorders meet criteria for Axis I diagnoses, most often major depressive disorder.

Personality disorders are defined in DSM-III-R as behaviors or traits that are characteristic of a person's recent and long-term functioning, that is, generally since adolescence or early adulthood. The constellation of behavior traits must cause either significant impairment in social or occupational functioning or subjective distress. It is important to note that these behaviors are traits and are not limited to episodes of illness, but are representative of long-term functioning. A personality disorder would not be diagnosed, for example, in a person who develops transient personality changes during an episode of depression.

The term *personality disorder* is sometimes considered pejorative, because many patients who receive this diagnosis have undesirable or unpleasant traits. These patients may be described as obnoxious, paranoid, overdramatic, or even criminal. These qualities lead to trouble getting along with other people, as well as difficulties in other spheres of life. Conversely, many patients with personality disorders, probably the majority, are not unpleasant or difficult to work with. These patients tend to be lonely, isolated, anxious, or dependent. Clearly, these latter character traits can also lead to interpersonal difficulties and unhappiness in life. What unites all patients with personality disorders, despite their heterogeneous character traits, is the way in which the disorder leads to pervasive problems in social and occupational adjustment. Many patients with personality disorders tend to be untroubled by their maladaptive traits, or are unaware of them. Other patients are acutely aware of their personality "problems," but seem powerless to change them. It is not surprising that personality disorder patients seek help for a variety of problems that occur in their life, including marital or work-related problems, depression, or substance abuse. Thus, it is rarely the personality disorder itself that brings the patient to seek professional help, although it may be the underlying problem. It is the task of the clinician to help the patient to recognize his or her maladaptive character traits as the source of ongoing troubles, and to help modify them if possible.

Because many traits characteristic of these patients are unpleasant, personality disorder patients in general have a bad reputation. Many mental health professionals have trouble dealing with these patients or refuse to treat them, and view treatment as necessarily long-term and complicated and the results frequently disappointing. However, most of these patients are not unpleasant or difficult to deal with, treatment is not always long-term, and treatment results are often rewarding. Personality disorders themselves are heterogeneous, so it is rarely useful to make generalizations about the entire category of personality disorder patients based on one's experience with a particular type of disorder (e.g., borderline personality).

Table 16-2. Prevalence (in percentages) of DSM-III personality disorders among psychiatric patients and screened control subjects

Disorder	Screened control subjects (n = 35)	Major depression (n = 78)	Obsessive-compulsive disorder (n = 37)	Panic disorder (n = 83)
Cluster A				
Paranoid	0	1	19	6
Schizoid	0	1	0	0
Schizotypal	3	9	19	0
Cluster B				
Histrionic	3	18	11	10
Narcissistic	3	0	5	0
Antisocial	0	1	0	1
Borderline	0	23	19	7
Cluster C				
Avoidant	0	15	27	20
Dependent	0	17	46	18
Obsessive-compulsive	3	6	30	8
Passive-aggressive	9	4	49	2

Source. Adapted from Pfohl B, Black DW, Noyes R, et al: Axis I and Axis II comorbidity findings: implications for validity, in Personality Disorders: New Perspectives on Diagnostic Validity. Edited by Oldham JM. Washington, DC, American Psychiatric Press, 1990, pp 145–161.

Epidemiology

It is difficult to know how widespread personality disorders are in the community, but surveys show that 10–20% of the general population may meet criteria for one or more disorders. The prevalence is far greater, however, in psychiatric samples, as demonstrated in Table 16-2, which is based on data collected at our hospital. In this table, the prevalence of personality disorder diagnosed using a self-report instrument (the Personality Diagnostic Questionnaire) is compared in four groups: normal control subjects and patients with major depression, obsessive-compulsive disorder (OCD), or panic disorder. Although the prevalence of specific personality disorders differs among the four groups, and no particular personality disorder is specific to Axis I pathology, prevalence is high in each of the three psychiatric disorders. In fact, in major depression, more than 50% of hospitalized patients have a personality disorder. There is great overlap among personality disorders as well, and most patients with personality disorder will meet criteria for more than one disorder.

Personality disorder traits are even more prevalent. Data from Iowa show that in the general community, nearly 30% of the general population, 8% of screened "normal" subjects (persons screened to exclude Axis I disorders), and nearly two-thirds of psychiatric outpatients have maladaptive personality traits (see Table 16-3).

Attention has recently focused on the importance of the comorbidity between personality disorders and Axis I disorders, because there are many differences between patients who have personality disorders and those who do not. For example, among depressed persons, patients with personality disorders tend to be younger, are more likely to be female, have a history of marital instability, report

Table 16-3. Prevalence (in percentages) of DSM-III personality traits in a community sample, psychiatric outpatients, and screened normal subjects

Traits	Community sample (n = 235)	Outpatient sample (n = 82)	Screened normal subjects (n = 40)
Any	29	67	8
Cluster A	13	32	7
Paranoid	1	1	5
Schizoid	1	4	3
Schizotypal	13	30	8
Cluster B	6	42	5
Narcissistic	0	0	0
Histrionic	4	28	5
Borderline	0	5	0
Antisocial	1	30	3
Cluster C	26	53	18
Avoidant	0	16	8
Dependent	15	43	10
Obsessive-compulsive	15	26	5
Passive-aggressive	0	4	0

Note. Numbers are not additive, as many patients have traits of several disorders.
Source. Adapted from Reich J, Yates W, Nguaguba M: Prevalence of DSM-III personality disorders in the community. Social Psychiatry and Psychiatric Epidemiology 24:12–16, 1989.

precipitating stressors, and have a history of nonserious suicide attempts. Depressed patients with personality disorders are also more likely to have an abnormal dexamethasone suppression test (DST) and are more likely to have a family history of alcoholism and antisocial personality. These findings suggest that depressed patients with personality disorders may form an important subgroup that differs genetically and chemically from depressed patients with primary depressive illness. The presence of a personality disorder also predicts a poor response to antidepressant medication. These interesting findings also seem to be true, to some extent, for patients with panic disorder and OCD, and probably other diagnostic groups as well.

Age at onset of personality disorder tends to be in adolescence (or younger), so the disorder is established by young adulthood. Late-onset personality changes, in general, suggest the presence of a major mental illness (e.g., the prodrome of schizophrenia) or an organic mental disorder. By definition, antisocial personality is established before age 15. Sex distribution differs among the 11 personality disorders, and some (e.g., antisocial, schizoid, obsessive-compulsive personality) have a male preponderance, others (e.g., avoidant, dependent) a female preponderance. Others have a more equal distribution (e.g., borderline, schizotypal).

Personality disorders tend to be stable and enduring. There have been few long-term follow-up studies, which is not surprising because many of the different personality disorders have only recently been defined. Apparently, schizotypal, borderline, and antisocial personality are all stable on follow-up.

Etiology

Freud believed that fixation at certain stages of development led to certain personality types. Several of the DSM-III-R disorders derive from his oral, anal, and phallic character types. Fixation at the oral stage was felt to result in a personality characterized by demanding and dependent behavior (dependent and passive-aggressive personality disorders). Fixation at the anal stage led to a personality characterized by obsessionality, rigidity, and emotional aloofness (obsessive-compulsive personality disorder). Fixation at the phallic stage was believed to lead to shallowness and an inability to engage in intimate relationships (histrionic personality). These broad character types have, in fact, been supported by factor analytic studies, but there is little evidence that early childhood events or fixation at certain stages of development lead to specific personality patterns.

Genetic factors have been used to a limited extent to explain some of the personality disorders. Family and adoption studies suggest that schizotypal personality may be genetically related to schizophrenia. A twin study has recently supported this finding. Family and adoption studies have also confirmed a strong genetic factor in the etiology of antisocial and borderline personality disorders. There is less evidence available for the heritability of the other DSM-III-R personality disorders.

Neurobiological models have also been applied to personality disorders. Schizotypal personality has been associated with low platelet monoamine oxidase (MAO) activity and impaired smooth pursuit eye movement. Among borderline patients, low cerebrospinal fluid 5-hydroxyindoleacetic acid (5-HIAA) negatively correlated with measures of aggression and a past history of suicide attempts. Interestingly, depressed patients with personality disorder are less likely to be DST nonsuppressors than patients with depression alone.

Electroencephalograph (EEG) abnormalities have been reported in antisocial personality for many years. The most widely reported abnormality is slow-wave activity. A study on borderline patients reported that a high percentage (38%) had at least marginal EEG abnormalities, compared to 19% in a control group. Some authors have suggested that some borderline and antisocial patients might actually be manifesting characterologic changes associated with minimal brain dysfunction.

Cluster A Disorders

Paranoid Personality Disorder

Although paranoid personality was first described by Adolf Meyer, it has been little studied. Psychoanalysts have associated paranoid traits with the anal character and a reaction formation to and projection of homosexual impulses. However, there is no evidence that homosexuals are differentially affected with paranoid personalities. Persons with paranoid personality disorder have a pervasive and unwarranted tendency to interpret the actions of others as deliberately demeaning or threatening. This

Table 16-4. DSM-III-R criteria for paranoid personality disorder

A. A pervasive and unwarranted tendency, beginning by early adulthood and present in a variety of contexts, to interpret the actions of people as deliberately demeaning or threatening, as indicated by at least four of the following:

1. Expects, without sufficient basis, to be exploited or harmed by others
2. Questions, without justification, the loyalty or trustworthiness of friends or associates
3. Reads hidden demeaning or threatening meanings into benign remarks or events, e.g., suspects that a neighbor put out trash early to annoy him or her
4. Bears grudges or is unforgiving of insults or slights
5. Is reluctant to confide in others because of unwarranted fear that the information will be used against him or her
6. Is easily slighted and quick to react with anger or to counterattack
7. Questions, without justification, fidelity of spouse or sexual partner

B. Occurrence not exclusively during the course of schizophrenia or a delusional disorder.

misperception occurs in various contexts and may be indicated by various behaviors. These behaviors and the full criteria for the disorder are listed in Table 16-4.

Some researchers have hypothesized that paranoid personality disorder may lie along a spectrum of schizophrenic disorders, providing a manifestation of a common genetic predisposition. Paranoid features have been described to occur premorbidly in persons with delusional disorder. A behavioral model has been theorized in which suspiciousness and mistrust are learned, leading to withdrawal, testing of others, and ruminative suspiciousness. Paranoid patients tend to fulfill their suspicious prophecies by inducing in others a tendency to be overly cautious and deceptive.

Patients with paranoid personality rarely seek treatment, probably due to their suspiciousness of everyone, including therapists. It is probably best to use a supportive approach, listening patiently to a person's accusations and complaints, while being open, honest, and respectful. Once rapport has been established, alternative explanations of the person's misperceptions might be advanced. Group therapy should probably be avoided, due to the paranoid patient's tendency to make misinterpretations. Suspiciousness may suggest to the clinician that antipsychotic medications are indicated, but their usefulness has not been studied in this disorder.

Schizoid Personality Disorder

Schizoid personality disorder was originally described to characterize the premorbid seclusiveness of schizophrenic patients and the eccentricity of their relatives. Over the years, the term has been used to include almost all persons with problems in achieving intimacy. The concept was again narrowed in DSM-III, when odd, eccentric persons were placed into a new category, schizotypal personality, and persons who were isolated due to an unwillingness to confront rejection were placed in another new category, avoidant personality. Schizoid personality disorder is now restricted to persons with a profound defect in the ability to form personal rela-

Table 16-5. DSM-III-R criteria for schizoid personality disorder

A. A pervasive pattern of indifference to social relationships and a restricted range of emotional experience and expression, beginning by early adulthood and present in a variety of contexts, as indicated by at least four of the following:

1. Neither desires nor enjoys close relationships, including being part of a family
2. Almost always chooses solitary activities
3. Rarely, if ever, claims or appears to experience strong emotions, such as anger and joy
4. Indicates little if any desire to have sexual experiences with another person (age being taken into account)
5. Is indifferent to the praise and criticism of others
6. Has no close friends or confidants (or only one) other than first-degree relatives
7. Displays constricted affect, e.g., is aloof, cold, rarely reciprocates gestures or facial expressions, such as smiles or nods

B. Occurrence not exclusively during the course of schizophrenia or a delusional disorder.

tionships and respond to others in a meaningful way. The diagnostic criteria for schizoid personality are listed in Table 16-5. The following case example illustrates schizoid personality.

Michael, a 24-year-old, was transferred to the psychiatric ward after receiving treatment for a gunshot wound to the head as a result of a suicide attempt. Michael had suffered spells of depression in the past and according to his family had been depressed for several weeks before shooting himself. On transfer, however, it was apparent that Michael was no longer depressed, and he believed there was no reason to remain in the hospital.

During his stay, a great deal was learned about Michael. According to his family, he had always been considered odd and eccentric, was isolative, and had no friends that the family was aware of. He had not done well in school and had dropped out before graduating from high school. He had never dated and admitted having no interest in sexual activity with either sex, preferring solitary masturbation. Further, Michael was not particularly close to any of his family members, and although he lived with his elderly father, he showed no interest or emotion in describing their relationship. Although of average intelligence, Michael had never been able to persist with a job and, as a result, had never had significant employment. He preferred to stay home and read or watch television. In fact, Michael was so unmotivated, and so isolated from the community, that he had never bothered to obtain a driver's license.

Despite his seclusive nature and emotional aloofness, Michael believed that his only problem was his occasional bouts of depression. He neither complained about his social isolation and emotional aloofness nor accepted the fact that these symptoms could be part of his underlying problem. He had no interest in changing his ways and refused referral for psychotherapy.

Schizoid patients are characterized by the absence of close relationships, including their family of origin, choosing solitary activities, rarely experiencing strong emotions, having little desire for sexual experience with another person, indifference to praise or criticism, having no close friends or confidants other than first-degree relatives, and displaying constricted affect. The diagnosis is not made in persons with schizophrenia or delusional disorder.

Apparently, schizoid personality is rare in clinical settings. This presumed rarity may be due to the overly restrictive criteria of DSM-III, which have since been revised, allowing for the diagnosis of other personality diagnoses as well. Little is known about the treatment of this disorder, and most persons with this condition probably do not seek professional help or probably do so only when seeking help for depression, substance abuse, or other problems. Most schizoid patients undoubtedly lack the insight or motivation for individual psychotherapy and probably would find the intimacy of group therapy too threatening. If the patient is motivated, behavior techniques may be helpful, such as graded exposure to various social tasks. For example, the clinician might encourage the patient to start by attending a concert, then to join a bridge club, and eventually to enter a dance class.

Schizotypal Personality Disorder

Schizotypal personality disorder was created in the development of DSM-III based on its presumed genetic relatedness to schizophrenia. The Danish Adoption Study had revealed that relatives of schizophrenic patients often had a cluster of schizophrenia-spectrum traits, a fact noted much earlier by both Kraepelin and Bleuler. Early precedents for this disorder included Bleuler's simple and latent schizophrenic subtypes. These diagnoses were applied to persons who displayed mild or attenuated symptoms of schizophrenia, but who were nonpsychotic.

Schizotypal personality is characterized by a pattern of peculiar behavior, odd speech and thinking, and unusual perceptual experiences. Schizotypal patients tend to be socially isolated and have idiosyncratic speech, unusual (i.e., "magical") beliefs, mild paranoid tendencies, inappropriate or constricted affect, and undue social anxiety. The complete criteria are found in Table 16-6.

Because the disorder is relatively new, little is known about its distribution, natural history, or treatment. In one community survey that used a self-report instrument for diagnosis, schizotypal personality was the most common of the 11 personality disorders studied, affecting approximately 5% of the respondents.

Treatment of the schizotypal patient will often center on issues that led the person to seek treatment. These problems may include feelings of alienation or isolation, mild feelings of paranoia or suspiciousness, or feelings of alienation due to paranoid ideation or ideas of reference. A supportive approach has been recommended, whereas exploratory and group psychotherapies are felt to be overly threatening. Social skills training may be useful in helping eccentric, odd persons to feel more comfortable with others.

Low-dose antipsychotics have been recommended to alleviate some of the intense anxiety and cognitive symptoms such as odd speech and unusual perceptual experiences; this approach has some empirical support. However, any enthusiasm for using these medications must be tempered by their tendency to induce troublesome and potentially irreversible side effects. Antipsychotics should not routinely be used in these patients.

Table 16-6. DSM-III-R criteria for schizotypal personality disorder

A. A pervasive pattern of deficits in interpersonal relatedness and peculiarities of ideation, appearance, and behavior, beginning by early adulthood and present in a variety of contexts, as indicated by at least five of the following:

1. Ideas of reference (excluding delusions of reference)
2. Excessive social anxiety, e.g., extreme discomfort in social situations involving unfamiliar people
3. Odd beliefs or magical thinking, influencing behavior and inconsistent with subcultural norms, e.g., superstitiousness, belief in clairvoyance, telepathy, or "sixth sense," "others can feel my feelings" (in children and adolescents, bizarre fantasies or preoccupations)
4. Unusual perceptual experiences, e.g., illusions, sensing the presence of a force or person not actually present (e.g., "I felt as if my dead mother were in the room with me")
5. Odd or eccentric behavior or appearance, e.g., unkempt, unusual mannerisms, talks to self
6. No close friends or confidants (or only one) other than first-degree relatives
7. Odd speech (without loosening of associations or incoherence), e.g., speech that is impoverished, digressive, vague, or inappropriately abstract
8. Inappropriate or constricted affect, e.g., silly, aloof, rarely reciprocates gestures or facial expressions such as smiles or nods
9. Suspiciousness or paranoid ideation

B. Occurrence not exclusively during the course of schizophrenia or a pervasive developmental disorder.

Cluster B Disorders

Antisocial Personality Disorder

Antisocial personality is the oldest and best validated of the 11 personality disorders and was first recognized in the 19th century as "moral insanity." The term was used to describe immoral or guiltless behavior that was not accompanied by impairments in reasoning. Other labels have included *psychopathic personality* and *sociopathic personality*. The disorder is characterized by a pattern of socially irresponsible, exploitative, and guiltless behavior, as evidenced by failure to conform to the law and to sustain consistent employment and tendencies to exploit and manipulate others for personal gain, to deceive, and to fail to develop stable relationships. Although the current criteria for the diagnosis of antisocial personality have been criticized for their "Chinese menu" approach and their failure to include psychological traits such as guiltlessness, egocentricity, incapacity for love, lack of remorse, and failure to learn from past experience, they have proved to be both reliable and valid. In fact, lack of remorse has now been included as a criterion in DSM-III-R. The diagnostic criteria are listed in Table 16-7.

The following case example illustrates a patient with an antisocial personality disorder and the personal and interpersonal difficulties that arise from the disorder.

Emily, a 34-year-old woman, was admitted to the hospital because of her cocaine abuse and suicidal wishes. In a lengthy, rambling, and confusing interview, a lifelong history

Table 16-7. DSM-III-R criteria for antisocial personality disorder

A. Current age at least 18.

B. Evidence of conduct disorder with onset before age 15, as indicated by a history of three or more of the following:
  1. Was often truant
  2. Ran away from home overnight at least twice while living in parental or parental surrogate home (or once without returning)
  3. Often initiated physical fights
  4. Used a weapon in more than one fight
  5. Forced someone into sexual activity with him or her
  6. Was physically cruel to animals
  7. Was physically cruel to other people
  8. Deliberately destroyed others' property (other than by fire-setting)
  9. Deliberately engaged in fire-setting
  10. Often lied (other than to avoid physical or sexual abuse)
  11. Has stolen without confrontation of a victim on more than one occasion (including forgery)
  12. Has stolen with confrontation of a victim (e.g., mugging, purse-snatching, extortion, armed robbery)

C. A pattern of irresponsible and antisocial behavior since the age of 15, as indicated by at least four of the following:
  1. Is unable to sustain consistent work behavior, as indicated by any of the following (including similar behavior in academic settings if the person is a student):
    a. Significant unemployment for 6 months or more within 5 years when expected to work and work was available
    b. Repeated absences from work unexplained by illness in self or family
    c. Abandonment of several jobs without realistic plans for others
  2. Fails to conform to social norms with respect to lawful behavior, as indicated by repeatedly performing antisocial acts that are grounds for arrest (whether arrested or not), e.g., destroying property, harassing others, stealing, pursuing an illegal occupation
  3. Is irritable and aggressive, as indicated by repeated physical fights or assaults (not required by one's job or to defend someone or oneself), including spouse- or child-beating
  4. Repeatedly fails to honor financial obligations, as indicated by defaulting on debts or failing to provide child support or support for other dependents on a regular basis
  5. Fails to plan ahead, or is impulsive, as indicated by one or both of the following:
    a. Traveling from place to place without a prearranged job or clear goal for the period of travel or clear idea about when the travel will terminate
    b. Lack of a fixed address for a month or more
  6. Has no regard for the truth, as indicated by repeated lying, use of aliases, or "conning" others for personal profit or pleasure
  7. Is reckless regarding his or her own or others' personal safety, as indicated by driving while intoxicated, or recurrent speeding
  8. If a parent or guardian, lacks ability to function as a responsible parent, as indicated by one or more of the following:
    a. Malnutrition of child
    b. Child's illness resulting from lack of minimal hygiene
    c. Failure to obtain medical care for a seriously ill child
    d. Child's dependence on neighbors or nonresident relatives for food or shelter
    e. Failure to arrange for a caretaker for young child when parent is away from home
    f. Repeated squandering, on personal items, of money required for household necessities
  9. Has never sustained a totally monogamous relationship for more than 1 year
  10. Lacks remorse (feels justified in having hurt, mistreated, or stolen from another)

D. Occurrence of antisocial behavior not exclusively during the course of schizophrenia or manic episodes.

of emotional disturbance was unraveled. She grew up in a chaotic household where she was both physically and sexually abused for many years by her father. As a youngster, she developed delinquent behaviors such as shoplifting and vandalism and was sent to a state mental hospital for 1 year at age 14.

At the hospital, despite various therapies, her behavior failed to improve. She was reported to have violent outbursts requiring physical restraints. During her teen years, she became sexually promiscuous and had at least one abortion before age 15. She lied frequently to her parents and talked back to her teachers at school. She ran away many times and skipped school frequently, and she was soon smoking marijuana, drinking on weekends, and using a variety of other illicit substances. Later, as an adult, she admitted to using aliases, moving from place to place for no particular reason, and engaging in activities including drug distribution, shoplifting, stealing, and prostitution.

She reported that she had been depressed much of her life, but had never had a clinical depression. Recently, she had been freebasing cocaine, which stopped 24 hours before admission, after which she developed nausea, vomiting, and diarrhea. She reported that many of her family members were "just like" her, including her father, a brother, and two sisters. One brother was a convicted felon and was currently in prison.

At interview, the patient was cooperative and superficially pleasant. She wore heavy makeup and had a tattoo of a flower on her right hand. She appeared to enjoy talking about her past exploits and showed no remorse for the problems that she had caused to either herself or others. She admitted to using drugs, but had no insight into the pervasive character disturbance underlying her many problems. She cooperated with ward activities, but after several days left against medical advice, having come to the conclusion that she no longer needed help. Several other hospitalizations had ended similarly.

Family and twin studies suggest that antisocial personality disorder has a hereditary basis. The disorder appears to be genetically related to alcoholism, and of course, the disorder is frequently complicated by alcohol abuse. It has been hypothesized that low cortical arousal and reduced level of inhibitory anxiety may contribute to an impulsive sensation-seeking life-style.

Antisocial patients are prone to various complications including major depression, suicide attempts, alcoholism and other substance abuse, and felonious behavior. These problems present a continuous challenge to the therapist charged with caring for the antisocial patient. Unfortunately, long-term follow-up studies, including one in progress in Iowa, show that the disorder is stable and enduring—even into the 60s and 70s. A common myth is that the disorder "burns out" or attenuates by age 40; it is true that after 40 years the antisocial person has fewer legal problems and is less troublesome to the community, but other characteristics of antisocial personality generally persist, including marital instability, substance abuse, impulsiveness, poor temper control, and failure to honor financial obligations. About 5% of antisocial patients commit suicide, and deaths from accidents (i.e., car wrecks) are common.

According to the Epidemiologic Catchment Area study, about 3% of men and 1% of women in the general population are antisocial. Onset occurs by definition before age 15. Prevalence varies with the setting, but in jails and prisons, the prevalence may reach 75%.

Treatment of antisocial patients is extremely difficult due to their lack of empathy and insight. Long-term behaviorally oriented inpatient programs have been recommended, although there are no data to support this approach. Correctional facilities may be the best means of controlling antisocial patients who engage in criminal activity. Occasional antisocial patients have recurrent rage attacks or episodes of anger that are poorly controlled and may respond to lithium carbonate, carbamazepine, or propranolol. These medications have not been systematically studied in the antisocial patient, however.

Borderline Personality Disorder

Borderline personality disorder was introduced in DSM-III, although the concept has a long history, and was created in an effort to characterize persons with instability in numerous areas, including their self-identity, interpersonal relationships, and mood. Many of these features would have been included in the DSM-II disorder "emotionally unstable personality." Early conceptualizations of borderline personality considered it to be a variant of schizophrenia, and the term *borderline schizophrenia* was developed to describe persons who have had transient episodes of psychosis during periods of regression or during psychotherapy. These patients were later separated from schizotypal patients on the basis of factor analytic study.

The disorder is of great interest to psychoanalysts. Kernberg, for example, uses the term *borderline personality organization* to describe his broad diagnostic concept and diagnoses borderline personality on the basis of presence of identity diffusion, primitive defense mechanisms such as splitting (i.e., exaggerated dichotomies of good and evil, black and white), and the maintenance of reality testing except in the perception of self and others. Unfortunately, reliable diagnosis is very difficult to achieve with these psychological criteria.

As currently conceptualized, borderline personality disorder represents a pervasive pattern of mood instability, unstable and intense interpersonal relationships, impulsivity, inappropriate or intense anger or lack of control of anger, recurrent suicide threats or gestures or self-mutilating behavior, marked and persistent identity disturbance, chronic feelings of emptiness or boredom, and frantic efforts to avoid real or imagined abandonment. Sydenham's quotation at the beginning of the chapter captures the essence of borderline personality. See Table 16-8 for the complete set of criteria.

Although the diagnosis identifies a large group of patients and tends to overlap with most other personality disorders, especially histrionic, antisocial, and schizotypal personality disorders, borderline personality disorder appears to have some descriptive and construct validity. Family studies have shown that borderline personality disorder is common in first-degree relatives and has been associated with certain biochemical and psychophysiologic abnormalities such as shortened rapid eye movement (REM) latency, abnormal dexamethasone suppression, and an ab-

Table 16-8. DSM-III-R criteria for borderline personality disorder

A pervasive pattern of instability of mood, interpersonal relationships, and self-image, beginning by early adulthood and present in a variety of contexts, as indicated by at least five of the following:

1. A pattern of unstable and intense interpersonal relationships characterized by alternating between extremes of overidealization and devaluation
2. Impulsiveness in at least two areas that are potentially self-damaging, e.g., spending, sex, substance use, shoplifting, reckless driving, binge eating (Do not include suicidal or self-mutilating behavior covered in 5.)
3. Affective instability: marked shifts from baseline mood to depression, irritability, or anxiety, usually lasting a few hours and only rarely more than a few days
4. Inappropriate, intense anger or lack of control of anger, e.g., frequent displays of temper, constant anger, recurrent physical fights
5. Recurrent suicidal threats, gestures, or behavior, or self-mutilating behavior
6. Marked and persistent identity disturbance manifested by uncertainty about at least two of the following: self-image, sexual orientation, long-term goals or career choice, type of friends desired, preferred values
7. Chronic feelings of emptiness or boredom
8. Frantic efforts to avoid real or imagined abandonment (Do not include suicidal or self-mutilating behavior covered in 5.)

normal thyrotropin-releasing hormone (TRH) test, abnormalities often found in major depression.

Some researchers have argued that borderline personality is a variant of mood disorder, as evidenced by its association with depression in family studies, follow-up, and drug research. In this sense, the chronic mood instability creates a personality disturbance, and not vice versa. It can be argued, however, that borderline patients may simply be sensitive to developing depressions either because of a psychosocial predisposition (e.g., history of verbal and sexual abuse during childhood) or biological vulnerability.

Treatment of borderline patients is controversial, ranging from Kernberg's recommendation for intensive, interpretive, and confrontational psychotherapy focusing on the transference relationship, to emphasis on a supportive and problem-solving approach. Borderline patients are reported to form intense transference, and countertransference itself can be a problem, as borderline patients tend to stimulate intense feelings of frustration, guilt, or anger in their therapists. Family or group psychotherapy may be used to dilute the transference. Cognitive-behavior techniques may be effective in correcting dysfunctional attitudes and ambivalent perceptions of others and oneself. Behavior techniques may also be useful in managing self-mutilating and other impulses.

Pharmacologic approaches have also been advised, but no one treatment has emerged as being superior. Low-dose antipsychotics may be helpful in treating cognitive distortions; lithium carbonate may be useful in treating mood swings; MAO inhibitors may be useful in treating dysphoria secondary to interpersonal rejection. In one study, four treatments were compared, including an antipsychotic (trifluoperazine), carbamazepine, alprazolam, and a MAO inhibitor (phenelzine).

Table 16-9. DSM-III-R criteria for histrionic personality disorder

A pervasive pattern of excessive emotionality and attention seeking, beginning by early adulthood and present in a variety of contexts, as indicated by at least four of the following:

1. Constantly seeks or demands reassurance, approval, or praise
2. Is inappropriately sexually seductive in appearance or behavior
3. Is overly concerned with physical attractiveness
4. Expresses emotion with inappropriate exaggeration, e.g., embraces casual acquaintances with excessive ardor, uncontrollable sobbing on minor sentimental occasions, has temper tantrums
5. Is uncomfortable in situations in which he or she is not the center of attention
6. Displays rapidly shifting and shallow expression of emotions
7. Is self-centered, actions being directed toward obtaining immediate satisfaction; has no tolerance for the frustration of delayed gratification
8. Has a style of speech that is excessively impressionistic and lacking in detail, e.g., when asked to describe mother, can be no more specific than, "She was a beautiful person."

All treatments were somewhat effective, except for alprazolam, which caused disinhibition and anger dyscontrol.

Because self-mutilating behavior and frequent suicide attempts are a problem in borderline patients, physicians should be cautious in prescribing any medication, particularly if it can be potentially fatal in overdose. Borderline personality is a stable disorder in long-term follow-up studies and is associated with poor outcome and a suicide rate exceeding 5%.

Histrionic Personality Disorder

Histrionic personality takes its name from hysteria, a disorder first characterized in the 19th century associated with conversion, phobias, anxiety, and somatization. Hysterical features, or a self-dramatizing, attention-seeking nature, were felt to be associated with hysteria. Hysterical personality was included in DSM-II and was renamed histrionic personality in DSM-III so as not to be confused with hysteria (renamed somatization disorder). See Chapter 12 for a discussion of the relationship between hysteria and histrionic personality.

According to DSM-III-R, persons with histrionic personality exhibit a pattern of excessive emotionality and attention seeking. Typical behaviors include excessive concern with appearance and wishing to be the center of attention. The full set of criteria are listed in Table 16-9. These persons are often gregarious and superficially charming, but they can be manipulative, vain, and demanding.

Although the cause of histrionic personality is unknown, the disorder has been linked through family studies to somatization disorder and antisocial personality. Research has suggested that histrionic and antisocial personalities may be sex-typed phenotypic variants of the same underlying genetic diathesis. It has also been suggested that histrionic personality is a sex-biased diagnosis that merely describes a caricature of stereotypic femininity.

Interventions have not been clearly studied, but psychoanalytic psychotherapy

Table 16-10. DSM-III-R criteria for narcissistic personality disorder

A pervasive pattern of grandiosity (in fantasy or behavior), lack of empathy, and hypersensitivity to the evaluation of others, beginning by early adulthood and present in a variety of contexts, as indicated by at least five of the following:

1. Reacts to criticism with feelings of rage, shame, or humiliation (even if not expressed)
2. Is interpersonally exploitative: takes advantage of others to achieve his or her own ends
3. Has a grandiose sense of self-importance, e.g., exaggerates achievements and talents, expects to be noticed as "special" without appropriate achievement
4. Believes that his or her problems are unique and can be understood only by other special people
5. Is preoccupied with fantasies of unlimited success, power, brilliance, beauty, or ideal love
6. Has a sense of entitlement: unreasonable expectation of especially favorable treatment, e.g., assumes that he or she does not have to wait in line when others must do so
7. Requires constant attention and admiration, e.g., keeps fishing for compliments
8. Lack of empathy: inability to recognize and experience how others feel, e.g., annoyance and surprise when a friend who is seriously ill cancels a date
9. Is preoccupied with feelings of envy

has a long tradition in the treatment of this and related syndromes and for that reason is considered by some the treatment of choice. However, others advocate a more supportive, problem-solving approach, or a cognitive approach to deal with distorted thinking (i.e., inflated self-image). An interpersonal approach may focus on conscious (or unconscious) motivations for seeking out disappointing lovers and being unable to commit oneself to a stable meaningful relationship. Group therapy may be useful in addressing provocative and attention-seeking behavior. As patients may not be aware of their behaviors, it may be helpful for others to point these traits out to them. A condition that may be related, *hysteroid dysphoria*, described in depressed women who have a history of sensitivity to rejection in relationships, is reportedly responsive to MAO inhibitors (e.g., phenelzine).

Narcissistic Personality Disorder

The category narcissistic personality was created during the development of DSM-III and has long been of interest to psychoanalysts. Narcissistic personality is characterized by grandiosity, lack of empathy, and hypersensitivity to evaluation by others. The criteria are listed in Table 16-10.

This relatively new disorder has met with various criticisms. Some have argued that it is not a distinctive syndrome because narcissistic traits are common in varying degrees in most personality disorder patients, that the criteria tend to ignore more subtle and indirect manifestations (e.g., dependency conflicts), and that the overlap with other disorders such as borderline personality adds to its lack of distinctiveness. Some clinicians believe that the diagnosis can only be made on the basis of the emerging transferential relationship in psychoanalytic psychotherapy.

Little is known about the treatment of this condition, although insight-oriented psychotherapy has been recommended. Other experts have recommended a more supportive approach. Narcissistic patients are often very difficult to work with, tend to devalue the therapist, and may abruptly terminate therapy.

Table 16-11. DSM-III-R criteria for avoidant personality disorder

A pervasive pattern of social discomfort, fear of negative evaluation, and timidity, beginning by early adulthood and present in a variety of contexts, as indicated by at least four of the following:

1. Is easily hurt by criticism or disapproval
2. Has no close friends or confidants (or only one) other than first-degree relatives
3. Is unwilling to get involved with people unless certain of being liked
4. Avoids social or occupational activities that involve significant interpersonal contact, e.g., refuses a promotion that will increase social demands
5. Is reticent in social situations because of a fear of saying something inappropriate or foolish, or of being unable to answer a question
6. Fears being embarrassed by blushing, crying, or showing signs of anxiety in front of other people
7. Exaggerates the potential difficulties, physical dangers, or risks involved in doing something ordinary but outside his or her usual routine, e.g., may cancel social plans because he or she anticipates being exhausted by the effort of getting there

Cluster C Disorders

Avoidant Personality Disorder

Avoidant personality disorder was also introduced in DSM-III and represents a variant of what had previously been termed *schizoid personality*. Another predecessor was *inadequate personality*, a term used to describe persons who were failures in a number of spheres of life (e.g., interpersonal relationships, occupation).

Avoidant personality behavior tends to be inhibited, introverted, and anxious. Persons with avoidant personality disorder tend to show low self-esteem, hypersensitivity to rejection, apprehension and mistrust, social awkwardness, timidity, social discomfort, and self-conscious fears of being embarrassed or acting foolish. Table 16-11 lists the criteria.

A current issue is whether avoidant personality represents a dimension along a spectrum of anxiety disorders, similar to the way borderline personality has been linked to mood disorders and schizotypal personality to schizophrenia. Clearly, many features of avoidant personality are indistinguishable from social phobia, and the two frequently overlap. Perhaps avoidant personality disorder involves a genetic predisposition to chronic anxiety.

Several psychotherapeutic strategies have evolved for the treatment of avoidant personality. Group therapy may be helpful in learning to overcome social anxiety in developing interpersonal trust. Assertiveness and social skills training may be useful, as well as systematic desensitization used to treat anxiety symptoms, shyness, and introversion. Cognitive techniques have been recommended to help correct dysfunctional thinking. Anxiolytics are often helpful during periods in which the patient is attempting to reverse previously avoided behavior. It is probably wise to limit the use of anxiolytics to short periods (i.e., weeks or months).

Table 16-12. DSM-III-R criteria for dependent personality disorder

A pervasive pattern of dependent and submissive behavior, beginning by early adulthood and present in a variety of contexts, as indicated by at least five of the following:

1. Is unable to make everyday decisions without an excessive amount of advice or reassurance from others
2. Allows others to make most of his or her important decisions, e.g., where to live, what job to take
3. Agrees with people even when he or she believes they are wrong, because of fear of being rejected
4. Has difficulty initiating projects or doing things on his or her own
5. Volunteers to do things that are unpleasant or demeaning in order to get other people to like him or her
6. Feels uncomfortable or helpless when alone, or goes to great lengths to avoid being alone
7. Feels devastated or helpless when close relationships end
8. Is frequently preoccupied with fears of being abandoned
9. Is easily hurt by criticism or disapproval

Dependent Personality Disorder

Dependent personality was a subtype of the DSM-I passive-aggressive personality and was not included in DSM-II. Psychoanalysts have suggested that dependent personality results from fixation at the oral stage of development. The disorder is a pattern of relying excessively on others for emotional support. Typical behaviors are listed with the criteria (Table 16-12).

Dependent personality disorder has not been well studied, and it has been questioned whether it is sufficiently distinct from other disorders, such as passive-aggressive personality, to stand alone. Additionally, dependent personality appears to be diagnosed more frequently in women, suggesting a sex bias. Chronic illnesses (both psychiatric and physical) may predispose to its development.

Recommended treatment includes insight-oriented psychotherapy, group therapy, and if applicable, marital counseling. Assertiveness training, social skills training, cognitive-behavior psychotherapy, and other approaches may be helpful in selected patients.

Obsessive-Compulsive Personality Disorder

Obsessive-compulsive personality disorder is felt by psychoanalysts to represent a fixation at the anal stage of development, characterized by the triad of obstinacy, parsimony, and orderliness. It was originally thought that this disorder predisposed to OCD. Although early studies showed that OCD patients were likely to have a premorbid obsessional personality, it is incorrect to assume that obsessive-compulsive personality and OCD lie along a continuum; they do not. The relationship between obsessive-compulsive personality disorder and OCD is further discussed in Chapter 11.

Obsessive-compulsive personality represents a lifelong pattern of perfectionism and inflexibility typically associated with overconscientiousness and constricted emotions. The diagnostic criteria are listed in Table 16-13. Obsessive-compulsive

Table 16-13. DSM-III-R criteria for obsessive-compulsive personality disorder

A pervasive pattern of perfectionism and inflexibility, beginning by early adulthood and present in a variety of contexts, as indicated by at least five of the following:

1. Perfectionism that interferes with task completion, e.g., inability to complete a project because own overly strict standards are not met
2. Preoccupation with details, rules, lists, order, organization, or schedules to the extent that the major point of the activity is lost
3. Unreasonable insistence that others submit to exactly his or her own way of doing things, or unreasonable reluctance to allow others to do things because of the conviction that they will not do them correctly
4. Excessive devotion to work and productivity to the exclusion of leisure activities and friendships (not accounted for by obvious economic necessity)
5. Indecisiveness: decision making is either avoided, postponed, or protracted, e.g., the person cannot get assignments done on time because of ruminating about priorities (do not include if indecisiveness is due to excessive need for advice or reassurance from others)
6. Overconscientiousness, scrupulousness, and inflexibility about matters of morality, ethics, or values (not accounted for by cultural or religious identification)
7. Restricted expression of affection
8. Lack of generosity in giving time, money, or gifts when no personal gain is likely to result
9. Inability to discard worn-out or worthless objects even when they have no sentimental value

personality disorder patients are prone to depression, particularly as they get older. Commonalities exist with the "type A" personality described by Rosenman (characterized by intense ambition and competitiveness), which has been identified as a cardiovascular risk factor.

Obsessive-compulsive personality disorder patients are difficult to treat. They tend to intellectualize and may be insightful, but develop little feeling. Paradoxical strategies have been recommended, such as suggesting that the patient become even more perfectionist or rigid. Cognitive techniques may be effective in addressing the illogic of the obsessive-compulsive patient's rigid severe beliefs and moral standards. Thought stopping may be helpful for ruminations.

Passive-Aggressive Personality Disorder

Passive-aggressive personality disorder has a long history and was included in DSM-I. Persons with this personality have a tendency to be passively and indirectly resistant to authority, demands, obligations, and responsibilities. This behavior is manifested by dawdling, procrastination, and forgetting. These persons tend to be complaining and whiny, argumentative, discontent, and disgruntled. They tend to express their anger indirectly through resistant and negativistic behavior. The disorder is characterized by a pervasive pattern of passive resistance to demands for adequate social and occupational performance such as that due to procrastination, working deliberately slowly, and avoiding obligations by claiming to have forgotten them. The criteria are listed in Table 16-14.

Treatment for these patients is difficult because they whine, complain, and are

Table 16-14.   DSM-III-R criteria for passive-aggressive personality disorder

A pervasive pattern of passive resistance to demands for adequate social and occupational performance, beginning by early adulthood and present in a variety of contexts, as indicated by at least five of the following:

1. Procrastinates, i.e., puts off things that need to be done so that deadlines are not met
2. Becomes sulky, irritable, or argumentative when asked to do something he or she does not want to do
3. Seems to work deliberately slowly or to do a bad job on tasks that he or she really does not want to do
4. Protests, without justification, that others make unreasonable demands on him or her
5. Avoids obligations by claiming to have "forgotten"
6. Believes that he or she is doing a much better job than others think he or she is doing
7. Resents useful suggestions from others concerning how he or she could be more productive
8. Obstructs the efforts of others by failing to do his or her share of the work
9. Unreasonably criticizes or scorns people in positions of authority

often unpleasant. Insight-oriented approaches and supportive approaches have been recommended. Social skills and assertiveness training may be helpful. Paradoxical approaches may at times be effective by capitalizing on the patient's oppositionalism.

Recommendations for management of personality disorders

1. Some patients with personality disorders can be difficult, unpleasant, and manipulative. Understand this fact from the outset.

2. Patients have enduring, long-term problems, and therapy may be long-term as well. Decades of maladaptive behavior cannot be easily understood or reversed.

3. Maintain a professional distance from the patient. You are not a friend or a collaborator, you are the therapist.

   - Avoid becoming overinvolved with patients, doing favors (i.e., giving out home telephone number), relating your problems, etc.

4. Establish ground rules for therapy, e.g., that you are willing to see the person regularly, at a specified time.

   - Spell out what the patient should do or who is to be called in a crisis (e.g., who is on-call).
   - Spell out consequences of self-damaging acts (e.g., hospitalization, referral to another therapist).

5. Avoid fantasies of becoming a "savior" to your patient. If the personality disorder has been enduring, the patient has undoubtedly seen other therapists without success. Why should you be the exception?

6. Seek support for yourself from peers or supervisors. Personality disorder patients can be a handful, and you will likely need advice or consultation now and then.

Bibliography

Akhtar S, Thompson JA: Full review: narcissistic personality disorder. Am J Psychiatry 139:12–20, 1982

Akiskal HS, Chen SE, Davis GC, et al: Borderline: an objective in search of a noun. J Clin Psychiatry 46:41–48, 1985

Black DW, Bell S, Hulbert J, et al: The importance of Axis II in patients with major depression—a controlled study. J Affective Disord 14:115–122, 1988

Brinkley JR, Beitman BD, Friedel RO: Low dose neuroleptic regimens in the treatment of borderline patients. Arch Gen Psychiatry 36:319–326, 1979

Cadoret RJ, O'Gorman TW, Troughton E, et al: Alcoholism and antisocial personality. Arch Gen Psychiatry 42:161–167, 1985

Cleckley H: The Mask of Sanity. St. Louis, MO, CV Mosby, 1941

Cowdry RW, Gardner D: Pharmacotherapy of borderline personality disorder. Arch Gen Psychiatry 45:111–119, 1988

Kernberg O: Severe Personality Disorders. New Haven, CT, Yale University Press, 1984

Lewis G, Appleby L: Personality disorders: the patients psychiatrists dislike. Br J Psychiatry 153:44–49, 1988

Liebowitz M, Stone M, Turkat I: Treatment of personality disorders, in Psychiatry Update: American Psychiatric Association Annual Review, Vol 5. Edited by Frances AJ, Hales RE. Washington, DC, American Psychiatric Press, 1986, pp 356–393

McGlashan TH: Schizotypal personality disorder. Arch Gen Psychiatry 43:329–334, 1986

Perry JC, Flannery RB: Passive-aggressive personality disorder—treatment implications of a clinical typology. J Nerv Ment Dis 170:164–173, 1982

Pfohl B, Stangl D, Zimmerman M: The implication of DSM-III personality disorders for patients with major depression. J Affective Disord 7:309–319, 1984

Pfohl B, Black DW, Noyes R, et al: Axis I and Axis II comorbidity findings: implications for validity, in Personality Disorders: New Perspectives on Diagnostic Validity. Edited by Oldham JM. Washington, DC, American Psychiatric Press, 1990, pp 145–161

Pollack J: Obsessive-compulsive personality. Journal of Personality Disorders 1:248–262, 1987

Pope HG, Jonas JM, Hudson JI, et al: The validity of DSM-III borderline personality disorder. Arch Gen Psychiatry 40:23–30, 1983

Pope HG, Hudson JI, Zubenko GS, et al: Schizoid personality disorder among psychiatric inpatients. McLean Hospital Journal 9:1–9, 1986

Quitkin FM, Klein DF: A follow-up of treatment failure: psychosis and character disorder. Am J Psychiatry 124:499–505, 1967

Reich J: Sex distribution of DSM-III personality disorders in psychiatric outpatients. Am J Psychiatry 144:485–488, 1987

Reich J, Yates W, Nguaguba M: Prevalence of DSM-III personality disorders in the community. Social Psychiatry and Psychiatric Epidemiology 24:12–16, 1989

Siever LJ, Coccaro ER, Zemishlany Z, et al: Psychobiology of personality disorders: pharmacologic implications. Psychopharmacol Bull 23:333–336, 1987

Soloff PH, Ansom G, Nathan RS: The dexamethasone suppression test in patients with borderline personality disorders. Am J Psychiatry 139:1621–1623, 1982

Tarnepolsky A, Berelowitz M: Borderline personality—a review of recent research. Br J Psychiatry 151:724–734, 1987

Thompson DJ, Goldberg D: Hysterical personality disorder. Br J Psychiatry 150:241–245, 1987

Torgerson S: The oral, obsessive, and hysterical personality syndromes: a study of hereditary and environmental factors by means of the twin method. Arch Gen Psychiatry 37:1272–1277, 1980

Torgerson S: Genetic and nosologic aspects of schizotypal and borderline personality disorders: a twin study. Arch Gen Psychiatry 41:546–554, 1984

Tucker L, Bauer S, Wagner S, et al: Long-term hospital treatment of borderline patients. Am J Psychiatry 144:1443–1448, 1987

Widiger TA, Frances A, Spitzer RL, et al: The DSM-III-R personality disorders: an overview. Am J Psychiatry 145:786–795, 1988

Zanarini MC, Gunderson JG, Marino MF, et al: Childhood experiences of borderline patients. Compr Psychiatry 30:18–25, 1989

Zanarini MC, Gunderson JG, Frankenburg FR, et al: Discriminating borderline personality disorder from other Axis II disorders. Am J Psychiatry 147:161–167, 1990

Zimmerman M, Coryell W: DSM-III personality disorder diagnosis in a non-patient sample. Arch Gen Psychiatry 46:682–689, 1989

Self-assessment Questions

1. What are the Greek temperaments and why are they still useful descriptively?
2. How are the personality disorders defined? What is the difference between trait and disorder?
3. Why is the term *personality disorder* considered pejorative?
4. How common are personality disorders? Which ones are more common in men? women? Are these disorders stable?
5. What are Freud's character types? How well do they correspond to present-day categories?
6. What evidence is there for a genetic or biological origin for the personality disorders? Which personality disorders?
7. Describe the three personality disorder clusters.
8. How do schizoid and schizotypal personality differ? How do these two categories differ from avoidant personality?
9. Are medications useful in treating Cluster A disorders? Which medications?
10. For which disorders might social skills training or assertiveness training be useful?
11. What is the polythetic approach to diagnosis? Why has it been criticized, using antisocial personality as an example?
12. What are the antecedents of borderline personality? What biological abnormalities have been found in these patients? Why is transference a problem with treatment of borderline patients? Are medications of any value?
13. What features characterize the Cluster C disorders? What are the general treatment recommendations for these disorders? How does obsessive-compulsive personality differ from obsessive-compulsive disorder?

Chapter 17
Sexual Disorders

Lolita, light of my life, fire of my loins. My sin, my soul.
Lo-lee-ta.

Vladimir Nabokov, Lolita

Two categories of sexual disorders are included in DSM-III-R: *sexual dysfunctions*, which involve either a disturbance of sexual arousal or a disturbance of psycho-physiologic performance, and *paraphilias*, which involve culturally inappropriate or dangerous patterns of sexual arousal, such as exhibitionism. To these categories we have added the *gender identity disorders* (e.g., transsexualism), which are grouped with disorders of infancy, childhood, or adolescence in DSM-III-R, because these disorders usually have their onset during those formative years. Sexual dysfunction is probably very common, although its full extent is unknown, due to the sensitive and private nature of sexual relations. Paraphilias are less common, but are more problematic, because they may lead to public arrest and incarceration. Gender identity disorders are less common still, but remain of interest to psychiatrists and other mental health professionals. The psychosexual disorders are listed in Table 17-1.

Sexual Dysfunction Disorders

DSM-III-R has identified four major categories of sexual dysfunction: sexual desire disorders, sexual arousal disorders, orgasm disorders, and sexual pain disorders. There are two residual categories, sexual dysfunction not otherwise

355

Table 17-1.   Psychosexual disorders

Sexual Disorders	
Sexual dysfunctions	**Paraphilias**

Sexual dysfunctions

Sexual desire disorders

- Hypoactive sexual desire disorder
- Sexual aversion disorder

Sexual arousal disorders

- Female sexual arousal disorder
- Male erectile disorder

Orgasm disorders

- Inhibited female orgasm
- Inhibited male orgasm
- Premature ejaculation

Sexual pain disorders

- Dyspareunia
- Vaginismus
- Sexual dysfunction not otherwise specified (NOS)

Paraphilias

- Exhibitionism
- Fetishism
- Frotteurism
- Pedophilia
- Sexual masochism
- Sexual sadism
- Transvestic fetishism
- Voyeurism
- Paraphilia NOS

Other sexual disorders

- Sexual disorder NOS

Gender Identity Disorders

- Gender identity disorder of childhood
- Transsexualism
- Gender identity disorder of adolescence or adulthood, nontranssexual type
- Gender identity disorder NOS

specified (NOS) and other sexual disorders, for a miscellaneous group of disorders that are not classifiable as any of the more specific disorders. The categories tend to correspond to the different phases of the sexual response cycle (see Tables 17-2 and 17-3).

According to DSM-III-R, the normal human sexual response cycle consists of four stages:

Stage 1—an appetitive phase lasting minutes to hours characterized by sexual fantasies and the desire to have sex.

Stage 2—an excitement phase consisting of 1) an early phase lasting minutes to hours characterized by physiological arousal, penile erection in males, and vaginal lubrication, nipple erection, and vasocongestion of the external genitalia in females; and 2) a late phase lasting seconds to minutes characterized by the appearance of drops of fluid at the head of the penis in males, and a tightening of the outer third of the vagina and breast engorgement in females.

Stage 3—orgasm that typically lasts 5–15 seconds, and in males is accompanied by ejaculation and involuntary muscular contractions of the pelvis, and in females by contractions of the outer third of the vagina and involuntary pelvic thrusting. Females may have multiple orgasms, but males have an obligatory refractory period before another orgasm is possible.

Table 17-2. Relationship of sexual dysfunction to stage of the sexual response cycle

Stage	Disorders
Appetitive	Hypoactive sexual desire disorder Sexual aversion disorder
Excitement	Male erectile disorder (impotence) Female sexual arousal disorder
Orgasm	Inhibited female orgasm (anorgasmia) Inhibited male orgasm Premature ejaculation

Stage 4—the resolution phase, consisting of relaxation, detumescence, and a sense of well-being.

Disorders of the Appetitive Phase

Hypoactive sexual desire disorder and *sexual aversion disorder* correspond to the appetitive phase of the sexual response cycle.

In *hypoactive sexual desire disorder*, there is a persistent or recurrent deficiency or absence of sexual fantasy and desire that is not due to major depression or another major Axis I disorder, such as schizophrenia (because these disorders are commonly associated with a low sex drive). The disorder is common among married couples, and more women are affected than men. In one study, 35% of women and 16% of men reported having no desire for sexual activity at least for some temporary period. (See Table 17-4 for additional findings from this study.) In another study of gynecology clinic patients, 12% of the women reported having little sexual interest.

The disorder may be primary or due to stressful situations that are temporary. In the latter case, low sex drive may result from overwork, lack of privacy, lack of opportunity for sex, lack of proper education about sex, or religious taboos. Before making a diagnosis, a clinician must take into account factors that affect

Table 17-3. Other sexual dysfunction disorders

Sexual pain disorders	Sexual disorder NOS
Dyspareunia Vaginismus	Preoccupation with size of genitals Ego-dystonic homosexuality
Sexual dysfunction not otherwise specified (NOS)	
Postcoital headaches Masturbatory pain Orgasmic anhedonia	

Table 17-4. Frequency of self-reported sexual problems

Problem	Women (%)	Men (%)
Sexual dysfunctions—women		
Difficulty getting excited	48	
Difficulty reaching orgasm	46	
Difficulty maintaining excitement	33	
Inability to have orgasm	15	
Reaching orgasm too quickly	11	
Sexual dysfunctions—men		
Ejaculating too quickly		36
Difficulty maintaining an erection		9
Difficulty having an erection		7
Difficulty ejaculating		4
Inability to ejaculate		0

Source. Adapted from Frank E, Anderson C, Rubinstein D: Frequency of sexual dysfunction in "normal couples." N Engl J Med 229:111–115, 1978.

sexual functioning, including age, sex, and the context of a person's life (e.g., it may be culturally appropriate for a nun to report a lack of sexual desire).

Sexual aversion disorder, on the other hand, represents a persistent and recurrent aversion to and avoidance of genital contact with a sexual partner and is not due to obsessive-compulsive disorder, major depression, or another serious Axis I disorder. It is believed that many persons with this disorder have been sexually victimized in the past and harbor unpleasant memories and beliefs about sexual activity.

Disorders of the Excitement Phase

The sexual arousal disorders include *male erectile disorder* (impotence) and *female sexual arousal disorder.*

Primary impotence occurs when a man has never been able to achieve an erection sufficient for vaginal insertion. With *secondary impotence,* the man has successfully achieved vaginal penetration at some time during his life, but is later unable to do so. Primary impotence is rare, but secondary impotence is reported in up to one-fifth of all men. Among men treated for sexual disorders, more than 50% have this problem.

Female sexual arousal disorder occurs in up to one-third of all married women and leads to partial or complete failure to attain or maintain the lubrication-swelling response characteristic of the excitement phase, or the total lack of sexual excitement and pleasure. The disorder may be due to physical factors, such as dyspareunia, and may be associated with anorgasmia.

Disorders of Orgasm

The disorders of orgasm include *inhibited female orgasm* (anorgasmia), *inhibited male orgasm,* and *premature ejaculation.* In women, this disorder is manifested by the absence of orgasm after a normal sexual excitement phase that the clinician judges to be adequate in focus, intensity, and duration. Inhibited male orgasm, also called *retarded ejaculation,* occurs when a man only achieves ejaculation during intercourse with great difficulty, if at all.

Premature ejaculation is a common disorder, reported by more than one-third of married men, and is the second most frequent complaint among men seeking help for sexual disorders. The diagnosis is made when the man has persistent or recurrent ejaculation with minimal sexual stimulation, or before, upon, or shortly after vaginal penetration and before the man wishes to ejaculate. Because women can experience multiple orgasms in a short period, there is no corresponding disorder in women.

Sexual Pain Disorders

The sexual pain disorders include *dyspareunia,* or painful intercourse in men or women, and *vaginismus* in women, in which involuntary muscle contractions occur in the outer one-third of the vagina sufficient to prevent penile insertion. Dyspareunia should not be diagnosed when an organic basis for the pain is found, or in women if it is caused exclusively by vaginismus or lack of lubrication. Although dyspareunia is uncommon among men, it is a frequent complaint of women evaluated for sexual therapy and is common, at least temporarily, among women who have had pelvic surgery, or who have recently undergone childbirth.

Other Sexual Dysfunctions

Less common sexual dysfunctions include *postcoital headaches*— i.e., headaches that occur immediately after intercourse, *orgasmic anhedonia*—a condition in which there is no physical sensation of orgasm even though ejaculation may have occurred, and *masturbatory pain*—in which pain is experienced with masturbation in the absence of physical abnormality. The latter disorder is usually caused by a small vaginal tear, Peyronie's disease of the penis, or some other physical disorder.

Etiology of Sexual Dysfunction Disorders

Sexual dysfunction may be caused by psychological or physical factors, or sometimes a combination of the two. For example, lack of desire can result from chronic stress, anxiety, or depression or may result from medications that either depress the central nervous system or decrease testosterone production. Prolonged abstinence from sex itself may suppress sexual desire. Major physical stresses, such as illness or surgery, especially when they alter body image (e.g., mastectomy, ileostomy), may also depress sexual desire.

Impotence may be caused by both physical and psychological conditions (see Table 17-5). Recent studies have shown that impotence in up to 75% of men evaluated in medical clinics has a physical cause, including cardiovascular disease (e.g., atherosclerotic disease), renal disorders (e.g., chronic renal failure), liver

Table 17-5. Causes of male erectile disorder (impotence)

Medical illness	Psychiatric illness
Acromegaly	Anxiety disorders
Addison's disease	Major depression
Diabetes mellitus	Organic mental disorders
Hyperthyroidism	Schizophrenia
Hypothyroidism	
Klinefelter's syndrome	**Drugs**
Multiple sclerosis	Alcohol
Parkinson's disease	Antiandrogens
Pelvic surgery or irradiation	Anticholinergics
Peripheral vascular disease	Antidepressants
Pituitary adenoma	Antihypertensives (especially centrally
Spinal cord injury	acting ones)
Syphilis	Antipsychotics
Temporal lobe epilepsy	Barbiturates
	Benzodiazepines
	Marijuana
	Narcotics
	Stimulants

disease (e.g., cirrhosis), malnutrition, diabetes mellitus, multiple sclerosis, traumatic spinal cord injury, abuse of alcohol and other addictive drugs, psychotropic medication, prostate surgery, and pelvic irradiation.

In determining the origin of impotence, it is important to obtain a record of spontaneous erections at times when the man does not plan to have intercourse (e.g., morning erections or erections with masturbation). If erections occur at these times, a psychological cause is likely. Evaluation of possible physical causes of impotence may include 1) recording of nocturnal penile tumescence, 2) measuring blood pressure in the penis with a penile plethysmograph or Doppler flow meter, and 3) measuring pudendal nerve latency time. Other laboratory tests used in the evaluation may include a glucose tolerance test, thyroid function and liver tests, prolactin, luteinizing hormone (LH), and follicle-stimulating hormone (FSH) measures to rule out metabolic or endocrinologic causes of impotence, such as diabetes mellitus. Invasive tests (e.g., penile arteriography, infusion cavernosography, or radioactive xenon penography) are used in evaluating the rare patient who is a candidate for vascular reconstructive surgery.

Anorgasmia may result from physical causes, such as medication or surgery, but may also be associated with psychological factors. Psychological factors may include fears of impregnation, rejection by the sex partner, depression, or cultural factors (e.g., women in the past were commonly told by their mothers that sex was not to be enjoyed, but endured).

Inhibited male orgasm (i.e., retarded ejaculation) is relatively uncommon and must be differentiated from *retrograde ejaculation,* in which ejaculation occurs but the seminal fluid passes backward into the bladder. Both retrograde and retarded ejaculation are most likely physiologic and due to medication, genitourinary surgery (e.g., prostatectomy), or neurologic disorders involving the lumbosacral section of the spinal cord. Medications that may be responsible include centrally acting antihypertensives (such as guanethidine or alpha-methyldopa) or antipsychotics, particularly the phenothiazines (e.g., chlorpromazine, thioridazine). Older men, however, may not ejaculate at every sexual encounter, but perhaps only every second or third time. The nonoccurrence of ejaculation in this population should not necessarily be construed as abnormal.

Clinical Management of Sexual Dysfunction Disorders

Psychoanalytic psychotherapy has slowly given way to "dual" sex therapy pioneered by Masters and Johnson. Their sex therapy includes both partners, because the sexual problem affects both persons in a relationship, and the principles apply to both heterosexual and homosexual couples. Therapy may begin with a review of the psychological and physiological aspects of sexual functioning, and an evaluation of the couple's attitudes about sexual behavior and of their ability to communicate. After the sexual disturbance is diagnosed, suggestions are made for specific sexual activity that the couple is expected to carry out in private. Sex is emphasized as a natural and healthy behavior that enhances a couple's relationship. Brief sex therapy focuses on correcting dysfunctional behavior, not interpreting presumed underlying dynamics. These treatment methods may be used for a variety of disorders and are modified depending on whether the sexual problem represents a disorder of the appetitive, excitement, or orgasmic stage of the sexual response cycle.

As an example of sex therapy for male erectile disorder, the couple is prohibited from engaging in sexual activity other than that prescribed by the therapist. Exercises may focus on increasing sensory awareness of erogenous zones, so that couples can learn to give and receive bodily pleasure (i.e., "sensate focus"). Sensate focus exercises are a technique in which the patient engages initially in nongenital, nondemand caressing with his or her partner with the focus on the patient's own pleasure and concentration on sexual feelings. At this stage, intercourse is prohibited so that couples can learn to separate pleasure from intercourse.

Genital stimulation is eventually included in the exercises; couples are instructed to try various positions for intercourse, but not to worry about completing the act. In time, the couples gain confidence, improve their communicative skills, and learn to give and receive pleasure without the pressure of intercourse. Without that pressure, the man gradually is able to have erections and to successfully complete vaginal intercourse and have a satisfactory orgasm.

Specific instructions are altered depending on the presenting complaint. For example, in the case of inhibited male orgasm, the woman may be instructed to self-insert her partner's penis. In anorgasmia, therapy may first involve training the woman to have an orgasm by masturbation, before treating the couple. Vaginismus may require individual therapy, relaxation techniques (e.g., progressive muscle relaxation), or the use of Hegar's dilators. The size of the dilators is slowly increased over 3–5 days to gradually enlarge the vaginal opening. The "squeeze method" has been advocated for treating premature ejaculation. The woman is instructed to squeeze the head of her partner's glans penis before ejaculation. This action effectively aborts the ejaculation so that the couple may prolong the excitement phase (i.e., foreplay). Alternatively, men may benefit from 1% dibucaine (Nupercaine) ointment applied to the coronal ridge and frenulum of the penis to reduce stimulation. A case example of inhibited male orgasm and its treatment is illustrated below.

> Robert, a 34-year-old bank officer, had been happily married for 6 months, but reported that he was now having trouble achieving orgasm. Although he had no sexual experience before marriage, he and his more experienced wife quickly developed a satisfying sexual relationship. They both had versatile sexual interests and were both able to achieve orgasm with adequate stimulation.
>
> Robert reported that for the past month he had been having difficulty achieving orgasm even though foreplay was mutually stimulating and he readily became erect. Although he was able to reach orgasm through masturbation, he was unable to achieve orgasm with vaginal intercourse, despite trying a variety of positions.
>
> An evaluation found no evidence of an anxiety disorder or major depression, nor evidence of a physical disorder. Although Robert had denied any recent change in his marital relationship, he disclosed to the therapist a deep-seated fear that he was unworthy of his new mate and felt that he could not satisfy her sexually. The therapist met with the couple, recommended that Robert abstain from masturbation, and prescribed sensate focus exercises to be tried initially without intercourse and suggested that as intercourse was attempted the wife take a dominant role. Learning that he could give and receive pleasure without the pressure of intercourse apparently allowed Robert and his wife to experience intercourse and to each achieve a satisfactory orgasm.

Recommendations for treatment of the sexual dysfunction disorders

1. Learn to take a sexual history without shame or embarrassment. Patients will detect your anxiety, which will only serve to increase their own.

2. Don't apologize for asking intimate questions. How couples behave sexually is important to assess.
   - Most couples will be surprisingly forthcoming about describing their sex life.

3. Both members of the couple need to participate in the therapy, which may be used with equal success in heterosexual and homosexual couples.

4. The principles of "dual" sex therapy are relatively simple to learn and emphasize education about sexual functioning, assisting couples to communicate better, and correcting dysfunctional attitudes about sex that one or both partners may hold.

5. Therapy involves "homework" assignments that assist the couple in learning to increase sensory awareness. Techniques may include self-masturbation, "sensate focus" exercises, special coital techniques, and learning to separate pleasure from physiologic response (e.g., erection).

Paraphilias (Sexual Deviations)

The paraphilias are disorders characterized by a disturbance in the object of sexual gratification, or in the expression of sexual gratification. Common paraphilias

Table 17-6. Paraphilias (sexual deviations)

Preferential sex act	Behavior of gratification
Exhibitionism	Exposing self to others
Fetishism	Use of inanimate object (e.g., shoe)
Frotteurism	Rubbing against nonconsenting persons
Pedophilia	Preferring prepubertal children
Sexual masochism	Enjoying pain and humiliation
Sexual sadism	Inflicting pain on others
Transvestism	Cross-dressing
Voyeurism	"Window peeping"
Paraphilia not otherwise specified	
Telephone scatologia	Obscene phone calls
Necrophilia	Dead persons
Partialism	Focusing on one part of the body (e.g., feet) to the exclusion of all else
Zoophilia (bestiality)	Animal contacts
Coprophilia	Feces
Klismania	Enemas
Urophilia	Urine
Hypoxophilia	Desire to achieve altered state of consciousness secondary to hypoxia
Oralism	Focusing on oral-genital contact to the exclusion of intercourse

include *exhibitionism*, in which there is repeated exposing of the genitals to unprepared strangers for the purpose of achieving sexual gratification; *fetishism*, in which inanimate objects are the preferred or only means of achieving sexual excitement; *pedophilia*, in which repeated sexual activity with prepubertal children is the preferred or exclusive method of obtaining sexual release (for example, the character Humbert Humbert in Nabokov's *Lolita*); *transvestic fetishism*, in which a person experiences sexual excitement while dressed in the clothes of the opposite sex; and *voyeurism*, in which observing the sexual activity of others is the preferred means of sexual arousal. There are other paraphilias as well, although most are significantly less common, such as sexual sadism, sexual masochism, frotteurism, and necrophilia. Various paraphilias are listed in Table 17-6.

Paraphilias have been known throughout recorded time, but have been subject to classification and study only in recent years. DSM-III-R provides specific criteria for eight paraphilias and a residual category for other disorders. To be considered paraphiliac, sexual activity must be characterized by a preference for the use of nonhuman objects in achieving sexual arousal, by imposed sexual humiliation or suffering, or by the sexual involvement of nonconsenting partners, such as children.

Sexual deviations are currently viewed as having three aspects. First, the behavior does not conform to the generally accepted views of what is normal, although the accepted view of normality is not identical in each society, nor has it been during each period in history. Second, the behavior may cause harm to another person involved in the sexual behavior, for example, intercourse with young children, or extreme forms of sexual sadism. Third, the behavior may result in suffering experienced by the individual himself. This suffering may result from societal attitudes in which the person sees himself at odds with his sexual urges and his own moral standards, and his awareness of distress caused to another person by his sexual practices. A case example of a person with a paraphilia follows.

Frank, a 38-year-old mechanic, presented to the emergency room requesting help. He had left his wife 3 days earlier, fearing that another arrest for indecent exposure would humiliate his family and friends. His story soon unfolded.

At age 10, he had lost a testicle in an accident—a fact that was known to his classmates, and he was teased endlessly, leading to feelings of insecurity and inadequacy. He began to masturbate at age 12 and was soon masturbating up to five times daily. Although he could not remember when, he soon began to masturbate in public settings—not out in the open—but in areas where he might be discovered. He found the challenge of avoiding detection sexually exciting. He would usually masturbate where he could observe women, such as in shopping centers, libraries, or even in his parked car where he could watch women walk by. Although he denied genital exposure, he admitted that occasionally women would "accidentally" observe him masturbating, adding to his excitement. His masturbation had a compulsive quality and he felt powerless to stop.

The behavior continued over a 25-year period, leading to several arrests for indecent exposure. Feeling guilty, and wishing to make amends, Frank sought psychotherapy after each arrest, but would soon drop out. One psychiatrist prescribed thioridazine to dampen his sex drive, but it only caused retrograde ejaculation. Another physician recommended that he read pornography and masturbate in private. Although he denied other paraphiliac behaviors and called pedophilia "disgusting," he admitted two episodes of exhibitionism, first at age 18 to a girl sitting next to him in class, and during his honeymoon. Although socially awkward with women, and not dating until age 21, Frank married at age 23 and had a stable marriage and a satisfying sexual relationship with his wife. He admitted, however, that he preferred masturbation in public to sexual relations with his wife.

Frank was admitted to the hospital for further evaluation. Physical examination confirmed an absence of the right testicle, but was otherwise normal. Serum testosterone was 288 ng/dl (normal serum levels 200–800 ng/dl). Treatment was started with medroxyprogesterone acetate. At a follow-up visit 1 month later, his serum testosterone had fallen to 41 ng/dl. He had been able to resist masturbating in public and no longer had spontaneous erections. He felt that he could control his behavior. Six months later, he chose to discontinue the medication and within 1 month had returned to his old ways.

Epidemiology

The paraphilias are relatively uncommon in psychiatric practice, probably due to the furtiveness and secrecy surrounding most of them. Most cases are noted only if treatment is sought, or if there are legal entanglements. The true prevalence is unknown due to lack of adequate information. The best available statistics are legal, and not medical. Nearly 80,000 persons are arrested annually on sex-related charges in the United States, excluding forcible rape. These estimates are biased toward impulsive individuals and paraphilias that are considered to be dangerous or a public nuisance. Of legally identified cases, pedophilia is the most common paraphilia, probably because of its unsavory nature and the greater effort spent in apprehending pedophiles. Exhibitionism is commonly reported, possibly because it may involve repeated public display to young girls. Sexual masochism and sadism are underrepresented in crime statistics, because it is unlikely that these disorders would come to public attention unless a tragedy occurred (e.g., autoerotic suffocation). Many of these disorders, such as fetishism, would scarcely be reported at all, because the activity takes place between consenting adults or by a lone individual. Furthermore, many individuals who are comfortable with their paraphilias are completely underrepresented in all samples.

Etiology

For centuries, variations of the sexual act were regarded as offenses against nature, God, or the law, rather than disorders that doctors should study and treat. The systematic study of the paraphilias began in the 1870s with the work of Krafft-Ebing, Hirschfeld, Ellis, and others. In 1886, Krafft-Ebing, a Viennese psychiatrist, compiled the first systematic account of sexual deviations in his book *Psychopathia Sexualis*. Krafft-Ebing considered the sexual deviations due mainly to heredity and believed they could be modified by social and psychological factors. Freud, also active at this time, attempted to explain sexual deviations as failures of the developmental processes during childhood. Psychoanalysts have devoted much attention to sexual deviations, and recent psychoanalytic literature follows this tradition.

Much of the recent work on paraphilias has focused on learning theory in both initiating and maintaining the disorder. In this model, paraphiliac persons learn that their fantasies and urges are inappropriate. Attempting to suppress these desires, they inadvertently use paraphiliac fantasies during masturbation, which intensifies their interest, and pairs the fantasy with the positive experience of orgasm. The paraphiliac arousal strengthens, control breaks down, and the fantasy is acted on. Once this process becomes entrenched, it is likely to reoccur. Learning theory does not explain all cases of paraphilia, but behavior techniques have proved valuable in their treatment, regardless of etiology.

Paraphiliac acts may also represent poor impulse control, resulting from a major mental disorder such as schizophrenia or an organic mental disorder such as dementia. Persons with antisocial personality disorder sometimes commit paraphiliac acts to gratify their immediate needs, although a true paraphilia may not exist. Many antisocial persons do have paraphilias, however.

Research has recently implicated familial transmission and abnormal hypothalamic-pituitary-gonadal axis dysfunction in pedophilia, but there has been almost no other neurobiological research into other paraphilias.

Clinical Description, Course, and Outcome of Specific Paraphilias

Paraphilias are usually established in adolescence and occur almost exclusively among men, although cases are described in women. Most paraphiliac patients are heterosexual, not homosexual, contrary to popular belief. These demographic features appear to be true for persons with fetishism, pedophilia, exhibitionism, and voyeurism. Most paraphiliac patients have a variety of sexual behaviors and may meet criteria for several paraphilias simultaneously, and many have other psychiatric disorders as well (e.g., substance abuse, mood disorders, personality disorders).

The *fetishist* often uses objects of gratification such as rubber garments, women's underclothing, and high-heeled shoes. Contact with the object causes sexual excitement, which is usually followed by masturbation. These individuals may spend considerable time seeking their desired objects. There are no reliable follow-up data, but the disorder tends to start in adolescence or young adulthood and may diminish when satisfying heterosexual relationships are established. A case example of fetishism follows.

> A 41-year-old attorney had his law license suspended after admitting to breaking into and entering more than 100 homes in his small town to obtain women's underwear for sexual gratification. He would generally enter houses through unlocked doors or would jimmy a lock with a credit card or knife. Once inside the house, he would search for the undergarments to use later in solitary acts of masturbation. He was finally caught at a neighbor's home, after he had entered a back door that was unlocked and was found searching for the neighbor's underwear. He was discovered by the woman's husband who reported him to the police. He was charged with criminal trespass.

Transvestic fetishism (transvestism) often begins at puberty. Persons may start by putting on only a few garments. In time, individuals may dress entirely in the clothes of the opposite sex. Transvestites experience erections when cross-dressing and may masturbate. As they gain confidence, the clothes may be worn in public. Although data are limited, the disorder may continue for years, but become less severe as the sexual drive declines.

The *pedophile* chooses a child of the same or opposite sex as a sexual partner. Although the condition may begin at any age, most pedophiles seen by physicians are middle-aged, but the preference probably starts much earlier. Prognosis has not been reliably studied, but probably depends on the length of the history of pedophiliac behavior, frequency of the behavior, absence of other social and sexual relationships, and the underlying personality.

Exhibitionists make up about one-third of sexual offenders referred for treatment and generally involve two groups of men—those with an inhibited temperament who struggle with their urges and often expose a flaccid penis, and those with aggressive traits who often expose an erect penis and masturbate. If the behavior begins in middle or advanced age, the behavior may be an indication of an organic mental disorder. Exhibitionists who repeat are likely to persist for years, according to evidence from the courts. In keeping with clinical impression, the evidence suggests that the reconviction rate for indecent exposure is low after the first conviction, but high after a second conviction.

Voyeuristic activities in adolescence are often an expression of sexual curiosity. The behavior is often replaced by direct sexual experience, although voyeurism may persist. A typical case of voyeurism follows.

A 27-year-old law student pleaded guilty to five counts of criminal trespass after admitting that he had spied on women in dormitory showers several times over a 6-month period. He had been arrested near the dormitory one morning after students had caught him spying on the women's shower. He had been seen lying on the floor outside the shower looking through the ventilation grate and was chased out of the dormitory by women who had found him there.

Residents of the dorm had banded together and would watch for him daily from 5 to 9 A.M., believing that he would repeat his act. The "peeper" was well known at the dorm for his voyeurism and for making a nuisance of himself.

Although *homosexuality* has traditionally been included with the sexual deviations, most psychiatrists now believe it to be an alternate form of sexual behavior that should be of little concern to physicians, other than as a risk factor for various diseases such as herpes or acquired immunodeficiency syndrome (AIDS). In fact, members of the American Psychiatric Association voted in 1973 to remove homosexuality from its list of mental disorders. Currently, homosexuality is not considered a mental disorder, unless the patient is chronically distressed by it (i.e., ego-dystonic homosexuality), although most homosexuals will experience a transient phase where they are disturbed or distressed by their sexual orientation. Ego-dystonic homosexuality is classified in DSM-III-R as a sexual disorder NOS.

Clinical Management of the Paraphilias

Great strides have been made in the treatment of the paraphilias in the last two decades. Behavioral interventions have become the mainstay of treatment. Methods have been developed to reduce deviant arousal patterns through masturbatory satiation or covert sensitization, and to generate arousal to nondeviant themes through masturbatory conditioning. Social skills training is useful to help the patient communicate more effectively with appropriate adult partners. Cognitive techniques have been useful in helping the paraphiliac patient to restructure faulty cognitions used to justify behavior (e.g., the pedophile erroneously interprets a child's docility as an expression of desire) and learn to correct these misperceptions through cognitive therapy. Relaxation training may help reduce the anxiety and stress that frequently precede paraphiliac behavior. A follow-up study of 194 child molesters treated with behavior modification techniques showed an 82% success rate (defined as no recidivism) at 12 months posttreatment. Although these results are encouraging, it is not known whether they may be generalized to the other paraphilias, and to persons not motivated by threats of arrest or imprisonment.

Reports on the use of antiandrogen medications (e.g., medroxyprogesterone [Depo-Provera], cyproterone) indicate promising results for the treatment of repeat offenders. These medications work peripherally to reduce serum testosterone levels and on the central nervous system to reduce sexual drive. These medications are primarily useful in carefully selected patients whose hypersexuality is uncontrolled or dangerous. Unfortunately, sustained use is necessary, as relapse generally follows discontinuation of the medication. The long-term risk of these medications has not been adequately studied, and because there may be a risk of liver disease or cancer, these medications should be used with caution and the patient's health carefully monitored. Other drug therapy, including antipsychotic or antidepressant medication, will be indicated for treatment of accompanying schizophrenia or major depression, if the paraphilia is associated with those disorders.

Recommendations for treatment of paraphilias

1. The history is of utmost importance in treating the paraphiliac. The therapist must learn where and when the behavior occurs, who or what the desired object is, and what occurs in the presence of the object.

   - Most paraphiliacs have a variety of abnormal behaviors, and the therapist is safe to assume that there is more there than initially disclosed by the patient.

2. Paraphiliacs are notoriously difficult to treat, but behavior therapy techniques may offer the best hope for success. The purpose of these techniques is to reduce deviant arousal patterns and to generate new arousal to nondeviant themes.

   - Methods may include masturbatory satiation and conditioning, social skills training, cognitive restructuring, etc.

3. Antiandrogens are promising treatments for severe, repeat offenders whose actions are uncontrolled or dangerous. Do not casually prescribe these medications.

4. You may wish to refer difficult patients to therapists who have experience in treating these disorders.

Gender Identity Disorders

Four gender identity disorders have been defined in DSM-III-R: *gender identity disorder of childhood, transsexualism, gender identity disorder of adolescence or adulthood—nontranssexual type,* and *gender identity disorder NOS.*

In the nontranssexual form of gender identity disorder, there is an absence of preoccupation with changing one's sex. Gender identity disorder NOS is a residual category that is used when a patient manifests an identity disturbance that cannot be classified in one of the other categories, e.g., an adult with transient stress-related cross-dressing. Because there is little information about the frequency, course, or outcome of gender identity disorder of childhood or the nontranssexual type of gender identity disorder of adolescence or adulthood, the discussion will focus on transsexualism.

The essential feature of transsexualism is the desire to be a member of the opposite sex. According to DSM-III-R, the transsexual typically manifests persistent discomfort and a sense of inappropriateness about his or her assigned sex and persistent preoccupation with getting rid of his or her primary and secondary sex characteristics and acquiring the sex characteristics of the opposite sex. The person must have reached puberty. The diagnostic criteria for transsexualism are listed in Table 17-7.

Table 17-7. DSM-III-R criteria for transsexualism

A. Persistent discomfort and sense of inappropriateness about one's assigned sex.

B. Persistent preoccupation for at least 2 years with getting rid of one's primary and secondary sex characteristics and acquiring the sex characteristics of the other sex.

C. The person has reached puberty.

The true prevalence of transsexualism is not known, but is estimated at 1 in 30,000 men and 1 in 100,000 women. A case example follows.

William, a 25-year-old convict, was referred to the hospital for evaluation of gender dysphoria. He had recently filed a lawsuit requesting that the state fund sex-reassignment surgery, as well as allow him to wear women's clothing, transfer to a women's prison, and have hormone injections, all of which the corrections officials had refused.

William reported that he had never felt comfortable with his gender and had decided years earlier that he needed an operation. As a child, he was effeminate, enjoyed playing house, and when playing house, assumed feminine roles such as the mother or sister. He also liked games typically associated with girls such as hopscotch and jump rope and was not very good at team sports. He began to cross-dress at age 9 and said that he felt more comfortable and natural dressed as a girl. He wished he had been born a girl and told us that he was unhappy with his male genitals, stating: "I can't stand them. I don't consider them mine."

When in his early 20s, William began to cross-dress full-time and for a 5-month period lived as a woman, calling himself Julie. William never had a desire for heterosexual relations, although he had experimented. He was able to perform sexually with a woman and have an orgasm, but "didn't like it." While experiencing sexual intercourse, William would fantasize about himself being made love to as a woman. He had had considerable homosexual experience, with over 100 different partners by his count, and had reported having had several long-term relationships (5–6 months in duration). He would generally assume a passive role, for example, performing oral sex on others or being the receptive partner of anal sex, but not the reverse. He refused to allow any of his partners to touch his genitals and would not allow mutual masturbation.

William had read widely about transsexualism and had written to many different medical centers for information. Imprisonment had been difficult for William, for he claimed that other inmates would make fun of his personal habits, including shaving his chest, arms, legs, and axilla. He had attempted to mutilate his genitals on three occasions and several months before his evaluation had managed to lacerate his penis with a piece of glass and had required sutures.

In addition to his gender dysphoria, William had a lifelong history of disciplinary and behavior problems and as a young boy had been placed in detention for a period. He also had a history of abusing both alcohol and marijuana and had had many runins with the law for shoplifting, theft, and writing bad checks. He also had had many psychiatric hospitalizations, mostly for depression or after suicide attempts. None of his suicide attempts had been medically serious, however.

At the time of evaluation, William was noted to cross his legs in an effeminate manner, was limp-wristed, and had long, greasy hair parted down the middle, covering half of his face in a Veronica Lake sort of way. There was no evidence of mood disturbance, but he exhibited a nervous giggle. No formal thought disorder, hallucinations, or delusions were present, and although somewhat guarded during the interview, he summarized everything with the words, "It's all a confused mess."

Although the diagnosis of transsexualism is easily made, it is important to rule out schizophrenia, transvestism, and effeminate homosexuality. In schizophrenia, a desire to change one's anatomic sex is generally part of a complex delusional system. Transvestites who cross-dress may occasionally come to feel that sex-reassignment surgery is a natural extension of their cross-dressing. Effeminate homosexuals, on the other hand, might request a sex change to make themselves more appealing to potential sex partners.

Transsexualism generally begins in childhood (before puberty is reached, the appropriate diagnosis is gender identity disorder of childhood). In boys, early features of transsexualism may include overidentification with the mother, overtly feminine behavior (e.g., playing with dolls), little interest in usual male pursuits (e.g., disliking sports), and peer relationships primarily with girls. Tomboyishness, on the other hand, will be found in young female transsexuals, but the behavior is more acceptable in society than feminine behavior in boys and tends to draw less attention.

DSM-III-R has divided transsexuals into three types—*asexual, homosexual,* and *heterosexual*—based on sexual orientation. The asexual person has a history of either no sexual activity or limited pleasure derived from the genitals. The homosexual transsexual reports sexual arousal from same-sex partners. The heterosexual transsexual reports arousal from opposite-sex partners. A category also exists for persons whose sexual orientation is unknown.

Depression is a frequent complication among transsexuals, as is substance abuse and personality disorder. Many transsexuals meet criteria for borderline personality disorder, as evidenced by their often unstable mood, persistent identity problems, self-mutilation, and angry outbursts. Self-mutilation may include damage to genitals, including autocastration in extreme cases. These acts are generally not suicide attempts, as they are aimed at forcing physicians to deal with the transsexualism.

As transsexuals age, they will eventually seek medical help, requesting hormonal therapy and sex-reassignment surgery. A new birth certificate designating the new sexual status will be sought after surgery. By the time they present for surgery, many transsexuals will have been living as a member of the opposite sex for years, and in fact, many clinics offering surgery will demand that patients have lived as members of the opposite sex for more than 1 year before surgery.

Treatment of transsexualism presents a vexing problem to the psychiatrist. Transsexuals will plead for surgery, yet studies suggest that the outcome in terms of social and occupational adjustment is no better with surgery than with psychotherapy.

Many sex-reassignment clinics around the United States and elsewhere offer medical and surgical treatment to the transsexual. The male-to-female transsexual is prescribed hormones (e.g., estradiol, progesterone) to create breasts and feminine contours, undergoes electrolysis to remove hair, and has surgery to remove the testes and penis and to create an artificial vagina. The female-to-male transsexual undergoes mastectomy, hysterectomy, and oophorectomy, is prescribed testosterone to help develop muscle mass and deepen the voice, and may have an artificial penis constructed. Clearly, male-to-female sex-reassignment surgery is more successful, as a penis capable of erection and ejaculation has yet to be constructed. Male-to-female transsexuals have good cosmetic results and many are able to achieve orgasm.

Psychotherapeutic strategies include individual and group sessions aimed at promoting acceptance of the transsexual's anatomic sex, developing the ability to experience pleasure from his or her genitals, and helping him or her to make a successful adjustment in other spheres of life, including social and occupational functioning. Although 70–80% of patients who undergo sex-reassignment surgery are usually pleased with the outcome of surgery and their new anatomical contours, psychological problems, such as an underlying severe personality disorder, endure. The patient who was unstable before surgery is the same person after surgery, despite the body changes.

Bibliography

Abel GG, Blanchard EB: The role of fantasy in the treatment of sexual deviation. Arch Gen Psychiatry 30:467–475, 1974

Berlin FS, Meinecke CF: Treatment of sex offenders with anti-androgenic medication. Am J Psychiatry 138:601–607, 1981

Fagan PJ, Wise TN, Derogatis LR, et al: Distressed transvestites—psychometric characteristics. J Nerv Ment Dis 176:626–632, 1988

Frank E, Anderson C, Rubinstein D: Frequency of sexual dysfunction in "normal couples." N Engl J Med 229:111–115, 1978

Fuller AK: Child molestation and pedophilia—an overview for the physician. JAMA 261:602–606, 1989

Gaffney GR, Berlin FS: Is there a gonadal dysfunction in pedophilia? A pilot study. Br J Psychiatry 145:657–660, 1984

Gaffney GR, Lurie SF, Berlin FS: Is there familial transmission of pedophilia? J Nerv Ment Dis 172:546–548, 1984

Green R: Gender identity in childhood and later sexual orientation: follow-up of 78 males. Am J Psychiatry 142:339–341, 1985

Grob CS: Female exhibitionism. J Nerv Ment Dis 173:253–256, 1985

Hawton K: Sex Therapy: A Practical Guide. New York, Oxford University Press, 1985

Herman J, LoPiccolo J: Clinical outcome of sex therapy. Arch Gen Psychiatry 40:443–449, 1983

Krafft-Ebing RV: Psychopathia Sexualis, English adaptation of 12th German Edition. Translated by Rebman FJ. Brooklyn, NY, Physicians and Surgeons Book Co., 1927

Lothstein LM: Sex reassignment surgery: historical, bioethical and theoretical issues. Am J Psychiatry 139:417–426, 1982

Masters WH, Johnson VE: Human Sexual Inadequacy. Boston, MA, Little, Brown, 1970

Meyer JK, Reter DJ: Sex reassignment follow-up. Arch Gen Psychiatry 36:1010–1015, 1979

Rooth G: Exhibitionism, sexual violence, and pedophilia. Br J Psychiatry 122:705–710, 1973

Segraves RJ: Effects of psychotropic drugs on human erection and ejaculation. Arch Gen Psychiatry 46:275–284, 1989

Smith RS: Voyeurism: a review of the literature. Arch Sex Behav 5:585–609, 1975

Steiner BW (ed): Gender Dysphoria: Development, Research, and Management. New York, Plenum, 1984

Walz TH, Blum NS: Sexual Health in Later Life. Lexington, MA, Lexington Books, 1987

Wise TN: Fetishism, etiology and treatment: a review from multiple perspectives. Compr Psychiatry 26:249–256, 1985

Self-assessment Questions

1. What are the three types of psychosexual disorders?
2. What are the four stages of the sexual response cycle as defined in DSM-III-R?
3. What are the disorders of the appetitive phase?
4. What are the causes of male erectile disorder (impotence)?
5. Describe "dual" sex therapy.
6. How common are paraphilias?
7. How can learning experiences lead to paraphiliac behavior?
8. Is homosexuality a sexual deviation?
9. What are the antecedent behavioral characteristics of transsexuals?
10. What are the treatments for transsexuals?

Chapter 18
Eating Disorders

O! that this too too solid flesh would melt.

William Shakespeare, Hamlet

Many persons believe that the eating disorders are relatively new, brought on by the stress of modern society and its near obsession with youth, beauty, and slimness. Nonetheless, the eating disorders have ancient roots. Bulimia, generally a cycle of excessive binge eating and purging, has as its precursor the banquets of Roman Sybarites. At these banquets, guests ate with gluttonous abandon, and then vomited in order to eat more. Many early Christian saints were observed to have episodes of severe starvation and binge eating. Saint Catherine of Siena is an example of the "fasting saints." However, it was not until 1868 that William Gull, an English physician, formally described anorexia nervosa as a disorder of starvation in the pursuit of thinness.

The eating disorders now share the limelight with the news-of-the-day, as the media appear fascinated by them. Perhaps this attention is due to the association between eating disorders and celebrity; for example, singer Karen Carpenter died tragically from the complications of anorexia nervosa, and actress Jane Fonda has admitted to a decades-long problem with bulimia.

Definition

Anorexia nervosa and bulimia nervosa comprise the two major eating disorders, according to DSM-III-R. They are included with the disorders of infancy, child-

Table 18-1. DSM-III-R criteria for anorexia nervosa

A. Refusal to maintain body weight over a minimal normal weight for age and height, e.g., weight loss leading to maintenance of body weight 15% below that expected; or failure to make expected weight gain during period of growth, leading to body weight 15% below that expected.

B. Intense fear of gaining weight or becoming fat, even though underweight.

C. Disturbance in the way in which one's body weight, size, or shape is experienced, e.g., the person claims to "feel fat" even when emaciated, believes that one area of the body is "too fat" even when obviously underweight.

D. In females, absence of at least three consecutive menstrual cycles when otherwise expected to occur (primary or secondary amenorrhea). (A woman is considered to have amenorrhea if her periods occur only following hormone, e.g., estrogen administration.)

hood, and adolescence because they usually have an onset during those formative years.

Anorexia nervosa is characterized by a refusal to maintain body weight and weight loss of at least 15% of original body weight; intense fear of gaining weight or becoming fat even though underweight; a disturbance in the way in which one's body shape is experienced; and, in women, absence of three consecutive menstrual cycles (Table 18-1).

Bulimia nervosa, on the other hand, consists of recurrent episodes of binge eating and a feeling of lack of control over eating during the binges; regular purging through vomiting, use of laxatives or diuretics, strict dieting or fasting, or vigorous exercise; an average of two binge episodes weekly for 3 months; and persistent overconcern with body shape and weight (Table 18-2).

Although the two disorders differ, patients with either one share an intense preoccupation with body weight and shape. Additionally, there is considerable diagnostic overlap between the two disorders, and their natural histories tend to intertwine. A residual category (eating disorder not otherwise specified) is used to categorize the patient with a disturbance of eating that does not fulfill criteria for either anorexia or bulimia. A woman with features of anorexia nervosa but who still menstruates would fit this category.

Table 18-2. DSM-III-R criteria for bulimia nervosa

A. Recurrent episodes of binge eating (rapid consumption of a large amount of food in a discrete period of time).

B. A feeling of lack of control over eating behavior during the eating binges.

C. The person regularly engages in either self-induced vomiting, use of laxatives or diuretics, strict dieting or fasting, or vigorous exercise in order to prevent weight gain.

D. A minimum average of two binge eating episodes a week for at least 3 months.

E. Persistent overconcern with body shape and weight.

The discrepancy between weight and perceived body image is key to the diagnosis of anorexia. Underweight persons, who are normally concerned about their weight, recognize that their weight is low and possibly harmful and express a desire to gain weight. Anorexic patients, on the other hand, delight in their weight loss and express a fear of gaining weight. The requirement that the anorexic patient be 15% underweight for body height emphasizes severity, and amenorrhea (in women) adds to the specificity of the diagnosis.

Bulimic patients are generally able to hide their binge eating and purging behaviors and often have normal weight.

Epidemiology

There has been some concern that eating disorders are increasing in prevalence, and several investigators have suggested that anorexia nervosa is more common than just 20 years ago. It seems more likely, however, that increasing public awareness has simply led to the recognition of the disorder. Also, as treatments have become available, patients may be more likely to seek help. Estimates from high school and college populations yield a prevalence among women of approximately 1% for anorexia nervosa, and up to 4% for bulimia nervosa. For both disorders, the frequency for men is about one-tenth that for women. Individual symptoms characteristic of eating disorder, such as binge eating, purging, or fasting, are far more common than the disorders themselves. It is not known why women are more likely to be affected than men, but the differences are probably not artifactual because population surveys confirm what clinicians have noted.

The typical age at onset of eating disorders falls during adolescence or young adulthood. Studies comparing anorexic and bulimic patients generally find an earlier age at onset among anorexic patients (early teens) compared with bulimic patients (late teens, early 20s).

Eating disorders are thought to be more prevalent in the higher socioeconomic classes. Anorexia nervosa, in particular, is uncommon in poorly developed countries and is rare among blacks in the United States. Eating disorders are also overrepresented in certain occupations that require rigorous control of body shape (e.g., modeling, ballet).

The following case example illustrates a patient who developed anorexia nervosa first and later achieved normal weight complicated by bulimia nervosa.

Mary, a 36-year-old registered nurse, has a 16-year history of abnormal eating behaviors. Now at normal weight and having regular periods, she has frequent binge episodes followed by spontaneous vomiting.

Mary grew up in a competitive, upper-middle-class family. The middle of five children, Mary always felt unloved and ignored by her parents, who she felt favored other children. She had frequent temper outbursts during her childhood and teen years. Despite these problems, she performed well in school, was active in clubs, was a cheerleader, and had many friends. Still, Mary felt insecure and unattractive, and dated little.

At age 20, she and a friend toured Europe together and, to save money, would skip meals. In fact, both felt they could afford to lose some weight, although Mary then weighed about 120 pounds (height 5 feet, 3 inches). On her return from Europe, she weighed less than 85 pounds. Her family was concerned about her scarecrow-like appearance, but Mary was pleased with her weight loss, as she felt she now was attractive. In fact, she believed she still weighed too much and could afford to lose more weight.

Over the next 5 years, her weight fluctuated, but she remained considerably underweight. Her family became concerned about her eating habits. She refused to eat meals with her family, adopted a vegetarian diet, and was constantly found in the kitchen preparing high-calorie snacks of sugar, condensed milk, or other sweets. Her mother noted that cakes, cookies, and other desserts prepared for the family would mysteriously disappear, or a cake might be found with all the frosting having been removed. Mary eventually moved out into her own apartment. Her brother remembers running into her at a grocery store and finding in her shopping cart only diet soda, a single head of lettuce, and several bags of candy.

Her family had noticed vomiting behaviors. Early on, Mary had learned how to induce vomiting with her fingers, but later vomiting became spontaneous. She would keep empty jars in her room to hold her vomit. After she had moved out, several jars were found under her bed, some of them moldy. Also, she made frequent trips to the bathroom to vomit and rarely cleaned up, leaving a visible trail of vomit in the unflushed toilet.

Always active, she became obsessed with exercise. She took up jogging before it became popular and eventually was jogging 10 miles daily. She took great pride in her running and was able to place high in several marathons. The running continued at a high level until bone spurs and an old back injury flared up so that she had to cut back on her running. A new routine developed involving a reduced amount of running, followed by biking 10 miles, then swimming for 45 minutes. Mary was so busy with her exercise routine that her social life became very constricted. She had little time for friends and seemed to have lost interest in dating. Despite her routine, she lived independently, maintained a full-time job, and attended school part-time, eventually getting a bachelor's degree in nursing.

When Mary was 25, her mother talked her into seeing a physician for evaluation of her thinness, but the physician, who was not familiar with distorted eating behavior, told her mother that Mary's thinness and abnormal behaviors were simply an idiosyncrasy. Mary later sought help from a counselor for relationship problems, but has never sought help specifically for an eating disorder. Although intelligent and a registered nurse, she still denies that she has an eating disorder.

Etiology and Pathophysiology

Psychological, genetic, and biological mechanisms have been used to explain the etiology of eating disorders. Psychological theories have stressed the importance of phobias, proposing that anorexia nervosa represents a phobic avoidance in response to food and an association with sexual tensions generated during puberty. Psychodynamic formulations have suggested that anorexic patients have fantasies of oral impregnation. It is unclear how bulimia nervosa fits either of these models.

Social theories stress the importance of conforming to the American ideal of youth, beauty, and slimness, and that this preoccupation with body shape and image may lead to eating disorders in vulnerable persons.

Studies of hereditary influences have shown that anorexia nervosa tends to run in families (e.g., 6–10% of female relatives suffer the condition), as do mood disorders and substance abuse. Twin studies also tend to confirm a genetic predisposition. For example, in one study of 34 twin pairs and one set of triplets, 9 of 16 monozygotic twin pairs but only 1 of 14 dizygotic twin pairs were concordant for anorexia nervosa.

Biological theories tend to focus on the role of the hypothalamus, a region of the brain concerned with the regulation of essential body functions, such as appetite, weight, temperature regulation, and general homeostasis. Support for a hypothalamic disturbance comes from neurotransmitter studies showing increased corticotropin-releasing factor (CRF) in the cerebrospinal fluid of anorexic patients. The occurrence of amenorrhea before weight loss also suggests a hypothalamic disturbance. There is also evidence of central neurotransmitter system dysregulation affecting dopamine, serotonin, and norepinephrine. Support for reduced norepinephrine activity and turnover is the most consistent finding in both anorexia and bulimia. Further research is needed to pin down the disturbances.

Clinical Findings

The anorexic person quickly develops a repertoire of behaviors in the pursuit of weight loss. These behaviors may include extreme dieting, adoption of unusual diets or vegetarianism, and refusal to eat meals with family members or in restaurants. Anorexic patients often show an unusual interest in food that belies their fear of gaining weight. This interest may include collecting and clipping recipes, preparing elaborate meals for friends and relatives, and developing an interest in nutrition. The person with weight loss may become of concern to friends and relatives, but will insist that her weight is not abnormal, and in fact, that she is *still* overweight. Many patients begin to abuse laxatives, diuretics, or stimulants in an effort to enhance their weight loss.

Anorexic patients may develop an intense, almost obsessive interest in physical exercise and conduct a strict workout routine. In fact, many ballet dancers and female athletes (e.g., marathon runners) have anorexia nervosa. Eating disorders have also been found in male athletes, especially wrestlers.

Anorexic patients with bulimic behavior, and bulimic patients, tend to carry out their binge eating and purging in private. These patients may consume enormous amounts of food, for example, an entire cake, a quart of ice cream, and cookies. Families may be unaware of binge eating, but observe that their food bill is increasing, or that special foods, such as those high in calories or carbohydrates, seem to disappear. The binge may first bring the patient relief from tension, which is followed by guilt and feelings of disgust. The patient then induces vomiting, often at first by placing the fingers in the throat, but later vomiting at will. Some patients abuse emetics, such as ipecac. Many bulimic patients, perhaps as many as 10%, steal food by shoplifting or other means.

Other unusual food-related habits may develop. Patients may be observed to play with the food on their plate at mealtime, cut meat into tiny pieces, or buy large amounts of candy at stores. When these behaviors are pointed out to patients, they tend to deny them.

According to clinical lore, patients with anorexia nervosa tend to have above-average scholastic achievement, are highly perfectionist, and come from families that are achievement oriented. Many anorexic patients have relatively poor sexual adjustment, which has suggested to some clinicians that anorexia represents an attempt to prolong childhood and escape the responsibilities of adulthood. In fact, anorexic patients tend to have delayed sexual development and diminished interest in sex accompanying the onset of their illness. Amenorrhea precedes the onset of obvious weight loss in one-fifth of patients.

Physical manifestations of the eating disorders tend to center around the eating behaviors manifested by the patient. Anorexic patients may develop profound weight loss that may make them look emaciated or cadaverous. With severe weight loss, other physical changes may develop, including hypothermia, dependent edema, bradycardia, hypotension, and lanugo hair. Anorexic patients may complain of sensitivity to cold weather and chronic constipation. Hormonal abnormalities also occur in anorexia, including elevated growth hormone and plasma cortisol levels and reduced gonadotropin levels. Thyroxine (T_4) and thyroid-stimulating hormone (TSH) levels may be normal, but triiodothyronine (T_3) levels may be reduced.

Bulimic patients, on the other hand, may develop calluses on the dorsal surface of their hands (resulting from the irritation caused by placing fingers down the throat), dental erosion and caries, and in some cases, esophageal erosion.

Medical complications in these patients may include hypocalcemia or hypokalemic alkalosis in those who engage in self-induced vomiting, or in those who abuse laxatives and diuretics. Other electrolyte disturbances may result in weakness, lethargy, or cardiac arrhythmias. Serum transaminase levels may become elevated, reflecting fatty degeneration of the liver. Elevated serum cholesterol levels and carotenemia may both develop, reflecting malnutrition. Parotid gland enlargement and elevated serum amylase levels may develop in bulimic patients. In severely ill bulimic patients, esophageal tears may develop from repeated vomiting and can be life threatening. Medical complications of the eating disorders are summarized in Table 18-3.

Course and Outcome

Prognosis in the eating disorders varies from full recovery to malignant weight loss and rapid death. Long-term follow-up studies of anorexic patients show death rates of nearly 7% after a 10-year follow-up, which is significantly higher than expected. Additionally, long-term studies show that although many anorexic patients may be much improved, many continue to display characteristic symptoms of the illness,

Table 18-3. Medical complications of eating disorders

Physical manifestations

- Amenorrhea
- Sensitivity to cold
- Constipation
- Low blood pressure
- Bradycardia
- Hypothermia
- Lanugo hair

- Hair loss
- Petechia
- Carotenemic skin
- Parotid gland enlargement[a]
- Dental erosion, caries[a]
- Pedal edema
- Dry skin

Endocrine abnormalities

- Increased growth hormone levels
- Increased plasma cortisol levels and loss of diurnal variation
- Reduced gonadotropin levels (LH, FSH, impaired response to LHRH)
- Low T_3, high T_3RU, impaired TRH responsiveness[a]
- Abnormal glucose tolerance test
- Abnormal dexamethasone suppression test[a]

Laboratory abnormalities

- Dehydration[a]
- Hypokalemia[a]
- Hypochloremia[a]
- Alkalosis[a]
- Leukopenia
- Elevated serum bicarbonate[a]

- Elevated transaminases
- Elevated serum cholesterol
- Carotenemia
- Elevated BUN[a]
- Elevated amylase levels[a]

Note. LH = luteinizing hormone. FSH = follicle-stimulating hormone. LHRH = luteinizing hormone–releasing hormone. T_3 = triiodothyronine. TRH = thyrotropin-releasing hormone. BUN = blood urea nitrogen.
[a] Seen in patients who binge/purge.

such as a distorted body image. Less than one-quarter of these patients have a good psychological outcome (which is indicated by no abnormal eating behaviors and the person being well-adjusted). Poor outcome is generally associated with longer duration of illness, older age at onset, prior psychiatric hospitalizations, poor premorbid adjustment, and comorbid personality disorder.

Differential Diagnosis

The differential diagnosis for anorexia nervosa and bulimia nervosa includes other psychiatric disorders. Schizophrenia may be accompanied by bizarre eating habits, but they are usually related to psychosis. Major depressive disorder may be accompanied by poor appetite and significant weight loss, but the weight loss is not associated with a distorted body image. Obsessive-compulsive disorder (OCD) may be characterized by ritualistic eating behaviors resulting in weight loss, but the weight loss is not accompanied by a distorted body image or fear of gaining weight. The majority of patients with anorexia or bulimia will also fulfill criteria for another psychiatric disorder, most commonly major depressive disorder, or a personality disorder, such as borderline personality. A few anorexic patients will fulfill diagnostic criteria for OCD as well.

Clinical Management

There are two fundamental goals in the treatment of the eating disorder patient. The first, and probably the most important, goal is restoring the patient's nutritional state. In the anorexic patient, this goal will mean restoring weight to within a normal range, and in the bulimic patient, ensuring that metabolic balance is achieved. The second goal is to modify the patient's distorted eating behavior, so that the patient is able to maintain weight within a normal range, and to reverse or at least attenuate binge eating, purging, and other abnormal behaviors. Treatment can usually be conducted on an outpatient basis, but many patients will need hospitalization. Indications for hospitalization include starvation and severe weight loss, hypotension or hypothermia, or electrolyte imbalance. The depressed patient with suicidal ideations or psychosis will also need to be hospitalized. Other reasons for hospitalization include failure of outpatient treatment, as indicated by failure to gain weight, or failure to reverse severe binge-purge cycles.

Treatment of the eating disorder patient generally involves behavior modification of the eating disturbance combined with individual psychotherapy. The purpose of behavior therapy is to restore normal eating behavior. In the hospital, this goal is accomplished through strict protocols that set specific weight goals for anorexic patients (e.g., expectations for daily average weight gain) and target certain abnormal behaviors for correction (e.g., reducing the number of vomiting episodes for bulimic patients). Positive reinforcement is used to help patients achieve the specific goals outlined in a treatment contract that is agreed to by the patient. For example, patients who are able to achieve their weight goals are rewarded with special privileges, such as a pass with a family member. Patients who do not achieve their targeted goals will have their privileges reduced.

Patients should be weighed daily, early in the morning after emptying their bladder and while wearing only a hospital gown. Daily fluid intake and output should be recorded. To prevent vomiting after meals, patients should be observed for several (at least 2) hours after meals, even if it means that attendants must accompany them to the bathroom. Generally, it is advisable to start patients on a diet providing about 500 calories more than the amount required to maintain present weight and to increase calorie intake slowly. At first, to prevent discomfort at meals, it may be advisable to spread meals out over six feedings during the day. Patients who are significantly underweight or who are having trouble gaining weight may need tube feedings.

Medication may be indicated in the treatment of selected patients. Tricyclic antidepressants, monoamine oxidase inhibitors, trazodone, and fluoxetine have been shown to decrease both binge eating and purging behaviors, although they have no specific role in treating anorexia nervosa. An antidepressant may be useful in the anorexic patient with a superimposed major depression, although treatment of depression in anorexic patients with antidepressants has not specifically been studied. Some success has been demonstrated with cyproheptadine (Periactin) in helping patients to gain weight, particularly among anorexic patients who have no history of bulimia. Other medications have been used, including the phenothiazines (e.g., chlorpromazine) and the benzodiazepines (e.g., lorazepam). These medications have been used most successfully to reduce the anxiety that accompanies early refeeding efforts, especially when tube feedings are needed.

Individual psychotherapy that is practical and goal oriented is probably the best approach to follow with an eating disorder patient. Efforts at altering abnormal eating behavior in patients with insight-oriented therapy have been disappointing. Family therapy may be helpful, particularly when the patient is living at home and the eating behavior has been perpetuated by disturbed family interactions, or the disturbed eating behavior has created problems among the family members.

Most patients with eating disorders will not seek treatment on their own and will deny their illness. Patients are typically brought unwillingly to a physician by their family or friends, and may resist hospitalization or leave the hospital against medical advice. In the hospital, the anorexic or bulimic patient has a reputation for being critical and manipulative. The eating disorder protocol is usually the focus of criticism. Typically, these patients will make repeated requests to get the physician to modify the protocol. This behavior soon becomes a vicious cycle, for as soon as one modification is agreed to, requests for other changes follow. The safest approach is to simply refuse any modifications once the behavior protocol has been set.

Recommendations for treatment of eating disorders

1. An empathic relationship should be encouraged. This goal may be difficult to achieve, because patients with eating disorders may be manipulative and unmotivated and may lack insight.

2. A commonsense approach is probably best for many outpatients.
   - Develop simple targets for behavior modification.
   - Use antidepressants in patients with binge eating/vomiting who do not respond to behavioral measures.

3. Use a strict, vigorous behavior protocol with inpatients.
   - Set the goals and then do not change them. Trivial changes in the protocol will open a Pandora's box.

4. Look carefully for comorbidity. Eating disorder patients are highly likely to have comorbid major depression, substance abuse, or a personality disorder.
   - Remember, the presence of a personality disorder complicates treatment of most all psychiatric disorders, including eating disorders.

5. Family therapy is especially helpful with patients who still live at home, or whose behavior has created problems within the family.

Bibliography

Crisp AH, Hsu LKG, Harding B, et al: Clinical features of anorexia nervosa: a study of 102 cases. J Psychosom Res 24:179–191, 1980

Devlin MJ, Walsh BT, Kral JG, et al: Metabolic abnormalities in bulimia nervosa. Arch Gen Psychiatry 47:144–148, 1990

Drewnowski A, Hopkins SA, Kessler RC: Prevalence of bulimia nervosa in the U.S. college student population. Am J Public Health 78:1322–1325, 1988

Fairburn C: A cognitive-behavioral approach to the treatment of bulimia. Psychol Med 11:707–711, 1981

Fava M, Copeland PM, Schweiger U, et al: Neurochemical abnormalities of anorexia nervosa and bulimia nervosa. Am J Psychiatry 146:963–971, 1989

Halmi KA, Eckert E, LaDeut J, et al: Anorexia nervosa: treatment efficacy of cyproheptadine and amitriptyline. Arch Gen Psychiatry 43:177–181, 1986

Holland AJ, Hall A, Murray R, et al: Anorexia nervosa study of 34 twin pairs and one set of triplets. Br J Psychiatry 145:414–419, 1984

Hudson JI, Pope HG, Jonas JM, et al: Phenomenologic relationship of eating disorders to major affective disorder. Psychiatric Res 9:345–354, 1983

Hughes TL, Wells LA, Cunningham CJ, et al: Treating bulimia with desipramine. Arch Gen Psychiatry 43:182–186, 1986

Liebman R, Minuchin S, Baker L: An integrated treatment program for anorexia nervosa. Am J Psychiatry 131:432–435, 1974

Logue CM, Crowe RR, Bean JA: A family study of anorexia nervosa and bulimia. Compr Psychiatry 30:179–188, 1989

Mitchell JE, Pyle RL, Eckert ED: A comparison study of antidepressants in structured, intensive group psychotherapy in the treatment of bulimia nervosa. Arch Gen Psychiatry 47:149–157, 1990

Pope HG, Hudson JI, Jonas JM, et al: Bulimia treated with imipramine: a placebo controlled double blind study. Am J Psychiatry 140:554–558, 1983

Pope HG, Keck PE, McElroy S, et al: A placebo controlled study of trazodone in bulimia nervosa. J Clin Psychopharmacol 9:254–259, 1989

Steinhausen HC, Glanville K: Follow-up studies of anorexia nervosa: review of research findings. Psychol Med 13:239–249, 1983

Yates WR, Sieleni B, Reich J, et al: Comorbidity of bulimia nervosa and personality disorder. J Clin Psychiatry 50:57–59, 1989

Self-assessment Questions

1. How do bulimia nervosa and anorexia nervosa differ? How do they overlap?
2. What are the sociodemographic characteristics of eating disorder patients?
3. What are some of the theories about the cause of anorexia nervosa?
4. What are typical clinical findings in anorexia and bulimia?
5. What potential medical complications may result from anorexia nervosa? from bulimia nervosa?
6. What are the major goals in the treatment of eating disorders?

Chapter 19
Adjustment Disorders

. . . whether 'tis nobler in the mind to suffer the slings and arrows of outrageous fortune or to take arms against a sea of troubles, and, by opposing, end them.

William Shakespeare, Hamlet

Stress is a common problem that each of us has to deal with on a regular basis. Whether one is a homemaker caring for small children or a bank president, stressful situations arise nearly daily. The homemaker may need to calm a colicky child and clean up a mess her other child has created in the kitchen. The bank president may have to reprimand an errant employee, and handle the consequences of his wife learning about his surreptitious affair with his secretary. In these examples, both the people involved and the circumstances differ tremendously, but serve to illustrate the universality of stressful events.

Most of us learn to handle everyday stressful situations. Some persons, however, do not learn and develop symptoms of emotional distress, such as depression, anxiety, or impaired work ability. These symptoms may be of sufficient severity to require brief periods of psychiatric care, usually on an outpatient basis. Persons with these problems often represent the "walking wounded"—the wife of an abusive alcoholic, the person rejected by a lover or spouse, the teenager failing in school, etc.

The term *adjustment disorder* was introduced in DSM-III to describe conditions in which a person develops psychological symptoms in reaction to stressful events, such as the situations noted above. The concept of adjustment disorders had been included in DSM-I under "transient situational personality disorders" and in DSM-II under "transient situational disturbances." These categories were used to describe

Table 19-1.   DSM-III-R criteria for adjustment disorder

A. A reaction to an identifiable psychosocial stressor (or multiple stressors) that occurs within 3 months of onset of the stressor(s).

B. The maladaptive nature of the reaction is indicated by either of the following:
1. Impairment in occupational (including school) functioning or in usual social activities or relationships with others
2. Symptoms that are in excess of a normal and expectable reaction to the stressor(s)

C. The disturbance is not merely one instance of a pattern of overreaction to stress or an exacerbation of one of the mental disorders previously described.

D. The maladaptive reaction has persisted for no longer than 6 months.

E. The disturbance does not meet the criteria for any specific mental disorder and does not represent uncomplicated bereavement.

superficial maladjustment to difficult situations or to newly experienced environmental factors in the absence of serious underlying personality defects. These disorders could be of any severity, including those of psychotic proportions.

In DSM-III, specific criteria for adjustment disorders were enumerated. The maladaptive reaction had to occur within 3 months of the psychosocial stressor, the diagnosis could be made in addition to another mental disorder but could not be part of a characterologic pattern, and the disturbance could not be an exacerbation of an existing mental disorder, such as major depression. DSM-III also prohibited psychotic disturbances from being categorized as adjustment disorders.

In DSM-III-R, the definition has remained the same, except that it is now specified that a maladaptive reaction cannot persist longer than 6 months (Table 19-1).

There are eight classifications of adjustment disorder, depending on the predominant symptoms that develop in response to the stressor, such as depressed mood, anxious mood, or disturbance of conduct (Table 19-2). A residual category, adjustment disorder not otherwise specified, exists for reactions that do not fit into any specific category, for example, a patient responding to a new diagnosis of acquired immunodeficiency syndrome (AIDS) with denial and noncompliance with the treatment regimen. A case example illustrating adjustment disorder follows.

Carol, a 34-year-old housewife, was admitted to the hospital after a tricyclic antidepressant overdose. According to Carol, she had felt well until earlier that day when she learned that she had lost a battle for custody of her 13-year-old daughter to her ex-husband. After the ruling, Carol became upset, anxious, sad, and tearful. That evening, feeling desperate, Carol gulped a handful of nortriptyline tablets that she had in her medicine chest, which had been prescribed months earlier for migraine. When her current husband returned home from work, she told him what she had done. He called an ambulance, which brought her to the hospital emergency room where she underwent charcoal lavage. She had no history suggesting emotional instability.

As the story unfolded, Carol explained that her current husband had been accused of fondling her daughter, an allegation that had been reported to local social service agencies, bringing about her daughter's placement in foster care. Although Carol denied

Table 19-2.   Types of adjustment disorder

Adjustment disorder with depressed mood
Adjustment disorder with anxious mood
Adjustment disorder with mixed emotional features
Adjustment disorder with disturbance of conduct
Adjustment disorder with mixed disturbance of emotions and conduct
Adjustment disorder with work (or academic) inhibition
Adjustment disorder with withdrawal
Adjustment disorder with physical complaints
Adjustment disorder not otherwise specified

that her husband had ever touched her daughter inappropriately, she conceded that such an allegation was serious and would be taken into account by a judge in determining custody. The crisis having passed, the patient reported that she was no longer depressed nor suicidal and that she would now be in an appropriate frame of mind to work with her lawyer in an attempt to regain custody of her child.

Epidemiology

Because the definition of adjustment disorder keeps changing, and due to the loose nature with which the diagnosis is applied, it is difficult to know how widespread it is, or in whom it occurs. It is likely that adjustment disorders are common, and according to one report, nearly 5% of psychiatric patients in Monroe County, New York, in 1971 had a diagnosis of adjustment reaction of adult life. Another report found that 5% of patients on an inpatient service had the diagnosis of adjustment disorder. It is likely that the percentage of psychiatric outpatients receiving this diagnosis may be closer to 10%. On consultation services at general hospitals, the frequency of this diagnosis approaches 20%.

The diagnosis is probably more common in women, singles, and young persons. Among adolescents, common symptoms seen are of the behavioral or acting-out type, whereas adults typically manifest mood or anxiety symptoms.

Etiology

According to DSM-III-R, adjustment disorders must occur in reaction to identifiable psychosocial stressors. As a result of this definition, adjustment disorder is one of the few diagnoses in which a cause-and-effect relationship is presumed. Clearly, most persons who experience psychosocial stressors do not develop psychiatric symptoms, a finding that suggests that individuals who develop an adjustment disorder may have an underlying vulnerability.

The question of why certain stressors produce illness in some persons and not in others was of interest to Freud, who believed that unpleasant childhood experiences led to fixation at certain stages of development that could trigger a regression when sufficient stress was applied. To draw an analogy, if enough pressure is applied

Table 19-3. Types of precipitants occurring in adjustment disorder

Adolescents		Adults	
Stressor	**%**	**Stressor**	**%**
School problems	60	Marital problems	25
Parental rejection	27	Separation or divorce	23
Alcohol and/or drug problems	26	Move	17
Parental separation or divorce	25	Financial problems	14
Girlfriend/boyfriend problems	20	School problems	14
Marital problems in parents	18	Work problems	9
Move	16	Alcohol and/or drug problems	8
Legal problem	12	Illness	6
Work problem	8	Legal problems	6
Other	60.2	Other	81.3

Source. Adapted from Andreasen NC, Wasek P: Adjustment disorders in adolescents and adults. Arch Gen Psychiatry 37:1166–1170, 1980.

to a bone, it will fracture, but depending on age, sex, and physical well-being, the amount of pressure will differ from person to person. So it is with adjustment disorders: each person will have his or her own "breaking point," depending on the amount of stress applied, underlying constitution, personality structure, and temperament. DSM-III suggested that underlying personality disorders or organic mental disorders may increase a person's vulnerability to developing an adjustment disorder, but DSM-III-R makes no such statement.

Clinical Findings

Adjustment disorder patients are typically in their 20s, but these disorders may occur at any age. Different subtypes of adjustment disorder reflect the varied symptoms that can occur, which typically include *depressed mood,* manifested by dysphoria, tearfulness, and hopelessness; *anxious mood,* manifested by psychic anxiety, palpitations, jitteriness, or hyperventilation; *mixed emotional features,* such as a combination of depression and anxiety or other emotions; *disturbance of conduct,* in which rights of others are violated or age-appropriate societal norms and rules are disregarded, such as vandalism, reckless driving, or fighting; *mixed disturbance of emotions and conduct,* manifested by emotional symptoms such as depression or anxiety, in addition to a disturbance of conduct such as truancy or vandalism; *work disturbance* (or academic inhibition), manifested by difficulty functioning on the job or in school; *withdrawal,* manifested by socially withdrawn behavior that is not typical for the person; or *physical complaints,* manifested by somatic symptoms such as low-back pain or fatigue.

In one study of adjustment disorders, the frequency of various stressors considered to have provoked patients' symptoms was determined (Table 19-3). Few of the listed stressors can be considered "overwhelming," and in many cases, the stressors were multiple, recurrent, or continuous. Among adolescents, school problems were the most common stressor. Parental rejection, alcohol and drug problems, and parental separation or divorce were also quite common. Among adults, the most common stressors were marital problems, separation or divorce, moving, and financial problems. Many of the stressors were chronic. For example, among the adolescents, nearly 60% of the stressors had been present for a year or more, and only 9% had been present for 3 months or less. Among adults, stressors showed more variation, but 36% had been present for a year or more and nearly 40% for 3 months or less.

Course and Outcome

By definition, adjustment disorders persist no longer than 6 months. Presumably, if a disturbance lasts longer, it would probably meet criteria for another disorder, such as generalized anxiety disorder, major depression, or dysthymia. DSM-III specified that the disorder eventually remits after the stressor ceases, or, if the stressor persists, when a new level of adaptation is achieved. This statement is not included in DSM-III-R.

In a 5-year follow-up of 100 patients given this diagnosis, 79% of adults were well at follow-up, with 8% having had an intervening problem. The rest (21%) had a current mental illness (e.g., schizoaffective disorder, major depression, alcoholism). Comparable figures for the adolescents were 57% well at follow-up, with 13% having had an intervening problem. An additional 43% had a current mental illness (e.g., schizophrenia, major depression, schizoaffective disorder, bipolar disorder, antisocial personality, alcoholism, drug abuse). Two adults and one adolescent had committed suicide. These findings suggest that in adults, adjustment disorders have relatively homogeneous good outcome, but that the disorder is less valid among adolescents. Because the diagnosis of adjustment disorder is relatively nonpejorative, some clinicians consider it particularly useful for younger patients, as it avoids stereotyping patients with a harsher, more severe diagnosis and avoids leading to self-fulfilling prophecies.

In another follow-up study, adjustment disorders were associated with increased risk of suicide, perhaps reflecting the tendency of some persons to become severely dysphoric, or to develop frank major depression.

Differential Diagnosis

With the variety of symptoms possible in adjustment disorders, their differential diagnosis is necessarily broad, including mood disorders such as major depression, anxiety disorders such as panic disorder or generalized anxiety disorder, or conduct disorders in the child or adolescent. Personality disorders should also be considered, as they are frequently associated with mood instability and behavior problems. The personality disorder patient typically reacts in maladaptive ways to stressors; therefore, an additional diagnosis of adjustment disorder cannot be justified, unless the new reaction differs from the patient's usual pattern of maladaptation. Schizophrenic disorders are often heralded by the development of social withdrawal, work or academic inhibition, or dysphoria and need to be differentiated from adjustment disorders. Other DSM-III-R disorders that are believed to occur in reaction to a stressor must also be considered, including brief reactive psychosis, in which a person develops psychotic symptoms in response to a stressor, and posttraumatic stress disorder, which develops after a traumatic event that is judged to be outside the range of usual human experience (e.g., war).

The patient being evaluated for an adjustment disorder needs to have a thorough physical examination and mental status examination to rule out alternative diagnoses.

Clinical Management

The treatment of adjustment disorders has not been systematically evaluated. However, individual psychotherapy that gives the patient an opportunity to review the meaning and significance of the psychosocial stressor is often helpful in assisting the patient to adapt to the stressor if it is ongoing, or understand the stressor if it has passed. Group approaches can be useful in patients who have experienced similar stressors, such as patients who have been diagnosed with AIDS. In group situations, the supportive atmosphere provided by persons who have experienced or are experiencing the same stressor can be enormously helpful in assisting the individual to adapt.

Pharmacologic interventions may be helpful, particularly when somatic symptoms, such as insomnia, are prominent. A patient with an adjustment disorder with depressed mood and exhibiting initial insomnia may benefit from a hypnotic (e.g., flurazepam 15–30 mg) at bedtime for a few days. A patient experiencing an anxious mood may benefit from a brief course (e.g., days to weeks) of diazepam (e.g., 5 mg three times a day). If the disorder persists, it is worthwhile to review the diagnosis. At some point, an adjustment disorder with depressed mood, for example, may develop into a major depressive disorder, which would best respond to antidepressant medication.

Recommendations for management of adjustment disorders

1. Adjustment disorders frequently evolve into other better defined disorders, such as major depression.
   - Be alert to changes in mental status and in symptoms.

2. A true adjustment disorder is transient. Tincture of time and simple supportive psychotherapy may be all that is necessary.

3. Patients with common psychosocial stressors (e.g., a diagnosis of cancer or AIDS, chronic back pain, or breakup of a relationship) often benefit from attending support groups with others who have also experienced the same stressor.

4. Benzodiazepines are short-term solutions only and should be prescribed with the idea of making the patient more comfortable.
   - If long-term therapy is needed, the patient probably has something else (e.g., generalized anxiety disorder).

Bibliography

Andreasen NC, Hoenk PR: The predictive value of adjustment disorders: a follow-up study. Am J Psychiatry 139:584–590, 1982

Andreasen NC, Wasek P: Adjustment disorders in adolescents and adults. Arch Gen Psychiatry 37:1166–1170, 1980

Black DW, Warrack G, Winokur G: The Iowa Record-Linkage Study, III: excess mortality among patients with 'functional' disorders. Arch Gen Psychiatry 42:82–88, 1985

Chess S, Thomas A: Origins in Evolution of Behavior Disorders. New York, Brunner/Mazel, 1984

Fabrega H, Mezzich JE, Mezzich AC: Adjustment disorder as a marginal or transitional illness category in DSM-III. Arch Gen Psychiatry 44:567–572, 1987

Looney JG, Gunderson EKE: Transient situational disturbances: course and outcome. Am J Psychiatry 135:660–663, 1978

Self-assessment Questions

1. What was the evolution of the adjustment disorder diagnosis from DSM-I to DSM-III-R?
2. How common are adjustment disorders, and what are their typical precipitants and manifestations?
3. What is the differential diagnosis for adjustment disorders?
4. How do the precipitants differ between adolescents and adults?
5. What is the treatment for adjustment disorders?

Section III
Special Topics

Chapter 20
Suicide

The thought of suicide is a great consolation; by means of it one gets successfully through many a bad night.

Friedrich Nietzsche

Suicide, or self-inflicted death that is intentional rather than accidental, remains a serious public health problem that is the eighth leading cause of death for adults and the second leading cause of death for persons between ages 15 and 24 in the United States. Nearly 30,000 suicides occur annually, or about 12.5 suicides per 100,000 of the U.S. population. The effects of a suicide are devastating; the death affects not only surviving friends and family members, but also the victim's physician, because most people who commit suicide communicate their suicidal intentions to, and see, physicians in the period before they die. Thus, suicide is a problem with which clinicians must familiarize themselves. They must be prepared to educate patients and family members about risk for suicide, to assess risk for suicide in their patients, and to act appropriately to intervene with suicide plans in order to prevent suicides.

Suicide is a complex human behavior with biological, sociological, and psychological roots. It is not a behavior that lends itself readily to simple formulations, such as one that appeared recently in a local newspaper that reported the unfortunate suicide of a middle-aged executive fired from his post as vice-president of a Fortune 500 firm. He committed suicide several years after the firing, while heavily involved in an expensive lawsuit contesting the job loss. The article implied that the fired executive killed himself because of the job loss and that the company was responsible. Clearly, the job loss may have played a role in the man's suicide,

393

but little mention was made of other factors, including a lengthy history of recurrent depression, chronic alcoholism, and an unstable marriage—factors that were later disclosed. The job loss may have been the straw that broke the camel's back, but most people who are fired from jobs do not kill themselves; other factors must have also played an important role in the suicide.

Epidemiology

Nearly 1% of the general population of the United States will die as a result of suicide. Suicide rates are specific for age, sex, and race. For example, in the United States, rates for men increase steadily with age and peak after age 75 years; rates for women are curvilinear and peak in the 40s. Nearly three times as many men take their lives as do women, and blacks are less likely than whites to commit suicide. An alarming trend in suicide rates has been the dramatic rise in the rate among young men and women. It is possible that increasing rates of drug abuse or the "cohort effect" (discussed later in the chapter) may account for some of this rise, but the reason for much of the increase remains a mystery.

Suicide rates differ geographically as well. Within the United States, rates are highest in the West and lowest in the middle Atlantic states. Among European countries, rates are highest in Hungary, where the rate hovers around 40 suicides per 100,000 of the population. Rates tend to be low in Mediterranean countries, particularly those with large Catholic populations. For religious reasons, Catholics are much less likely than Protestants to commit suicide.

Suicide rates tend to peak during the spring and fall and are evenly distributed throughout the week, unlike homicides, which tend to peak on Friday evenings. Rates tend to be high in times of economic depression, such as the Great Depression of the 1930s, and low in times of war. Among occupations, professionals are associated with the greatest risk for suicide. Physicians especially are at high risk, and, in contrast to suicide statistics in general, female physicians are at higher risk than male physicians. Married persons are less likely to commit suicide than single, widowed, or divorced persons. It is not clear whether social class affects suicide rates, but some studies suggest that rates are highest in both the highest and lowest social classes.

Etiology

Nearly all persons who commit suicide have a diagnosable mental illness at the time of death, a fact repeatedly confirmed in study after study. The largest diagnostic group among suicide completers is depression (50%), followed by alcoholism (30%), and the remainder of the diagnoses are split among schizophrenia, anxiety disorders, drug dependence, and other conditions. About 5% of suicide completers have serious physical illnesses at the time of suicide that may have contributed to the death; suicide rates are high in people suffering from brain trauma, epilepsy, multiple

Table 20-1. Risk of suicide among nine diagnostic groups

Diagnosis	Standardized mortality ratio[a]
Organic mental disorders	2.4
Schizophrenia	37.8
Schizoaffective disorder, schizophreniform disorder	33.3
Mood disorders	28.2
Neurotic disorders (e.g., anxiety, somatoform, dissociative disorders)	29.4
Depressive neurosis (dysthymic disorder)	31.3
Personality disorders	13.0
Alcohol/drug abuse/dependence	18.8
Adjustment disorders	14.3

Source. Adapted from Black DW, Warrack G, Winokur G: The Iowa Record-Linkage Study, I: suicide and accidental death among psychiatric patients. Arch Gen Psychiatry 42:71–75, 1985.
[a] Ratio of observed to expected suicides based on comparisons with the general population. All are significantly greater than expectation except ratio for organic mental disorders. For example, a patient with schizophrenia is 37.8 times more likely to commit suicide than a member of the general population matched for age and sex.

sclerosis, Huntington's chorea, Parkinson's disease, acquired immunodeficiency syndrome (AIDS), and cancer. A study from New York showed that the suicide rate in patients with AIDS is nearly 60 times that of the general population.

In about 5% of suicides, there is no evidence of mental or physical illness. Many have argued that these suicides are "rational," i.e., based on a logical appraisal of the need for death; for example, a very elderly man recently widowed, who feels it is time to die. It is likely that most of these apparently rational suicides are actually irrational, but information was simply unavailable to confirm the presence of a mental illness because the person who died was socially isolated and informants could not be interviewed. It still may be argued that many suicides are logical, and many philosophers, such as Nietzsche, have argued passionately on its behalf. Of the 900 suicides in Jonestown, Guyana, for example, it is unlikely that all were mentally ill. Many probably committed suicide for reasons that had to do with their religious beliefs, not mental illness.

Mental illness clearly predisposes to suicide, and individual disorders are associated with high rates of suicide. Nearly 15% of persons with mood disorders will commit suicide, as will 2–4% of chronic alcoholic patients and 10% of schizophrenic patients. A few psychiatric disorders, such as obsessive-compulsive disorder, are not associated with increased rates of suicide. Table 20-1 presents a comparison of nine diagnostic categories and their relative risk for suicide posthospitalization compared with rates in the general population (i.e., standardized mortality ratio). Clearly, among psychiatric patients, the risk for suicide is much higher than in the general population. Psychiatric and/or medical illnesses are usually necessary for suicide to occur, but are not sufficient, since most mentally ill persons do not commit suicide.

Suicide tends to be familial. Large kindreds, such as the Old Order Amish in Pennsylvania, show that suicide tends to cluster in certain families and is multigenerational. In these large pedigrees, suicides tend to occur in families rife with unipolar and bipolar affective disorders. Twin studies have demonstrated higher concordance for suicide among monozygotic twins compared with dizygotic twins, suggesting that suicide may be genetic, as well as familial, at least to some degree. Further, the Danish Adoption Study was able to demonstrate high prevalence of suicide among biological relatives of probands who had killed themselves.

Methods of Suicide

Firearms are the most popular method for committing suicide, followed by poisoning, hanging, and other methods. Men are more likely to use violent means such as firearms or hanging, which may explain why men are more successful than women in killing themselves. Women prefer less violent means such as poisoning by overdose, although women are beginning to choose more lethal methods.

Biology of Suicide

Suicide may be biologically mediated, at least to some extent. High levels of cerebrospinal fluid 5-hydroxyindoleacetic acid (5-HIAA) have been found in suicide completers, as has decreased imipramine binding in postmortem frontal cortex tissue samples. Follow-up studies have also shown that many suicide completers have had abnormal dexamethasone suppression tests, suggestive of hypothalamic-pituitary-adrenal axis hyperactivity. Suicide completers have also been found to have high levels of urinary metabolites of cortisol and to have enlarged adrenal glands. All of these measures are abnormal in severe depression; they may indicate depression rather than risk of suicide.

Clinical Findings

Suicide is an act of desperation. Suicidal persons frequently convey their discontent to others, and nearly two-thirds communicate their suicidal intentions to others. Depression is the most common psychiatric diagnosis leading to suicide, and suicide may occur during all phases of a depressive episode. A common belief is that suicide risk is highest in a depressed patient who is recovering and has regained sufficient energy to kill himself or herself. Actually, the suicidal urge waxes and wanes during the course of a depressive episode. One of the strongest correlates of suicidal behavior is hopelessness, a finding independent of psychiatric diagnosis.

Suicide completers tend to be socially isolated. Approximately 30% have a history of suicide attempts, but only one in six leaves a suicide note. Many who plan a suicide will prepare wills, give away possessions, and purchase burial plots; therefore, clinicians should be alert to these behaviors. Nearly 40% of suicide completers have alcohol in their bloodstream at the time of death, suggesting that alcohol may have disinhibited them enough to give them the courage to complete the suicide, and almost 90% of alcoholic persons have alcohol in their bloodstream at the time of death. A patient remains at high risk for suicide in the posthospitalization period. Although depressed patients may appear to be significantly improved at the time of hospital discharge, a person may relapse quickly and enter another episode of depression. Recently discharged patients need close follow-up.

Events that appear to trigger suicide differ by age and diagnostic group. Triggering events in adolescents or young adults often include relationship problems, whereas in older persons the event may be financial or health related. Among alcoholic persons who commit suicide, more than 50% have a history of interpersonal loss (usually of a sexual partner) within the year before suicide. This is not the case among depressed persons.

Youth Suicide

Suicide rates have been increasing in both males and females between ages 15 and 24 years. In fact, studies have shown that recent cohorts (i.e., groups of persons in the population with similar characteristics, such as being born in the same decade) have higher suicide rates than older cohorts. It is difficult to determine why rates should be increasing in this age-group, but other data seem to show that the prevalence of depression is increasing in each successive cohort as well. Drug abuse has become a serious problem for society at large, and for young persons in particular. This problem may be leading to higher rates of suicide. Studies of youthful suicide completers have shown that suicide is more frequently associated with drug and alcohol abuse than in adults, but is also associated with depression and behavior problems.

Teenagers are more prone to the effects of peer pressure than adults, and this may be reflected in suicide "clusters." It has been suggested that media depictions of suicide, such as televised movies that create sympathetic portrayals of suicide victims, tend to be followed by an increased rate in both suicide attempts and completed suicides.

Suicide Attempts

Suicide attempts are intentional acts of self-injury that do not result in death. They are easily 5–20 times more frequent than completed suicides, perhaps more so because most suicide attempts are not reported to authorities. Two-thirds of suicide attempters are female, unlike suicide completers, who are more commonly male. Suicide completers may be any age, but attempters are usually younger than age 35 years. Whereas suicide completers suffer predominantly from depression or alcoholism, suicide attempters suffer from depression (one-third), alcoholism (one-third), and other disturbances including somatization disorder and antisocial personality, which are relatively uncommon among suicide completers. In fact, up to 40% or more of attempters have personality disorders. Attempters generally use

Table 20-2.   Differences between suicide completers and attempters

Variable	Completers	Attempters
Sex	Male	Female
Age	Older	Younger
Diagnosis	Depression, alcoholism, schizophrenia	Depression, alcoholism, personality disorder
Planning	Careful	Impulsive
Lethality	High (e.g., firearms)	Low (e.g., poisoning)
Availability of help	Low	High

ineffective means (80% of attempts are from overdoses), and the attempts tend to be impulsive rather than planned and are typically designed to fail. Differences between suicide attempters and completers are summarized in Table 20-2.

The typical picture of a suicide attempter is that of an angry young woman just rejected by her boyfriend, who rushes to the bathroom, grabs a bottle of pills out of the medicine cabinet, and gulps the pills in the presence of her boyfriend. With great fanfare, she is taken to the emergency room where her stomach is lavaged. Suicide attempts are often emotionally cathartic, so that the patient may feel a sense of relief afterward. The suicide attempter usually regrets having done such a "stupid" thing. Some attempters will admit that the attempt was an effort to gain attention, or to hurt a loved one, or to win back a former lover.

Research has shown that the more serious the attempt, the more closely the suicide attempter resembles the suicide completer in terms of risk factors. Suicide attempters remain at risk for future attempts, and 1–2% will die annually after the attempt. Ultimately, 10% of attempters will complete suicide.

Prevention of Suicide

To prevent something, we must know what causes it. Because we do not know what causes suicide, it is only through an awareness of its risk factors that we can hope to have any impact on altering suicide rates. Demographic, social, and clinical risk factors associated with suicide are presented in Table 20-3. Even though these

Table 20-3.   Risk factors for suicide

- Being a psychiatric patient
- Being male, although the gender distinction is less important among psychiatric patients than among the general population
- Age: risk increases as men age, but peaks in the middle years for women
- Race: whites are at higher risk than nonwhites
- Psychiatric diagnosis: depression, alcoholism, schizophrenia
- History of prior suicide attempts
- Recent interpersonal loss (among alcoholic patients)
- Feelings of hopelessness and low self-esteem
- Timing: early in the posthospital discharge period
- Adolescents: a history of drug abuse, behavior problems, or depression

risk factors are well established, researchers have been unable to create statistical models that are able to predict suicide in groups at risk (e.g., hospitalized patients) with any degree of accuracy.

The assessment of suicide risk includes a thorough psychiatric history, family history, and mental status examination. The clinician must be alert to the possibility of suicide in any psychiatric patient, especially those who are depressed or have a depressed affect. In these patients, the assessment will focus on vegetative signs and cognitive symptoms of depression, death wishes, suicidal ideation, and suicide plans. Most suicidal patients are willing to discuss their thoughts with a physician if asked, but only one in six clinicians asks his or her patients about suicide. An unfortunate myth is that asking a patient about suicide will give the patient ideas that he or she has not already had. A physician *must* ask about suicide. Suicidal thoughts are common in depression. Patients are often fearful or feel guilty about having these thoughts so giving the patient an opportunity to discuss suicidal thoughts may in fact provide some relief. Specific questions that should be asked of the patient include

1. Are you having any thoughts about harming yourself?
2. Are you having any thoughts about taking your life?
3. Have you developed a plan for committing suicide? What is your plan?

The physician should also assess the patient's history of suicidality:

1. Have you ever had thoughts of killing yourself?
2. Have your ever attempted suicide? Could you tell me about the attempt?

The issue of suicide should be approached in a slow and deliberate manner, after having developed some rapport and trust with the patient. Because suicidal thoughts may fluctuate, physicians must reassess suicide risk with each patient contact. Patients who have developed well-thought-out plans and have the means to carry them out require surveillance, usually in a hospital on a locked psychiatric unit. It may be necessary to obtain a court order for hospitalization if the suicidal patient refuses voluntary hospitalization. Although a suicidal patient may plead with the doctor, family, or friends not to enter the hospital, it is not fair to entrust the patient's loved ones with the responsibility of protecting the patient. Most people are not sufficiently prepared or educated to handle a suicidal person.

Once the suicidal patient is hospitalized, the nursing staff will need to make sure that all sharp objects, belts, and other potentially lethal items are taken from the patient and that those patients at risk for elopement are carefully watched. Occasionally, patients will need seclusion. The physician will need to document the case carefully in the chart, noting signs and symptoms of depression and risk of suicide, protective measures taken, and treatment interventions.

Once the safety of the patient has been ensured, the task of treating the underlying illness can begin. Treatment will depend on the diagnosis. Antidepressant medication or electroconvulsive therapy (ECT) will be helpful in the treatment of depressed patients, although lithium carbonate and antipsychotics will be appropriate additions to the treatment of bipolar and psychotically depressed patients, respectively. Antipsychotics will be helpful in the suicidal schizophrenic patient. ECT is often specifically recommended for treatment of the suicidal depressed patient because it tends to have a quicker onset of action than antidepressant medication.

If the patient is treated on an outpatient basis, close follow-up is absolutely essential, including frequent physician visits for assessment of depression and suicide risk, for psychotherapeutic support, and for frequent prescriptions of medication to avoid the problem of having large amounts of pills on hand. Family members can be helpful in monitoring the medication. Family members should be told to remove all firearms from the home.

Recommendations for management of the suicidal patient

1. Always ask depressed patients about suicidal thoughts and plans. You will not plant ideas that were not there merely by asking.

- Reassess risk of suicide at every visit with depressed patients.

2. Hospitalize suicidal patients, even if it means hospitalizing them against their will. Patients who do not have suicidal plans and have supportive families who can monitor them can probably be managed at home.

3. In the hospital, *write* suicide precautions in the doctors' orders, or one-on-one protection if needed. Document signs and/or symptoms carefully.

4. In the outpatient, monitor suicide risk frequently, write frequent small prescriptions, and consider using a newer antidepressant that has a higher therapeutic index (e.g., fluoxetine, bupropion).

- Have the family remove all firearms from the home.

5. Remember that even though the risk factors are known, it is not possible to predict who will commit suicide.

- Simply use good clinical judgment, provide close follow-up, and prescribe effective treatments.

Bibliography

Barraclough B, Bunch J, Nelson B, et al: A hundred cases of suicide: clinical aspects. Br J Psychiatry 125:355–373, 1974

Beck AT, Steer RA, Kovacs M, et al: Hopelessness and eventual suicide. Am J Psychiatry 142:559–563, 1985

Black DW, Winokur G: Suicide and psychiatric diagnosis, in Suicide Over the Life Cycle. Edited by Blumenthal S, Kupfer D. Washington, DC, American Psychiatric Press, 1990, pp 135–153

Black DW, Warrack G, Winokur G: The Iowa Record-Linkage Study, I: suicide and accidental death among psychiatric patients. Arch Gen Psychiatry 42:71–75, 1985

Egeland JA, Sussex JN: Suicide and family loading for affective disorder. JAMA 254:915–918, 1985

Fawcett TJ, Scheftner W, Clark D, et al: Clinical predictors of suicide in patients with major affective disorders: a controlled prospective study. Am J Psychiatry 144:35–40, 1987

Goldstein R, Black DW, Winokur G, et al: The prediction of suicide: sensitivity, specificity, and predictive value of a multivariate model applied to suicide in 1,906 affectively ill patients. Arch Gen Psychiatry (in press)

Miles CP: Conditions predisposing to suicide: a review. J Nerv Ment Dis 164:231–246, 1977

Murphy GE, Wetzel RD: The lifetime risk of suicide and alcoholism. Arch Gen Psychiatry 47:383–392, 1990

Phillips DP, Carstonson LL: Clustering of teenage suicides after television news stories about suicide. N Engl J Med 55:685–689, 1986

Pokorny AD: Prediction of suicide in psychiatric patients. Arch Gen Psychiatry 40:249–257, 1983

Rich CL, Young D, Fowler RC: San Diego Suicide Study, I: young versus old subjects. Arch Gen Psychiatry 43:577–582, 1986

Robins E: The Final Months: A Study of 134 Persons Who Committed Suicide. New York, Oxford University Press, 1981

Robins E, Murphy GE, Wilkinson RH, et al: Some clinical considerations in the prevention of suicide based on a study of 134 successful suicides. Am J Public Health 49:888–899, 1959

Schmidtke A, Hafner H: The "Werther" effect after television films: new evidence for an old hypothesis. Psychol Med 18:665–676, 1988

Shafii M, Steltz-Lenarsky J, Derrick AM, et al: Comorbidity of mental disorders in the post-mortem diagnoses of completed suicide in children and adolescents. J Affective Disord 15:227–233, 1988

Stanley M, Mann JJ: Biologic factors associated with suicide, in American Psychiatric Press Review of Psychiatry, Vol 7. Edited by Francis AJ, Hales RE. Washington, DC, American Psychiatric Press, 1988, pp 344–352

Self-assessment Questions

1. Why is suicide a major health problem?
2. What are the common risk factors for suicide?
3. How do completed suicides differ from attempted suicides?
4. What is a "rational" suicide?
5. Are there different risk factors for suicide among youth?
6. How should the suicidal patient be managed in the hospital? as an outpatient?

Chapter 21

Acquired Immunodeficiency Syndrome (AIDS)

It is the responsibility of every citizen to be informed about AIDS and to exercise the appropriate preventive measures.

C. Everett Koop

One of the most fascinating (and alarming) stories in medicine during this century has been the development of the acquired immunodeficiency syndrome (AIDS). Although the syndrome was not recognized until the early 1980s, there is evidence that it may have existed in the United States for up to two decades before its recognition. From the physician's perspective, a unique aspect is that we have been able to watch a very serious new disease evolve over a short period. Because the disease is nearly always fatal and has such striking social and economic costs, it has gained far more attention that other relatively new epidemics, such as genital herpes. Although by the late 1980s, the incidence (i.e., new cases) appeared to have peaked, the prevalence continues to grow as new cases become evident. In 1989, it was estimated that in the United States, over 1.5 million persons had been infected with the virus and that over 60,000 had died of AIDS. By 1992, between 300,000 and 450,000 persons will have contracted AIDS. It is now the number one killer of men between ages 30 and 50 in New York City and is straining budgets everywhere, especially as treatments are allowing these patients to live longer.

Etiology and Pathophysiology

The disease is transmitted by a slow retrovirus referred to as *human immunodeficiency virus* (HIV). The virus specifically binds to receptors on the surface of cells of the human immune system. Once bound, the virus gains entry to the cell. HIV infects a number of human cells, but its hallmark is the progressive destruction of helper, or T_4, lymphocytes. Once inside the cell, the enzyme *reverse transcriptase* copies the viral RNA into DNA, which then inserts itself into the nuclear DNA of the human cell. HIV can remain latent for months or years after incorporation into the human cell genome. After a period of latency, the virus becomes active, makes copies of itself, and bursts out of the human cell, killing it and preparing to infect more cells.

As patients develop lower and lower T_4 counts, they become progressively more susceptible to acquiring opportunistic infections (e.g., *Pneumocystis carinii*, toxoplasmosis) or certain types of cancer (e.g., Kaposi's sarcoma). Besides devastating the immune system, HIV is a neurotropic virus. Early in the course of the infection, the virus enters the central nervous system (CNS), probably carried there by macrophages. In the CNS, HIV infects astrocytes and glial cells, causing a variety of psychiatric and neurologic complications.

The virus is transmitted from person to person through exchange of body fluids (e.g., semen, blood) and through intravenous use of contaminated syringes and needles. In the United States, homosexual men compose the largest risk group and make up 70–80% of reported cases. Intravenous-drug abusers account for the next largest group (10–20%). Heterosexuals infected through sexual intercourse, newborns infected via placental transmission, and recipients of HIV-contaminated blood transfusions, including persons with hemophilia, make up the rest of reported cases. The virus is not transmitted through the kinds of casual contact that people sharing a home engage in, such as touching, hugging, kissing, sharing the same dishes, etc.

The serum test used to detect HIV is known as the enzyme-linked immunosorbent assay (ELISA). If the result is positive, the serum is then subjected to the more accurate Western blot test, because false positives may occur with ELISA. Persons should not be notified of a positive result until the Western blot test has been performed. In some states, all positive results are reported to public health authorities.

Clinical Findings

Clinical manifestations of persons infected with HIV range widely. The initial stage of the infection is represented by HIV seropositivity, i.e., the detectable presence of antibodies to HIV in serum. Although the incubation period from exposure to HIV and development of seropositivity may range from months to years, many, if not most, patients who are seropositive will develop AIDS. The actual percentage is unknown, but appears to be increasing now that long-term follow-up studies are being conducted.

Persons who do not meet diagnostic criteria for AIDS, but test positive for HIV antibodies and exhibit some of the clinical symptoms of AIDS such as generalized lymphadenopathy, night sweats, or fever, are defined as having AIDS-related complex (ARC). About one-fourth to one-half of ARC patients develop AIDS within 3 years. Other ARC patients may continue to be symptomatic or may become symptom free. Although ARC patients and HIV-seropositive patients without symptoms do not have AIDS, they are infected with HIV and are carriers of the disease.

The diagnosis of AIDS is made when a person who is HIV positive develops an opportunistic infection such as *Pneumocystis carinii, Toxoplasma gondii,* or Kaposi's sarcoma (see Table 21-1 for the case definition of AIDS). The initial symptoms of AIDS generally include persistent generalized lymphadenopathy, shortness of breath and coughing, yeast infections, fatigue, recurrent diarrhea, and unexplained weight loss. In some patients, depression, cognitive impairment, or psychosis may antedate other symptoms. Pneumocystis carinii pneumonia, the most common disease in AIDS patients, is usually the initial diagnosis. Symptoms include the gradual onset of a nonproductive cough, low-grade fevers, and chest pain. Kaposi's sarcoma is diagnosed in about 40% of AIDS patients and is particularly virulent, leading to rapid spread and death, usually within 2 years. The stages of HIV infection are summarized in Table 21-2.

There are no effective treatments for the underlying immune disturbance of AIDS. Treatment of AIDS patients generally consists of efforts to treat opportunistic infections. Numerous drugs, including zidovudine (azidothymidine or AZT), are being studied for their ability to inhibit reverse transcriptase, which inhibits HIV replication, diminishing the total viral "load." AZT is currently approved for use in patients with AIDS and has been shown to improve longevity and quality of life and may delay progression from ARC to the full-blown disease. AZT has also been demonstrated to ameliorate cognitive impairment in some individuals.

Psychiatric Manifestations

Although early explanations of psychiatric morbidity among HIV-positive and AIDS patients emphasized the emotional repercussions of developing AIDS, the focus has now turned to primary CNS infection with HIV. In fact, about 10% of AIDS patients present with neurologic or psychiatric symptoms, and as the disease progresses, up to 60% of patients develop a neuropsychiatric syndrome. The most frequent CNS manifestation is the *AIDS dementia complex,* or AIDS encephalopathy. Typical symptoms include memory impairment, poor concentration, disorientation or confusion, social withdrawal, and psychomotor agitation. Depression and, in some instances, mood elevation, are also seen. Occasionally, patients develop psychosis, characterized by hallucinations and delusions. Psychiatric manifestations are listed in Table 21-3.

In the early stages of AIDS dementia, symptoms may be mild, and patients may be aware of diminishing mental functioning, particularly as they will have read

Table 21-1. Case definition of AIDS

A case of AIDS is defined as an illness characterized by one or more of the following "indicator" diseases, depending on the status of laboratory evidence of HIV infection, as shown below:

1. Without laboratory evidence regarding HIV infection (i.e., HIV tests inconclusive or not performed) and the patient has no other underlying cause of immunodeficiency (e.g., long-term corticosteroid therapy, certain cancers, congenital immunodeficiency syndrome).

   - Kaposi's sarcoma in patients younger than age 60 years
   - Primary lymphoma of the central nervous system in patients younger than age 60 years
   - Pneumocystis carinii pneumonia
   - Unusually extensive mucocutaneous herpes simplex infection
   - Cryptosporidium enterocolitis with diarrhea persisting more than 1 month
   - Extrapulmonary cryptococcosis
   - Candidiasis of the esophagus, trachea, bronchi, or lungs
   - Cytomegalovirus disease of an organ other than the liver, spleen, or lymph nodes in a patient older than age 1 month
   - Progressive multifocal leukoencephalopathy
   - Toxoplasmosis of the brain affecting a patient older than age 1 month
   - Lymphoid interstitial pneumonia and/or pulmonary lymphoid hyperplasia affecting a child younger than age 13
   - Mycobacterium avium complex or Mycobacterium kansasii disease, disseminated

2. With laboratory evidence for HIV infection, regardless of the presence of other causes of immunodeficiency and any disease listed above or below (2A or 2B) indicates a disease of AIDS.

   A. Indicator disease is diagnosed definitively:

      - Bacterial infections, multiple or recurrent pneumonia, affecting a child younger than age 13 years (e.g., septicemia, pneumonia, meningitis)
      - Coccidioidomycosis, disseminated
      - HIV encephalopathy
      - Histoplasmosis, disseminated
      - Isosporiasis with diarrhea persisting more than 1 month
      - Kaposi's sarcoma at any age
      - Primary lymphoma of the brain at any age
      - Other non-Hodgkin's lymphoma of B cell or unknown immunologic phenotype and involving certain histologic types
      - Any mycobacterial disease, disseminated
      - Disease caused by Mycobacterium tuberculosis, extrapulmonary
      - Salmonella septicemia, recurrent
      - HIV wasting syndrome (i.e., "slim disease")

   B. Indicator disease is diagnosed presumptively:

      - Candidiasis of the esophagus
      - Cytomegalovirus retinitis with loss of vision
      - Kaposi's sarcoma
      - Lymphoid interstitial pneumonia or pulmonary lymphoid hyperplasia affecting a child younger than age 13 years
      - Mycobacterial disease
      - Pneumocystis carinii pneumonia
      - Toxoplasmosis of the brain affecting a patient older than age 1 month

3. With laboratory evidence against HIV infection:

   A. Other causes of immunodeficiency are excluded; and

   B. The patient has had either:

      - Pneumocystis carinii pneumonia diagnosed by a definitive method; or
      - Any of the other diseases indicative of AIDS listed in Section 1 diagnosed by a definitive method; and a T helper/inducer lymphocyte count <400 mm^3

Source. From Centers for Disease Control: MMWR 36:45–65, 1987.

Table 21-2. Stages of HIV infection

Stage	Seropositivity	Clinical findings	Course
Initial exposure	Seropositivity develops after a variable latency period (months to years)	Usually none; a person may have experienced a mild viral syndrome (e.g., malaise, anorexia, nausea) shortly after exposure	May develop into ARC or AIDS; may remain asymptomatic
AIDS-related complex (ARC)	Present	No opportunistic infections or cancers, but may exhibit generalized lymphadenopathy, skin rashes, fatigue, night sweats, fever, weight loss, etc.	May progress to AIDS, may remit, or may fluctuate with periods of remission or exacerbations
AIDS	Present	Opportunistic infections develop (e.g., *Pneumocystis carinii*, toxoplasmosis, cryptococcus), cancers (e.g., Kaposi's sarcoma, non-Hodgkin's lymphoma), progressive multifocal leukoencephalopathy, HIV wasting syndrome, etc.	Almost uniformly fatal; some long-term survivors are reported, however

Table 21-3. Psychiatric manifestations of AIDS and AIDS-related complex

Dementia	Depression
Delirium	Adjustment disorders
Personality changes	Generalized anxiety
Psychosis	Hypochondriasis

about AIDS. Awareness of these symptoms may lead to depression, anxiety, and frustration. A patient may become angry about his or her inability to deal with simple matters, such as balancing a checkbook. As the dementia progresses, cognitive impairment becomes more pronounced; muteness, incontinence, seizures, and coma may occur, leading eventually to death.

Psychological aspects of AIDS extend to the "worried well," e.g., homosexual and bisexual men, or persons in other risk groups, who have not had symptoms of AIDS but who are at risk for the disease. Many of the "worried well" develop significant psychological distress, especially symptoms of anxiety or depression (e.g., dysphoria, panic attacks, free-floating anxiety, phobic symptoms, hypochondriasis). Because of their risk for illness, some persons develop excessive somatic preoccupation and fear of disease. Like the hypochondriac, these patients may misinterpret normal or new bodily sensations. Many tests are conducted without relief of their anxiety, and frequent reassurance is demanded from the doctor, who finds their preoccupation difficult to allay. Although some of these psychological reactions are probably normal given the situation, some persons do suffer sufficiently to disrupt their social and occupational functioning and can benefit from treatment.

The following case example illustrates some of the symptoms that may be seen in the HIV-seropositive patient.

Lynn, a 23-year-old man, was admitted to the hospital after trying to take his life with an overdose of diazepam. Lynn lived at home with his parents and, after taking the pills, told his mother, who brought him to the hospital. At the emergency room, he was alert but lethargic. His stomach was lavaged, and he was admitted to the psychiatric service for evaluation and treatment.

Lynn had grown up in a small midwestern farming community. He had been somewhat effeminate as a boy and was picked on by his peers, but otherwise developed normally, had friends, and behaved in school. Although he had always been attracted to other boys and had always felt that he was a homosexual, Lynn had "come out of the closet" only recently. Before "coming out," Lynn had hid his sexual orientation from his friends and family members and had even dated and gone steady with a girl. After "coming out," he tried to fit in with what he thought was a gay life-style, by dressing colorfully, wearing a single earring, and frequenting gay bars in nearby communities. He had had a series of one-night stands and short-lived affairs, and had had an assortment of sexual experiences with dozens of young men. Lynn eventually developed a stable monogamous relationship.

A year before his hospitalization, Lynn sought HIV testing and was found to be positive. His lover was also positive. Lynn felt devastated by this knowledge, became depressed, and felt hopeless about his future. To help deal with these feelings, Lynn had sought out individual counseling and saw a therapist on a regular basis. He also joined a local support group for persons with AIDS or AIDS-related illnesses. These measures seemed to help, but he was constantly reminded of what his future held as members of the support group would stop coming, and the group would later learn of that person's death. He also read widely about AIDS and had learned of its devastating effects on the mind and body. An attractive young man, Lynn had always worked out and felt physically fit. He didn't want to think of himself as deformed or debilitated.

On the night before admission, Lynn was feeling particularly sorry for himself and had been out partying with several of his friends. After returning home, he started to ruminate about his HIV seropositivity, how alone and isolated he felt, and the devastating complications that he faced in the future. He knew that his mother had been treated for "nervous" problems in the past and found a bottle containing diazepam that had been prescribed for her. Not knowing its effect, but knowing that it was a tranquilizer, he gulped the contents of the bottle thinking that it would kill him. Within a few minutes, he had a change of mind and informed his parents of what he had done, and he was brought to the hospital.

At the hospital, Lynn admitted to having poorly adjusted to his HIV seropositivity. Initially, he admitted that he had denied the result and, in fact, to "prove" that he was healthy, had engaged in several sexual escapades, which he now regretted, knowing that he placed these persons at risk for AIDS. He had also become overly concerned about physical symptoms and was constantly seeking reassurance from his doctors. He also became dysphoric and had spontaneous crying spells. Despite these psychological symptoms, he had not developed vegetative symptoms of depression, such as weight loss, anorexia, or fatigue. At the hospital, Lynn was diagnosed as having an adjustment disorder with depressed mood and within days had returned to his normal level of functioning.

Psychological reactions to having AIDS are similar to those reported in patients with terminal cancer. In both situations, patients may deny that they are ill and express disbelief in their diagnosis. Depression and anxiety, feelings of hopelessness and uncertainty, and suicidal ideation may occur as the disease progresses. Intense anger may be directed at the medical establishment because of its inability to provide a cure, and the government for not providing a more helpful response. Psychological issues such as uncertainty about the implication of an AIDS diagnosis, social isolation, abandonment by friends or lovers, and guilt over life-style may come up.

Psychiatric consultations are frequently sought for AIDS patients, usually for depression. Although suicidal ideation is common in AIDS patients, self-destructive behavior is generally found in patients who are clinically depressed or in those with a preexisting personality disorder, such as borderline personality. The suicide rate in AIDS patients is more than 60 times that expected, so the presence of suicidal ideation merits great attention.

Psychotic symptoms may occur as a result of CNS infection with HIV. In one study, 2 of 46 patients with AIDS-related dementia had presented with predominantly psychotic symptoms and an additional 5 developed prominent psychotic symptoms later in the course of the illness, for a combined prevalence of 15%. In these patients, the duration of psychosis ranged from several days to several months before presentation, and the most common symptom was either a persecutory, grandiose, or somatic delusion. Auditory hallucinations were also common, as were anxiety, agitation, formal thought disorder, mood disturbance, bizarre behavior, and cognitive impairment.

On initial neurological examination, nearly one-half of HIV-positive patients have minor motor disturbances such as hyperreflexia, increased tone, tremor, and mild ataxia. Cerebrospinal fluid tends to be normal except when cryptococcal meningitis is found to be the etiology of the psychosis (e.g., increased number of cells, positive India ink test). Computerized tomography (CT) or magnetic resonance imaging of the brain are normal in more than one-half of patients at the time of initial evaluation. The remainder have evidence of cortical atrophy. An abnormal electroencephalogram (EEG) consisting of predominantly diffuse cortical slowing has been reported in approximately 50% of the patients—the same patients who have atrophy on CT scan. Patients with an abnormal CT scan or EEG are noted to follow a more rapidly progressive downhill course.

Clinical Management

Monitoring of mental status and evaluating cognitive impairment is an important part of the overall management of AIDS patients, in view of the common psychiatric and CNS sequelae. Depressive symptoms and suicide risk need to be assessed at each visit. Many patients will benefit from supportive psychotherapy, where issues such as guilt associated with previous sexual practices or drug abuse, social isolation, and acknowledgment of illness along with associated fear or anger can be addressed. Stress management (e.g., relaxation training) and problem-solving techniques may also benefit these patients.

Patients who develop psychiatric syndromes can benefit from medication. Anxiolytics (e.g., benzodiazepines) may be helpful to patients with generalized anxiety or adjustment disorders, and antidepressants may be useful for patients with a major depression or panic disorder. Antipsychotics will be helpful in treating the patient who develops hallucinations or delusions. Electroconvulsive therapy may be useful in depressed or manic AIDS patients not responding to medication.

Patient management should also include educating the patient about AIDS, providing information about etiology and modes of transmission, and practical precautions regarding safe sex and safe needle use by drug abusers. Support groups organized by local AIDS outreach organizations can be especially helpful in buttressing social support. Public health agencies may need to help patients obtain financial and physical assistance.

Caring for the AIDS Patient

The problems of caring for the AIDS patient extend beyond the medical and psychiatric complications. Due to the nature of the illness and the life-style of the patient, caregivers may have a difficult time providing appropriate care. Health care workers may need to confront their own prejudices toward the high-risk groups in order to offer the highest standard of care. Many doctors believe that AIDS patients deserve their illness and are less deserving of sympathy than, for example, a cancer patient. These views should not be tolerated.

Group discussions among caregivers to ventilate their feelings and frustrations may be valuable. Caregivers may have difficulty caring for these patients because of the issues of treating young individuals with fatal illnesses. Caregivers must also understand modes of transmission and help to counsel patients on how to reduce their high-risk behaviors so as to minimize any future transmission of HIV.

Recommendations for management of AIDS patients

1. Acceptance and a nonjudgmental attitude are essential in the care of patients infected with HIV.

   - There is no excuse for blaming or belittling the patient for his or her predicament.
   - The caregiver needs to separate personal beliefs about the patient's life-style (e.g., attitudes toward homosexuality, drug abuse) from care of the patient.

2. Be alert to neuropsychiatric symptoms that can signal involvement of the central nervous system, including neurologic signs (e.g., tingling, numbness, weakness) and psychiatric symptoms (e.g., depression, mania, confusion).

3. AIDS patients need emotional support, especially since many will have lost their traditional supports after having revealed simultaneously their homosexuality (or drug addiction) and their development of a fatal and communicable illness.

   - Many patients need practical assistance in solving everyday problems. Many will need to be referred to social service agencies.
   - The therapist must also help the patient deal with issues of death and dying in a realistic and humane way.
   - Support groups are available in most communities for AIDS and AIDS-related complex patients, as well as for the "worried well."

4. Many patients will benefit from specific treatment for depression, anxiety, or psychosis (e.g., antidepressants, anxiolytics, antipsychotics).

5. Educate yourself, other staff members, and the patient about AIDS and its transmission.

   - Despite great publicity and major national educational efforts, some persons (including medical personnel) stubbornly cling to inaccurate beliefs (e.g., AIDS can be transmitted by casual contact).

Bibliography

Atkinson JH, Grant I, Kennedy CJ, et al: Prevalence of psychiatric disorders among men infected with human immunodeficiency virus. Arch Gen Psychiatry 45:859–864, 1988

Centers for Disease Control: MMWR 36:45–65, 1987

Curran JW, Morgan WM, Hardy AM: The epidemiology of AIDS: current status and future prospects. Science 229:1352–1357, 1985

Dilley JW, Ochitill HN, Pearl M, et al: Findings in psychiatric consultations with patients with acquired immune deficiency syndrome. Am J Psychiatry 142:82–86, 1985

Faulstich ME: Psychiatric aspects of AIDS. Am J Psychiatry 144:551–556, 1987

Navia BA, Choo ES, Petito CK: The AIDS dementia complex, II: neuropathology. Ann Neurol 19:525–535, 1986

Navia BA, Jordan BD, Price RW: The AIDS dementia complex, I: clinical features. Ann Neurol 19:517–524, 1986

Nichols SE, Ostrow DG (eds): Psychiatric Implications of Acquired Immune Deficiency Syndrome. Washington, DC, American Psychiatric Press, 1984

Ostrow DJ: Psychiatric consequences of AIDS: an overview. Int J Neurosci 32:669–676, 1987

Rabkin JG, Harrison WM: Effect of imipramine on depression and immune status in a sample of men with HIV infection. Am J Psychiatry 147:495–497, 1990

Schmitt FA, Bigley JW, McKinnis R, et al: Neuropsychological outcome of zidovudine (AZT) treatment of patients with AIDS and AIDS-related complex. N Engl J Med 319:1573–1578, 1988

Self-assessment Questions

1. What is HIV?
2. What are the diagnostic criteria for AIDS?
3. What neuropsychiatric symptoms have been reported in patients with AIDS?
4. What symptoms affect the "worried well"?
5. How does prejudice affect the caregiver?

Chapter 22

Disorders of Childhood and Adolescence

Children sweeten labors, but they make misfortunes more bitter. They increase the cares of life, but they mitigate the remembrance of death.

Francis Bacon

As any 17-year-old will testify, the distinction between childhood and adulthood is arbitrary, often ludicrous, and frequently fluctuating in response to the needs of someone invoking the distinction. Psychiatric nosology and classification are no exception to this rule. Many of the disorders described in other chapters (not classified among childhood disorders in DSM-III-R) occur rather frequently in children. Mood disorders and anxiety disorders are especially common. Schizophrenia often arises during adolescence and occasionally during childhood. In inner cities, "crack" is traded on the grade school playground. Children and adolescents display signs and symptoms of personality disorder. Indeed, the dementias may be the only "adult" disorder from which children are exempt.

Nevertheless, DSM-III-R nosology does set aside a group of disorders that are considered to be relatively specific to children and adolescents, in that they typically arise during that period of life, rather than simply occurring during childhood and adolescence. The overall summary of this group of disorders appears in Tables 22-1 (Axis I disorders) and 22-2 (Axis II disorders). In general, most of the disorders listed in these tables do indeed manifest their first symptoms before patients are

413

Table 22-1.   DSM-III-R Axis I disorders usually first evident in infancy, childhood, or adolescence

Disruptive behavior disorders

- Attention-deficit hyperactivity disorder
- Conduct disorder
- Oppositional defiant disorder

Anxiety disorders of childhood or adolescence

- Separation anxiety disorder
- Avoidant disorder of childhood or adolescence
- Overanxious disorder

Eating disorders

- Anorexia nervosa
- Bulimia nervosa
- Pica
- Rumination disorder of infancy
- Eating disorder not otherwise specified

Gender identity disorders

- Gender identity disorder of childhood
- Transsexualism
- Gender identity disorder of adolescence or adulthood, nontranssexual type
- Gender identity disorder not otherwise specified

Tic disorders

- Tourette's disorder
- Chronic motor or vocal tic disorder
- Transient tic disorder
- Tic disorder not otherwise specified

Elimination disorders

- Functional encopresis
- Functional enuresis

Speech disorders not elsewhere classified

- Cluttering
- Stuttering

Other disorders of infancy, childhood, or adolescence

- Elective mutism
- Identity disorder
- Reactive attachment disorder of infancy or early childhood
- Stereotypy/habit disorder
- Undifferentiated attention-deficit disorder

in their late teens or early 20s. Nearly all these disorders have a clear childhood onset, with the possible exception of some of the eating disorders.

The disorders listed in Tables 22-1 and 22-2 are both diverse and numerous. Some are not very common (e.g., elective mutism), some are discussed in other chapters (e.g., gender identity disorders in Chapter 17, and eating disorders in Chapter 18), and some are seen more frequently in pediatric clinics than in child

Table 22-2. DSM-III-R Axis II disorders usually first evident in infancy, childhood, or adolescence

Mental retardation

- Mild mental retardation
- Moderate mental retardation
- Severe mental retardation
- Profound mental retardation
- Unspecified mental retardation

Passive developmental disorders

- Autistic disorder
- Pervasive developmental disorder not otherwise specified

Specific developmental disorders

- Academic-skills disorders
  Developmental arithmetic disorder
  Developmental expressive writing disorder
  Developmental reading disorder
  Language and speech disorders
  Developmental articulation disorder
  Developmental expressive language disorder
  Developmental receptive language disorder
- Motor-skills disorder
  Developmental coordination disorder
- Specific developmental disorder not otherwise specified

Other developmental disorders

- Developmental disorder not otherwise specified

psychiatry clinics (e.g., encopresis and enuresis). To permit more complete coverage of the most important disorders, this chapter selectively reviews only some of those listed in Tables 22-1 and 22-2, those that are most frequently seen in child psychiatry clinics and inpatient units. These include the disruptive behavior disorders, anxiety disorders, Tourette's disorder, mental retardation, autism, and the academic-skills disorders.

As Tables 22-1 and 22-2 indicate, the disorders of childhood may be classified either on Axis I or Axis II of DSM-III-R. As in the remainder of DSM-III-R, the fundamental distinction between Axis I and Axis II is that the disorders listed on the latter axis not only generally begin in childhood, but also persist in stable form into adult life.

Special Aspects of the Assessment of Children

Although there are many continuities between adult and child psychiatry, there are also important differences in emphasis and approach, for example, in techniques of assessment, the importance of flexible "norms" or criteria, involvement of family or significant others, an increased role of nonphysicians in the health care team, and the frequent occurrence of comorbidity. These aspects of assessment must be kept in mind when attempting to evaluate the presence or absence of the various disorders listed in Tables 22-1 and 22-2.

Assessment of Children

"Childhood" disorders can be diagnosed in individuals ranging from infants through those in their late teens or early 20s. Obviously, standard approaches to interviewing and assessment (described in Chapter 3) will not apply well to infants, children, or young teenagers. Standard techniques for the psychiatric assessment of adults, which may be applicable to patients in their late teens and are applicable to patients in their early 20s, emphasize the use of questioning, self-report, and introspection. These approaches require verbal skills not yet achieved in the maturational process of children, the capacity to separate and step back from oneself to describe feelings and behavior, and the ability to form abstractions about cognition, behavior, and emotions. For example, young children may not be able to respond to questions about concepts such as depression, loneliness, or anger. The interviewer will often need to talk to children at a much more concrete level, asking questions such as

1. Do you feel like crying a lot?
2. What kinds of things make you feel like crying?
3. Do you ever want to hit people?
4. Who do you feel like hitting?
5. Who are your best friends?
6. How often do you see them?
7. What kinds of things do you do together?
8. Do they like you?

In addition to interviewing, playing games with children will often give the clinician some insight as to their ability to function interpersonally, to tolerate frustration, and to focus attention. Imaginative play, with dolls that can represent important figures in the child's life, may also give some sense as to feelings toward and relationships with others. Direct observation of activity level, motor skills, verbal expression, and vocabulary are also fundamental components of assessment.

Application of Norms and Criteria

In assessing children, the clinician must have a good sense of what is normal for a given child at a given age, as well as an awareness that "norms" may vary widely. Younger clinicians, who are completing medical school or a residency, usually have not had the experience of rearing their own children or of watching a large number of younger siblings develop. Thus, they must get their sense of "norms" from textbooks, from observing many children, or from recalling their own experiences in the process of growing up. The latter approach may be particularly helpful in the assessment of teenagers, although the average medical student or physician must recognize that he or she is likely to be much more "uptight," obsessional, and compliant with authority than the average child. Nevertheless, remembering one's own "growing pains" will often help to increase empathy with the frustrations and struggles that many adolescents are experiencing and seeking help with.

Having a sense of what is "normal" or "abnormal" for a given child, in a given family, and in a given social and intellectual environment can be extremely difficult. For example, a typical "normal" 10-year-old will have an IQ of 100, be able to read at a fourth-grade level, be able to perform addition and subtraction and some multiplication, and be able to throw, catch, and kick a ball with at least some accuracy. Some "normal" children will have an IQ of only 85, however, whereas others will have an IQ of 160. These children will clearly differ a great deal from one another in their school performance.

Boys and girls also have quite different levels of maturation both physically and mentally, and these differences are especially pronounced in younger children. Boys and girls also have different maturational tasks as they go through puberty and enter adolescence, and consequently, they will experience different stresses. Success and failure will also mean different things to an inner-city child than to a child from an affluent background.

Particularly in the area of child psychiatry, clinicians are likely to be asked over and over, "Is this child normal?" or "Is this behavior normal?" The clinician who experiences some doubt, ambiguity, and difficulty in answering these questions easily is definitely normal. Coming up with facile judgments about normality is probably an indication that the clinician has not been thinking hard enough or has too simple and authoritarian a notion of what constitutes normality. Extreme cases are simple, of course, but most are likely to be in the "murky middle."

Involvement of Family and Significant Others

Clinicians who work with children usually need to work with their families and significant others as well. The degree of family involvement will vary, of course, depending on the age of the child. In the case of very young children, the parents are likely to be the primary informants and probably will be important recipients of treatment as well, since they are likely to need both psychological support and assistance in learning behavior techniques to manage their child's behavior. For grade school children, involvement of family members remains essential, but the child becomes an increasingly important protagonist in both assessment and treatment. Teenagers, who are going through important maturational changes as they move into adulthood, are usually brought to the forefront of the assessment and treatment process, although the family will also provide resources much of the time.

Deciding about maintaining complete confidentiality, versus sharing information, becomes a crucial issue in the assessment of teenagers. In general, teenagers should be assured that the things they tell the clinician will end there, unless the teenager gives permission to share the information or can be encouraged to bring it out in a family or group setting. The assurance of confidentiality is important in establishing a bond of trust between teenager and clinician, because the patient otherwise is likely to see the therapist as a potentially antagonistic authority figure.

Although this advice may seem easy in principle, it in fact places a great burden of responsibility on the clinician, because he or she is likely to hear things that parents would want to know about and that he or she instinctively feels should be discussed with them, such as suicidal thinking, sexual experimentation, lying, cheating, or drug use. Only in situations dangerous to the child, such as a clear risk of suicide, should the rule of confidentiality be broken. This rule should be explained to the parents in a tactful manner so that they do not feel excluded. Depending on circumstances, the clinician may also choose to see the parents independently. Alternatively, the clinician may refer the parents to another psychiatrist, psychologist, or social worker with whom he or she has a good working relationship. If the parents are referred elsewhere, maintaining some liaison in the continuing assessment and treatment process is quite important.

Involvement of Nonphysicians in the Health Care Team

Depending on the specific problem, the evaluation and treatment of children may require more knowledge and input than a single psychiatrist can provide. Child psychiatry is more difficult and complicated than adult psychiatry, because the problems of children tend to impinge on many different aspects of their lives, and treatment will often involve many of these different aspects. A child with some particular childhood disorder, such as attention-deficit hyperactivity disorder (ADHD), is likely to have difficulty with parents, siblings, school performance, and relationship with peers. Most people who must interact with the child are likely to find her high level of impulsivity, distractibility, and physical activity to be annoying and disruptive. The child will have a poor self-concept, and this will be produced in part by a sense of frustration and failure in all spheres of life.

In such instances, assessment will involve determining how well the child is functioning in these various domains. That is, the clinician will need to talk to the child and to observe him. In addition, however, the clinician will need to talk to the parents and perhaps the entire family. With the permission of the child and family, the clinician may need to talk to the child's teacher and to obtain some assessment of his performance in the classroom. School records, as well as the child's scores on tests of educational achievement, will be important aspects of assessment. Parents or teachers may also need to provide information about the child's interaction with his peers.

Because of the diversity of domains involved, many clinicians working in the area of child psychiatry like to operate in the context of a *health care team*. This team may be relatively small, involving a psychologist or social worker in addition to the psychiatrist. In larger settings, however, it will include a psychiatrist (who works primarily with the child in psychotherapy and the prescription of medication), a social worker (who works primarily with the family), an educational specialist (who assesses the child's educational achievement and assists in designing a nonfrustrating remedial program as needed), and a psychologist (who develops programs for behavior management, may do psychotherapy as needed, and may work with child, family, and school system as needed).

Comorbidity

Comorbidity, or the simultaneous occurrence of two or more diagnoses in the same patient, sometimes occurs in adults; for example, patients with depression often have problems with anxiety or substance abuse as well. Comorbidity tends to be the norm rather than the exception in children, however. For example, children with ADHD will often have an impairment in academic skills, such as specific disabilities in reading or arithmetic. They may also show symptoms of conduct disorder, oppositional defiant disorder, or anxiety disorder.

The clinician has to remain very alert to the likelihood of multiple problems and design the assessment and treatment plan accordingly. This aspect of child psychiatry also makes it somewhat more complex and difficult than adult psychiatry. On the positive side, however, is the hope that early intervention will prevent larger problems from developing or the addition of new diagnoses (e.g., substance abuse in addition to ADHD).

Testing in Child Psychiatry

Because of the complexity and ambiguity of child psychiatry, selected objective assessment measures may be quite useful. Psychological tests such as IQ tests may be helpful in determining a child's specific areas of strength and weakness, as well as the level of academic performance that she can be expected to achieve. Some diagnoses in child psychiatry depend on knowledge of the child's IQ, such as mental retardation or the academic-skills disorders. Some disorders of childhood, such as Tourette's disorder or autism, have an "organic" quality to them that suggests a need to rule out an associated or underlying disorder, such as seizures. Others, such as mental retardation, are often accompanied by various organic problems (e.g., seizures, congenital anomalies, metabolic disorders). In these instances, laboratory tests are useful in diagnosing the accompanying organic disorders or monitoring their progress.

Psychological and Educational Testing

Psychological and educational testing often plays a central role in the evaluation of children. Several tests commonly used in child psychiatry are listed in Table 22-3.

General intelligence. This may be assessed with the Stanford-Binet Intelligence Scale, the recently revised (1986) Wechsler Intelligence Scale for Children (WISC-R), and other well-validated instruments. The Stanford-Binet Intelligence Scale was one of the earliest IQ tests developed, and it is still appropriate for relatively

Table 22-3. Cognitive, psychological, and educational tests used in child psychiatry

Intelligence	Stanford-Binet Intelligence Scale, Wechsler Intelligence Scale for Children—Revised (WISC-R), Peabody Picture Vocabulary, Kaufman ABC, Wechsler Preschool and Primary Scale of Intelligence (WPPSI)
Educational achievement	Iowa Test of Basic Skills (ITBS), Iowa Test of Educational Development (ITED), Wide Range Achievement Test—Revised (WRAT-R), Woodcock-Johnson Psychoeducational Battery
Adaptive behavior	Vineland Adaptive Behavior Scale, Iowa Conner's Teacher Rating Scale
Perceptual-motor abilities	Draw-a-Person, Bender-Gestalt, Benton Visual Retention Test, Purdue Pegboard Test, Beery Developmental Test of Visual-Motor Integration
Personality	Thematic apperception test (TAT), Rorschach test

young children, because its bottom threshold is lower and does not require extensive acquisition of knowledge. The Kaufman ABC and a new Wechsler Preschool and Primary Scale of Intelligence (WPPSI) have also become available recently and are very appropriate for assessing young children.

The WISC-R has now become established as the standard test for assessing the intelligence of school-age children. As in the Wechsler Adult Intelligence Scale—Revised (WAIS-R), the WISC-R consists of a group of verbal scales (information, vocabulary, similarities, arithmetic, and comprehension, plus digit span) and a set of performance tests (picture completion, picture arrangement, block design, object assembly, coding, and mazes). Thus, verbal and performance IQs can be derived separately, as well as a full-scale IQ.

Examining the scores on individual WISC-R subtests gives clinicians a sense of the child's overall intellectual skills and weaknesses. The test is scaled to have a mean of 100 and a standard deviation of 15. Sixty-seven percent of children will have IQs that fall between 85 and 115, whereas 95% will fall between 70 and 130. Children from middle-class and culturally advantaged backgrounds tend to perform better on these tests. In such instances, the performance scales of the test may give a somewhat better indication of the child's "culture-free intelligence," although this clearly will not be helpful for those children who have performance deficits for some reason (e.g., visual-motor/perception difficulties). Interpretation of the WISC-R must be made within the context of each child's social background and educational opportunities.

The Peabody Picture Vocabulary test is a simpler and cruder test that is sometimes used to give a simple global measure of intelligence. Using pictures, it provides a measure of oral language comprehension, from which verbal intelligence can be inferred. In general, IQ based on the Peabody Picture Vocabulary tends to be an overestimate.

Educational achievement.   Several standardized educational achievement tests are often widely used in the public school systems. Two of the most widely used are the Iowa Test of Basic Skills (ITBS) and the Iowa Test of Educational Development (ITED). The former is typically used for younger children, whereas the latter has tests available for assessment until completion of high school. For the ITBS and the ITED, national, state, and school-specific norms are available; therefore, children's achievement can be assessed within their specific environmental context. These achievement tests provide scores for specific areas such as reading, language arts, study skills, arithmetic, and social studies. Evaluating the pattern of achievement can provide some index as to whether the child has an academic-skills disorder.

The ITBS and ITED are widely used group tests. If a specific concern is present, the child may also be referred for individual testing by an educational specialist, which will often involve the Wide Range Achievement Test—Revised (WRAT-R). The Woodcock-Johnson Psychoeducational Battery is also a widely used individual test to assess skills such as reading or arithmetic. Children may perform poorly on group tests due to inattention or other problems; therefore, group tests may underestimate the child's true abilities.

Adaptive behavior.   Various standard questionnaires can be used to assess adaptive behavior. The Vineland Adaptive Behavior Scales were originally developed to evaluate children with mental retardation, but they are now widely used to provide a standardized measure of adaptive skills for children with a broader range of problems, including those with normal intelligence. The Iowa Connor's Teacher Rating Scale was developed to assess the child's behavior in the classroom. It is specifically targeted to assessing behavior that tends to be associated with ADHD, such as impulsivity, physical activity, or impaired attention. It also has subscales to assess social withdrawal and aggressive behavior.

Perceptual-motor skills.   Various standardized tests are used to evaluate perceptual-motor skills. In the assessment of young children, the Draw-a-Person test is one of the most popular. The complexity and detail of the person drawn gives a crude indication of the child's maturity, and the drawing skills exhibited assess the child's ability to translate thoughts into a visual representation. The Bender-Gestalt and Benton Visual Retention Test assess the ability to copy a design or to recall it later, which are also fundamental aspects of perceptual-motor skills. The Purdue Pegboard Test is a somewhat pure test of manual dexterity, assessing the child's ability to place pegs in appropriate slots. The Beery Developmental Test of Visual-Motor Integration is popular with school systems.

Personality style and social adjustment.   These are typically evaluated in children through projective tests. The thematic apperception test (TAT) uses a series of cards depicting obscure figures in ambiguous situations; the child is asked to describe what is happening and tell a story about it. The Rorschach test is the famous "inkblot test." In this test, the child is shown cards containing inkblots that have ambiguous and suggestive shapes. The child is asked to identify and label what he sees and to indicate the basis for his perception. Although semistandardized scores can be applied, one of the most common applications of these tests is to provide a standardized structured stimulus to the child, using her response as an indication of interpersonal experiences, anxieties, fears, drives, and other important psychological components.

Other Tests

Other laboratory tests may also be useful in the assessment of children. The decision to order these tests will depend on the child's past history and the clinician's index of suspicion for finding an abnormality. For example, there is often comorbidity between seizure disorders and other childhood disorders, such as autism or mental retardation, and children with these diagnoses should probably be evaluated with an electroencephalogram (EEG). For other disorders, in which seizures sometimes occur or in which EEG abnormalities have been noted, such as conduct disorders or ADHD, an EEG may be appropriate if the history indicates a possibility of seizures.

Evaluation of children with mental retardation will typically include an assessment for possible causes of the mental retardation. Karyotyping may be used to evaluate for the "fragile X" syndrome, Down's syndrome, or XYY. Computerized tomography (CT) or magnetic resonance imaging (MRI) may be appropriate in such patients, as well as in patients suffering from autism or Tourette's disorder.

Physical Examination

A careful physical examination, incorporating some simple standardized neuropsychological tests, is also an important part of the evaluation. In addition to the standard physical examination, the clinician should carefully inspect the child for indications of congenital anomalies, such as a high-arched palate, low-set ears, single palmar creases, unusual carrying angle, webbing, abnormalities of the genitalia, or neuroectodermal anomalies. It is well recognized that congenital anomalies tend to occur together and that midline or neuroectodermal anomalies are more likely to be associated with central nervous system anomalies. The observation of any such anomalies provides an indication for CT or MRI.

The clinician should be attentive to assessment of neurological soft signs in children as well. A standardized repertoire should be developed for assessing graphesthesia, left-right discrimination, motor coordination, and simple perceptual-motor skills that can be evaluated at the bedside. For example, left-right discrimination can be examined systematically through a graded series of questions such as the following: "Hold up your right hand. Hold up your left foot. Put your right forefinger on your nose. Use your left forefinger to point to your right foot. Point to my right hand. Use your left forefinger to point to my left hand." Tongue twisters such as "Methodist-Episcopal" or "Luke Luck likes lakes" may be used to assess oral-motor coordination, and hopping, tandem, and rapid alternating movements are used to evaluate other motor skills. Fine motor skills are evaluated through drawing and writing. After assessing many children across a wide range of ages, the clinician will gradually develop a sense of what constitutes "normal" performance on such tests of soft signs for a given child of a given age. Extensive neurological soft signs may serve as an indicator for ordering a more extensive laboratory workup, involving an EEG or a brain scan.

Disruptive Behavior Disorders

The disruptive behavior disorders are the "staple" of child psychiatry. Children with these disorders are experienced as difficult to manage and therefore as disruptive by those around them, including parents, teachers, and often peers. Sometimes this group of disorders is referred to as involving *acting-out* behavior, meaning that the child expresses problems outwardly rather than holding them within. This group of behavior disorders is contrasted with the *internalizing* disorders such as the anxiety disorders, in which the child is considered to turn suffering inward. Although closer contact with many of the children who manifest disruptive behavior makes it clear that they may too suffer a great deal internally and may also experience considerable anxiety, this aspect of the disorder is not immediately obvious to those who must deal with them on a day-to-day basis. On superficial contact, these children may seem hard to love and even hard to like. The three major classes of disruptive behavior disorders include attention-deficit hyperactivity disorder (ADHD), conduct disorder, and oppositional defiant disorder.

Attention-Deficit Hyperactivity Disorder

ADHD has been recognized under various names for many years, and probably for many centuries. Children with this disorder are a caricature of "the active child." They are physically overactive, distractible, inattentive, impulsive, and hard to manage. Because they often show soft neurological signs and indices of slight delay in reaching developmental milestones, this disorder was originally referred to as "minimal brain dysfunction." Later, as it became apparent that no objective evidence could be marshaled for the minimal brain dysfunction, the disorder was referred to as "hyperactivity" and the patient as a "hyperactive child." These designations appear in the earlier DSM nomenclature. By the time DSM-III was developed, child psychiatrists had reached a consensus that the basic deficit in this disorder is one of attention. Thus, it came to be known as attention-deficit disorder (ADD), and clinicians could indicate whether hyperactivity was present or absent as well. By the time DSM-III-R was produced, clinicians had decided that this distinction was arbitrary and began to refer to the disorder as ADHD.

The DSM-III-R criteria for ADHD are summarized in Table 22-4. The criteria require that at least 8 from a group of 14 different symptoms be present for at least 6 months. These symptoms fall into three broad categories that characterize the overall syndrome: hyperactivity, difficulty focusing and maintaining attention, and

Table 22-4. DSM-III-R criteria for attention-deficit hyperactivity disorder

Note: Consider a criterion met only if the behavior is considerably more frequent than that of most people of the same mental age.

A. A disturbance of at least 6 months during which at least eight of the following are present:

1. Often fidgets with hands or feet or squirms in seat (in adolescents, may be limited to subjective feelings of restlessness)
2. Has difficulty remaining seated when required to do so
3. Is easily distracted by extraneous stimuli
4. Has difficulty awaiting turn in games or group situations
5. Often blurts out answers to questions before they have been completed
6. Has difficulty following through on instructions from others (not due to oppositional behavior or failure of comprehension), e.g., fails to finish chores
7. Has difficulty sustaining attention in tasks or play activities
8. Often shifts from one uncompleted activity to another
9. Has difficulty playing quietly
10. Often talks excessively
11. Often interrupts or intrudes on others, e.g., butts into other children's games
12. Often does not seem to listen to what is being said to him or her
13. Often loses things necessary for tasks or activities at school or at home (e.g., toys, pencils, books, assignments)
14. Often engages in physically dangerous activities without considering possible consequences (not for the purpose of thrill seeking), e.g., runs into street without looking

Note: The above-mentioned items are listed in descending order of discriminating power based on data from a national field trial of the DSM-III-R criteria for disruptive behavior disorders.

B. Onset before age 7 years.

C. Does not meet the criteria for pervasive developmental disorder.

Criteria for severity of attention-deficit hyperactivity disorder:

Mild: Few, if any, symptoms in excess of those required to make the diagnosis and only minimal impairment in school and social functioning.

Moderate: Symptoms or functional impairment intermediate between "mild" and "severe."

Severe: Many symptoms in excess of those required to make the diagnosis and significant and pervasive impairment in functioning at home and school and with peers.

---

impulsivity. The symptoms involving hyperactivity include fidgeting, difficulty sitting still, difficulty playing quietly, and talking excessively. Those involving attention include being easily distracted, difficulty following instructions, difficulty sustaining attention in tasks, shifting attention from one uncompleted activity to another, not listening, and losing things. Those involving impulsivity include difficulty waiting in turn, blurting out answers to questions, interrupting or intruding on others, and engaging in physically dangerous activities. Thus, four of the symptoms involve hyperactivity, six involve problems in focusing attention, and four involve impulsivity.

The actual manifestation of these symptoms will vary depending on the age of the child. Younger children (in the 4–6 years age range) will be "little terrors." They run from one part of the room to another, hop on furniture, knock objects off tables, explore the contents of visitors' handbags, talk incessantly, run outside without telling their mother where they are going, have difficulty learning to look both ways when crossing the street, lose and break toys, stay up late, wake up early, and generally exhaust their parents. When the child enters school and begins the task of learning, the difficulties in focusing attention become more obvious. The child may "miss" things that the teacher says, is unable to finish assignments, forgets pencils or notebooks, and answers the teacher's questions without holding up his hand and often without even waiting to have the question completed. He may annoy his schoolmates by pushing ahead in line, grabbing equipment on the playground, or violating the rules of games without seeming to be aware of them. The child may begin to fall behind peers in school and to develop a poor concept of himself. Teachers may complain about his behavior to his parents and request that help be sought.

The following is a relatively typical case example of a patient with ADHD.

Charlie was a 6-year-old boy brought in by his mother after a recent school conference in which it was pointed out that he seemed to be having difficulty in adjusting to first grade.

Charlie's mother described that he had always been a somewhat difficult child. He was the second of two, and his older sister Mary (age 9 years) had always been much quieter and more pliable. Charlie's mother had assumed that much of Charlie's disruptive behavior was due to the fact that "little boys tend to be more active." Whereas Mary had responded well to encouragement to put her toys away each evening and had kept their various components intact (i.e., puzzles in their boxes, Lincoln Logs in their containers), Charlie never seemed to be able to keep track of anything or put it away. He had been a whiny infant who had suffered from colic. Even as an infant he was irritable and overactive. He learned to crawl at age 7 months and was soon exploring the entire house, leaving a wake of emptied wastepaper baskets and disrupted cupboards behind him. He did not seem to be able to remember or follow through with parental instructions that he should keep his feet off the furniture, not walk on the tops of tables, or not run through the living room carrying melting chocolate Popsicles. As he learned to talk, he seemed to talk incessantly and to be continuously in need of attention from his parents. Attempts to ignore his attention-seeking behavior seemed to have little effect on him. His parents complained that he was a "perpetual-motion machine."

He began to attend preschool at age 4 years. Teachers at that time complained that he was disruptive and impulsive and seemed to have little consideration for the other children in the school. The same noisy attention-seeking behavior that occurred at home was noticed at the preschool. Similar complaints were registered by his teacher when he entered kindergarten the following year.

After 3 months of first grade, the patience of the public school system was already exhausted. Charlie's teacher complained that it was difficult to even get through a routine class day because of Charlie's behavior. He would not sit in his seat like the other children and would often get up and run around the room. He could not work on an assignment for more than 5 minutes without being distracted. He would also distract his classmates by talking to them when they were supposed to be working quietly. None of the teacher's efforts seemed to be effective in quieting or calming Charlie.

On initial evaluation, Charlie was noted to indeed be quite active. He entered the doctor's office with a firm, aggressive step. He jumped on his chair rather than sitting down, finally squirming himself into a sitting position, which he maintained for only 2 or 3 minutes. He then jumped up and began pulling books off the bookshelves, asking what they were for in a somewhat immature whiny tone of voice. When told that they belonged to the doctor and should be placed back on the shelf, he threw one or two on the floor and proceeded to the doctor's desk to examine the pens, pencils, and paperweights. Charlie's mother looked embarrassed and exasperated and tried to get him to sit back down.

An individual evaluation with Charlie alone, involving an attempt to put a puzzle together, indicated that Charlie indeed did have problems focusing his attention on a relatively simple task. He was given a five-piece puzzle that the average 6-year-old can complete quickly. Charlie put one piece in place and then lost interest, instead pounding another puzzle piece on the floor and then throwing the remainder across the room. He was unable to perform any tests of graphesthesia. When asked to write the first six letters of the alphabet, after five tries he completed four with one letter reversal and then lost interest. He also reversed the letter *r* when writing his name. He could not distinguish between right and left at any level. Otherwise, his physical examination was totally normal.

A decision was made to try Charlie on methylphenidate. Within 1 week, his mother related that the effects were "amazing." Almost immediately, his behavior improved, and he showed a distinct increase in his ability to focus attention and a decrease in impulsive overactive behavior. His teacher also noticed a distinct difference. He was able to complete the first grade with only minimal difficulty and was considered to have appropriate progress for his age in basic skills of learning to read and doing very simple arithmetic.

Epidemiology.   Because the definition of ADHD has changed over time, its prevalence is uncertain, but it is definitely common in preschool- and school-age children. Estimates range from 3 to 10%. It is far more common in boys than girls, with approximately a 3:1 sex ratio. The etiology and pathophysiology of ADHD are uncertain. Genetic, environmental, neurobiological, and social explanations have been proposed.

Etiology and pathophysiology.   ADHD runs in families. Not only does ADHD itself show familial aggregation, particularly in boys, but other psychiatric disorders tend to show familial aggregation with it as well. In particular, there appears to be an association with academic-skills disorders, mood disorder, substance abuse, and possibly "acting-out" personality disorders. Most of the existing evidence for familial aggregation is based on family studies. Twin studies have not been done. There may be a "gender threshold effect" in that girls with ADHD tend to have a stronger family history of ADHD than do boys.

Environmental explanations tend to stress the possibility of perinatal problems, including maternal nutrition, maternal substance abuse, obstetric complications during delivery, viral infections, and exposure to toxins. The possible role of such environmental factors is consistent with the higher prevalence of ADHD in boys, as well as the gender threshold effect described above, in that male children are more vulnerable to prenatal and perinatal injury. It is also consistent with the slight increase in soft signs that has been observed in children with ADHD.

Other neurobiological markers have also been evaluated in children with ADHD. There is no specific diagnostic marker, but various findings have been observed. A decrease in norepinephrine metabolites (3-methoxy-4-hydroxyphenylglycol [MHPG]) has been argued to support a catecholamine hypothesis, whereas low levels of homovanillic acid have been thought to support the possibility of hypo-dopaminergic function. Approximately 20% of ADHD children show EEG abnormalities, and sleep EEG studies show decreased rapid eye movement (REM) latency and increased delta latency; the latter finding is consistent with the clinical observation that these children tend to have difficulty falling asleep.

Psychosocial explanations stress the role of parental anxiety and inexperience, as well as failure to extinguish undesirable behavior through ignoring it (often difficult to do with hyperactive children). Parents may become uncertain of their parenting skills when faced with a child who seems so difficult to control or shape, thereby conveying uncertainty or anxiety to the child.

Course and outcome. The long-term course and outcome of ADHD is variable. Approximately one-half of the children diagnosed with this disorder have a good outcome, completing school on schedule with acceptable grades consistent with their family background and family expectations. For a time, it was assumed that most children with ADHD would "grow out of it." This does not seem to be the case in many individuals, however, and approximately one-half of the patients diagnosed as having ADHD during childhood continue to show some problems with attention and impulsivity as adults. In fact, a subset continue to need medication as adults, and a small number of individuals are occasionally diagnosed as having "adult attention-deficit disorder," or "adult ADD." These individuals are sometimes treated with psychostimulants (e.g., dextroamphetamine, methylphenidate) by psychiatrists.

Some patients with ADHD have a relatively poor outcome. Twenty-five percent subsequently meet criteria for antisocial personality as adults. Children given the diagnosis of ADHD also experience higher rates of substance abuse, more arrests, more suicide attempts, and more car accidents and complete fewer years of school. Problems with confidence and self-esteem may be prominent, because the disorder invites rejection by both parents and peers.

Differential diagnosis. A wide variety of disorders are included in the differential diagnosis of ADHD. In making a differential diagnosis, the clinician must also be aware that a child with this disorder may have comorbidity with other disorders common in childhood, such as seizure disorders, other disruptive behavior disorders (i.e., conduct and oppositional defiant), and academic-skills disorders. When any of these various disorders are present, it is often difficult to distinguish which is primary and which is secondary. Other disorders that may present with similar symptoms include childhood bipolar disorder, childhood depression, conduct disorder, a normal response to a pathological or abusive home environment (e.g., physical abuse or neglect by the parents), or a neuroendocrine abnormality such as thyroid disorder.

Clinical management.   The treatment for ADHD will often involve a combination of somatic therapy and behavior management.

A majority of children respond favorably to psychostimulants. Methylphenidate in a dosage of 10–60 mg per day is usually the first line of treatment, followed by dextroamphetamine in a dosage of 5–40 mg per day. If neither of these succeeds, another psychostimulant (pemoline) or tricyclic antidepressants (e.g., imipramine) may be used. Tricyclic dosages range from 25 to 100 mg per day. In general, methylphenidate and dextroamphetamine offer short-term effects, lasting 4–6 hours, whereas the effects of the antidepressants tend to last longer. Because psychostimulants may have long-term effects on weight gain and body size (i.e., to decrease or inhibit them), clinicians usually strive to use them in the lowest possible doses and, whenever possible, to restrict their use to periods of greatest need, such as during the school year. Sometimes it is possible to diminish or discontinue medication as the child enters puberty. Further information about the use of psychostimulants is found in Chapter 24.

Behavior and environmental management is also important. Parents will benefit from learning basic techniques of behavior management, such as the value of positive reinforcement and firm nonpunitive limit setting. They can also be taught techniques for reducing stimulation, thereby diminishing distractibility and inattentiveness. For example, young hyperactive children do better playing with only one friend than in groups. Noisy or complex toys should be avoided, as should toys that encourage impulsivity and aggression. The parent may wish to work closely with the child in completing homework tasks and to teach the child the value of working on tasks in the single, small increments that are best suited to his relatively short attention span, mastering one completely before going on to another.

Conduct Disorders

Conduct disorders are characterized by a pattern of behavior that violates the rights of others, such as stealing, lying, or cheating. In terms of both behavior and diagnostic criteria, conduct disorder can be considered to be a forerunner of antisocial personality as adults, because it involves similar antisocial behavior. Nevertheless, not all children who manifest conduct disorder develop antisocial personality as adults. With appropriate treatment and rehabilitation, many of these "juvenile delinquents" go on to lead acceptable and normal adult lives.

The DSM-III-R criteria for conduct disorder appear in Table 22-5. The presence of 3 from a list of 13 antisocial behaviors and a persistence of at least 6 months are required for diagnosis.

Table 22-5. DSM-III-R criteria for conduct disorder

A. A disturbance of conduct lasting at least 6 months, during which at least three of the following have been present:

1. Has stolen without confrontation of a victim on more than one occasion (including forgery)
2. Has run away from home overnight at least twice while living in parental or parental surrogate home (or once without returning)
3. Often lies (other than to avoid physical or sexual abuse)
4. Has deliberately engaged in fire-setting
5. Is often truant from school (for older person, absent from work)
6. Has broken into someone else's house, building, or car
7. Has deliberately destroyed others' property (other than by fire-setting)
8. Has been physically cruel to animals
9. Has forced someone into sexual activity with him or her
10. Has used a weapon in more than one fight
11. Often initiates physical fights
12. Has stolen with confrontation of a victim (e.g., mugging, purse-snatching, extortion, armed robbery)
13. Has been physically cruel to people

Note: The above items are listed in descending order of discriminating power based on data from a national field trial of the DSM-III-R criteria for disruptive behavior disorders.

B. If 18 or older, does not meet criteria for antisocial personality disorder.

Criteria for severity of conduct disorder:

Mild: Few, if any, conduct problems in excess of those required to make the diagnosis, and conduct problems cause only minor harm to others.

Moderate: Number of conduct problems and effect on others intermediate between "mild" and "severe."

Severe: Many conduct problems in excess of those required to make the diagnosis, or conduct problems cause considerable harm to others, e.g., serious physical injury to victims, extensive vandalism or theft, prolonged absence from home.

Individuals who manifest this delinquent behavior are further subdivided into several different types. *Group delinquents* manifest their antisocial behavior while accompanied by other members of their peer group. Children with this type of conduct disorder are able to feel loyalty and to have a sense of responsibility and an ethical code, although their code is not consistent with the majority of adult society. Because they have a sense of the value of social relationships, children with this type of conduct disorder are considered to have a better prognosis. The *solitary aggressive type* of conduct disorder is characterized by aggressive behavior toward others performed in isolation; children who display this type of conduct disorder do not feel loyalty or ties to others and appear to be lacking in any sense of "connectedness" or social responsibility. The *undifferentiated type* is a residual group for children who do not fall neatly into either of the other two types. As pointed out in DSM-III-R, this residual category may in fact be quite common.

There is continuing controversy about the fundamental defining features of conduct disorder, as well as the best ways to subclassify children and adolescents who manifest delinquent behavior. Two key dimensions have been noted. One dimension reflects the social skills and social interactions of the young person, emphasizing that it is better to have relationships and loyalties to peers than to be isolated and lacking in loyalty. The second dimension relates to the presence or absence of aggressive and violent behavior, suggesting that aggressive forms of delinquency (destroying property, using weapons, or cruelty to animals or humans) are a worse form of delinquency than behavior that involves passiveness or withdrawal (e.g., running away from home, being truant from school). Reflecting these dimensions, early classifications of conduct disorders divided them into socialized aggressive (equivalent to the group type), unsocialized aggressive (equivalent to the solitary aggressive type), socialized unaggressive (children who have friends and loyalties to peers, but run away or are truant), and unsocialized unaggressive (the withdrawn solitary child who is passively delinquent). These latter two are now compressed into the undifferentiated type of DSM-III-R.

As is the case for the adult equivalent of conduct disorder, antisocial personality, DSM-III-R criteria stress behavior in the definition of conduct disorder, as opposed to values, motives, or attitudes. Although the objective behavioral definition clearly improves reliability, some critics have expressed the concern that these behavioral definitions ignore the true "core phenomena" of delinquency and antisocial personality: shallowness of relationships and attachments, inability to feel for others, and an impaired capacity to feel guilt. The distinction between group delinquency and solitary aggressive behavior refines the definition to some extent, by stressing that young delinquents who commit antisocial acts as part of a gang are able to form some ties to others. Recent episodes of "wilding" make it clear, however, that "group delinquents" can commit senseless acts of violence that seem to indicate a fundamental and severe lack of moral sense.

Children and adolescents who present with signs and symptoms of conduct disorder are a very mixed group, and most clinicians regard this category as fundamentally quite heterogeneous, both with respect to etiology and with respect to outcome. The child seen in a psychiatry clinic for conduct disorder is usually brought in at someone else's request after committing some kind of socially unacceptable behavior, such as lying, cheating, stealing, fighting, or assaulting. Some children come from families where this type of behavior is not unusual, but others perform these acts in a more "middle-class" context, thereby shocking and dismaying their parents. The degree of parental support for the child, and assistance in helping her modify her behavior, will vary substantially.

The child typically is angry, sullen, and resentful when placed in the context of the "adult" world, with its pressures to conform, stay in school, and persist in conspicuously dull activities. School performance is usually average to poor. The child or adolescent will typically consider school work irrelevant or uninteresting, not complete homework, and often cut class to "joyride" with buddies, smoke pot, or drink beer. When with his peers, his anger and sullenness often disappear, and he seems to be having a good time. Beneath the veneer of anger, toughness, and rebellion, however, the child or adolescent may often have profound feelings of self-doubt and worthlessness, although he may be reluctant to discuss these with adults or with his peers. Some children with conduct disorder have experienced either physical or sexual abuse from their parents.

The following is a representative case history of a child with conduct disorder.

Heather, a 14-year-old girl, was brought to the child psychiatry clinic by her mother with the complaint that "Heather is getting out of hand. I just can't seem to discipline her anymore." Heather was the youngest of four children and the only girl in the family. She was the product of a normal pregnancy and delivery and had completed her developmental milestones on schedule. She had been an average student, but had taken a particular interest in sports as a child. Her three older siblings were all boys, and she tended to "tag along" after them and play with them and their friends whenever they would permit. Her brother Tom, with whom she was closest, was 3 years older. Heather was noted to be somewhat stubborn and moody as a child and was occasionally defiant, but otherwise had seemed completely normal.

Heather's father was a truck driver and was often away from the family, leaving the mother to rear the four children largely by herself. Heather's mother remained at home with the children until Heather was in second grade and then took a job as a clerk in a store. Both parents had completed high school and had similar expectations for their children. Although the two oldest boys had some problems with drinking, using drugs, and truancy, both were able to complete high school. Both had obtained jobs, married, and "settled down." Tom, a high school senior, was currently showing behavior similar to that of his older brothers, but his school performance was adequate and he appeared to be due for graduation in the spring, with plans to join the military thereafter.

Heather's parents had separated and divorced 3 years earlier. This appeared to bother Heather much more than the boys, because she had always been her father's "little girl." Her father had developed a relationship with a woman in another city, had moved away, saw the children infrequently, and was not dependable in child-support payments. Heather had not told her sixth-grade friends about the separation and divorce for many months, because she felt embarrassed and ashamed.

Heather's behavior problems began when she entered junior high. She began to enter puberty in the sixth grade, and by the seventh grade, her body was markedly feminized. Her mother reported that she seemed to react to this by "acting tougher instead of more like a girl." She started to hang out more with boys her own age or slightly older and began to smoke cigarettes secretly (although the evidence was smelled all over the house and on her clothes). Her grades, previously average, began to drop steadily. She also showed signs of increasingly devious behavior, lying to her mother about where she was going, returning at night well past predefined deadlines, and staying home "sick" without telling her mother (having called the school herself to report the "illness" in her mother's guise). Articles began to appear in the house that Heather could not afford, such as expensive costume jewelry and cosmetics. Heather's mother suspected her of having stolen these things, but Heather insisted that they were gifts from friends. Several times marijuana was found in Heather's room. Whenever Heather's mother confronted her, Heather became angry and ran out of the house. Several times she stayed away overnight without telling her mother of her whereabouts.

When interviewed alone, Heather was initially evasive and defensive, looking at the floor and answering questions very briefly. She was an attractive, slightly overweight, dark-haired girl attired in "conventional" teenage garb with a slightly "punk" touch (multiple earrings in her ears, leather boots, sleeveless T-shirt showing a nude couple embracing and bearing the logo "too drunk to fuck"). Eventually she admitted to most of the conduct abnormalities that her mother described.

As a consequence of this assessment, it was concluded that Heather was indeed having difficulties, but that fortunately she had many strengths: a relatively intact childhood, normal intelligence and a past history of adequate school performance, and a mother who appeared to genuinely care about her. Heather was seen in individual therapy on a weekly basis for 3–4 months, with a primary emphasis on supportive and relationship approaches. Heather responded well to this and began to talk freely about her difficulties in adjusting to the loss of her father, her experience of entering puberty, and her confusion about whether it was better to relate to her male peers (from whom she desperately desired love and approval) as a "tough girl" or as a "sexy girl." With Heather's permission, she was also seen jointly with her mother in family therapy, and on several occasions, her older brother joined as well. Tom was able to assist his mother by assuming the role of a surrogate father and encouraging his "little sis" to be more honest, to attend school regularly, and to behave in ways that he and his older brothers could be proud of. Heather responded well to this increased attention and support, and it was possible to terminate the therapy successfully at the end of the school year.

Epidemiology. Approximately 10% of boys and 2% of girls under age 18 years meet criteria for conduct disorder. The rate in girls may be increasing.

Etiology and pathophysiology. The etiology and pathophysiology of conduct disorder are almost certainly multifactorial. Family studies indicate that children with conduct disorder tend to come from families that have increased prevalence of antisocial personality, mood disorder, substance abuse, and learning disorders. Adopted children may also have higher rates of conduct disorder, consistent with reports that the adopted offspring of female felons have a high rate of antisocial behavior such as traffic violations or arrests for robbery, which suggests that there may be at least some genetic component to conduct disorder. Apart from a possible genetic component, no specific neurobiological factors have been identified in children with conduct disorders to any consistent degree, although a slight increase in neurological soft signs and psychomotor seizures has been observed.

Psychosocial factors probably play a major role in the development of conduct disorders. Psychosocial factors that have been shown to have some relationship to conduct disorders include parental separation or divorce, parental substance abuse, other forms of "poor parenting" (e.g., rejection, abandonment, abuse, inadequate supervision, inconsistent or excessively harsh discipline), and association with a delinquent peer group.

Differential diagnosis. Conduct disorders have considerable comorbidity with other childhood disorders. Among those that often coexist with conduct disorder are academic-skills disorders, ADHD, and mood disorders. These disorders will often be encountered as the clinician runs through a differential diagnosis for conduct disorder because these disorders are the most common from which conduct disorder must be distinguished. From 60 to 70% of children who present with ADHD also meet criteria for conduct disorder. At least 10% of children with conduct disorder have specific academic-skills disorders. In general, the greater the comorbidity, the more complicated the case, and the worse the outcome.

Course and outcome.   The long-term course and outcome of conduct disorders is variable. To some extent, outcome depends on the degree of socialization and aggressiveness. Children with the "socialized" types of conduct disorder tend to have a much better outcome, as do children who are less aggressive. As children get older, the severity of the conduct disorder worsens in that the teenager or young adult gets into increasingly serious problems that may eventually lead to incarceration.

Clinical management.   Treatment of conduct disorders will vary greatly, depending on the age of the child, the symptoms with which he presents, the extent of comorbidity, the availability of family supports, and the child's intellectual and social assets. A relatively mild case of conduct disorder, such as was represented by Heather in the case example above, will typically be treated with individual and family therapy. At the opposite extreme are those cases in which the child comes from a highly deviant family and is engaged in repeated antisocial acts that bring him to legal attention; such patients may require removal from the home and placement in a group home or perhaps even in a juvenile detention facility.

Children and adolescents with conduct disorder who have comorbid disorders such as hyperactivity or seizures will benefit from medication to treat the comorbid condition; apart from such indications, however, medications are not typically used to treat patients with conduct disorder. Limit setting, consistency, and other techniques for behavior management are essential components of the treatment of conduct disorder, both on the part of family members (when a supportive family is available) and on the part of the clinician. Testing limits and manipulating or defying "the system" are a fundamental component of conduct disorder, and the clinician must be prepared to react to this behavior with firmness, but preferably without annoyance or rejection.

Oppositional Defiant Disorder

Oppositional defiant disorder is a new diagnosis that was introduced in DSM-III-R. It attempts to provide a category for children and adolescents who demonstrate "difficult" behavior, but who do not have full-blown conduct disorder. As this category enjoys increasing use, it has become apparent that many youngsters who would have been diagnosed as having "good prognosis" or mild conduct disorder in DSM-III are now being placed in this category. The criteria for oppositional defiant disorder are summarized in Table 22-6.

There is clearly a fine line between "normal naughtiness" and oppositional defiant disorder. Most children at times lose their tempers, argue with their parents, refuse to clean their rooms, or fail to obey a curfew. Thus, the proviso is added that this behavior must be "more frequent than that of most people of the same mental age." Clearly, however, there will be great variation in the definition of "more

Table 22-6. DSM-III-R criteria for oppositional defiant disorder

Note: Consider a criterion met only if the behavior is considerably more frequent than that of most people of the same mental age.

A. A disturbance of at least 6 months during which at least five of the following are present:

1. Often loses temper
2. Often argues with adults
3. Often actively defies or refuses adult requests or rules, e.g., refuses to do chores at home
4. Often deliberately does things that annoy other people, e.g., grabs other children's hats
5. Often blames others for his or her own mistakes
6. Is often touchy or easily annoyed by others
7. Is often angry or resentful
8. Is often spiteful or vindictive
9. Often swears or uses obscene language

Note: The above items are listed in descending order of discriminating power based on data from a national field trial of the DSM-III-R criteria for disruptive behavior disorders.

B. Does not meet criteria for conduct disorder and does not occur exclusively during the course of a psychotic disorder, dysthymia, or a major depressive, hypomanic, or manic episode.

frequent," depending on who is rendering the judgment. Religiously conservative or authoritarian families are likely to be less tolerant of opposition and defiance than families in which there is an existing background of behavior abnormalities. Thus, to some extent, the appearance of children with this diagnosis in child psychiatry clinics may partially reflect a given family's threshold for accepting defiant behavior, a factor that must be taken into account in treatment planning. Unlike the conduct disorders, which specify that the child must have violated personal rights and social rules (thereby making it more likely that the child's deviant behavior has come to the attention of people outside the immediate family), oppositional defiant disorder is defined almost totally on the basis of annoying, difficult, and disruptive behavior.

Because this is a new disorder, very little is known about its epidemiology, etiology, pathophysiology, comorbidity, or treatment. By definition, it cannot coexist with conduct disorder, but it may coexist with ADHD. Common sense dictates that management will emphasize individual and family counseling, with treatment of comorbid hyperactivity (or possibly mood disorder) with medications as needed.

Anxiety Disorders

Separation Anxiety Disorder

The major anxiety disorder seen in children is *separation anxiety disorder*. This disorder represents a more severe and disabling form of a maturational experience

Table 22-7. DSM-III-R criteria for separation anxiety disorder

A. Excessive anxiety concerning separation from those to whom the child is attached, as evidenced by at least three of the following:

1. Unrealistic and persistent worry about possible harm befalling major attachment figures or fear that they will leave and not return
2. Unrealistic and persistent worry that an untoward calamitous event will separate the child from a major attachment figure, e.g., the child will be lost, kidnapped, killed, or the victim of an accident
3. Persistent reluctance or refusal to go to school in order to stay with major attachment figures or at home
4. Persistent reluctance or refusal to go to sleep without being near a major attachment figure or to go to sleep away from home
5. Persistent avoidance of being alone, including "clinging" to and "shadowing" major attachment figures
6. Repeated nightmares involving the theme of separation
7. Complaints of physical symptoms, e.g., headaches, stomachaches, nausea, or vomiting, on many school days or on other occasions when anticipating separation from major attachment figures
8. Recurrent signs or complaints of excessive distress in anticipation of separation from home or major attachment figures, e.g., temper tantrums or crying, pleading with parents not to leave
9. Recurrent signs or complaints of excessive distress when separated from home or major attachment figures, e.g., wants to return home, needs to call parents when they are absent or when child is away from home

B. Duration of disturbance of at least 2 weeks.

C. Onset before age 18 years.

D. Occurrence not exclusively during the course of a pervasive developmental disorder, schizophrenia, or any other psychotic disorder.

that all children normally have. Most infants and children experience fear at the possibility (or reality) of being separated from their parents. Once infants learn to recognize maternal and paternal faces and shapes, they also learn to cry when the parent leaves the room or hands them to a stranger. No doubt this pattern of behavior reflects some type of primal fear of loss or fear of the unknown. As the child grows older, she also experiences natural fears of being left with a babysitter, being sent to preschool, or entering kindergarten. Crying, tenseness, or physical complaints may appear and last for minutes, hours, or days in such situations.

As the DSM-III-R criteria (Table 22-7) specify, separation anxiety disorder is defined largely by the persistence of such symptoms or a long-enough duration to be considered pathological. Three from a list of nine characteristic symptoms must be present for at least 2 weeks. The characteristic symptoms include two types of worries (that some harm will come to the parents, or that the child will be lost or somehow separated from them), three types of behaviors (school refusal, sleep refusal, and "clinging"), two physiological symptoms (nightmares, physical complaints such as headache or nausea), and two specific types of behavior reflective of psychological distress (temper tantrums or crying, "checking" behaviors such as returning or calling home).

School Refusal

Perhaps the most important and clinically significant anxiety disorder observed in children is variously referred to as *school phobia, school refusal,* or *school absenteeism.* Although this particular anxiety disorder is classified among the adult disorders as a type of social phobia in DSM-III-R, it is in fact an important and common childhood anxiety disorder. In some cases, it may be related to separation anxiety disorder. Children with this problem develop a fear of going to school. It may begin with attendance at preschool or kindergarten, but more typically it develops during grade school or junior high. Typically, a child who has previously been going to school (albeit with some anxiety) begins to develop methods for staying home. He may display repeated episodes of "illness" such as headache or nausea. He may be truant, leaving home with the appearance of going to school and then returning home without his parents' knowledge or going to some other environment that he experiences as safe. He may simply refuse to go to school and only give some vague explanation such as "I don't like it." These various reasons explain why the problem is variously referred to as a phobia, absenteeism, or refusal. There is some controversy among child psychiatrists as to whether school refusal should be considered strictly a subset of separation anxiety disorder or should be defined more broadly to include all children who do not attend school, for whatever reason (e.g., truancy secondary to conduct disorder, avoidance of school as a complication of mood disorder, school avoidance secondary to a psychosis).

Once discovered, school avoidance should be thoroughly evaluated and treated as quickly as possible to prevent personal, social, and academic complications. The clinician should attempt to determine the reasons why the child does not wish to go to school. These reasons may be expressed overtly (e.g., "The kids make fun of me because I'm stupid," "I'm afraid that Jimmy Taylor will beat me up"), but often considerable investigation will be needed. The child's intellectual and school performance should be evaluated to determine whether there is indeed some problem with academic skills, which may make the child feel inferior and avoidant. Teachers and parents need to be consulted about the child's relationships with peers, and a specific effort should be made to determine whether there is a problem with teasing or bullying. Other situations that children often find stressful may occur on the playground, in the gym, or in the school lunchroom. Young teenagers may be embarrassed about the appearance of their bodies, or they may be afraid that others will not sit with them in the lunchroom or on the bus. Clearly, the child's own self-esteem and self-concept need to be examined, and parental behavior needs to be explored to determine whether it is contributing to the child's problem or even causing it. Anxious, fearful, controlling parents may be communicating their own fears about separation to the child. They may be setting academic or social expectations so high that the child feels doomed to failure at school.

Clinical management. Treatment of school avoidance will depend on the cause that has been identified. Often the child will need encouragement and support from several directions: at home, at school, and from the clinician. If specific

Table 22-8. DSM-III-R criteria for Tourette's disorder

A. Both multiple motor and one or more vocal tics have been present at some time during the illness, although not necessarily concurrently.

B. The tics occur many times a day (usually in bouts), nearly every day or intermittently throughout a period of more than 1 year.

C. The anatomic location, number, frequency, complexity, and severity of the tics change over time.

D. Onset before age 21 years.

E. Occurrence not exclusively during psychoactive substance intoxication or known central nervous system disease, such as Huntington's chorea and postviral encephalitis.

problems are identified with academic skills, remedial training should be initiated. Similar training may be appropriate for problems with athletic or social skills. Whatever the cause, however, it is important to impress on both child and family that the child *must* go to school regularly, and that absenteeism or refusal will not be tolerated.

Tourette's Disorder

Tourette's disorder is a condition that is characterized by the presence of multiple motor and vocal tics. By definition, there must be at least one form of vocal tic that has been present for at least 1 year. The vocal tics are most likely to cause psychological discomfort for the patient and to engage the attention of others. Vocal tics associated with Tourette's disorder most frequently consist of loud grunts or barks, but approximately 30% of the time they involve shouting words, and the words are sometimes obscenities such as "shit." Patients are aware that they are saying these phrases, are able to exert a mild degree of control over them, but ultimately have to submit to expressing them as an uncontrollable urge overwhelms them. Because of this awareness, they find the tics very embarrassing. Because the disorder is essentially unknown to the general public, the behavior is simply seen as inappropriate or bizarre. Motor tics include various phenomena such as blinking, nodding, tongue protrusion, sniffing, or even squatting or hopping. The criteria for Tourette's disorder appear in Table 22-8.

Tourette's disorder usually begins during childhood or early adolescence, and motor tics usually antedate vocal tics. Thus, grade school–age children may display motor tics and some barks or grunts. During late grade school or early junior high, vocalization of obscenities (coprolalia) begins to appear. Twenty percent of patients have a remission of motor and vocal tics during their third decade of life, and the majority of the remainder of patients with Tourette's disorder have a significant decrease in their symptoms as they grow older. Patients with Tourette's disorder may experience shame and embarrassment about their disorder, which may lead them to avoid public or social situations or even close interpersonal relationships.

Epidemiology. Tourette's disorder is relatively rare, affecting 0.4% of the population. It is more common in males than in females, with a 3:1 ratio. As with ADHD, a "gender threshold effect" has been observed; that is, females with Tourette's disorder appear to have higher genetic loading than male patients with Tourette's disorder, suggesting that there is a lower penetrance for the disorder in females.

Etiology and pathophysiology. Tourette's disorder appears to be highly familial. It appears to cotransmit with obsessive-compulsive disorder (OCD), and the obsessive-compulsive phenomena tend to be more prominent in females in affected families, whereas the males manifest full-blown Tourette's. These findings suggest that, in some instances, obsessive-compulsive behavior may be on a continuum with motor and vocal tic phenomena. The genetic pattern of transmission is not clear; in some families it appears to follow an autosomal dominant pattern, but not in all. The search for a "Tourette's gene" is underway at present.

Clinical management. For two decades, it has been clear that the symptoms of Tourette's disorder can be markedly improved through treatment with neuroleptic medication. Because neuroleptics exert a primary effect by blocking dopaminergic pathways in the brain, abnormalities in dopamine transmission are the most commonly hypothesized neurochemical abnormality. Because of the prominent motor component, investigators suspect that the primary abnormalities may lie within nigrostriatal projections, but, given the complex feedback loops of the dopamine system (described in Chapter 5), many other localizations are also possible.

The evaluation of a patient presenting with Tourette's disorder should stress a comprehensive neurological evaluation to rule out other causes for the tics. The patient should be examined for stigmata of Wilson's disease, and a family history obtained to evaluate the possibility of Huntington's chorea. An EEG is useful to rule out the possibility of seizure disorder. The patient should also be evaluated for other psychiatric conditions. Comorbidity with ADHD may occur, as may symptoms of mood disorder, anxiety disorders, or OCD.

The treatment of Tourette's disorder primarily stresses the use of neuroleptics. Haloperidol has been used for many years as the first-line treatment; dosages are lower than those used to treat psychosis and tend to range from 1 to 5 mg per day. Pimozide, used for decades in Europe, is also effective; dosages of 8–10 mg per day are used (maximum dosage is 0.3 mg/kg body weight per day, or a total of 20 mg/day).

Although the treatment of Tourette's disorder stresses the use of medications, it is also important to educate the family about the disorder and assist them in providing psychological support to the patient. Because of the social embarrassment that it produces, Tourette's disorder has a potential for serious long-term social complications, and supportive psychotherapy to the patient or family may assist in minimizing these problems.

Autistic Disorder

The film *Rain Man*, through its sympathetic portrayal of a person suffering from autism, has done much to help increase public understanding of this particular disorder. Although Raymond Babbit is not a perfectly typical autistic person because he is cognitively very gifted in specific isolated areas, he is not atypical. He displays all the characteristic features of autism: impaired social interactions, impaired ability to communicate, and a restricted repertoire of activities and interests.

Individuals with autism are usually noted to be developing abnormally relatively soon after birth. Within the first 3–6 months of their lives, their parents may note that they do not develop a normal pattern of smiling or responding to cuddling. As they grow older, they do not progress through developmental milestones such as learning to say words or speak sentences. Instead, they seem aloof, withdrawn, and detached. Instead of developing patterns of relating warmly to their parents, they may instead engage in self-stimulating behavior such as rocking or head banging. By age 2 or 3 years, it is usually clear that there is something severely wrong, and the features of the disorder continue to become more obvious over time as the child fails to develop normal verbal or interpersonal communication. Children with this disorder are referred to as "autistic" because they appear to be withdrawn and self-absorbed. Most of the defining features of autistic disorder reflect this autistic pattern of thinking, speaking, feeling, and behaving.

DSM-III-R criteria for autistic disorder appear in Table 22-9. The criteria require that at least 8 from a list of 16 items be present. The criteria provide an excellent comprehensive description of the symptoms of this disorder.

The impairment in social interaction is usually the first obvious sign of the disorder and persists throughout life. The child appears to lack the ability to bond to parents or others. In severe cases, the child seems totally withdrawn. In milder cases, the child displays some interaction, but lacks warmth, sensitivity, and awareness. Interactions, when they occur, tend to have a detached and mechanical quality to them. Displays of love and affection do not occur, nor does the child (or autistic adult) appear to respond to such displays from others. Likewise, the verbal impairments range from the complete absence of verbal speech to mildly deviant speech and language patterns. Even in patients who develop good facility in verbal expression, the speech has an empty, repetitive quality to it, and intonations may be singsong and monotonous. The child or adult seems to lack the capacity to engage in conversation with others, sometimes talking spontaneously without an audience, and at other times replying irrelevantly or inappropriately. There is an intense and rigid commitment to maintaining specific routines, and the child tends to become quite distressed if routines are interrupted. The child may have to sit in a particular chair, dress in a particular way, or eat particular foods.

Most autistic patients (70%) show some evidence of mental retardation, but others have normal intelligence, and some have very specific talents or abilities, particularly in areas of music or mathematics. IQ testing tends to show considerable

Table 22-9. DSM-III-R criteria for autistic disorder

At least 8 of the following 16 items are present, including at least two items from A, one from B, and one from C.

Note: Consider a criterion to be met only if the behavior is abnormal for the person's developmental level.

A. Qualitative impairment in reciprocal social interaction as manifested by the following:
   (The examples with parentheses are arranged so that those first mentioned are more likely to appear to younger or more handicapped, and the later ones to older or less handicapped, persons with this disorder.)

   1. Marked lack of awareness of the existence or feelings of others (e.g., treats a person as if he or she were a piece of furniture; does not notice another person's distress; apparently has no concept of the need of others for privacy)
   2. No or abnormal seeking of comfort at times of distress (e.g., does not come for comfort even when ill, hurt, or tired; seeks comfort in a stereotyped way, e.g., says "cheese, cheese, cheese" whenever hurt)
   3. No or impaired imitation (e.g., does not wave bye-bye; does not copy mother's domestic activities; mechanical imitation of others' actions out of context)
   4. No or abnormal social play (e.g., does not actively participate in simple games; prefers solitary play activities; involves other children in play only as "mechanical aids")
   5. Gross impairment in ability to make peer friendships (e.g., no interest in making peer friendships; despite interest in making friends, demonstrates lack of understanding of conventions of social interaction, for example, reads telephone book to uninterested peer)

B. Qualitative impairment in verbal and nonverbal communication, and in imaginative activity, as manifested by the following:
   (The numbered items are arranged so that those first listed are more likely to apply to younger or more handicapped, and the later ones to older or less handicapped, persons with this disorder.)

   1. No mode of communication, such as communicative babbling, facial expression, gesture, mime, or spoken language
   2. Markedly abnormal nonverbal communication, as in the use of eye-to-eye gaze, facial expression, body posture, or gestures to initiate or modulate social interaction (e.g., does not anticipate being held, stiffens when held, does not look at the person or smile when making a social approach, does not greet parents or visitors, has a fixed stare in social situations)
   3. Absence of imaginative activity, such as playacting of adult roles, fantasy characters, or animals; lack of interest in stories about imaginary events
   4. Marked abnormalities in the production of speech, including volume, pitch, stress, rate, rhythm, and intonation (e.g., monotonous tone, question-like melody, or high pitch)
   5. Marked abnormalities in the form or content of speech, including stereotyped and repetitive use of speech (e.g., immediate echolalia or mechanical repetition of television commercial); use of "you" when "I" is meant (e.g., using "You want cookie?" to mean "I want a cookie"); idiosyncratic use of words or phrases (e.g., "Go on green riding" to mean "I want to go on the swing"); or frequent irrelevant remarks (e.g., starts talking about train schedules during a conversation about sports)
   6. Marked impairment in the ability to initiate or sustain a conversation with others, despite adequate speech (e.g., indulging in lengthy monologues on one subject regardless of interjections from others)

C. Markedly restricted repertoire of activities and interests, as manifested by the following:

   1. Stereotyped body movements, e.g., hand-flicking or -twisting, spinning, head-banging, complex whole-body movements
   2. Persistent preoccupation with parts of objects (e.g., sniffing or smelling objects, repetitive feeling of texture of materials, spinning wheels of toy cars) or attachment to unusual objects (e.g., insists on carrying around a piece of string)

(continues)

Table 22-9.   DSM-III-R criteria for autistic disorder—*Continued*

3. Marked distress over changes in trivial aspects of environment, e.g., when a vase is moved from usual position
4. Unreasonable insistence on following routine in precise detail, e.g., insisting that exactly the same route always be followed when shopping
5. Markedly restricted range of interests and a preoccupation with one narrow interest, e.g., interested only in lining up objects, in amassing facts about meteorology, or in pretending to be a fantasy character

D. Onset during infancy or childhood.

Specify if childhood onset (after age 36 months).

scatter, and there is a tendency for patients with autism to perform better on performance scales than on verbal scales.

Epidemiology.   Autism is relatively rare and has a prevalence of approximately 10–15 in 10,000. It is more common in males than in females, with a ratio of 3:1 or 4:1. The onset of autism usually occurs in early childhood, and problems are typically noted during the 1st or 2nd year of life.

Course and outcome.   Autism is associated with relatively severe morbidity. It is a chronic, lifelong disorder. Some children do show some improvement as they mature, although others may in fact worsen. Very few individuals with autism (2–3%) are able to progress normally through school or to live independently. Follow-up studies of a group of autistic individuals diagnosed in childhood and reevaluated in adulthood indicate that most autistic patients show some improvement with social interaction over time, but even the most functional never achieve normality. Nearly all of the defining features of the disorder tend to persist into adulthood, including social aloofness, language abnormalities, and rigid and ritualistic behavior. Good prognostic features include higher IQ and better language and social skills.

Etiology and pathophysiology.   The pathophysiology and etiology of autism are uncertain, but the preponderance of evidence indicates that this disorder is due almost totally to some type of brain abnormality. The disorder is familial, with some suggestion of an autosomal recessive inheritance. The concordance rate in monozygotic twins has been estimated at 36% in comparison to 0 in dizygotic twins, further supporting a genetic component that is not totally penetrant. A "fragile X" chromosome has been noted in a small number of autistic patients, but, apart from this finding, data are not available to assist in defining the genetic anomaly more specifically.

The neurochemistry and cerebral localization of autism have not been determined. Abnormalities in both the dopamine system and the serotonin system have been reported. MRI studies have identified anomalies suggestive of a neurodevelopmental defect. Positron-emission tomography (PET) studies have failed to show any specific regional abnormalities in glucose utilization.

Children who present with symptoms suggestive of autism should receive a comprehensive psychiatric and physical examination, with emphasis on neurological evaluation as well. As in the case of Tourette's disorder, children should be screened for metabolic disorders such as Wilson's disease or phenylketonuria, and karyotyping should also be done. Because these children present with profound social withdrawal, hearing and vision should be checked to rule out sensory defects as a cause. Because a substantial number of children with autism have a comorbid seizure disorder (25%) or develop one eventually, an EEG should also be obtained. IQ testing will assist in assessing the child's intellectual strengths and weaknesses.

Differential diagnosis. The major differential diagnoses include childhood psychosis, mental retardation, and congenital deafness, blindness, or language disorders. The distinction between childhood psychosis and mental retardation can be quite difficult, particularly in children who have low intelligence. The major distinction between autism and childhood schizophrenia turns on the presence or absence of overt psychotic symptoms (delusions and hallucinations), which typically do not occur in autism, but are difficult to assess in the noncommunicative child. Mentally retarded children typically have pervasive intellectual impairments, whereas autistic children tend to have a much more uneven profile of functional intellectual abilities on the WISC-R and may be normal to superior in some areas.

Clinical management. The treatment of autism requires assistance and support in the many different areas of functioning in which these children are impaired. Once the diagnosis is firmly made, the disorder should be described and explained to the parents, making it clear that their child suffers from a neurodevelopmental disease and not from a psychological disturbance that they have caused through poor parenting. They should be apprised of the relatively poor long-term prognosis, but assured that some gains can probably be made. Guidelines for behavior management should be provided, so that the parents can assist in reducing the rigid and stereotyped behaviors and improving language and social skills.

Children with autism will usually require special education or specialized day care programs that also emphasize improvement in social and language skills. Medications are often used as adjuncts to these supportive and behavioral approaches. Those children who have seizures will require anticonvulsants. Among other medications, neuroleptics (e.g., haloperidol, in low doses ranging from 1 to 10 mg per day) have been empirically observed to decrease aggressive and self-stimulating behavior.

Mental Retardation

Mental retardation is a disorder characterized by subnormal intelligence accompanied by deficits in adaptive functioning. The specific IQ cutoff point used to

Table 22-10.   DSM-III-R criteria for mental retardation

A. Significantly subaverage general intellectual functioning: an IQ of 70 or below on an individually administered IQ test (for infants, a clinical judgment of significantly subaverage intellectual functioning, since available intelligence tests do not yield numerical IQ values).

B. Concurrent deficits or impairments in adaptive functioning, i.e., the person's effectiveness in meeting the standards expected for his or her age by his or her cultural group in areas such as social skills and responsibility, communication, daily living skills, personal independence, and self-sufficiency.

C. Onset before age 18 years.

define mental retardation is 70; individuals with an IQ below 70 are more than two standard deviations below the population mean. People with IQs between 70 and 85 (one standard deviation below the mean) are considered to have borderline intellectual functioning. Many, but not all, individuals with IQs below 70 have problems in coping with social and economic demands or exhibit other abnormalities in social adjustment.

The criteria for mental retardation, which appear in Table 22-10, summarize this definition. They also require an onset before age 18 years. In general, mental retardation is typically observed and diagnosed long before age 18 years and usually is considered to be present from very early in life. For example, a 13-year-old who sustains a head injury in a car accident is considered to have an organic mental disorder, not mental retardation.

Mental retardation is divided into four broad categories: mild, moderate, severe, and profound. Children with *mild mental retardation* have IQs between approximately 50 and 70. They represent the majority of cases of mental retardation, constituting approximately 85% of individuals with IQs below 70. Children with IQs in this range are considered to be "educable," and they are usually able to attend special classes and to work toward the long-term goal of being able to function in the community and to hold some type of job. They usually can learn to read, write, and perform simple arithmetic calculations.

Children with *moderate mental retardation* have IQs ranging between 35 and 50 (between three and four standard deviations below the population mean) and constitute approximately 10% of the mentally retarded population. They are considered to be "trainable," in that they can learn to talk, to recognize their name and other simple words, to perform activities of self-care such as bathing or doing their laundry, and to handle small change. They require management and treatment in special education classes. The ideal long-term goal for these individuals is care in a sheltered environment such as a group home.

Individuals with severe and profound mental retardation constitute the smallest groups. *Severe mental retardation* is defined as an IQ between 20 and 35 and *profound mental retardation* as an IQ below 20. Individuals with IQs in this range are considered to be untrainable and almost invariably require care in institutions, usually beginning relatively early in life.

Epidemiology. Mental retardation is very common, affecting between 1 and 2% of the population. Mental retardation is more common in males, with a male-to-female ratio of approximately 2:1. Mild mental retardation is more common in lower social classes, but moderate, severe, and profound mental retardation are equally common among all social classes.

Etiology and pathophysiology. The pathophysiology and etiology of mental retardation are heterogeneous. Mental retardation is almost certainly a syndrome that represents a final common pathway produced by various factors that injure the brain and affect its normal development. Down's syndrome (trisomy 21) is the most common cause of mental retardation; pure genetic defects and inborn errors of metabolism account for approximately 5% of cases; examples include Tay-Sachs disease, "fragile X" syndrome, and untreated phenylketonuria. In addition to these clearly defined genetic causes, a substantial proportion of cases of mental retardation probably also reflect polygenic inheritance, possibly interacting with various environmental factors such as nutrition or psychosocial nurturance.

Various prenatal factors may also affect fetal development and lead to neurodevelopmental anomalies. The high rate of Down's syndrome in infants born to older mothers is a prime example. Other prenatal factors that may affect fetal development include maternal substance abuse, exposure to other toxins such as radiation, or maternal illnesses such as diabetes, toxemia, or rubella. Perinatal and early postnatal factors may also contribute. Examples include traumatic deliveries that cause brain injury, malnutrition, exposure to toxins, infections such as encephalitis, or head injuries occurring during infancy or early childhood.

Psychosocial factors obviously contribute to some of these "biological" factors, and some psychosocial factors may also contribute independently to mental retardation. Malnutrition, exposure to toxins such as lead, increased likelihood of maternal infection due to inadequate immunization, and poor prenatal and perinatal care are more likely to occur in children born in impoverished environments. Poverty, teenage pregnancy, and substance abuse may produce a self-perpetuating familial pattern of mild mental retardation in inner cities and other pockets of social deprivation.

Course and outcome. The long-term outcome of mental retardation is variable. The severe and profound forms are often characterized by progressive deterioration and ultimately premature death, as early as the teens or early 20s (e.g., as in Tay-Sachs disease). Individuals with mild and moderate forms of mental retardation have a somewhat reduced life expectancy, but active intervention may enhance their quality of life. Like all children, children with mental retardation grow and develop, and they may show maturational spurts that could not be predicted at an earlier age. Typically, mentally retarded children progress through normal milestones, such as sitting, standing, talking, and learning numbers and letters in similar patterns to normal children, but at a slower rate. The educable and trainable mentally retarded person will be able to learn to read, write, and calculate at some level, as long as appropriately structured educational settings are provided.

Differential diagnosis. As in other childhood disorders, the differential diagnosis of mental retardation (particularly mild mental retardation) can be complex, due to the frequent comorbidity of childhood disorders. The differential diagnosis includes ADHD, academic-skills disorders, autism, and childhood psychoses or mood disorders, but all these conditions can occur with mental retardation. Seizure disorders are also very common in children with mental retardation.

Children in whom mental retardation is suspected should be thoroughly evaluated with a careful physical and neurological examination, EEG, and CT (or MRI if available), as well as IQ testing.

Clinical management. The treatment of mental retardation is similar to that of other serious chronic childhood disorders such as autism. After a thorough evaluation, a comprehensive program should be developed to determine the best situation in which to place and treat the child, taking the needs and abilities of both the child and the parents into account. Decisions may range from care in the home (supplemented by family support and special education), through placement in a foster or group home, to long-term institutionalization. Because the majority of mentally retarded children are in the mild range, most will remain at home, at least initially. Because the parents in some of these families will themselves suffer from mental retardation, ongoing evaluation through social service agencies may be helpful and even necessary to ensure that the child's needs are being adequately met. Whatever their own intellectual resources, the parents of mentally retarded children are confronted with a host of burdens and stresses and will benefit from both supportive counseling and training in behavior techniques to assist in the management of their child's behavior problems.

Comorbid conditions such as seizures will require medical management. Intellectual evaluation will assist in determining the appropriate educational placement for the child, but this should be subjected to periodic review. At this stage, it is still not clear whether mildly mentally retarded children benefit more from placement in regular school programs ("mainstreaming") or from placement in special settings where education is tailored to their specific needs. To a large extent, however, mainstreaming is currently the dominant trend.

Academic-Skills Disorders

The academic-skills disorders, formerly referred to as specific learning disabilities, are characterized by an inability to achieve in a specific area of learning (reading, writing, or arithmetic) at a level consistent with the person's overall IQ. Typically, individuals with these disorders have normal intelligence (although it may be borderline or high), but have a specific inability to learn at least one of these academic skills, and sometimes several.

Table 22-11. DSM-III-R criteria for developmental reading disorder

A. Reading achievement, as measured by a standardized, individually administered test, is markedly below the expected level, given the person's schooling and intellectual capacity (as determined by an individually administered IQ test).

B. The disturbance in A significantly interferes with academic achievement or activities of daily living requiring reading skills.

C. Not due to a defect in visual or hearing acuity or a neurologic disorder.

The DSM-III-R criteria for *developmental reading disorder* appear in Table 22-11. The definitions for *developmental expressive writing disorder* and *developmental arithmetic disorder* are similar. In each case, the diagnosis is made on the basis of educational testing that indicates that the individual is performing markedly below a level expected on the basis of the person's IQ. For example, a 14-year-old with developmental reading disorder ("developmental dyslexia") may be observed to have an IQ of 110 and to be reading at a third-grade level.

These disorders are relatively common. A specific disability in reading affects 2–8% of school-age children; although the rates for writing and arithmetic disabilities are not known, they are probably high as well. These disorders are two to four times more common in boys than in girls.

Specific learning disabilities tend to be familial, but not uniformly or consistently. They are assumed to represent a neurodevelopmental defect or cerebral injury affecting the particular brain region involved in developing the academic skill. For example, in the case of some developmental reading or writing disorders, the language regions in the brain (i.e., Broca's area, Wernicke's area, or the left hemisphere) are thought to be affected.

If not diagnosed and treated early and aggressively, academic-skills disorders are extremely handicapping. Although children with these disorders typically have normal intelligence, they quickly come to view themselves as failures because of their inability to progress academically in a particular area. They may come to regard themselves as "stupid" and to be rejected by their peers.

The frustration associated with an impairment in academic skills can lead to various complications, such as truancy, school refusal, conduct disorder, mood disorder, or substance abuse. Consequently, it is important to identify the condition early and treat it aggressively. Rather than being causal, academic-skills disorders may also be comorbid with these conditions, as well as with ADHD. In this instance, it is also important to recognize the multiple disorders and to treat both (or all) of them appropriately.

Educational intervention proceeds on two fronts. The child or teenager usually needs remedial instruction to shore up skill deficits, and the development of "attack" skills that will assist in learning strategies to compensate for the neural deficits that underlie the condition. With steady sympathetic educational support, most children with these specific learning disabilities are able to develop acceptable skills in reading, writing, or arithmetic.

Recommendations for management of child and adolescent disorders

1. In assessing children and adolescents, be imaginative and meet each patient on his or her own terms.
   - Play games to evaluate problem-solving and motor skills.
   - Use dolls and toys with young children to create "pretend" situations that will provide insight about personal and social interactions.

2. Remember that normal maturational levels are highly variable in children and adolescents.

3. Remember that children and adolescents often do not have a level of cognitive development suitable for the insight-oriented and introspective approaches used with adults.

4. Establishing rapport with adolescents is difficult, but may be crucial to creating a "therapeutic alliance."
   - Find out what the patient is interested in and relate to him or her through these interests.

5. Don't preach or judge.

6. Remember that the basic maturational task of adolescents is to disengage themselves from their parents, become independent, and define their own identities; reliance on peers is an important "crutch" for adolescents in this transitional period.

7. Remain neutral; try not to criticize either parents or peers.

8. Most work with adolescents will carry an inevitable transference component; the adolescent's first reaction will be to see you as a parent; you need to try to work this toward a therapeutic advantage, or at least to prevent it from being a therapeutic handicap.

9. It is best to strike a balance between being perceived as a "good parent" or a "good peer," but this cannot and should not (usually) be achieved by attacking the real parent or real peer.

10. Because the parents and peers of adolescents may vary in quality, you need to be flexible, insightful, and creative in dealing with transference components.

11. Be aware of the pervasiveness of comorbidity in childhood and adolescent disorders.
    - The more diagnoses there are, the more complicated the management.
    - Drugs used for one condition may work at cross-purposes with another (e.g., psychostimulants prescribed for attention-deficit hyperactivity disorder [ADHD] may worsen Tourette's disorder; anticonvulsants prescribed for seizures may be sedative and affect school performance or worsen ADHD).
    - Because comorbid disorders often interact with one another, identifying one that is crucial and highly treatable may have a major impact on outcome (e.g., aggressive assistance with academic-skills disorders may prevent the worsening of mild conduct disorders or school phobias).

12. Be prepared to use a team approach and to combine a variety of assessment and therapeutic techniques when working with most children and adolescents.
    - Disorders often impinge on many aspects of the child's life, e.g., relationship with parents, relationships with peers, educational achievement.
    - Special skills not possessed by M.D.'s may be needed for management (e.g., consultation with an education specialist).
    - Use of cotherapists is often helpful in working with the patient and his or her family, since both need to feel that their special needs are recognized and receiving support and assistance.

Bibliography

Anderson JC, Williams S, McGee R, et al: DSM-III disorders in preadolescent children—prevalence in a large sample from the general population. Arch Gen Psychiatry 44:69–76, 1987

August GJ, Stewart MA: Is there a syndrome of pure hyperactivity? Br J Psychiatry 140:305–311, 1982

August GJ, Stewart MA: Familial subtypes of childhood hyperactivity. J Nerv Ment Dis 171:362–368, 1983

August GJ, Stewart MA, Holmes CS: A four-year follow-up of hyperactive boys with and without conduct disorder. Br J Psychiatry 143:192–198, 1983

Baroff GS: Mental Retardation—Nature, Cause and Management. New York, Hemisphere Publishers, 1986

Behar D, Stewart MA: Aggressive conduct disorder: the influence of social class, sex and age on the clinical picture. J Child Psychol Psychiatry 25:119–124, 1984

Berg I: School phobia in children of agoraphobic women. Br J Psychiatry 128:86–89, 1976

Biederman J, Munir K, Knee D, et al: High rate of affective disorders in probands with attention deficit disorder and in their relatives—a controlled family study. Am J Psychiatry 144:330–333, 1987

Brown W, Miller TP, Jenkins RL: The fallacy of radical nonintervention. Annals of Clinical Psychiatry 1:55–57, 1989

Campbell M, Green WH, Deutsch SI: Child and Adolescent Psychopharmacology. Beverly Hills, CA, Sage, 1985

Cantwell DP: Classification in Psychiatry, Vol 2. Edited by Michels R, Cavenar JO, Brodie HKH, et al. Philadelphia, PA, JB Lippincott, 1985, pp 1–15

Cantwell DP, Baker L: Developmental Speech and Language Disorders. New York, Guilford, 1987

Cohen D, Donnellan A, Rhea P (eds): Handbook of Autism and Pervasive Developmental Disorders. New York, John Wiley, 1987

Cohen D, Bruun R, Leckman J: Tourette's Syndrome. New York, John Wiley (in press)

Deutsch CK, Swanson JM, Bruell JH, et al: Overrepresentation of adoptees in children with the attention deficit disorder. Behav Genet 12:231–238, 1982

Famularo R, Fenton T: The effect of methylphenidate on school grades in children with attention deficit disorder without hyperactivity—a preliminary report. J Clin Psychiatry 48:112–114, 1987

Gittleman R: Anxiety Disorders of Childhood. New York, Guilford, 1986

Green WH, Campbell M, Hardesty AS, et al: A comparison of schizophrenic and autistic children. J Am Acad Child Psychiatry 4:399–409, 1984

Kanner L: Autistic disturbances of affective contact. Nervous Child 2:217–250, 1943

Kelso J, Stewart MA: Factors which predict the persistence of aggressive conduct disorder. J Child Psychol Psychiatry 27:77–86, 1986

Last CG, Francis G, Hersen M, et al: Separation anxiety and school phobia—a comparison using DSM-III criteria. Am J Psychiatry 144:653–657, 1987

Lewis DO, Pincus JH, Shanok SS, et al: Psychomotor epilepsy and violence in a group of incarcerated adolescent boys. Am J Psychiatry 139:882–887, 1982

Pauls DL, Leckman JF: The inheritance of Gilles de la Tourette's syndrome and associated behaviors. N Engl J Med 315:993–997, 1986

Popper C: Child and adolescent psychopharmacology, in Psychiatry, Vol 2. Edited by Michels R, Cavenar JO. Philadelphia, PA, JB Lippincott, 1985, pp 1–23

Popper CW: Disorders usually first evident in infancy, childhood, or adolescence, in The American Psychiatric Press Textbook of Psychiatry. Edited by Talbott JA, Hales RE, Yudofsky SC. Washington, DC, American Psychiatric Press, 1988, pp 649–735

Porrino LJ, Rapoport JL, Behar D, et al: A naturalistic assessment of the motor activity of hyperactive boys, I: comparison with normal controls. Arch Gen Psychiatry 40:681–687, 1983

Puig-Antich J: Major depression and conduct disorder in prepuberty. J Am Acad Child Psychiatry 21:118–128, 1982

Rapoport JL, Buchsbaum MS, Weingartner H, et al: Dextroamphetamine—its cognitive and behavioral effects in normal and hyperactive boys and normal men. Arch Gen Psychiatry 37:933–943, 1980

Rapoport JL, Conners CK, Reatig N: Rating scales and assessment instruments for use in pediatric psychopharmacology research. Psychopharmacol Bull 21:713–1125, 1985

Rumsey JM, Andreasen NC, Rapoport JL: Thought, language, communication, and affective flattening in autistic adults. Arch Gen Psychiatry 43:771–777, 1986

Shapiro E, Shapiro AK, Fulop G, et al: Controlled study of haloperidol, pimozide, and placebo for the treatment of Gilles de la Tourette's syndrome. Arch Gen Psychiatry 46:722–730, 1989

Stewart MA, Behar D: Subtypes of aggressive conduct behavior. Acta Psychiatr Scand 68:178–185, 1983

Stewart MA, deBlois S: Diagnostic criteria for aggressive conduct disorder. Psychopathology 18:11–17, 1985

Stewart M, Kelso J: A two-year follow-up of boys with aggressive conduct disorder. Psychopathology 20:296–304, 1987

Stewart MA, deBlois CS, Cummings C: Psychiatric disorder in the parents of hyperactive boys and those with conduct disorder. J Child Psychol Psychiatry 21:283–292, 1980

Tsai L, Stewart MA, August G: Implication of sex differences in the familial transmission of infantile autism. J Autism Dev Disord 11:165–173, 1981

Self-assessment Questions

1. What is the fundamental distinction between Axis I and Axis II disorders of childhood and adolescence?
2. Describe some techniques that are useful in assessing younger children and establishing rapport with them.
3. Describe some techniques that are useful in assessing adolescents and establishing rapport with them.
4. List the various types of non-M.D. clinicians who may be helpful in assessing and managing children and adolescents; describe how they might help.
5. Give four examples of conditions that often are comorbid in children and adolescents.
6. What IQ range defines children within one standard deviation of the population mean of 100? What percentage of children fall in this range? What IQ range encompasses children between one and two standard deviations from the mean? What percentage of children fall in this range? List the IQ levels

that are used to define borderline intelligence and mild, moderate, severe, and profound mental retardation.

7. Discuss the distinction between autism, mental retardation, and academic-skills disorders.
8. List three well-recognized causes of mental retardation.
9. Why is it important to obtain IQ testing and educational testing in some children and adolescents? Give three examples where the use of such testing may be crucial either to establishing a diagnosis or to planning treatment.
10. List three disorders of childhood or adolescence that may be comorbid with a seizure disorder and for which an EEG may be a useful laboratory assessment procedure.
11. List three disorders of childhood or adolescence for which karyotyping may be useful.
12. Describe four simple tests to assess "soft neurological signs" in children.
13. List the three broad categories of symptoms used to define ADHD, and give several examples of each. Describe the long-term course and outcome of ADHD. Identify two medications commonly used to treat ADHD and specify the appropriate dosage range.
14. Describe the two basic dimensions that occur in conduct disorders. What are the three subtypes of conduct disorder, and how do they relate to these basic dimensions? What is the prevalence and sex ratio for conduct disorder? What is the long-term course and outcome of conduct disorder? Give two different case examples of conduct disorder, and describe appropriate treatment for each.
15. Describe the clinical features of Tourette's disorder. What is the hypothesized pathophysiology and etiology of this disorder? How common is it? Describe two pharmacologic strategies for treating Tourette's disorder.
16. Describe the three major domains that are abnormal in autism, and give examples of signs and symptoms within these domains. How common is autism? What is its long-term course and outcome? What methods are used to treat it?
17. Describe oppositional defiant disorder and discuss its relationship to conduct disorder.
18. Describe separation anxiety disorder and discuss its relationship to school refusal (phobia, avoidance). List three factors that may predispose to the development of school avoidance. Describe three approaches to treating school avoidance.
19. Define academic-skills disorders and list the three skills that are commonly affected. How common is developmental dyslexia, and what is its sex ratio?
20. Why do you think most disorders of childhood and adolescence are more common in boys than in girls? (The answer to this one is not really included in the chapter, and if you can come up with a definitive answer, you may be on your way to winning a Nobel prize.)

Section IV
Treatments

Chapter 23
Psychosocial Treatments

The mind is its own place, and can make
A hell of heaven, a heaven of hell

John Milton, Paradise Lost

Although the use of medication has become increasingly important in psychiatry, clinicians who care for patients suffering from the broad range of mental illnesses must also develop a high level of skill in talking with their patients, listening to their problems, instilling confidence and a sense of support, helping them have insight into abnormal patterns of behavior, and assisting them in learning new ways to correct or alter maladaptive or painful behavior, emotions, and attitudes. Because psychiatrists deal with diseases that are especially human, involving thoughts, feelings, and relationships, it is essential that they maintain a humanistic, empathic, and caring attitude toward their patients and that they become skilled in treating patients with therapies directed at the mind in addition to the brain.

This chapter provides a brief overview of the major classes of psychotherapy that are employed by specialists who care for the mentally ill. Many of these psychosocial treatments require extensive experience and training, on a scale that is outside the range of description of a single chapter. Students who wish to explore specific types of psychosocial treatments in more detail may wish to read material cited in the Bibliography at the end of this chapter or to obtain additional training in psychotherapy under the supervision of skilled clinicians.

The various psychosocial treatments that are often used for major mental illnesses include behavior therapy, cognitive therapy, the individual psychotherapies that draw on psychodynamic principles, group therapy, family therapy, and social skills

Table 23-1.   Types of psychosocial therapy

- Behavior therapy

- Cognitive therapy

- Individual psychotherapy

    Classical psychoanalysis
    Psychodynamic psychotherapy
    Insight-oriented psychotherapy
    Relationship psychotherapy
    Supportive psychotherapy

- Group therapy

- Family therapy

- Social skills training

training. The major classes of psychosocial treatments are summarized in Table 23-1.

Behavior Therapy

The theoretical underpinnings of behavior therapy derive from British empiricism, Pavlov's studies of conditioning, and subsequent research on stimulus-response relationships conducted by other leading behaviorists such as Skinner, Wolpe, and Eysenck. The behaviorist stresses the importance of working with objective observable phenomena, usually referred to as behavior, including physical activities such as eating, drinking, talking, or completing the serial-sequential activities that lead to habit formations and social interactions. In contrast to psychodynamic psychotherapies, discussed below, the therapist using behavior techniques will not necessarily help the patient in understanding emotions or motivations. Instead of working on the patient's thoughts and feelings, the behavior therapist works on *what the patient does.* Indeed, some clinicians using behavior approaches argue that changing a patient's behavior may lead to substantial changes in how the patient thinks and feels and that correcting pathological behavior may be more effective than correcting pathological emotions. The motto for this approach is "Change the behavior, and the feelings will follow."

Behavior therapies are particularly effective for disorders that have clearly abnormal behavior patterns in need of correction. These disorders include alcohol and drug abuse, eating disorders, anxiety disorders, and, particularly, phobias and obsessive-compulsive behavior. A general knowledge of the principles of behaviorism may be useful in dealing with a broad range of patients, however, including patients with dementias, psychoses, adjustment disorders, childhood disorders, or personality disorders.

The concept of conditioning is fundamental to the various behavior therapies. Two types of conditioning have been described: classical (Pavlovian) and operant. Early in the 20th century, the Russian physiologist Pavlov described the first controlled experiments with conditioning. He demonstrated that through pairing stimuli, such as striking a bell at the same time that dogs were given food, he could eventually "condition" the animals to produce a "conditioned reflex" in the absence of the original triggering stimulus. For example, if the two stimuli (food and the ringing of a bell) were paired frequently enough, the dog would eventually learn to salivate when hearing the bell alone. In this model, the food is regarded as the unconditioned stimulus, the bell as the conditioned stimulus, and salivation in response to the bell as the conditioned reflex.

The concept of stimulus pairing can obviously be used both to explain the development of psychopathology and to create behavior therapies through conditioning patients to alter their response patterns.

The study and use of operant conditioning involve examining responses that are produced within the subject, rather than produced by some outside stimulus. Operant conditioning seeks to understand the forces that trigger and modify specific behaviors, rather than beginning with a predetermined conditioned stimulus. Operant responses, as compared with conditioned reflexes, are voluntary. For example, a young child sitting in a high chair quickly learns that banging a spoon on his tray gets his mother's attention and is likely to produce gratification of some desire, such as more milk in his cup or another piece of toast. By varying the amount of banging, he may also learn that if he bangs too much his mother may become annoyed, take away his spoon, and remove him from his high chair before a dessert is provided. Thus, the child learns to change both his behavior and his environment in relation to the responses that his behavior elicits in a manner that is under his voluntary control.

The study of operant conditioning has created an enormous experimental literature that explores the various ways that learning occurs and that behaviors are reinforced or extinguished. The concepts of positive and negative reinforcement are fundamental. A positive reinforcer (e.g., giving a reward) is one that strengthens the response, whereas a negative reinforcer (e.g., giving a punishment) diminishes the response. An extensive behavioral literature now suggests that positive reinforcement is more effective in sustaining behavior than negative reinforcement, that failure to provide reinforcements will usually extinguish a behavior, and that variable and unpredictable schedules of reinforcement may be more effective in maintaining behavior than fixed regular reinforcements. For example, pathological gamblers receive the positive reinforcement of winning only occasionally, but continue to gamble and are rarely deterred by threats of punishment or even punishment itself, such as loss of their financial assets, or even incarceration. If they won every time they gambled, they would very likely lose interest eventually, and likewise they would lose interest if they never won at all.

Some of the established forms of behavior therapy that use these principles are listed in Table 23-2. They include relaxation training, systematic desensitization,

Table 23-2. Established forms of behavior therapy

Relaxation training
Systematic desensitization
Flooding
Behavior modification techniques

flooding, and behavior modification. Obviously, however, these principles can also be used to shape the behavior of patients (and one's children, colleagues, or friends) in spontaneous or creative ways.

Relaxation Training

Relaxation training is used to teach patients control over their body and mental state. Relaxation training is a simple and straightforward procedure; patients are instructed to move through the muscle groups of the body and make them tense and then completely relaxed. Through this procedure, patients learn how to achieve voluntary control over their feelings of tension and relaxation. Relaxation training can be done simply through providing patients with an instructional audiotape that can be listened to in order to practice the techniques on their own. Relaxation training can be used in isolation to help patients suffering from anxiety or various problems involving pain (e.g., headache, low back pain), or it can be used in conjunction with systematic desensitization.

Systematic Desensitization

Systematic desensitization is a behavior technique that involves teaching patients how to reduce or control the fear elicited by specific stimuli. This technique is particularly useful for patients suffering from specific fears, such as agoraphobia or the various social phobias. The therapist may use any one of a variety of techniques to train patients to reduce their tense and anxious response to the feared stimulus. For example, the therapist may ask the agoraphobic person to imagine what it is like to leave the house and go to the shopping mall where he or she typically develops panic attacks, thereby leading the patient to experience the panic attack; the patient is then encouraged to use relaxation techniques to diminish the sensation of panic and place it under voluntary control. Progressively, the patient will be able to enter the feared situation, such as actually going to the shopping mall, and use relaxation techniques while in the feared setting. In complex and difficult situations, the therapist may need to lead the patient gradually into a sense of control, through developing a hierarchy of stimuli that increasingly approximate the feared stimulus—e.g., moving from imagination, to photographs, to photographs plus recorded noises, to the actual situation itself.

Flooding

Flooding involves teaching patients to extinguish anxiety produced by a feared stimulus through placing them in continuous contact with the stimulus and helping them learn that the stimulus does not in fact lead to any feared consequences. For example, a patient with a disabling fear of riding on airplanes may be forced to take repeated flights until the fear is extinguished. The patient with a fear of snakes may be requested to go to the zoo and stand in front of the snake cage, until her anxiety is completely gone. A patient with compulsions triggered by some external stimulus may be asked to actually seek out the stimulus; for example, a patient with a hand-washing ritual triggered by touching doorknobs may be requested to repeatedly handle doorknobs, until the anxiety and subsequent rituals produced by the stimulus are extinguished.

A variant of flooding, also used to treat obsessions and compulsions, is referred to as *paradoxical intention*. The therapist asks the patient to perform the rituals regularly and to keep a daily record of the rituals; when encouraged to perform them, the patient gradually becomes aware of their inherent ludicrousness and their ineffectiveness as a method for reducing anxiety and therefore is able to voluntarily abandon them.

Behavior Modification Techniques

Behavior modification techniques tend to use the concept of reinforcement as a way of shaping behavior and in particular to reduce or eliminate undesirable behavior and to replace it with healthier behaviors or habits. Behavior modification techniques are especially appropriate for disorders of impulse control, such as alcoholism, substance abuse, eating disorders, and conduct disorders.

Individual programs of behavior modification must be designed to suit the particular patient, using stimuli that are specific positive and negative reinforcers for that individual. For example, the long-term goal for a patient with anorexia nervosa is weight gain. Intermediate goals are to become less preoccupied with food and body image. Patients with anorexia nervosa typically enjoy exercise. A particular anorexic person may also enjoy reading mystery novels and chewing gum. A specific program would be developed for such a patient, in which she would be provided with three regular well-balanced meals per day and told that access to her specific preferred pleasures would be contingent on going to the dining room for meals, eating them, and demonstrating a regular pattern of weight gain. A schedule of reinforcers would be developed to encourage her compliance with eating regularly. For example, she might be restricted to her room initially between meals and given no access to exercise, mystery novels, or chewing gum. After she gains 5 pounds, she will be allowed to leave her room. After she gains an additional 5 pounds, she will be given access to mystery novels. After the gain of an additional 5 pounds, she will be allowed access to chewing gum. After she reaches her desired target weight (involving a total weight gain of 20 pounds), she will be allowed to exercise regularly. To be permitted to continue exercising, however, she must maintain her target weight for 2 weeks while exercising as much as she desires. If her weight drops, positive reinforcers will gradually be removed until the weight gain is re-established. In such a program, negative reinforcers, such as tube feeding, may also be built in. As mentioned above, however, it is well recognized that these negative reinforcers are much less effective than the positive reinforcers.

Different mixtures of behavior modification techniques are required for different disorders. For example, a similar program to the one above, but involving a different schedule of reinforcers and different targets might be appropriate for the obese patient. Behavior modification programs for patients with substance abuse are more likely to stress teaching the patient the various stimuli that tend to trigger cravings, such as diminishing the pent-up irritation of a long day at work by dropping by the bar and socializing with "the boys." The patient would be taught instead to substitute other positive reinforcers in their place, such as dropping by an exercise spa and releasing hostility by hitting a punching bag or some other enjoyable form of physical activity, followed by drinking copious amounts of a favorite nonalcoholic beverage with a new set of friends developed through contacts with Alcoholics Anonymous (AA).

Combining Therapies

Originally, proponents of behavior therapy were "purists," and they tended to denigrate the admixture of other types of psychotherapy or the use of medications. Increasingly, however, various types of therapy may be combined. Thus, the treatment of panic disorder and agoraphobia may involve the use of antidepressants or alprazolam along with systematic desensitization. Behavior therapy may also be combined with psychodynamic psychotherapy; for example, a patient with anorexia nervosa may benefit from a behavior modification program and from efforts to help her understand the underlying fears that make her seek a bodily appearance that most people find quite unattractive. A patient with comorbid anxiety and depression may benefit from a program of relaxation training, cognitive therapy, and antidepressant medication.

Cognitive Therapy

The theoretical support for cognitive therapy derives from various sources, including cognitive psychology, Freudian psychodynamic theory, and some aspects of behaviorism. The theory and techniques of cognitive therapy have been developed principally by Aaron Beck. The techniques of cognitive therapy are based on the assumption that "cognitive structures" or "schemata" shape the way people react and adapt to a variety of situations that they encounter in their lives. An individual's particular cognitive structures derive from various constitutional and experiential factors (e.g., physical appearance, loss of a parent early in life, previous achievements or failures at school or with friends); each person has his own specific set of cognitive structures that determines how he will react to any given stressor in any particular situation. A person develops a psychiatric syndrome, such as anxiety or depression, when these schemata become overactive and predispose him to developing a pathological or negative response.

The most widespread use of cognitive therapy is for the treatment of depression. In this instance, the individual is typically found to have schemata that lead to negative interpretations. Beck has designated the three major cognitive patterns observed in depression as the *cognitive triad*. These consist of a negative view of oneself, a negative interpretation of experience, and a negative view of the future. Patients with these cognitive patterns are predisposed to react to situations by interpreting them in the light of these three negative sets. For example, a woman who has applied for a highly competitive job and not received it, and whose perceptions are shaped by such negative sets, may conclude, "I didn't get it because I'm not really bright, in spite of my good school record, and the employer was able to figure that out" (negative view of self). "Trying to find a decent job is so hopeless that I might as well just give up trying" (negative view of experience). "I'm always going to be a failure. I'll never succeed at anything" (negative view of the future).

The techniques of cognitive therapy focus on teaching patients new ways to change these pathological schemata. Cognitive therapy tends to be relatively short-term and highly structured. Its goal is to help patients restructure negative cognitions so that they can perceive reality in a less distorted way and learn to react accordingly.

The actual practice of cognitive therapy combines a group of behavior techniques with a group of cognitive restructuring techniques. The behavior techniques include various homework assignments and a graded program of activities designed to teach patients that their negative schemata are incorrect and that they are in fact able to achieve small successes and interpret them as such. For example, the woman described above who failed to obtain the job might be asked to keep a record of her daily activities during the course of a week. Together, therapist and patient would then review this diary and (in the context of other information about her) develop a set of assignments to be completed during the next week. The diary of activities might indicate a very limited range of social contacts, based on the patient's fear and expectation of rejection. The patient might be assigned to make at least five social contacts during the course of the week by talking to neighbors, phoning friends, and going out on at least one social engagement. These activities would also be recorded in a diary and reviewed the following week with the therapist, including the patient's notes about her responses to the various contacts. She would be helped to see that she tended to initiate each contact with a negative hypothesis or expectation, which typically was disconfirmed by her actual experience. Instead of experiencing rejection, the contacts were largely affirmative. As therapy progresses, and confidence builds, the assignments are gradually made more difficult, until the patient has achieved an essentially normal level of behavior and expectation. The diary serves as a comforting reminder to the patient that, based on past experience, negative hypotheses are typically disconfirmed. The patient will, of course, have some negative experiences; the therapist will also assist in her understanding that such negative experiences are not a consequence of her own deficiencies and that even negative experiences can be surmounted.

These behavior techniques are complemented with various cognitive techniques that assist the patient in identifying and correcting the dysfunctional schemata

Table 23-3.   Typical cognitive distortions treated through cognitive therapy

Distortion	Definition
Arbitrary inference	Drawing an erroneous conclusion from an experience
Selective abstraction	Taking a detail out of context and using it to denigrate the entire experience
Overgeneralization	Making general conclusions about overall experiences and relationships based on a single instance
Magnification and minimization	Altering the significance of specific events in a way that is structured by negative interpretations
Personalization	Interpreting events as reflecting on the patient when they have no relationship to him or her
Dichotomous thinking	Seeing things in an all-or-none way

that shape the patient's perception of reality. These techniques involve identifying various cognitive distortions that the patient is prone to make and "automatic thoughts" that intrude into the patient's consciousness and produce negative attitudes. Six typical cognitive distortions, identified by Beck, are listed in Table 23-3.

Arbitrary inference involves drawing an erroneous conclusion from an experience. For example, if the patient's hairdresser suggests that she may want to try a new hairstyle, the patient assumes that the hairdresser believes she is becoming older-appearing and unattractive. *Selective abstraction* involves taking a detail out of context and using it to denigrate the entire experience. For example, while playing tennis, the patient may hit the ball out of the court, losing it in a grassy area, and reach the conclusion: "That just proves I'm a lousy tennis player." *Overgeneralization* involves making general conclusions about overall experiences and relationships based on a single interaction. For example, after a disagreement with another employee at his current (less desirable) job, the patient concludes: "I'm a failure. I can't get along with anybody." *Magnification* and *minimization* involve altering the significance of specific small events in a way that is structured by negative interpretations. For example, the significance of a success may be minimized (e.g., a good grade on an exam is considered to be trivial because the exam was easy), and the significance of a failure is maximized (e.g., losing a tennis game is seen as indicating that the patient will never succeed at anything). *Personalization* involves interpreting events as reflecting on the patient herself when they in fact have no specific relationship to her. For example, a frown from a grouchy traffic policeman is seen as a recognition of the patient's overall lack of skill as a driver and general worthlessness. *Dichotomous thinking* represents a tendency to see things in an all-or-none way. For example, an A student with high expectations receives a B in a course and concludes: "That just proves it. I'm really a terrible student after all."

In addition to these erroneous interpretations, patients are also often troubled with various *automatic thoughts* that spontaneously intrude into their flow of consciousness. The specific automatic thoughts vary from one individual to another, but involve negative themes of self-denigration and failure (e.g., "You're so stupid," "You never do anything right," or "People wouldn't want to talk to you"). These thoughts intrude spontaneously and produce an accompanying dysphoric affect. Patients are encouraged to identify these automatic thoughts and to learn ways to counteract them. Such techniques include replacing them with counterthoughts that are positive, testing the beliefs that are expressed in the thoughts through behavior techniques described above, and identifying and testing the assumptions behind the thoughts.

The goal of the cognitive component of cognitive therapy is to identify and restructure the various negative schemata that shape patients' perceptions. This approach is achieved in a manner analogous to the behavior techniques. Patients are encouraged to do homework, to complete assignments in which they identify the occurrence of dysfunctional cognitions, and to steadily test and correct them. The therapist will also review these aspects of patients' diaries and help them identify an organized program for restructuring cognitive sets, providing ample empathy and positive reinforcement.

Cognitive therapy is particularly effective for patients suffering from depression. Its techniques can also be adapted to treat the broad range of anxiety disorders through identifying cognitive schemata characterized by fear. It may either be used alone for the treatment of relatively mild psychopathology or in conjunction with medications for patients with more severe disorders.

Individual Psychotherapy

The term *individual psychotherapy* covers a broad range of psychotherapeutic techniques, including behavior therapy and cognitive therapy, which are usually done individually (i.e., a single therapist working with a single patient). It also includes individual psychodynamic psychotherapy, the historical roots of which derive from Freudian psychodynamic approaches. In addition, however, simpler, briefer approaches to individual psychotherapy have been developed, which may draw either directly or indirectly on psychodynamic approaches. At present, there are countless "schools of psychotherapy" that offer a variety of approaches. The student with particular interest in this topic can easily spend years learning about its various aspects. The description below is designed to provide a very simple and selective overview of this complex topic.

Classical Psychoanalysis and Psychodynamic Psychotherapy

Psychoanalysis was originally developed by Freud during the early 20th century. The technique arose originally from Freud's experience in attempting to treat patients with hysterical conversion symptoms, such as pains and paralyses. Following the lead of Charcot, his initial efforts involved the use of hypnosis. He observed, however, that this treatment was not always effective and that there was a high recurrence and relapse rate. He began to suspect that these conversion symptoms reflected some sort of painful early psychological experience that had been repressed. Instead of hypnosis, he began to experiment with the technique of having the patient lie down and relax while he placed his hand on her forehead and encouraged her to talk about whatever came into her mind and to release the repressed thoughts.

This treatment was developed at a time when Victorian puritanism and hypocrisy still reigned supreme, and even Freud must have been astonished at the thoughts that flowed from his patients' minds, covering a variety of sexual fantasies and experiences. Based on his many years of experience applying this approach, initially to conversion symptoms, but subsequently to a broad range of symptoms including anxiety disorders and even psychoses, Freud developed a systematic theory to describe the structure and operations of the human psyche. Basic concepts include stages of psychosexual development (oral, anal, phallic, and genital), the structure of conscious and unconscious thoughts (primary versus secondary process thinking), the structure of drives and motivations (id, ego, and superego), the symbolism inherent in dreams, theories of infant sexuality, and a host of other concepts that the lay person associates with "Freudianism."

Subsequent psychoanalysts have elaborated and modified Freud's original work in various ways, such as the development of theories of ego psychology, or expanding understanding of the mental mechanisms involved in defense, coping, and adaptation. These various ideas and theories are major resources for clinicians trained in either psychoanalysis or psychodynamic psychotherapy. Use of these approaches requires extensive experience and training under the supervision of a qualified psychoanalyst.

Classical psychoanalysis at present is used only in relatively special situations and settings. The form of treatment is best adapted to individuals who are fundamentally healthy and who have sufficient adaptive resources to go through the intensive process of self-scrutiny required by psychoanalysis. Typical reasons for seeking psychoanalysis include difficulties in relationships or persistent and recurrent anxiety, although neither should be so severe as to be incapacitating.

The core component of classical psychoanalysis is the development of a transference neurosis. That is, the patient transfers to the therapist all the thoughts and feelings that he experienced during early life; through this transference, he is able to make conscious the various unconscious drives and emotions that are troubling him and ultimately to modify and heal them, as the analyst makes appropriate "interpretations" during the course of the psychoanalysis. The patient is typically asked to lie on a couch and to free-associate, saying whatever comes into his mind without any type of censorship. The analyst sits behind the patient, remaining a relatively shadowy and neutral figure in order to encourage the development of transference. (If the analyst becomes too human or "real," then transference cannot develop.) To maintain an appropriate level of intensity, the patient must be seen four to five times per week for 50-minute sessions. The process typically requires 2–3 years. Because the analyst becomes a repository of large quantities of intimate and highly personal information, it is essential that she be both psychologically and ethically trustworthy. Analysts must go through an extensive period of psychoanalysis themselves to understand their own psychological vulnerabilities, and in particular the nature of the countertransference that they are likely to develop in relation to their patients.

Psychodynamic psychotherapy employs many of the concepts embodied in psychoanalytic theory, but these concepts are used in ways that make them more suitable for the treatment of larger numbers of patients. Treatment is not necessarily less intensive, in the sense of attempting to focus on and correct problems, but it does not involve the relatively rigidly defined techniques (e.g., use of the couch) that characterize classical psychoanalysis.

Psychodynamic psychotherapy is used to treat patients with a broad variety of problems, including personality disorders, sexual dysfunctions, somatoform disorders, anxiety disorders, and mild depression. Psychodynamic psychotherapy is typically conducted face-to-face. Depending on the frequency and duration of therapy, a transference neurosis may or may not occur. The therapist attempts to help the patient in a neutral but empathic way. The patient is encouraged to review early relationships with parents and significant others, but may also focus on the here and now. As in classical psychoanalysis, the patient is expected to do the bulk of the talking, while the psychodynamic psychotherapist occasionally interjects clarifications to assist the patient in understanding the underlying dynamics that shape his behavior. Psychodynamic psychotherapy typically involves sessions from one to two times a week and may involve 2–5 years of treatment.

Insight-Oriented and Relationship Psychotherapy

Insight-oriented psychotherapy and relationship psychotherapy are two other variants of psychotherapy that may be somewhat less intensive or long-term.

Insight-oriented psychotherapy draws on many basic psychodynamic concepts, but focuses even more on interpersonal relationships and here-and-now situations than does purely psychodynamic psychotherapy. Patients are typically seen once a week for 50 minutes, and during the sessions, they are encouraged to review and discuss relationships, attitudes toward themselves, and early life experiences. The therapist maintains an involved and supportive attitude and occasionally assists patients with interpretations that will help them achieve insights. This form of psychotherapy does not encourage transference, regression, and abreaction. Instead of reexperiencing and reliving, patients are encouraged to achieve an intellectual understanding about the mainsprings of their behavior that will assist them in changing it as needed.

In *relationship psychotherapy*, the therapist assumes a more active role. The stress is on achieving a "corrective emotional experience," with the therapist serving as a loving and trustworthy surrogate parent who assists the patient in confronting unrecognized needs and unresolved drives.

The patient is typically seen once per week, and the therapy may last from 6 months to several years, depending on the patient's problems and level of maturity. As in insight-oriented psychotherapy, the content of the sessions focuses primarily on current situations and relationships, with some looking backward to early life experiences. Although the patient may achieve insight, the most important component of this type of psychotherapy is provided through the empathic and caring attitude of the therapist.

Supportive Psychotherapy

Supportive psychotherapy is used to help patients get through difficult situations. Components of supportive psychotherapy may be incorporated into any of the other types of psychotherapy described above or below, with the exception of classical psychoanalysis.

In conducting supportive psychotherapy, the therapist maintains an attitude of sympathy, interest, and concern. Patients describe and discuss the various problems that they are confronting, which could range from marital discord through psychotic experiences such as persecutory delusions. Supportive psychotherapy is appropriate for the broad spectrum of psychiatric disorders, ranging from adjustment disorders through the psychoses and even dementia or delirium.

As in relationship psychotherapy, the therapist may function much like a healthy and loving parent who provides the patient with encouragement and direction as needed. The goal of supportive therapy is to help patients cope with difficult situations, experiences, or periods of adjustment. Patients typically describe their problems, and the therapist counters with encouragement or even specific advice. The therapist may suggest specific techniques that patients can use in coping with their problems, such as developing new interests or hobbies, trying new activities that may expand range of social contacts, achieving emancipation from parents by moving into independent living circumstances, or developing more organized study habits to improve school performance. The psychotic patient may be taught to refrain from discussing delusional ideas, except to the therapist. The alcoholic patient may receive praise and encouragement for "staying dry," while also receiving suggestions about ways to increase self-esteem by achieving mastery and control, such as through improving skills in a particular sport, or developing a new creative hobby. As the above examples indicate, the clinician involved in conducting supportive therapy needs to tailor the therapy sessions to the individual needs of each particular patient.

Supportive psychotherapy is typically done weekly, often in conjunction with other treatments, particularly the somatic therapies. It may be relatively brief, as when it is used for crisis intervention in adjustment disorders. On the other hand, it may be very long-term, although less frequent than weekly when used as a treatment modality for patients with more chronic or protracted mental illnesses such as schizophrenia, recurrent mania or depression, or various anxiety disorders.

Defense and Coping Mechanisms

Defense and coping mechanisms are techniques that people use to help themselves deal with difficult situations or emotional experiences. These techniques are divided into defense mechanisms (which are considered less mature and more primitive

Table 23-4.   Common defense and coping mechanisms

Defense mechanisms (immature)	Coping mechanisms (mature)
Denial	Sublimation
Projection	Religiosity
Regression	Humor
Repression	Altruism
Splitting	Mastery and control
Reaction formation	
Undoing	
Isolation	
Displacement	

and therefore less healthy) and coping mechanisms (which represent a higher adaptive level and are considered to represent mature ways to cope with life's stresses and problems) (Table 23-4). The clinician can observe these mechanisms in operation in various medical settings, ranging from the emergency room to the recovery room. Understanding these mechanisms assists the clinician in providing most types of psychosocial treatments for psychiatric patients, and in providing general medical care.

Clinicians who do supportive therapy, as well as other therapies that draw on psychodynamic concepts, need to be familiar with various defense and coping mechanisms that patients may use to adapt and survive. Therapy may involve supporting and enhancing healthy and useful mechanisms and assisting the patient in substituting these for less healthy ones.

Defense Mechanisms

Defense mechanisms are used to ward off or avoid painful feelings and thoughts that are difficult to confront. They are usually considered to be neurotic and immature.

Denial is characterized by ignoring an undesirable situation or piece of information and behaving as if it did not exist. For example, a man with established coronary artery disease may insist that he feels fine and refuse to comply with instructions to diet, lose weight, stop smoking, and exercise. A manic patient may refuse to admit the presence of periods of pathological euphoria.

Projection involves attributing to others unwanted ideas or feelings that are experienced within oneself. Archetypally, this mechanism involves attributing to others the negative emotions that one has toward them; for example, a paranoid patient who feels angry with his doctor (an unacceptable emotion) believes instead that the doctor is angry toward him and is tormenting him by insisting that he take medication. On a more everyday level, projection is often seen as a mechanism by which people refuse to accept responsibility for their own mistakes, and instead place the blame on others. For example, a man who is having difficulty at work because of procrastination and failure to meet deadlines says to himself: "It isn't my fault. They're all being too demanding. If only my co-workers would be more helpful, I'd be able to get my work done."

Regression is withdrawal to a more primitive level of adaptation in response to some overwhelming stressor. For example, a woman with a mild dementia may be able to cope at a minimal but acceptable level, but regresses into an infantile state characterized by inability to feed herself or maintain her toilet habits when confronted with the death of the husband who has supported her for the past 50 years. A 40-year-old woman in intensive psychotherapy may relate to her therapist in a childlike dependent way, treating the therapist as if he is a father (a regression that may be appropriate in the context of intensive psychodynamic therapy).

Repression involves suppressing from awareness emotions and memories that are experienced as painful. For example, a patient dying from cancer may go through a period when he feels quite cheerful, even though he is consciously aware that his illness is terminal, simply because he feels an uncontrollable need to ward off the recognition of his inevitable and impending death.

Splitting involves keeping emotions and past experiences in stereotyped univalent "logic-tight compartments," preventing recognition and integration of the nuances and complexities of relationships and experiences. For example, a woman who feels angry with her mother for divorcing her father and remarrying may be unable to develop a much-needed reconciliation, because she has "split away" the "good affects" (based on the genuine periods of happiness that she shared with her mother) and can recognize only the "bad affects" of anger and estrangement.

Reaction formation involves substituting an opposite attitude and experience for one that is experienced as psychologically painful. For example, a patient with hemophilia may take up motorcycle racing and skydiving as a way of counteracting the painful fact of his disease. A patient with obsessive-compulsive personality disorder, who feels angry that his meticulousness and diligence are not recognized by his boss, may maintain an air of affection and cheerfulness toward the boss.

Undoing involves the substitution of one behavior for another, in an effort to change or modify the initial behavior. It is particularly common in obsessive-compulsive disorder and is thought to reflect the patient's basic ambivalence and indecisiveness. For example, a person may become angry with a supervisor or teacher and reflect this anger by making a critical comment; then later he may try to "undo" this behavior by performing an opposite one, such as giving the supervisor or teacher a small gift or praising him in some way.

Isolation (intellectualization) is a defense technique for coping with painful affects; the affect is separated from its content, often by treating it objectively rather than experientially. Thus, a patient who is prone to experience intense anxiety about some topic, such as sexuality or emotional intimacy, will avoid placing himself in situations where he will be forced to confront this anxiety. Instead, he may pursue research on the mating habits of frogs or bees. In a clinical therapy setting, this defense is most commonly noted when the patient talks about problems in an intellectual, overabstract manner and has difficulty describing, recalling, or experiencing actual feelings.

Displacement involves the resolution of a conflict about some particular relationship or event by shifting the emotion attached to it onto some other relationship or event. For example, a woman who feels intense anger toward her father or her husband because of neglect or mistreatment may direct her anger toward her young male child (or even her female child), because she feels unable to express it directly to her husband or father because she perceives them as more powerful.

Coping Mechanisms

Coping mechanisms are considered to be on a somewhat higher adaptational level. Although these may also be mechanisms that ward off unpleasant or unconscious emotions and experiences, they are usually productive and helpful to both the patient and those around him.

Sublimation involves using past experiences or emotions that are traumatic or unpleasant or basic "id drives" in a way that is both anxiety reducing and not injurious to society. For example, a person with high levels of sexual energy may choose to work long hours.

Religiosity involves making painful past experiences more acceptable by experiencing them as part of God's will; for example, a dying patient may come to terms with her impending death by seeing it as simply part of a universal pattern ordained by God.

Humor involves counteracting painful affects by countering them with their alternative and seeing the comic side of the human situation; sometimes the comedy may be "black," but other times it may be light and positive. Making jokes in the anatomy lab, the operating room, or the military trenches are all examples.

Altruism involves taking a negative experience and turning it into a socially useful or positive one. For example, a reformed alcoholic patient may obtain great satisfaction by helping others in the context of Alcoholics Anonymous.

Mastery and control involve gaining a sense of control over a painful situation by confronting it directly and developing techniques that prevent the person from feeling overwhelmed. For example, a medical student confronted with an enormous mass of information and responsibility (which makes her feel psychologically threatened and powerless) will throw herself intensively into her work, eventually reducing anxiety and increasing sense of self-worth and internal strength by learning as much as she can. Some individuals choose to go into medicine as a way of gaining mastery and control: having experienced illness or death within their immediate family, they may seek to gain control over it by choosing a profession that works toward reducing illness and death.

Group Therapy

Whereas most of the above types of psychosocial therapy derived originally from a theoretical or conceptual framework, group therapy derives largely from practical considerations, although it is not without theoretical underpinnings. Group therapy provides a highly effective way for clinicians to follow and monitor relatively large numbers of patients. It also provides patients with a social environment or even surrogate peer group that will help them learn new and constructive ways to interact with others in a controlled and supportive environment.

There are many different kinds of group therapy. The types vary depending on the individuals who compose the group, the problems or disorders that they are confronting, the setting in which the group meets, the type of role that the group leader takes, and the therapeutic goals that have been established.

In many hospital settings, a group therapy program is established for inpatients. Such groups are typically led by a physician, nurse, social worker, or some combination thereof. In very large inpatient hospital settings, several groups may run concurrently and be composed of patients with similar types of problems. For example, one group might consist of relatively high-functioning individuals with personality problems or depression. Another group might consist of patients with severe mood and psychotic disorders, and yet another group might consist of individuals with eating disorders. Such groups provide patients with a forum to share their problems, diminish their sense of isolation and loneliness, learn new techniques to cope with their problems either through other patients or through the group leader, and provide support, inspiration, and hope. Such groups may also assist patients in improving interpersonal and social skills; for example, patients with schizophrenia and other psychoses may improve their social skills in relating to others, while patients with personality disorders may receive useful feedback from other group members concerning behavior that is counterproductive.

In many clinical settings, such inpatient groups are supplemented by outpatient or aftercare groups in which patients receive continued follow-up, pursuing goals similar to those described above, but in the more stressful environment of the "real world." These outpatient groups represent an attempt to consolidate and support the learning and skills that have already been developed in the inpatient setting.

Some groups are oriented largely toward providing support. Such groups may or may not have a professional leader. Examples of such support groups include Alcoholics Anonymous, family support groups such as those organized by chapters of the Alliance for the Mentally Ill (AMI; an organization composed of the family members of patients with serious mental illnesses), support groups for individuals who conceive of themselves as minorities in a particular setting (e.g., female professionals, female medical students, black students), groups composed of Vietnam veterans, or groups composed of individuals who have experienced some serious medical illness or difficult surgery (e.g., patients with diabetes, women who have experienced mastectomies, individuals receiving dialysis). Such groups provide a forum for sharing information, with members giving one another encouragement and support and instilling hope through diminishing feelings of isolation.

Groups are also constituted to conduct group psychotherapy. Such groups are typically under the leadership of a therapist with extensive experience in group psychotherapy, often conducted with a cotherapist. These groups aim to achieve goals similar to those of insight-oriented or interpersonal psychotherapy, but within the context of a group setting. Psychotherapy groups are typically more highly structured than the other types of groups described earlier. The group leaders will take an active role in organizing each session, will often prescribe exercises within the session, will establish ground rules for membership within the group (e.g., no tardiness, regular attendance), will resolve conflicts between members of the group, and will assume responsibility for providing summaries of each session and access to videotapes of the sessions. Patients are typically carefully screened before being admitted to a psychotherapy group, to ensure that they will be able to participate at an effective level. Such groups are particularly helpful for individuals suffering from the same sorts of problems that lead them into individual psychotherapy, such as interpersonal and relationship problems, anxiety, mild depression, and personality disorders.

Yalom, one of the major leaders of the group therapy movement in the United States, has enumerated various factors that summarize the therapeutic mechanisms that occur during the process of group therapy. These include instilling hope, developing socializing skills, imitative behavior, catharsis, interpersonal learning, imparting of information, behaving altruistically through attempting to help other members of the group, experiencing a corrective recapitulation of the primary family group, developing a sense of group cohesiveness, diminishing feelings of isolation ("universality"), and learning through feedback how one's behavior affects others ("interpersonal learning").

Marital Therapy and Family Therapy

Some problems for which patients seek treatment clearly also involve other people. A man may present with feelings of depression and inadequacy because his wife has returned to work and is requesting that he assume his "fair share" of household duties and child care, a situation that he finds demeaning and inappropriate. A young teenager may present with mild symptoms of "acting-out" behavior, such as truancy from school and experimenting with alcohol, and indicate that he is seeking support from peers because he is having difficulty coping with his parents' inappropriately high expectations and overprotective "smothering." In such situations, although the patient may come in initially as an "individual case," the clinician will usually rapidly assess the need for seeing the patient within the context of the larger family unit, which might be husband and wife in the first example (marital counseling) or the parents and child in the second (family therapy).

Marital counseling and family therapy may be done by psychiatrists, but are also often done by psychologists, social workers, or nurses. Depending on the specific problems of the presenting individual, family therapy or marital counseling may be done in addition to individual therapy and medication management. Both of these types of therapy are usually relatively short-term, lasting from weeks to months, and both are oriented toward identifying and resolving specific and clearly identifiable problems as quickly as possible. All physicians should have at least a superficial familiarity with these types of therapy, since they must recognize that nearly all their patients live within the context of a family. In specific instances, the internist, pediatrician, or family physician will need to recognize the need for family therapy or marital counseling and refer the patient appropriately (usually through an additional screening and assessment by a psychiatrist, who will evaluate the need for a referral or will conduct the treatment herself).

Marital Therapy

Marital therapy involves seeing a husband and wife (or in contemporary society, an unmarried or homosexual couple) in order to help them stabilize and improve their relationship. Depending on the commitment of the two partners, there are many variations to marital therapy. Ideally, both partners are willing and cooperative participants who are anxious to initiate change. Sometimes, however, seeking marital therapy has been precipitated by a crisis; one of the partners may have lost interest in the relationship (and may or may not want to "get out"), whereas the other is hanging on tight and trying to "save" the relationship. In this instance, one possible outcome might be the eventual decision to end the relationship, and therapy might turn into divorce mediation and counseling; if children are involved, what began as marital therapy might turn into family therapy as the couple attempts to work out an equitable arrangement in the context of the larger number of people who will be affected. In some instances, a dysfunctional sexual relationship between the couple will become apparent, and the couple may wish referral to a sex therapy clinic for treatment of impotence or anorgasmia.

An individual conducting marital therapy must take care to maintain an atmosphere of fairness, neutrality, and impartiality. Either of the partners will be particularly sensitive to the possibility that the therapist may "take sides" and treat him or her unfairly. The sex of the therapist may seem quite significant to either of the partners, even though the therapist may feel quite comfortable with his or her ability to be impartial. The women's movement has left both achievements and scars in its wake, sometimes causing individuals to conceptualize members of the opposite sex as potentially "the enemy." Women may feel that only a female therapist is able to understand their point of view and feel quite defensive if asked to work with a male therapist. Male partners may have similar attitudes or problems.

Marital counseling typically begins with identifying the specific problem. Each partner is asked to identify specific areas in which he or she would like to see change in the other. The therapist attempts to assist the couple in implementing changes in a gradual, graded way, attacking one problem at a time. Typically, in the early sessions, a single, salient problem is the focus of attention. For example, a wife may express feelings of being ignored, whereas a husband may complain of his wife's whining expressions of dependence. Each will identify specific target behaviors in the other that are in need of modification. They then contract with one another to modify these behaviors. Subsequent marital sessions focus on the steps that they have taken to achieve improvement and continuing work on additional new areas of concern that arise.

Graded behavior change of this type is the minimum component of marital therapy. Often couples will benefit as well from discussing their hopes and expectations of one another in the context of personal values, prior family experiences (i.e., role expectations about men and women, based on the behavior of their own parents), changing social norms about the roles of men and women, and needs for both intimacy and independence that occur within the context of male-female relationships.

Family Therapy

Family therapy tends to focus on the larger family unit—at a minimum, one parent and a child (in single-parent families), but more typically both parents (or a parent and stepparent, two separated parents, or other parental pairings depending on the family environment in which the child lives) and the child or one or several parents and the child plus siblings. Typically the "child" is brought in initially for treatment of a specific problem, such as school difficulties, hyperactivity, delinquency, or aggressive behavior. Often, it rapidly becomes clear that these problems exist in the overall context of the family setting. The family should not necessarily be regarded as dysfunctional, but because of changing circumstances or demands, the parents may have difficulty in determining methods for coping with the child's behavior or understanding why it is occurring.

As in marital therapy, it is important for the therapist to be fair and impartial in family therapy. In this instance, however, the therapist is not dealing with two potential equals, but rather a hierarchy in which parents are expected to assume some authority and responsibility for the behavior of their child. The degree of hierarchy will vary, depending on the age of the child, and for adolescents and teenagers one important problem may be the challenge that the child's growing independence is adding to this hierarchical structure.

As in marital therapy, behavioral approaches are a mainstay for family therapy. The therapist usually begins by focusing on here-and-now problems. Parents and child discuss openly the nature of the problem that has brought about the need for therapy. For example, a 12-year-old boy may be intermittently truant from school, tell lies about his activities, and seek out parties on the weekends where he has been known to drink beer occasionally. The child may complain of parental pressure and repeated criticism, whereas the parents express their fears about the child's unreliability and his poor school performance. As in marital therapy, graded areas of priority are identified and contracts made involving changes that both parents and child will implement. Parents are given tactful but explicit suggestions about the value of positive reinforcement instead of criticism as a way of modifying behavior, while the child is led to realize that some hierarchy and structure will remain in his life, although to a gradually lessening degree as he demonstrates mature and dependable behavior.

Family therapy may also be used as a means of helping families in which at least one member has a relatively serious mental illness, such as schizophrenia, mania, or recurrent depression. In this type of family therapy, it is important to work firmly within the medical model and to emphasize that the patient has an illness for which neither he nor the family can be considered responsible. This approach minimizes guilt, scapegoating, and castigation, and it permits both patient and family members to seek methods for coping with the symptoms of the illness that may be more consoling and constructive. A young schizophrenic patient living at home may need some assistance from his family in the development of social skills (see social skills training below), whereas family members may need assistance in learning ways to cope with outbursts of anger or periods of emotional disengagement and withdrawal. Families with high levels of involvement (referred to as high "expressed emotion") may need counseling on ways of being less intensely involved because it has been shown that in some instances high expressed emotion may be experienced as stressful by the schizophrenic patient and lead to relapse. Thus, families may need assistance in finding the right balance between providing needed support and encouragement and setting excessively high expectations. Education about the symptoms of the illness is also an important component of family therapy for both patient and family members.

Social Skills Training

Social skills training is a specific type of psychotherapy that focuses primarily on developing abilities in relating to others and in coping with the demands of daily life. It is used primarily for patients with severe mental illnesses such as schizophrenia, which are often accompanied by marked impairments in social skills.

Social skills training may be done initially on an inpatient basis, but the bulk of the effort is typically done with outpatients, because the long-term goal of social skills training is to assist patients in learning to live in the "real world." Social skills training is typically done by nurses, social workers, or psychologists. It may be done individually, but more typically is accompanied with some group work as well, and it may occur in the context of day hospitals or sheltered workshops.

The techniques of social skills training are also primarily behavioral. Specific problems are identified and addressed in a sequentially integrated manner. Severely handicapped patients may need assistance initially in grooming and hygiene. They may need encouragement in learning to shave and bathe daily, to keep their clothes laundered, or to eat regular meals. They may also need help in learning how to approach other people and to talk with them appropriately. At higher levels of functioning, patients may need assistance in learning how to apply for a job, complete job interviews, or relate to employers and co-workers. Because long-term institutional care is no longer available to most patients with psychotic illnesses, these individuals are literally being forced to learn to live in the community. Many cannot do so without receiving training and assistance in activities of daily living, such as grooming, managing money, or achieving at least a minimal level of social interaction with others. Although the development of such skills may seem elementary or minimal, for some patients it can lead to a substantial improvement in their quality of life.

Bibliography

Beck AT, Rush AJ, Shaw BF, et al: Cognitive Therapy of Depression. New York, Guilford, 1979

Beck AT, Emery G, Greenberg BL: Anxiety Disorders and Phobias: A Cognitive Perspective. New York, Basic Books, 1985

Bowen M: Family Therapy in Clinical Practice. New York, Jason Aronson, 1978

Corsini RJ (ed): Current Psychotherapies, 3rd Edition. Itasca, IL, FE Peacock, 1984

Davanloo H (ed): Short-term Dynamic Psychotherapy. New York, Jason Aronson, 1980

Fenichel O: The Psychoanalytic Theory of Neurosis. New York, WW Norton, 1945

Freud A: The Ego and the Mechanisms of Defense. New York, International Universities Press, 1965

Freud S: The dynamics of transference (1912), in the Standard Edition of the Complete Psychological Works of Sigmund Freud, Vol 12. Translated and edited by Strachey J. London, Hogarth Press, 1958, pp 97–108

Freud S: On beginning the treatment (1913), in the Standard Edition of the Complete Psychological Works of Sigmund Freud, Vol 12. Translated and edited by Strachey J. London, Hogarth Press, 1958, pp 121–144

Leff J, Vaughan C: Expressed Emotion in Families. New York, Brunner/Mazel, 1979

Nichols M: Family Therapy: Concepts and Methods. New York, Gardner Press, 1984

Satir V: Conjoint Family Therapy. Palo Alto, CA, Science and Behaviour Books, 1967

Vaillant GE: Theoretical hierarchy of adaptive ego mechanisms. Arch Gen Psychiatry 24:107–118, 1971

Vaillant GE: Adaptation to Life. New York, Little, Brown, 1977

Vaillant GE: An empirically derived hierarchy of adaptive mechanisms and its usefulness as a potential diagnostic axis, in Diagnosis and Classification in Psychiatry: A Critical Appraisal of DSM-III. Edited by Tischler G. New York, Cambridge University Press, 1987, pp 464–476

Vaillant GE, Bond M, Vaillant CO: An empirically validated hierarchy of defense mechanisms. Arch Gen Psychiatry 43:786–794, 1986

Weiner M: Practical Psychotherapy. New York, Brunner/Mazel, 1986

Yalom ID: Inpatient Group Psychotherapy. New York, Basic Books, 1980

Yalom ID: The Theory and Practice of Group Psychotherapy, 3rd Edition. New York, Basic Books, 1985

Self-assessment Questions

1. What is the difference between classical conditioning and operant conditioning?
2. What is the definition of a positive reinforcer? a negative reinforcer?
3. Describe four common techniques for conducting behavior therapy.
4. Describe cognitive therapy. What is the cognitive triad? What are "automatic thoughts"?

5. Describe classical psychoanalysis. How does it differ from psychodynamic psychotherapy? What is transference?
6. Describe the concept of a "corrective emotional experience" in psychotherapy.
7. Describe two different types of group therapy and enumerate some situations in which they would be appropriate.
8. Describe the role of the therapist in marital and family therapy.

Chapter 24
Somatic Treatments

The desire to take medicine is perhaps the greatest feature which distinguishes man from animals.

Sir William Osler

The modern treatment era in psychiatry began with the introduction of effective psychotropic medication in the early 1950s. Until that time, the mainstay of treatment had been psychotherapy, although prefrontal leukotomy and electroconvulsive therapy (ECT) had been recently introduced and were each accompanied by the excitement that any new treatment generates. Their limitations soon became apparent, and, in fact, after the introduction of antipsychotics and antidepressants, leukotomy fell into disuse, and the use of ECT became limited to a relatively small group of patients with severe illnesses (e.g., major depression).

Before the availability of these new somatic treatments, psychiatrists were greatly limited in their ability to help patients, and overcrowded mental hospitals were common. The introduction of medication revolutionized psychiatry and led to the era of deinstitutionalization, a period in which mental patients were released from state hospitals in large numbers to be cared for in the community. The wisdom of this movement is now being critically assessed.

Antipsychotics

Chlorpromazine was first introduced in 1952 by two French psychiatrists, Jean Delay and Pierre Deniker, after it had become clear that the drug had powerful

475

calming effects on agitated psychotic patients. Delay and Deniker soon discovered that the drug was especially effective in patients suffering from schizophrenia. Not only were agitated schizophrenic patients calmed, but the new drug seemed to eradicate or markedly diminish their terrifying hallucinations and troubling delusional thoughts.

Since chlorpromazine was introduced, many antipsychotics have been developed and marketed. Antipsychotics, with minor exceptions, are similar in action and efficacy and differ primarily in their side effects and potency. Antipsychotics ameliorate the symptoms of psychotic illnesses including hallucinations, delusions, bizarre behavior, disordered thinking, and agitation. Although they are collectively referred to as "major tranquilizers," this term is a misnomer because the drugs do not produce a state of tranquility in normal or psychotic persons, and in fact, in normal persons they produce a rather unpleasant state. The term *antipsychotic* is more appropriate in that the drugs are helpful in ameliorating symptoms of psychoses.

Although their use is primarily confined to schizophrenia and related illnesses (e.g., schizophreniform disorder, schizoaffective disorder), antipsychotics are also prescribed to psychotic patients with mood disorders and organic mental disorders. Additionally, antipsychotics have been used to control behavior in mentally retarded patients, patients with borderline personality disorder, and patients with organic disorders. They are also prescribed to patients with Tourette's disorder to diminish the frequency and severity of vocal tics. Because of their ability to induce irreversible neurologic damage (e.g., tardive dyskinesia), other indications requiring nonspecific sedation are probably not appropriate (e.g., generalized anxiety disorder).

There are nine classes of antipsychotic drugs, each differing in molecular structure. The *phenothiazines*, the most important class, have a three-ring nucleus but differ in the side chains that are joined to the nitrogen atom in the middle ring. The three phenothiazine subtypes differ by nature of the side chain, and include the aliphatics (e.g., chlorpromazine), the piperidines (e.g., thioridazine), and the piperazines (e.g., trifluoperazine). Other classes of antipsychotics include the *thioxanthenes* (e.g., thiothixene), the *dibenzoxazepines* (e.g., loxapine), the *butyrophenones* (e.g., haloperidol), the *dihydroindolones* (e.g., molindone), the *dibenzodiazepines* (e.g., clozapine), the *benzamides* (e.g., sulpiride, not available in the United States), the *rauwolfia alkaloids* (e.g., reserpine, no longer used to treat psychoses), and the *diphenylbutylpiperidines* (e.g., pimozide, used to treat Tourette's disorder).

Clozapine may be more effective than other antipsychotics; research has shown that up to 60% of treatment-refractory schizophrenic patients improve when treated with clozapine in trials of 1 year or more. Improvement in these patients may mean that they can be returned to the community and take part in day hospital programs or a sheltered workshop. However, adverse hematologic effects and its expense will limit the usefulness of clozapine.

Mechanism of Action of Antipsychotics

The potency of antipsychotic compounds correlates closely with their affinity for the dopamine 2 (D_2) receptor, blocking the effect of endogenous dopamine at these sites. An exception may be clozapine, which has weak affinity for D_2 receptors. Antipsychotics appear to exert their influence at mesocortical and mesolimbic dopaminergic pathways. Interestingly, although positron-emission tomography (PET) studies have demonstrated that antipsychotics block these receptors almost immediately, onset of antipsychotic action takes weeks to develop. Also, although all antipsychotics block these same receptors, a patient may respond to one antipsychotic but not to another. These observations suggest that antipsychotics have other effects in the brain that may actually be responsible for the antipsychotic action.

Although many side effects of these drugs can be directly attributed to their dopamine-blocking properties (i.e., extrapyramidal side effects, galactorrhea in women), these drugs also block noradrenergic, cholinergic, and histaminic receptors to different degrees, accounting for the unique side-effect profiles of each individual antipsychotic. See Table 24-1 for a comparison of commonly used antipsychotics.

Pharmacokinetics of Antipsychotics

Absorption of orally administered antipsychotics is variable, but clinical effects generally appear within 30–60 minutes. Intramuscular administration usually produces effects within 10 minutes because injectable antipsychotics have much greater bioavailability than oral medication. For example, intramuscular chlorpromazine is 4–10 times more bioavailable than an equivalent oral dose. Metabolism occurs almost entirely in the liver, largely by oxidation, so that these highly lipid-soluble agents are converted to water-soluble metabolites and excreted through the kidneys. Excretion of antipsychotics tends to be slow due to drug accumulation in fatty tissue. Most antipsychotic agents have a half-life of 24 hours or longer and have many active metabolites that have even longer half-lives. This has made it difficult to correlate blood levels with therapeutic response. As a result, no dose-response curve has ever been demonstrated for the antipsychotics. Haloperidol, which has no active metabolites, may have a therapeutic window (i.e., 9–15 ng/ml), however.

Antipsychotics also differ greatly in potency. For example, 100 mg of chlorpromazine is approximately equal therapeutically to 1.6 mg of haloperidol. The relative potency of the antipsychotics is listed in Table 24-1.

Use of Antipsychotics in Acute Psychosis

For the treatment of acute psychosis, a dosage of 300 mg of chlorpromazine (or its equivalent) orally per day is considered a minimal therapeutic dosage for the treatment of psychosis, and peak response usually occurs at 800 mg of chlorpromazine (or its equivalent) per day. Higher dosages do not add to therapeutic response and only increase the likelihood of side effects. In general, the acutely agitated psychotic patient can be started on 100 mg of chlorpromazine (or its equivalent) two or three times daily. The medication is increased at the rate of 100–200 mg of chlorpromazine (or its equivalent) per day to the upper limit of the recommended

Table 24-1. Common antipsychotic agents

Category	Drug (trade name)	Sedative potency	Orthostatic hypotensive potency	Anticholinergic potency	Extrapyramidal potency	Equivalent dosage (mg)	Dosage range (mg/day)
Phenothiazines							
Aliphatics	Chlorpromazine (Thorazine)	High	High	High	Low	100	50–1200
Piperidines	Mesoridazine (Serentil)	High	High	High	Low	50	50–400
	Thioridazine (Mellari)	High	High	Very high	Low	95	50–800
Piperazines	Fluphenazine (Prolixin)	Low	Low	Low	Moderate	2	2–20
	Fluphenazine decanoate	Low	Low	Low	Moderate	a	12.5–50 mg q 2 wk
	Perphenazine (Trilafon)	Low	Low	Low	Moderate	10	12–64
	Trifluoperazine (Stelazine)	Low	Low	Low	Moderate	5	5–40 +
Thioxanthenes	Thiothixene (Navane)	Moderate	Low	Low	High	5	5–60
Dibenzoxazepines	Loxapine (Loxitane)	Moderate	Moderate	Moderate	High	15	20–250
Butyrophenones	Haloperidol (Haldol)	Low	Low	Low	High	1.6	2–100
	Haloperidol decanoate	Low	Low	Low	High	a	50–150 mg q 4 wk
Dihydroindolones	Molindone (Moban)	Low	Low	Low	Low	10	50–400
Dibenzodiazepines	Clozapine (Clozaril)	High	Very high	High	Very low	50	200–900

a Long-acting ester; dosage not directly comparable with that of standard compounds.

dosage range or until intolerable side effects occur. One week after a stable dose is achieved, the medication can be given once daily, usually at bedtime. The uncontrollable patient should be given frequent, equally spaced doses of an antipsychotic every 2 hours until agitation is under control (i.e., "rapid neuroleptization"). Seldom is more than 1.5 g of chlorpromazine (or its equivalent) necessary in a 24-hour period.

In many patients, any improvement may be the result of sedation rather than antipsychotic activity. It may be more rational to sedate acutely psychotic or agitated patients with benzodiazepines to help control their behavior. Antipsychotics should be started simultaneously. Actual antipsychotic effect may take weeks to become apparent.

Maintenance Treatment With Antipsychotics

Once the patient has been stabilized on a dosage of antipsychotic and the target symptoms (e.g., hallucinations, agitation) are under control, the dosage may be gradually reduced to one-half to one-third the maximal dosage, but generally not falling below 300 mg per day of chlorpromazine (or its equivalent). Schizophrenic patients should receive maintenance therapy for at least 1 year after an initial psychotic episode. Chronic schizophrenic patients may need therapy longer, and in some patients, maintenance treatment will be indefinite. However, it is wise to reassess the need for antipsychotic medication every year or so.

An attempt should be made to withdraw the medication slowly (e.g., weeks and months). Should symptoms reoccur, the drug should immediately be reinstituted or the dosage increased. Some patients will remain well for months or years without medication, although controlled studies show that with maintenance treatment, patients are much less likely to relapse. Because the medications have long-acting metabolites, relapse may often not occur for months after the drug is withdrawn. Of course, the patient with tardive dyskinesia, a side effect discussed below, presents special problems, for the treatment of choice is to stop the offending antipsychotic. However, many patients will decompensate without the medication so that they (and their families) may choose to remain on the antipsychotic regardless of the tardive dyskinesia because life may be intolerable without medication. In this situation, there are no simple answers, and patients and their families need to be consulted. Further information about the use of antipsychotics in the treatment of schizophrenia is found in Chapter 7.

There are generally no good reasons to use antipsychotics as maintenance treatment in psychotic mood disorders. Instead, antidepressants or lithium should be used. An occasional patient with a psychotic mood disorder will benefit from continuing antipsychotic treatment, but as this indication has been poorly studied, the decision to use antipsychotics for maintenance will be based on trial and error. These caveats also apply to schizoaffective disorders.

For patients who are unable to take medication on a regular basis or who are noncompliant, long-acting preparations are available (e.g., fluphenazine decanoate, haloperidol decanoate). There is no universally accepted method for converting a patient from oral to long-acting dosage forms, and dosing with sustained-release preparations must be individualized. Usually, patients are started on a dose of 25 mg im fluphenazine decanoate (Prolixin) every 2 weeks or haloperidol decanoate 100 mg im each month, with the dosage being titrated upward or downward based on the patient's therapeutic response and side effects.

Rational use of antipsychotics

---

1. Adequate dosages should produce improvement in 4–6 weeks.
   - Improvement should be monitored by following target symptoms (e.g., hyperactivity, delusions, hostility).
   - If the patient doesn't improve, the dosage should be increased.

2. Each drug trial should last about 3 months.
   - If response is unsatisfactory, even after the dosage increase, then the drug should be discontinued.

3. There is no reason to use combinations of antipsychotics, particularly as combinations will serve to increase side effects without adding to efficacy.

4. Drug holidays, once advocated for reducing risk of tardive dyskinesia, are ineffective and only increase risk of relapse.

5. Because all antipsychotics (except clozapine) are equally effective, choice of drug depends only on side effects.
   - An agitated patient may do best with a sedating antipsychotic (e.g., chlorpromazine); an elderly patient may not tolerate anticholinergic side effects (e.g., with chlorpromazine).

6. Clozapine may benefit treatment-refractory patients, but its use is limited by its tendency to cause agranulocytosis and its cost (estimated at $9,000 per year).

Side Effects of Antipsychotics

Despite their effectiveness in managing psychotic syndromes, antipsychotics have a variety of potentially troublesome side effects. The severity of side effects differs from drug to drug and corresponds to its ability to affect a particular neurotransmitter system (e.g., dopaminergic, noradrenergic, cholinergic, histaminic). Extrapyramidal side effects mediated by dopamine blockade are the most troublesome. The antipsychotic clozapine appears unique in not causing these side effects.

The most dreaded complication of antipsychotics, *tardive dyskinesia,* is untreatable and often irreversible. Elderly patients, women, and patients with mood disorders appear to be more susceptible to developing tardive dyskinesia, and it has been reported to occur in up to 15% of all patients using antipsychotics for more than a year. It is generally advisable to use the lowest effective dosage of antipsychotic medication possible. Tardive dyskinesia consists of abnormal involuntary movements, usually of the mouth and tongue, although other parts of the body may become involved, including the trunk and extremities. In most patients with tardive dyskinesia, the movements are mild and tolerable, but some patients develop a more malignant form of the disorder that may be totally disabling.

Patients on chronic antipsychotic administration should be regularly monitored for the development of tardive dyskinesia. The Abnormal Involuntary Movement Scale (AIMS) has been developed to help clinicians and researchers rate the severity of tardive dyskinesia. A copy of this instrument is included in the Appendix.

Antipsychotic medications are also frequently associated with the development of *pseudoparkinsonism*. Although this side effect may take 3 or more weeks to develop, patients will develop the symptoms of the parkinsonian triad of tremor, rigidity, and hypokinesia. *Akathisia* is another side effect that may not appear immediately but typically has an onset in the first few weeks of treatment with antipsychotics. This condition consists of subjective feelings of anxiety and tension and objective fidgetiness and agitation. Patients will report that they feel compelled to pace, move around in their chairs, or tap their feet. Treatment for both pseudoparkinsonism and akathisia generally consists of reducing the dose of antipsychotic if possible, and/or adding to the medication regimen an antiparkinsonian drug (e.g., benztropine). Amantadine, a drug that potentiates the release of dopamine in the basal ganglia, has also been used to treat pseudoparkinsonism. Akathisia has been treated with beta-blockers (e.g., propranolol 40–160 mg daily in divided doses). Clonidine has also been used to treat akathisia with some success.

Another potential neurologic side effect is the *acute dystonic reaction*, which usually occurs during the first 4 days of treatment with antipsychotics. A dystonia is a sustained contraction of the muscles of the neck, mouth, tongue, or occasionally other muscle groups that is subjectively distressing and often painful. Acute dystonias usually respond dramatically to intravenous benztropine (i.e., 1–2 mg) or diphenhydramine (i.e., 25–50 mg). After the dystonia resolves, a 2-week course of benztropine 2 mg twice a day or another antiparkinsonian agent will usually prevent recurrences. Patients with a history of dystonic reactions can benefit from a week of prophylactic benztropine when restarted on antipsychotics.

The most common cardiovascular effect of the antipsychotics is *postural hypotension*, mediated by alpha-adrenergic blockade. This side effect is caused more frequently by low-potency compounds (e.g., chlorpromazine, thioridazine). Antipsychotics generally do not cause arrhythmogenic effects when used in standard dosages. Thioridazine and pimozide, however, can prolong the Q-T interval and predispose to ventricular tachyarrhythmia.

Low-potency antipsychotics may also induce *seizures*, especially at higher doses (e.g., >1 g chlorpromazine daily), but high-potency drugs (e.g., haloperidol) are usually safe. The drugs are not contraindicated in epileptic patients, as long as they are adequately treated with anticonvulsants.

Agranulocytosis, a side effect associated with the use of low-potency antipsychotics, is rare, and its incidence peaks during the first 2 months of treatment. The best prevention is clinical alertness for the appearance of malaise, fever, or sore throat early in the course of therapy; routine blood counts are usually not necessary. An exception is clozapine, which causes agranulocytosis at a higher rate, usually between weeks 6 and 24 of treatment. Due to this potentially fatal side effect, patients on clozapine must have weekly blood counts.

Other miscellaneous side effects of antipsychotics include nonspecific skin rashes, retinitis pigmentosa (especially with dosages of thioridazine greater than 800 mg per day), fever (with clozapine), pigmentary changes in the skin (i.e., blue, gray, or tan), weight gain, cholestatic jaundice (1% of patients treated with chlorpromazine), reduced libido, and inhibition of ejaculation (especially with thioridazine). Antipsychotics appear to be safe during pregnancy but as a general rule should be avoided if possible.

Antipsychotics commonly cause anticholinergic side effects, particularly low-potency compounds such as chlorpromazine. Anticholinergic side effects include dry mouth, urinary retention, blurry vision, and constipation. Anticholinergics may also exacerbate narrow-angle glaucoma. These side effects are best treated by reducing the dose of medication or switching to a more potent agent (e.g., haloperidol). Antiparkinsonian drugs (e.g., benztropine) used to treat extrapyramidal symptoms can exacerbate these side effects. If urinary retention continues to be a problem, small doses of bethanechol (Urecholine) (i.e., 15 mg three times daily) may help the patient empty his or her bladder more efficiently, and bulk laxatives will be helpful in lessening constipation.

All antipsychotics including clozapine have been reported to lead to the *neuroleptic malignant syndrome* (NMS), a rare idiosyncratic reaction that does not appear to be dose related. Usually considered a medical emergency, the syndrome is characterized by rigidity, high fever, delirium, and marked autonomic instability. There are no pathognomonic laboratory abnormalities, although elevations of creatinine phosphokinase and of liver enzymes are common. The muscle relaxant dantrolene and the dopamine agonist bromocriptine have been used to treat NMS, although some experts believe that merely stopping the offending agent and providing supportive care is just as effective. Although earlier reports suggested an alarming 20% mortality rate, the current estimated rate is about 4%. Once the patient has recovered, antipsychotics may be cautiously reintroduced after a 2-week wait, although an agent from a different antipsychotic class is advisable (e.g., chlorpromazine rather than haloperidol, if haloperidol caused the NMS).

Antidepressants

Not long after chlorpromazine appeared, the antidepressant imipramine was synthesized in an attempt by researchers to find additional compounds for the treatment of schizophrenia. It was soon learned, however, that whereas imipramine had little effect on hallucinations and delusions, it clearly alleviated depression in patients who were both psychotic and depressed. Thus, another class of drugs had been created: the tricyclic antidepressants (TCAs). Other modifications of the three-ring structure followed as other TCAs were produced, including amitriptyline and desipramine.

About the same time TCAs were being discovered, the antidepressant properties of the monoamine oxidase (MAO) inhibitors were being uncovered. In this case, iproniazid, an antibiotic used to treat tuberculosis, was noted to bring relief to depressed tuberculosis patients. Later work showed that the drug was also effective in relieving depression in a broad range of psychiatric patients. Although iproniazid is no longer used as an antidepressant, it has been succeeded by other more effective MAO inhibitors, such as phenelzine and tranylcypromine.

Other antidepressants have since been developed, some of which differ structurally from both the tricyclics and MAO inhibitors. All antidepressants, with minor exceptions, do not differ in efficacy, but differ primarily in their potency and side effects. Three groups of antidepressants are commonly recognized: the TCAs, the MAO inhibitors, and the newer or atypical agents. Although these medications are classified as antidepressants, and all are effective in relieving depressive symptoms, they are used to treat a wide variety of disorders. Hence, the term *antidepressant* is a misnomer.

Indications for Antidepressants

Antidepressants are useful in treating many different psychiatric disorders. The primary indication for antidepressants, however, is the treatment of depressive syndromes. The efficacy of antidepressants is unequivocal, and approximately 70% of patients treated with TCAs and 65% of patients treated with MAO inhibitors will respond to treatment within 6 weeks. (The placebo response rate in depression is approximately 25–40%.) Depressed patients with melancholic symptoms (e.g., diurnal variation, psychomotor agitation or retardation, terminal insomnia, pervasive anhedonia) appear to respond better to antidepressants than depressed patients without these features. Depressions that are secondary (i.e., depressions that follow, or complicate, other psychiatric disorders), accompanied by neurotic features (i.e., anxiety, somatization, hypochondriasis), or accompanied by personality disorders do not respond as well to antidepressants as depressions without these features. Depressed schizophrenic patients also tend not to respond to antidepressants.

Other disorders that are treated with antidepressants include the depressed phase of bipolar disorder, dysthymic disorder, panic disorder and agoraphobia, obsessive-compulsive disorder, selected patients with chronic pain, social phobia, generalized anxiety disorder, and certain childhood conditions (e.g., enuresis, school phobia). Antidepressants can also be used for maintenance therapy in unipolar depression. New indications for antidepressants include the treatment of bulimia and facilitation of withdrawal from cocaine.

MAO inhibitors have been recommended as the treatment of choice in cases of atypical depression. Patients with this condition usually have a mixture of anxiety and depression and often have reversal of diurnal variation (i.e., worse in evening), hypersomnia, mood lability, and hyperphagia. Clomipramine, a tricyclic, and fluoxetine, a newer antidepressant, have been shown to have antiobsessional properties and are of special value in the treatment of obsessive-compulsive disorder.

Mechanism of Action of Antidepressants

It is believed that antidepressants work as a result of their ability to alter levels of the central nervous system (CNS) neurotransmitters. TCAs affect both norepinephrine and serotonin levels by blocking their reuptake at the presynaptic nerve ending. These activities form the cornerstone of the so-called biogenic amine hypothesis of the mood disorders. The tertiary amines (e.g., amitriptyline, imipramine, doxepin) tend to block serotonin reuptake to a greater extent, whereas the secondary amines (e.g., desipramine, nortriptyline, protriptyline) tend to block norepinephrine reuptake.

MAO inhibitors inhibit MAO, an enzyme responsible for the oxidation of tyramine, serotonin, dopamine, and norepinephrine. Blocking this enzymatic process leads to an increase in CNS levels of norepinephrine and serotonin. Two types of MAO have been identified: MAO A, found in the brain, liver, gut, and sympathetic nerves, and MAO B, found in the brain, liver, and platelets. MAO A acts primarily on serotonin and norepinephrine, and MAO B acts primarily on phenylethylamine, and both act on dopamine and tyramine. It is thought that inhibitors of MAO A may be more effective as antidepressants.

The newer antidepressants also affect CNS neurotransmitter levels. Maprotiline and amoxapine primarily block reuptake of norepinephrine, whereas trazodone and fluoxetine are serotonin reuptake blockers. The mechanism of action of bupropion is unknown, although it does provide some dopamine receptor blockade.

Pharmacokinetics of Antidepressants

All antidepressants are metabolized by the liver. The TCAs and newer antidepressants all have active metabolites, but MAO inhibitors do not. There is as much as a 10-fold variation in steady-state plasma levels of TCAs among individuals, due primarily to individual variation in the way the liver metabolizes the drugs. In general, the medications are well absorbed orally, undergo an enterohepatic cycle, and develop peak plasma levels 2–4 hours after ingestion. TCAs are highly bound to plasma and tissue proteins and are fat soluble. Free TCA comprises about 1% of the total body load of antidepressants. All antidepressants are excreted by the kidney, and their half-lives range from several hours to more than 5 days for fluoxetine. Steady-state plasma levels are achieved after five half-lives; half-life in turn is dependent on metabolism of the drug by hepatic microsomal enzymes. Blood levels tend to be increased by drugs that inhibit the cytochrome P450 system, including chlorpromazine and other antipsychotics, disulfiram, cimetidine, estrogens, and methylphenidate. Fluoxetine has been shown to elevate TCA plasma levels. Fluoxetine has a particularly long half-life; therefore, women of childbearing age should be warned that when contemplating pregnancy, they should stop using the drug approximately 5 weeks before attempting to conceive.

Meaningful plasma blood levels are available for imipramine, nortriptyline, and desipramine. Plasma blood levels may be measured on other antidepressants but are not as yet clinically useful. Plasma levels should be obtained 12 hours after the last dose. Therapeutic ranges have been established for imipramine (the total for imipramine plus its metabolite desipramine) of greater than 240 ng/ml; for desipramine, plasma levels of between 110 and 160 ng/ml; and for nortriptyline, plasma levels of between 60 and 150 ng/ml.

Plasma levels should not be obtained routinely, particularly if the patient is doing well. Reasons for obtaining blood levels include failure to respond adequately, significant symptoms of toxicity, cases of suspected patient noncompliance, establishing a therapeutic window (e.g., with nortriptyline), and perhaps in patients with significant cardiac or other medical disease where it is desirable to keep the blood level at the lower range of the therapeutic value. Blood levels are also valuable in cases of drug overdose.

Side Effects of Antidepressants

The most common side effects of TCAs are sedation, orthostatic hypotension, and the anticholinergic side effects (e.g., constipation, urinary hesitancy, dry mouth, visual blurring). Each TCA differs somewhat in its propensity to cause these effects. (See Table 24-2 for a comparison of the antidepressants.) Tertiary amines (e.g., amitriptyline, imipramine, doxepin) tend to provide more prominent side effects. Tolerance usually develops to anticholinergic side effects and sedation, but TCAs should be used with caution in patients with prostate enlargement and narrow-angle glaucoma. The elderly should have their blood pressure carefully monitored, because drug-induced hypotension can lead to falls and resultant fractures.

Antihistamine effects include sedation and weight gain. Alpha-adrenergic blockade causes orthostatic hypotension and reflex tachycardia. Miscellaneous side effects of TCAs include sedation, tremors, pedal edema, myoclonus, restlessness or hyperstimulation, insomnia, nausea and vomiting, electroencephalograph changes, rashes or allergic reactions, confusion, and seizures. It is uncertain whether TCAs are teratogenic, but their use in the first trimester of pregnancy should be avoided if possible.

Cardiovascular side effects tend to be the most worrisome. All TCAs prolong cardiac conduction, much like quinidine or procainamide. In fact, trials have favorably compared imipramine with these Type I antiarrhythmics. Thus, TCAs carry the risk of exacerbating existing conduction abnormalities. Patients with low-grade abnormalities such as a first-degree atrioventricular (AV) block or right bundle-branch block should use these medications cautiously, with dosage increase accompanied by serial electrocardiogram (ECG). Patients with higher block (e.g., a second-degree AV block) should not take TCAs. Doxepin has been advocated as having less cardiovascular toxicity, but this recommendation was based on data in early studies that used inadequate dosages. In patients with cardiac conduction defects, the newer antidepressants that do not prolong cardiac conduction (e.g., trazodone, fluoxetine) should be used.

A withdrawal syndrome occurs in some patients who have been taking high doses of TCAs for weeks or months. If the medication is stopped abruptly, symptoms may begin within days, including anxiety, insomnia, headache, myalgia, chills,

Table 24-2. Common antidepressants

Category	Drug (trade name)	Sedative potency	Anticholinergic potency	Orthostatic hypotensive potency	Cardiac arrhythmogenic potency	Target dosage (mg/day)	Dosage range (mg/day)
Tricyclics							
Tertiary amines	Doxepin (Sinequan, Adapin)	Very high	Moderate	Moderate	Yes	200	75–300
	Amitriptyline (Elavil)	Very high	Very high	High	Yes	150	75–300
	Imipramine (Tofranil)	Moderate	Moderate	High	Yes	200	75–300
	Trimipramine (Surmontil)	High	Moderate	Moderate	Yes	150	75–300
	Clomipramine (Anafranil)	High	High	High	Yes	150	75–300
Secondary amines	Protriptyline (Vivactil)	Low	High	Low	Yes	30	15–60
	Nortriptyline (Pamelor)	Moderate	Low	Lowest	Yes	100	40–150
	Desipramine (Norpramin)	Low	Low	High	Yes	150	75–300
Monoamine oxidase inhibitors	Phenelzine (Nardil)	Low	Low	High	Low	60	30–90
	Tranylcypromine (Parnate)	Low	Low	High	Low	30–40	20–90
	Isocarboxazid (Marplan)	Low	Low	High	Low	30	10–30
Newer agents	Amoxapine (Asendin)	Low	Low	Moderate	Yes	200	75–300
	Maprotiline (Ludiomil)	Moderate	Low	Moderate	Yes	150	75–200
	Trazodone (Desyrel)	High	Very low	High	Low	400	300–600
	Fluoxetine (Prozac)	Very low	Very low	Low	Low	20	20–80
	Bupropion (Wellbutrin)	Very low	Very low	Low	Low	300	150–450

Table 24-3. Dietary instructions for patients taking monoamine oxidase inhibitors

Foods to avoid

- Cheese: All cheeses except for cottage cheese, farmer cheese, and cream cheese
- Meat and fish: Caviar, liver; smoked, dried, pickled, cured, or preserved meats and fish
- Vegetables: Overripe avocados; fava beans
- Fruits: Overripe fruits; canned figs
- Other foods: Yeast extracts
- Beverages: Chianti wine; beers that contain yeast

Foods to be used in moderation

- Chocolate
- Coffee

Medications to avoid

- Over-the-counter pain medications except for plain aspirin, acetaminophen, and ibuprofen
- Cold or allergy medications
- Nasal decongestants and inhalers
- Cough medications: plain guaifenesin elixir may be taken
- Stimulants and diet pills
- Sympathomimetic drugs
- Meperidine

Source. Adapted from Hyman SE, Arana GW: Handbook of Psychiatric Drug Therapy. Boston, MA, Little, Brown, 1987.

malaise, and nausea. This syndrome can usually be prevented by a gradual medication taper (e.g., 25–50 mg per week), or if this is not possible, small doses of an anticholinergic medication such as diphenhydramine (e.g., 25 mg two or three times daily) may help alleviate symptoms.

The MAO inhibitors have minimal anticholinergic or antihistamine effects. They are, however, potent alpha-adrenergic blockers, resulting in a high frequency of orthostatic hypotension. Other common side effects include sedation or hyperstimulation (e.g., agitation), insomnia, dry mouth, weight gain, and impotence in men and anorgasmia in women. The most serious side effect results from the concomitant ingestion of a MAO inhibitor and substances containing tyramine, leading to severe hypertension and (rarely) death or stroke. For this reason, patients must follow a special low-tyramine diet and must also be aware of potential interactions with prescribed and over-the-counter sympathomimetic medications. A list of foods and substances to be avoided when taking MAO inhibitors is found in Table 24-3.

In addition to interacting with foods, MAO inhibitors can interact with sympathomimetics (e.g., amphetamines) to produce a hypertensive crisis. MAO inhibitors also have a potentially lethal interaction with meperidine, the mechanism of which is not fully understood, but may have to do with serotonin agonism. If symptoms of a hypertensive crisis do occur (e.g., headache, nausea, vomiting), patients should be instructed to immediately seek medical attention. Patients can be treated with intravenous phentolamine (e.g., 5 mg). Patients who do not have easy access to medical care should be advised to carry a 10-mg tablet of nifedipine with them. Its alpha-blocking properties, which when taken sublingually act to lower blood pressure, make it a useful stopgap measure.

All physicians and dentists must be informed if their patients are taking these agents, especially if surgery or dental work is indicated, so that drugs that interact adversely with MAO inhibitors can be avoided. It is prudent to wait 2 weeks after discontinuing a MAO inhibitor before resuming a normal diet or the use of a TCA or other medications that may have an adverse interaction.

Newer antidepressant agents (e.g., trazodone, fluoxetine, bupropion) have little or no anticholinergic properties and none seem to cause cardiac toxicity or produce fatality in an overdose. Amoxapine and maprotiline, however, have mild anticholinergic side effects and can cause hypotension and cardiac arrhythmias. The major side effects of trazodone are postural hypotension, nausea, and sedation, and the major side effects of fluoxetine are nausea, vomiting, insomnia, and hyperstimulation (e.g., agitation, nervousness). A rare but troublesome side effect of trazodone is priapism. Men given this drug should be warned to report any abnormal erections to their physician immediately. If priapism or abnormal erection occurs, the drug should be discontinued immediately because priapism can lead to permanent erectile dysfunction.

Antidopaminergic effects such as dystonia, parkinsonism, and akathisia are rare side effects of antidepressants. However, amoxapine may give rise to these extrapyramidal side effects, because its major metabolite has antipsychotic properties. For these reasons, we do not recommend using amoxapine as a first-line treatment.

Use of Antidepressants

Treatment should begin with a TCA unless the patient has a history of good response to a MAO inhibitor, or cardiac conduction defects suggest that a MAO inhibitor or newer antidepressant should be used. If there is no contraindication, nortriptyline, imipramine, or desipramine should be used because meaningful plasma levels can be assessed. A typical patient may be started on 50 mg of imipramine at bedtime, increasing the dose by 50 mg every 3–4 days as tolerated up to 150 mg. If no therapeutic response is seen within a week of this dosage, the dosage should be increased to 200 mg. If no response occurs within 1 week, the dosage should be gradually increased to 300 mg. If the patient responds positively to medication, the treatment should be maintained for at least 16–20 weeks after maximal relief is obtained. Patients with recurrent depression may need to remain on medication chronically.

Recommended dosage ranges for the different antidepressants are found in Table 24-2. Although these dosages will work for most patients, some patients will be unable to tolerate dosages near the upper limits, and some patients may respond to dosages at the lower end of the range. Dosages must be individualized to the patient, and much skill and experience are needed to learn how to adjust medication properly. Dosing is key to the therapeutic efficacy of antidepressants.

If the depressed patient fails to respond to an antidepressant with 4 weeks of treatment at the target dosage shown in Table 24-2, an alternative TCA, a MAO inhibitor, a newer antidepressant, or ECT should be considered. A 2-week washout should precede the trial of a MAO inhibitor. If this regimen fails, lithium augmentation may be tried. Nonresponders to TCAs may benefit from the addition of lithium, which increases the likelihood of response in many patients. Response from lithium augmentation is often evident within a week at relatively low dosages (e.g., 300 mg three times daily).

Other agents have been used to augment the effect of TCAs, including triio-dothyronine (e.g., 25–50 μg daily), L-tryptophan (e.g., 0.5–2 g daily), and methylphenidate (e.g., 10–40 mg daily), but the effect of these agents in augmenting response has not been adequately studied. L-Tryptophan has recently been associated with the potentially fatal eosinophilic-myalgia syndrome and has been temporarily withdrawn from the market.

Some patients refractory to either TCAs or MAO inhibitors alone may respond to a combination of the two. However, precautions must be taken to avoid potentially dangerous complications such as a hypertensive crisis. Generally, the two drugs should be started together, preferably after a medication-free period (e.g., 2 weeks if the patient had been taking TCAs). The doses are gradually increased.

Rational use of antidepressants

1. Tricyclic antidepressants (TCAs) should be used initially; monoamine oxidase (MAO) inhibitors and newer antidepressants should be reserved for nonresponders to TCAs. Patients with conduction disturbances should be treated with trazodone, fluoxetine, or bupropion.

2. TCAs generally need to be administered as a single dose, usually at bedtime. MAO inhibitors are usually prescribed twice daily, but not at bedtime because they can cause insomnia. Bupropion, a new antidepressant, needs to be administered in two or three divided doses, due to its propensity to cause seizures.

3. Although side effects appear within days of starting a drug, therapeutic effects may require 2–4 weeks to become apparent.

4. Antidepressants should not be used in grief reactions (uncomplicated bereavement) or adjustment disorder with depressed mood due to their self-limiting nature.

5. TCAs should be tapered slowly (e.g., over weeks to months) due to their tendency to cause withdrawal reactions. There is no clinically significant withdrawal reaction from MAO inhibitors, but a taper over 5–7 days is probably wise. The newer agents should also be tapered, although there are insufficient data about any withdrawal syndromes they may cause.

6. Use of two different antidepressants simultaneously will not boost efficacy and will only worsen side effects. In rare cases, the combined use of a TCA and a MAO inhibitor is justified, but this should *never* be routinely done.

Antimanic Agents

By 1970, another major type of drug was added to the psychiatrist's therapeutic armamentarium—lithium carbonate, a naturally occurring salt. Its first use in medicine (in the form of lithium chloride) was as a salt substitute for people suffering hypertension who needed a low-sodium diet. Its use as a salt substitute was soon abandoned, after it was discovered to make some people sick. In the late 1940s, the Australian John Cade found that lithium seemed to sedate agitated psychotic patients. Later, it was learned that lithium was particularly effective in people suffering from mania and was free of many of the unwanted side effects of chlorpromazine. A Danish researcher, Mogens Schou, observed that not only was lithium effective in relieving the target symptoms of mania, but that it also seemed to have a prophylactic effect. Lithium is now the treatment of choice for acute mania and for the maintenance treatment of bipolar illness.

Carbamazepine, an anticonvulsant, is now being used for these indications, but has different side effects. Other compounds have been used to treat bipolar illness (e.g., sodium valproate, calcium channel blockers, clonidine), but are still considered experimental.

Lithium Carbonate

Despite much research, the precise mechanism of action of lithium is not known. Lithium has many effects on intracellular processes, such as inhibition of norepinephrine-sensitive adenylate cyclase, and these actions may be relevant to its efficacy. Research into its effects is ongoing.

The onset of action of lithium often takes 5–7 days to become fully apparent. Antipsychotics, which work more quickly, may be preferred when rapid behavior control is needed, although benzodiazepine-induced sedation has also been found to be effective. The usual plasma level of lithium for the treatment of acute mania is 0.9–1.4 meq/L, although individual patients may do well outside this range. Lithium is also the medication of choice for prophylaxis in bipolar patients.

Maintenance dosages may be smaller, aiming for a blood level in the range of 0.6–0.8 meq/L. Lithium has no proven role in the acute treatment of unipolar depression, although the bipolar depressed patient or patient with a family history of bipolar illness may respond to lithium alone. Lithium is also used to augment tricyclic antidepressants.

The most dramatic effect of lithium is in the prophylaxis of manic and depressive episodes in bipolar patients, although in these patients, lithium appears to work best at reducing the frequency and severity of manic episodes. Prevention of episodes with lithium is not absolute, and patients may still have breakthrough episodes. Lithium has also been shown to be as effective as antidepressants in preventing recurrences of depression in unipolar patients.

The use of lithium in the treatment of schizoaffective disorders and schizophrenia has not been adequately studied, although it is reported that about one-half of schizophrenic patients will show improvement if lithium is added to their antipsychotic. The response rate among schizophrenic patients may be higher if there is a strong affective component to their illness. Mood symptoms are the most likely symptoms to respond, but there may be some improvement in core schizophrenic symptoms (e.g., thought disorder, psychosis). It is probably worthwhile to conduct a trial of adding lithium to antipsychotics in treatment-refractory schizophrenic patients.

Other uses of lithium include treatment of alcoholic patients to enhance abstinence (discussed in Chapter 14) and treatment of aggression in patients with organic mental disorders, mental retardation, and personality disorders (especially borderline and antisocial personalities). These indications are based on case reports or small case series; thus, further study is needed before specific recommendations for the use of lithium in these situations can be made.

Pharmacokinetics. Lithium carbonate is administered orally as a salt, most commonly in the form of a 300-mg capsule. In liquid form, it is available as lithium citrate. Lithium carbonate is rapidly absorbed, and peak blood levels are obtained about 2 hours after ingestion. The elimination half-life is about 8–12 hours in acute mania and about 18–36 hours in euthymic patients. Lithium is not protein bound, nor does it have metabolites. It is almost entirely excreted through the kidney, but may be found in all body fluids (e.g., saliva, semen). Lithium levels may be monitored in any body fluid, but blood plasma levels 12 hours after the last dose are the most easily obtained. Slow-release preparations are available and indicated where there is gastrointestinal toxicity or where twice-daily dosing would enhance compliance. Lithium is usually administered two or three times daily in acute manic patients, whereas once-daily dosing with extended-release preparations is recommended in patients receiving the drug prophylactically. Some investigators believe that once-daily dosing offers some protection to the kidneys, but a single large daily dose often causes gastric irritation. Lithium carbonate is usually begun with 300 mg three times daily in the average individual and is then titrated by blood levels until a target level is achieved. Adjustments in dosage may be made every 3–5 days. Lithium may be discontinued abruptly without a characteristic withdrawal.

Side effects. Minor side effects of lithium occur frequently after initiating treatment. Approximately 50% of patients report thirst or polyuria, 40% tremor, 20% diarrhea, 20% weight gain, and 10% edema. Side effects tend to diminish over time, although 5–15% of patients undergoing long-term treatment may develop clinical signs of hypothyroidism. This side effect is more common in women and tends to occur during the first 6 months of treatment. If hypothyroidism develops, patients may be managed effectively with thyroid replacement. It is wise to obtain baseline thyroid assays before starting lithium, and thyroid-stimulating hormone (TSH) should be monitored on a semiannual basis, or whenever there is a clinical suspicion of abnormality. Thyroid dysfunction should reverse after lithium is discontinued.

Patients undergoing long-term lithium treatment may develop an increase in calcium, ionized calcium, and parathyroid hormone levels, although these elevations are usually clinically insignificant. High levels of calcium, however, can cause lethargy, ataxia, and dysphoria, symptoms that may be attributed to depression rather than hypercalcemia.

Patients commonly gain weight when treated with lithium and should be warned of this possibility. Lithium is excreted through the kidneys and is reabsorbed in the proximal tubule with sodium and water. If the body is experiencing sodium deficiency, the kidneys compensate by reabsorbing more sodium than normal in the proximal tubules, and lithium is absorbed along with sodium and poses the risk of lithium toxicity with hyponatremia. Thus, patients should be instructed to avoid becoming dehydrated due to exercise, fever, or other causes of increased sweating. Sodium-depleting diuretics (e.g., thiazides) should be avoided because they may increase lithium levels.

In some patients, lithium can cause nephrogenic diabetes insipidus, because it reduces the ability of the kidneys to concentrate urine. As a result, these patients produce large volumes of dilute urine, which may be clinically significant for some, particularly if output exceeds 4 liters per day. Significant polyuria may be difficult for some patients to tolerate, and if it is necessary to reduce urine output, diuretics, such as amiloride (e.g., 5 mg twice daily) or hydrochlorothiazide (e.g., 50 mg twice daily) may paradoxically reduce urine output. Lithium patients (rarely) may develop a nephrotic syndrome due to a glomerulonephritis. This complication typically reverses with discontinuation of lithium. Taken long-term, lithium can cause a small decrease in the glomerular filtration rate, although significant decreases are uncommon. The decrease is presumably due to a tubulo-interstitial nephropathy. It is thought that cumulative exposure to lithium causes this, so it is wise to maintain the lowest effective dose possible. Serum creatinine and urinalysis should be obtained at baseline and semiannually thereafter. If there is any evidence of proteinuria or a rise in creatinine, more elaborate tests should be performed. Edema is occasionally noted in patients and tends to be mild and transient.

About one-fourth of patients on lithium develop reversible, nonspecific T wave changes similar to those seen with hypokalemia. Arrhythmias are rare, but sinus node dysfunction has been reported. Many patients develop acne, and those with acne may have an exacerbation. Psoriasis may also be worsened. Lithium has been reported to cause hair loss in some patients.

Lithium induces a reversible leukocytosis with white counts of 13,000–15,000 mm^3. The increase is usually in neutrophils and represents a step-up of the total body count rather than demargination.

Parkinsonian symptoms may develop with lithium treatment, although these symptoms are unusual. Symptoms of pseudoparkinsonism may include cogwheeling, hypokinesis, or rigidity. Perceptual-motor slowing may develop in some patients, but there are no adverse effects on cognition.

Contraindications. Lithium is contraindicated in patients with severe renal disease such as glomerulonephritis, pyelonephritis, or polycystic kidneys because lithium is primarily excreted through the kidney and dangerous blood levels may result. In patients who have suffered myocardial infarction, lithium should be discontinued for at least 10–14 days. If treatment with lithium should occur during the postinfarct period, low dosages and cardiac monitoring may be necessary.

Lithium is also contraindicated in the presence of myasthenia gravis because it blocks the release of acetylcholine in therapeutic dosages. Because lithium may aggravate or cause parkinsonism, the parkinsonian patient should be closely monitored if lithium is administered. Lithium should be given cautiously in the presence of diabetes mellitus, ulcerative colitis, psoriasis, and senile cataracts. Because of the increased incidence of cardiovascular malformations in infants of mothers taking lithium (Ebstein's deformity), lithium should be discontinued during the first trimester of pregnancy. Because lithium is secreted in breast milk, mothers taking the drug should not breast-feed.

Carbamazepine

Carbamazepine (Tegretol) is an anticonvulsant used to treat complex-partial and tonic-clonic seizures that has a structure similar to the TCAs. It is used increasingly as an alternative to lithium carbonate in the treatment of bipolar illness. Carbamazepine has a therapeutic profile like lithium and appears effective in treating acute mania and may be effective as a prophylaxis for bipolar illness. There are some data to indicate that it has a role in the treatment of bipolar depression, but it does not have any known role in the treatment of unipolar depression.

Although the precise mechanism of action of carbamazepine is unknown, it has multiple effects on the CNS. Of particular theoretical interest is its dampening effect on kindling. In the process of kindling, repetitive stimuli may lead either to a behavioral or convulsive activity. In mood disorders, repeated biochemical or psychological stressors are thought to result in abnormal excitability of limbic neurons, which carbamazepine dampens through its antikindling action.

When used to treat mania, carbamazepine is reported to have comparable efficacy to chlorpromazine and lithium. There is generally a delay of 5–7 days before its full effect is apparent, and it may be combined with antipsychotics, especially when behavior control is necessary. Carbamazepine may be more effective in patients who cycle rapidly (i.e., more than three episodes per year) and who tend not to respond well to lithium. Although a dose-response curve has not been established, the usual custom is to aim for typical anticonvulsant blood levels of 8–12 µg/ml.

Side effects of carbamazepine include a skin rash in 10–15% of patients, which is a cause for discontinuation. Other side effects may include impaired coordination, drowsiness, dizziness, slurred speech, and ataxia. Many of these symptoms can be avoided by starting the drug slowly and avoiding a rapid escalation of dosage. A transient leukopenia with up to a 25% decrease in the white count occurs in 10% of patients. In some patients, a smaller reduction in the white count may persist as long as they are on the drug, but this is not a reason for discontinuation. In rare patients, aplastic anemia can develop, but the estimated prevalence of this complication is less than 1 per 50,000 patients exposed.

Carbamazepine should be started with 200 mg twice daily and increased to three times daily after 3–5 days. Blood levels should be determined 5 days later, 12 hours after the last dose. Most patients will require between 600 and 1,600 mg daily.

Before starting carbamazepine, the patient should have a complete blood count

(CBC) and an ECG. While the dose is being adjusted, a CBC should be obtained weekly for 4 weeks and, once the dosage is stabilized, every 3 months. The patient should be warned about the hematologic side effects, and any indication of infection, anemia, or thrombocytopenia (e.g., petechiae) should be investigated. Carbamazepine levels should be checked weekly during the first 4 weeks and every 3 months thereafter. Hyponatremia may be associated with carbamazepine; therefore, convulsions or undue drowsiness should be cause for obtaining serum electrolytes. Because carbamazepine has been linked with malformations similar to those seen with phenytoin, it should be avoided in pregnant women, especially during the first trimester.

If patients do not respond to lithium alone or carbamazepine alone, they may respond to their joint administration. Other pharmacologic alternatives that have been studied include clonazepam, clonidine, sodium valproate (an anticonvulsant), and calcium channel blockers (e.g., verapamil, diltiazem).

Rational use of antimanics

1. Lithium should be used initially (along with an antipsychotic in highly agitated patients). Carbamazepine should be used in lithium nonresponders.

2. A clinical trial of lithium in mania lasts 3 weeks at therapeutic blood levels (i.e., 0.9–1.4 meq/L). A trial of carbamazepine lasts 3 weeks, but blood levels have not been well correlated with response.

3. Lithium may be given as a single daily dose at bedtime if the amount is less than 1,200 mg. Lithium should be given with food to minimize gastric irritation.

4. Because there is no withdrawal syndrome, lithium can be abruptly withdrawn.

5. Carbamazepine may be combined with lithium safely and may be of value in lithium nonresponders. Carbamazepine is thought to be particularly effective in rapid cyclers (i.e., more than 3 episodes/year).

Anxiolytics

Anxiolytics are the most widely prescribed class of drugs, and include the barbiturates, the nonbarbiturate sedative-hypnotics (e.g., meprobamate), the benzodiazepines, and buspirone. Currently, only the benzodiazepines and buspirone can be recommended, due to their superior safety record. The use of anxiolytics probably peaked in the 1970s and has since dropped by about one-third, perhaps due to the increase in awareness of their abuse potential. There is still a great sense among the general population that these medications are overused by psychiatrists and other physicians. In fact, one study suggests that despite their reputation, benzodiazepines are generally prescribed for short periods, for rational indications, and are not overused by the vast majority of patients.

Rational use of anxiolytics

1. In general, the benzodiazepines should be used for limited periods (e.g., weeks to months) to avoid the problem of dependence, because most conditions they are used to treat are probably self-limiting.

   • Occasionally, certain patients will benefit from long-term benzodiazepine administration. This can be safely done, but the patient should be periodically assessed for its continuing need.

2. The benzodiazepines have similar clinical efficacy, so the choice of a specific agent will depend on its half-life, the presence of metabolites, and route of administration.

3. In most clinical situations, multiple daily dosing with benzodiazepines is not necessary for adequate effect and once- or twice-daily dosing may be sufficient.

   • A dose given at bedtime will eliminate any need for a separate hypnotic.
   • Short-acting agents (e.g., alprazolam) will be an exception, because their dosing interval is determined by their half-lives.

4. Buspirone is not effective on an as-needed ("prn") basis and is useful only for the treatment of chronic anxiety (e.g., generalized anxiety disorder).

Benzodiazepines

Benzodiazepines are an important class of drug with clear superiority over the barbiturates and nonbarbiturate sedative-hypnotics. They also have a higher therapeutic index, less toxicity, and fewer drug interactions. All benzodiazepines can serve as antianxiety agents, sedatives, muscle relaxants, and anticonvulsants. Their approved indications reflect subtle differences among them (e.g., side effects, potency) and marketing strategy. Common benzodiazepines are compared in Table 24-4.

Benzodiazepines are believed to exert their effects by binding to specific benzodiazepine receptors in the brain. The receptors are intimately linked to receptors for gamma-aminobutyric acid (GABA), a major inhibitory neurotransmitter. By

Table 24-4. Common benzodiazepines

Drug (trade name)	Rate of onset	Half-life (hours)	Equivalent dosage (mg)	Dosage range (mg/day)
Alprazolam (Xanax)	Intermediate	6–20	0.5	1–4
Chlordiazepoxide (Librium)	Intermediate	20–100	25.0	15–60
Clorazepate (Tranxene)	Rapid	30–100	7.5	15–45
Diazepam (Valium)	Rapid	30–100	5.0	5–40
Flurazepam (Dalmane)	Rapid	50–100	30.0	15–30 hs
Lorazepam (Ativan)	Intermediate	10–20	1.0	2–6
Oxazepam (Serax)	Slow	5–20	15.0	30–120
Prazepam (Centrax)	Slow	60–70	7.5	20–60
Temazepam (Restoril)	Intermediate	8–18	15.0	15–30 hs
Triazolam (Halcion)	Rapid	2–3	0.25	0.125–0.5 hs

Note. hs = at bedtime.

binding to benzodiazepine receptors, the drugs potentiate the actions of GABA, leading to a direct anxiolytic effect on the limbic system.

Indications. The benzodiazepines are indicated for treatment of anxiety syndromes, sleep disturbances, musculoskeletal disorders, seizure disorders, and alcohol withdrawal and for inducing anesthesia.

Benzodiazepines are useful in the treatment of generalized anxiety disorder, especially in persons with severe anxiety. Although some patients may need long-term maintenance treatment with benzodiazepines, this chronic use has been poorly studied, and it is probably wise to treat patients for a short period (e.g., weeks or months), withdraw the medication, and reevaluate. Many patients will need benzodiazepines for a relatively short period when their anxiety is most acute and most problematic. Patients with mild anxiety may not need medication and can probably be successfully managed with behavioral interventions (e.g., progressive muscle relaxation). Further information about the treatment of generalized anxiety disorder is found in Chapter 10.

Alprazolam has been shown to have an antipanic effect, a property that may be shared by other benzodiazepines. However, because of its abuse potential, it is probably best to use TCAs initially in treating panic disorder. Alprazolam also appears to work as an antidepressant in mild to moderate depression. Again, it is probably wise to use a traditional antidepressant in the initial treatment in patients with major depression.

Anxiety may also complicate depression. Although the depression should be treated with an antidepressant, accompanying anxiety is more quickly relieved by use of a benzodiazepine. In some patients, it is wise to combine an antidepressant with a benzodiazepine to provide quick symptomatic relief. When the antidepressant begins to take effect, the benzodiazepine can then be safely withdrawn.

Benzodiazepines are effective in alleviating "situational" anxiety. These situations, termed *adjustment disorders with anxious mood* in DSM-III-R, include conditions characterized by anxiety symptoms (e.g., tremors, palpitations) that appear to occur in reaction to a stressful event. Adjustment disorders are generally brief; therefore, treatment with benzodiazepines will be time limited.

Benzodiazepines have established efficacy in the short-term treatment of insomnia that is unrelated to identifiable medical or psychiatric illness. Most patients with insomnia do not require long-term treatment, and there are few hazards with well-monitored therapy of limited duration. Three benzodiazepines are indicated specifically for the treatment of insomnia—flurazepam, temazepam, and triazolam—although other anxiolytics are probably effective as well. Most patients with insomnia report difficulty falling asleep, and so rate of absorption is a critical determinant for the drug's efficacy in this form of insomnia. Of the three available hypnotics, flurazepam is the most rapidly absorbed, followed by triazolam and temazepam. Accumulation of compounds with long half-lives increases the likelihood of continued efficacy during repeated dosage and minimizes the probability that rebound insomnia will occur on discontinuation of the drug. The likelihood of daytime drowsiness and impairment of performance is increased, but partly offset by clinical adaptation or tolerance. Nonaccumulating hypnotics with short half-lives, such as triazolam, have a reduced likelihood of adverse daytime sequelae (e.g., morning grogginess).

Diazepam is approved for the treatment of muscle spasms or musculoskeletal disorders and is also used to treat spasticity associated with spinal cord injury. Its efficacy in these disorders probably results from its nonspecific sedative and anxiolytic effects, because patients with muscle spasm and low back pain commonly experience considerable anxiety or agitation that may exacerbate pain and spasm.

Parenteral diazepam remains the drug of choice for the treatment of status epilepticus. Lorazepam probably has similar efficacy, although onset of action may be slightly slower than that of diazepam. However, lorazepam's activity may last longer because its peripheral distribution is more limited. (Diazepam is extensively distributed in peripheral tissues.)

Clonazepam is used to treat certain seizure disorders in childhood. Its use is limited, however, by a relatively high incidence of side effects (e.g., sedation) and tolerance.

The alcohol withdrawal syndromes described in Chapter 14 are commonly treated with benzodiazepines, particularly chlordiazepoxide. Benzodiazepines are also used preoperatively before surgical or endoscopic procedures and as induction agents before the initiation of inhalation anesthesia. Benzodiazepines are a logical choice as induction agents before general anesthesia because they carry a low risk of cardiovascular and respiratory depression compared with barbiturates.

Pharmacokinetics. Benzodiazepines are rapidly absorbed from the gastrointestinal tract and, with the exception of lorazepam, are poorly absorbed intramuscularly. Several of the benzodiazepines are available for parenteral use (e.g., diazepam). Midazolam is a short-acting agent used to induce anesthesia and is not available orally. Benzodiazepines are metabolized chiefly by hepatic oxidation. Lorazepam, oxazepam, and temazepam, however, are metabolized by glucuronide conjugation and have no active metabolites, are relatively shorter acting, and therefore are the preferred benzodiazepines in the elderly.

There is a difference in half-lives between single-dose and steady-state kinetics. Rapid-onset drugs tend to be very lipophilic, a property that facilitates rapid transit of the blood-brain barrier. The drugs differ markedly in their half-lives. The drugs with longer half-lives accumulate more slowly and take a longer time to reach steady state. Washout of the drug is similarly prolonged. Drugs with shorter half-lives reach steady state much more rapidly, but also have less total accumulation. Drugs with long half-lives tend to have active metabolites. Because of the differences in metabolism and half-lives, the best therapeutic results are obtained when the needs of the patient and situation are taken into account. When prescribing, three parameters—half-life, presence of metabolites, and route of elimination—largely determine which drug should be selected. For example, in the elderly, the clinician would want to select a benzodiazepine with a short half-life and few metabolites and renal excretion, all in an effort to reduce the possibility that the drug would accumulate, leading to undesirable side effects, such as excessive sedation.

Side effects. CNS depression is the most common side effect with benzodiazepines. Specific manifestations depend on the sensitivity of the individual. Commonly reported side effects include drowsiness, excessive somnolence, impairment of intellectual function, reduced motor coordination, and impairment of memory and recall. When these symptoms complicate long-term therapy, they usually occur early in the course of therapy and gradually diminish due to adaptation or tolerance, or after reduction of dosage.

All benzodiazepines have a potential for abuse and addiction, although their tendency to produce these effects tends to be exaggerated in the media. Most patients who take these drugs benefit from them, even when they are taken for long periods, and evidence of drug abuse or excessive escalation of dosage is rare. True psychological addiction can occur, most commonly when high dosages are prescribed, but can occur with usual therapeutic dosages. Because physiologic dependence is more likely to occur with longer drug exposure, minimizing the duration of continuous treatment should reduce this potential.

Discontinuation of benzodiazepine treatment after long-term use will almost certainly lead to recurrence of symptoms, but these symptoms do not suggest addiction. Withdrawal symptoms seem to appear rapidly, reach a peak, and then wane over time. Symptoms of withdrawal may include tremulousness, sweating, sensitivity to light and sound, insomnia, abdominal distress, and systolic hypertension. Serious withdrawal syndromes and seizures are relatively uncommon. Symptom recurrence appears to have a more rapid onset after discontinuation of short-acting benzodiazepines, and the impact of drug discontinuation can be minimized by tapering rather than abruptly discontinuing treatment. A slow taper is particularly important for benzodiazepines with short half-lives. In fact, when discontinuing a short-acting benzodiazepine, it is often helpful to switch the patient to a long-acting medication before initiating a taper (e.g., from alprazolam to diazepam).

Patients should be advised to avoid alcohol when taking benzodiazepines, due to their tendency to interact and cause greater depression of the CNS together than either given alone.

The benzodiazepines appear to be safe during pregnancy, but as a rule should be avoided. Benzodiazepines are secreted in breast milk; therefore, mothers taking these drugs should be instructed not to breast-feed.

The least controversial aspect of benzodiazepines is their tremendous index of safety. When taken alone, massive quantities of benzodiazepines can be ingested with little or no hazard of prolonged or serious CNS depression. Fatal overdose with benzodiazepines taken alone is almost unheard of. Therapy of benzodiazepine overdose beyond the usual supportive measures is usually not necessary.

Buspirone

Buspirone is used primarily in treating generalized anxiety disorder. Structurally unlike other anxiolytics, buspirone is relatively nonsedating, does not alter seizure threshold, does not interact with alcohol, and is not a muscle relaxant. It does not interact with the benzodiazepine receptor, cannot be used to treat alcohol withdrawal, and, it appears, has little abuse potential. Buspirone is well absorbed orally and is metabolized by hepatic oxidation. Its half-life ranges from 2 to 11 hours.

Research shows that buspirone's effect on chronic anxiety is equal to that of diazepam, although its effects are not apparent for 1–2 weeks.

Agents Used to Treat Extrapyramidal Syndromes

Anticholinergics closely resemble atropine in their ability to block muscarinic receptors, and all are similar in action and effectiveness in alleviating antipsychotic-induced extrapyramidal syndromes (EPS), especially pseudoparkinsonism. Anticholinergics are believed to act by diminishing or eliminating EPS by reestablishing dopamine-acetylcholine equilibrium by blocking acetylcholine in the corpus striatum. An equilibrium of dopaminergic (inhibitory) and cholinergic (excitatory) neuronal activity in the corpus striatum is thought to be necessary for normal motor functioning. Antipsychotics cause dopamine reuptake blockage and an absolute decrease in dopamine and, hence, a relative increase in interneuronal acetylcholine, which results in EPS.

The anticholinergic benztropine should be started at dosages of 1–2 mg per day. Smaller dosages should be used with geriatric patients. The maximum allowable dosage is 6 mg per day of benztropine or its equivalent, because a delirium can occur at higher doses. Benztropine can be administered once daily, preferably at bedtime because it can cause sedation. Students should remember that the anticholinergic side effects (e.g., dry mouth, blurry vision, constipation, urinary hesitancy) of these medications are additive with those of the antipsychotics. Most of the anticholinergics are similar in action and efficacy. Their dosage range is compared in Table 24-5.

Parenteral benztropine (1–2 mg) or diphenhydramine (25–50 mg) works within minutes to alleviate acute dystonic reactions. Diazepam (5–10 mg iv) also seems to work. Benztropine is the preferred agent because it usually does not cause sedation.

Other agents commonly used to treat EPS include amantadine and propranolol. Amantadine acts to increase CNS concentrations of dopamine by blocking its reuptake and increasing its release from presynaptic fibers. This action is thought to restore the dopamine-acetylcholine balance in the striatum. Amantadine is primarily useful in treating the symptoms of pseudoparkinsonism, such as tremors, rigidity, and hypokinesia. One advantage of the drug is its lack of anticholinergic properties, so that it can be safely combined with antipsychotics without concern for the development of an anticholinergic delirium. Treatment is initiated at 100 mg daily and increased to 200–300 mg daily. Onset of action occurs within 1 week. Adverse effects include orthostatic hypotension, livedo reticularis, ankle edema, gastrointestinal upset, and (rarely) visual hallucinations.

Propranolol and other beta-blockers have been used successfully to treat aka-

Table 24-5. Common agents used to treat extrapyramidal syndromes

Category	Drug (trade name)	Dosage range (mg/day)	Comments
Anticholinergics	Benztropine (Cogentin)	0.5–6	Use 1–2 mg iv of benztropine or 25–50 mg iv of diphenhydramine for acute dystonia. Anticholinergics tend to work better at relieving the tremor of pseudoparkinsonism than the hypokinesia.
	Biperiden (Akineton)	2–6	
	Diphenhydramine (Benadryl)	12.5–150	
	Procyclidine (Kemadrin)	2.5–22.5	
	Trihexyphenidyl (Artane)	1–15	
Dopamine facilitators	Amantadine (Symmetrel)	100–300	Useful in situations in which anticholinergic side effects need to be avoided.
Beta-blockers	Propranolol (Inderal)	10–80	Works well for treating akathisia.

thisia, which is usually not alleviated with an anticholinergic. Propranolol (e.g., 10–20 mg three to four times daily), or its equivalent with another centrally acting beta-blocker, seem to work well. Clonidine has also been found to be an effective treatment of akathisia, but is not widely used for this indication.

In treating any EPS, the clinician should begin by reducing the dosage of the antipsychotic if at all possible, or switching to an antipsychotic with less tendency to cause EPS. If these steps fail, anticholinergics, amantadine, or propranolol can be useful adjuncts. It is important to remember that EPS are unpleasant, and reduce the likelihood that the patient will remain compliant with treatment. Agents used to treat EPS can make a significant difference to the patient's subjective comfort. Common agents used to treat EPS are summarized in Table 24-5.

Psychostimulants

Amphetamines were introduced for clinical use in the 1930s and were soon used for dozens of conditions. As their abuse potential became apparent, governmental regulations became highly restrictive so that medical use of these agents today has been confined to a few specific indications (e.g., narcolepsy, childhood attention-deficit hyperactivity disorder [ADHD], refractory obesity). However, interest remains strong for the use of psychostimulants for the treatment of various other psychiatric disorders.

Amphetamine is an indirect-acting sympathomimetic agent that exerts a host of pharmacologic effects including CNS stimulation, anorexia, vasoconstriction, and hyperthermia. Development of tolerance has been documented for certain effects, such as anorexia, although not for CNS stimulant properties. The D isomer is more active than the L form, is highly lipophilic, and is rapidly absorbed from the intestine. Onset of clinical effects is rapid, and peak plasma levels following oral dosages are achieved in 1–3 hours. Excretion is by both renal excretion and hepatic biotransformation. Plasma half-life is about 12 hours. Amphetamine exerts its action through direct neuronal release of dopamine and norepinephrine and the blockade of catecholamine reuptake.

Methylphenidate is structurally related to amphetamine and has similar pharmacologic actions, although it is a somewhat milder stimulant. An oral dose is rapidly absorbed, peaks in the plasma in about 2 hours, and has a half-life of about 2 hours. Pemoline is structurally different from amphetamine and is a very mild CNS stimulant with minimal sympathomimetic activity. Its half-life is about 13 hours, and it peaks in the plasma in about 3 hours. The mode of excretion is primarily renal. The drug has little or no abuse potential.

The main psychiatric use for these drugs is the treatment of ADHD in children, although as noted earlier in the chapter, psychostimulants have also been used in the treatment of refractory depression, particularly as agents to augment the effects of TCAs. They have also been used with some success in treating depression in the elderly and the medically ill, but have not been adequately studied for these indications.

Table 24-6.   Common psychostimulants used to treat attention-deficit hyperactivity disorder

Drug (trade name)	Half-life (hours)	Dosage range in mg/kg/day (mg/day)	Comments
Dextroamphetamine (Dexedrine)	6–7	0.3–1.25 (5–40)	Associated with growth retardation
Methylphenidate (Ritalin)	2–4	0.6–1.7 (10–60)	Most commonly used and best studied; high dosages (>1 mg/kg) may impair cognitive performance
Pemoline (Cylert)	Acute: 2–12 Chronic: 14–34	0.5–3.0 (37.5–112.5)	May take weeks for effects to become apparent; less abuse potential

Parents, teachers, and clinicians rate 75% of children with ADHD to be improved on stimulants, compared to 40% of placebo-treated children. Stimulants tend to decrease physical activity, particularly during times when children are expected to be less active such as during school, decrease vocalization and noise and disruptive activity, and improve handwriting. Stimulants improve compliance with adult commands, improve attention span and short-term memory, and reduce distractibility and impulsivity. Common psychostimulants used to treat ADHD are listed in Table 24-6.

Stimulant medication should be initiated at a low dosage and titrated weekly according to response and side effects within the recommended range. Stimulants should be given after meals to reduce the likelihood of suppressing appetite. Beginning therapy with a morning dose may be useful in assessing drug effect because morning and afternoon school performance may then be compared. The need for medication on weekends or after school needs to be determined on an individual basis. Pulse and blood pressure should be taken initially and at times of dosage change. Weight should be followed during the initial titration and weight and height measured several times annually.

Common side effects that usually disappear within 2 or 3 weeks of use or from a reduction in dosage include anorexia, weight loss, irritability, abdominal pain, and insomnia. Occasional patients may develop mild dysphoria and social withdrawal at higher dosages. Children may (rarely) develop a mild to moderate depression requiring discontinuation of stimulants. A major concern has been the possibility of stimulant-induced growth retardation, and in fact, this side effect appears to be greater with dextroamphetamine than with methylphenidate or pemoline. The effect on growth reaches clinical significance in a small proportion of patients and can be minimized by using drug holidays. This effect is probably due to the effect of stimulants on cartilage metabolism. A potentially serious side effect is the development of motor or vocal tics, which may persist after the withdrawal of medication. Stimulants should be used with great caution in patients with a personal or family history of tics or Tourette's disorder and should be discontinued if tics develop.

Other miscellaneous side effects include dizziness, nausea, nightmares, dry mouth, constipation, lethargy, anxiety, hyperacusis, and fearfulness. Rebound effects consisting of excitability and overtalkativeness approximately 5 hours after a dose are commonly found as the last dose of the day wears off or for up to several days after the sudden withdrawal of high dosages of stimulants.

Further information about the use of stimulants in children with ADHD is found in Chapter 22.

Electroconvulsive Therapy

Electroconvulsive therapy (ECT) is a procedure in which an electric current is applied across scalp electrodes to induce a grand mal seizure. Interestingly, the treatment developed when the erroneous observation was made that schizophrenic patients improved after spontaneous seizures. The procedure was introduced in 1938 in Italy by Cerletti and Bini to replace less reliable convulsive therapies that used liquid chemicals or gasses. ECT is presently one of the oldest medical treatments available, a fact that attests to its safety and efficacy. Its mechanism of action remains a mystery, although it is known to produce multiple effects on the CNS, including the downregulation of beta-receptors, a property that ECT has in common with antidepressants. No alternative therapy has been demonstrated to be more effective than ECT in the treatment of depression.

Indications for ECT

When introduced, ECT was used indiscriminately and administered to patients with all types of problems and diagnoses. It soon became clear, however, that certain types of patients responded much better than others. Patients with mood disorders and certain forms of schizophrenia seemed to respond best. ECT is now used almost exclusively for the treatment of depression, and nearly 80% of patients who receive ECT are depressed. Because not all depressed persons need this treatment, ECT is generally held in reserve for depressed patients who fail one or more trials of antidepressant medication, patients at high risk for suicide, and patients who are debilitated by their failure to take in adequate food and fluids, and who may be at risk for cardiovascular collapse.

For antidepressant nonresponders, ECT is an excellent alternative, and it is reported that approximately 70–80% of drug nonresponders receiving ECT will improve. Patients at high risk for suicide and in need of rapid treatment should receive ECT because it tends to work more quickly than antidepressant medication. Further, research has shown that certain depressive symptoms are associated with a good response to ECT. These symptoms include psychomotor agitation or retardation, nihilistic, somatic, or paranoid delusions, and acute onset of illness. ECT has never been very useful in patients with chronic illnesses or in patients

Table 24-7. Indications for electroconvulsive therapy (ECT)

- Medication-refractory depression
- Suicidal depression
- Depression accompanied by refusal to eat or take fluids
- Depression during pregnancy
- History of positive response to ECT
- Catatonic syndromes
- Acute forms of schizophrenia
- Mania unresponsive to medication
- Psychotic or melancholic depression unresponsive to medication

afflicted with neurotic tendencies (e.g., anxiety, somatization, hypochondriasis) or personality disorders.

Mania refractory to medication also responds well to ECT. In the past, it was suggested that mania required between 12 and 20 ECT sessions, but research shows that mania responds to the same number of sessions as depression. Unilateral and bilateral ECT treatments are probably equally effective in mania as in depression, although some investigators believe that bilateral treatments are more effective. Predictors of response to ECT include mixed manic and depressive symptoms and severe manic behavior.

Occasionally, schizophrenic patients are treated with ECT, particularly when there is a superimposed secondary depression or a catatonic syndrome. Anecdotally, catatonia often responds with fewer than five treatments, and we have seen catatonic patients respond to a single treatment. Patients with schizophrenia of less than 18 months in duration and who have not adequately responded to antipsychotic medication may respond to ECT, but once the illness has become chronic, ECT is of little value. Indications for ECT are summarized in Table 24-7.

Pre-ECT Workup

Although ECT is classified as a surgical procedure, it is relatively uncomplicated. Routine chemistries including a CBC, serum electrolytes, urinalysis, ECG, chest X ray, and a physical examination are performed to rule out physical disorders that may contraindicate ECT. Spine films are no longer routine, but may be of value in documenting the condition of the vertebrae before ECT, especially in the elderly or patients with arthritis. The only absolute contraindication for ECT is increased intracranial pressure, because a physiologic rise in cerebrospinal fluid pressure during treatment could lead to herniation. Relative contraindications include recent myocardial infarction, coronary artery disease, cardiac failure, hypertensive cardiovascular disease, bronchopulmonary disease, and venous thrombosis.

ECT Procedure

Patients are not allowed food or fluids after midnight to minimize risk of aspiration. At the ECT site, patients are anesthetized with a short-acting anesthetic (e.g., methohexital), receive oxygen to prevent hypoxia, receive atropine to reduce secretions and bradyarrhythmias, and receive succinylcholine as a muscle relaxant to attenuate convulsions. After the patient is anesthetized, electrodes are placed on the scalp. Although bitemporal electrode placement is still widely used, unilateral placement on the nondominant hemisphere is becoming more popular as it has been found to reduce memory impairment after treatment. The majority of studies on ECT have found the two forms of treatment equally effective, although some investigators question this finding.

After placement of the electrodes, a brief stimulus is applied. The amount of electricity applied is approximately equivalent to that required to light a 20-watt bulb for 2 seconds. A brief pulse of electrical stimulus is usually used, rather than a continuous sinusoidal waveform because, in theory, the brief pulse causes less cognitive impairment. Stimulation usually produces a 30- to 60-second tonic-clonic seizure. This seizure is accompanied by a period of bradycardia, with a fall in blood pressure lasting about 60 seconds, followed by tachycardia and a rise in blood pressure. A rise in cerebrospinal fluid pressure parallels the rise in blood pressure. The use of anesthesia in ECT attenuates these responses. Minor arrhythmias are frequent but rarely a problem.

Most depressive patients receive a series of 6–10 treatments, although the exact number is individualized. In the past, extra treatments were often administered to reduce the risk of relapse, but research has shown that this practice is ineffective.

Side Effects of ECT

As with any medical or surgical procedure, ECT is associated with adverse effects. During treatment, these effects can include brief episodes of hypotension or hypertension, bradyarrhythmias, and tachyarrhythmias; in most cases, these effects are not serious. Fractures were widely reported to occur during ECT-induced seizures in the past, but are uncommon now due to the use of muscle relaxants. Other possible adverse effects include prolonged seizures (which are easily terminated with intravenous diazepam), laryngospasm, and prolonged apnea due to pseudocholinesterase deficiency, a rare genetic disorder. Immediately after treatment, patients often experience transient confusion. Headache, nausea, and muscle pain may also be experienced after the ECT treatment.

The most troublesome long-term effect of ECT is memory impairment, which has led to the concern that ECT may cause brain damage. Several groups of investigators have looked at memory loss and cognitive impairment, and their findings are consistent in showing that the complaints of memory loss are often associated with continuing or untreated depression. Also, ECT can cause a retrograde amnesia involving a short period before and during the hospitalization and can sensitize patients to the normal process of forgetting. Thus, patients who have undergone ECT may be more aware of minor memory disturbance than patients not having had such treatment. There is little evidence that ECT affects anterograde memory and subsequent learning. Thus, although ECT may cause a limited retrograde amnesia, there is no lasting effect on anterograde memory. Furthermore, not all patients experience amnesia, and modifications in ECT, including unilateral electrode placement and brief-pulse stimulation, help minimize any memory loss that occurs.

Acceptance of ECT

Surveys of patients receiving ECT have generally found high acceptance levels. In one study, nearly 80% of patients felt they were helped by ECT and 80% said they would not be reluctant to have it again. A substantial minority reported approaching treatment with anxiety, but in retrospect, over 80% found it no more anxiety producing than a dental appointment.

Amobarbital Sodium (Amytal) Interview

Amobarbital sodium, thiopental, or pentobarbital have been used for many years to produce a sedated state during which an interview ("Amytal interview") may be conducted that is of value both diagnostically and therapeutically. Despite its long history, indications for the Amytal interview are not well established, nor is its value adequately demonstrated.

The technique consists of administering 200–500 mg of amobarbital sodium intravenously at a rate of 25–50 mg per minute. The interviewer talks with the patient as the drug is being administered and halts the drug temporarily when the desired level of sedation is obtained (i.e., when lateral nystagmus appears at light sedation and slurred speech develops during a deeper state of sedation). The interview should continue for 30–60 minutes, or until sufficient material has been produced for diagnostic purposes, or therapeutic goals have been reached.

One of the indications for the Amytal interview is in the evaluation of mute patients. Patients whose muteness is due to a functional illness, such as a catatonic syndrome, often recover spontaneously and begin to speak. The speech may reveal a formal thought disorder, hallucinations, or delusions that are useful in diagnosing the underlying disorder. When the sedation wears off, the muteness will return. Occasional patients are immobilized by acute anxiety or panic and may talk about their concerns when sedated. Psychogenic amnesia, psychogenic fugue states, and conversion disorders are often temporarily relieved by amobarbital sodium; useful information may then be obtained (e.g., the amnesic patient may reveal his or her name and address). The interview has also been felt to be helpful in separating organic from functional cognitive impairment. Patients who are confused or disoriented from an organic process tend to worsen with amobarbital sodium, but patients whose impairment is due to a functional illness, such as major depression, will often temporarily improve.

There are several medical and psychiatric contraindications for use of the Amytal interview. Medical contraindications include a history of barbiturate allergy or addiction, severe liver, renal, or cardiac disorders, and upper respiratory infections. A thorough history, physical examination, and screening laboratory examination should identify these conditions. It is unwise to use the interview in paranoid patients, who may misinterpret its use, nor should it be used in unwilling patients because cooperation is key to the procedure. Overeager patients are poor candidates for the interview because they may use the test for their own (possibly manipulative) purposes, or may have unrealistic expectations for the procedure.

Bibliography

Addonizio G, Susman VL, Roth SB: Neuroleptic malignant syndrome: review and analysis of 115 cases. Biol Psychiatry 22:1004–1020, 1987

Adler LA, Angrest B, Peselow E, et al: Clonidine in neuroleptic induced akathisia. Am J Psychiatry 144:235–236, 1987

American Psychiatric Association Task Force on the Use of Laboratory Tests in Psychiatry: Tricyclic antidepressants—blood level measurements and clinical outcome: an APA task force report. Am J Psychiatry 142:155–162, 1985

Black DW, Winokur G, Nasrallah A: ECT in unipolar and bipolar disorders: a naturalistic evaluation of 460 patients. Convulsive Therapy 2:231–237, 1986

Black JL, Richelson E, Richardson JW: Antipsychotic agents: a clinical update. Mayo Clin Proc 60:777–789, 1985

Busto U, Sellers EM, Naranjo CA, et al: Withdrawal reaction after long-term therapeutic use of benzodiazepines. N Engl J Med 315:854–859, 1986

Chiarello RJ, Cole JO: The use of psychostimulants in general psychiatry: a reconsideration. Arch Gen Psychiatry 44:286–295, 1987

Clary C, Schweizer E: Treatment of MAOI hypertensive crisis with sublingual nifedipine. J Clin Psychiatry 48:249–250, 1987

Cole JO: Psychopharmacology update: medication and seclusion in restraint. McLean Hospital Journal 10:37–53, 1985

Cole JO, Chiarello RJ, Merzela PC: Psychopharmacology update: long-term pharmacotherapy of affective disorders. McLean Hospital Journal 11:106–138, 1986

Consensus Conference: Electroconvulsive therapy. JAMA 254:2103–2108, 1985

Cooper GL: The safety of fluoxetine—an update. Br J Psychiatry 153 (suppl 3):77–86, 1988

Crowe RR: Electroconvulsive therapy—a current perspective. N Engl J Med 311:163–167, 1984

Delva N, Letemendia F: Lithium treatment in schizophrenic and schizoaffective disorders. Br J Psychiatry 141:387–400, 1982

Dilsaver SC: Antidepressant withdrawal syndromes: phenomenology and pathophysiology. Acta Psychiatr Scand 79:113–117, 1989

Fawcett J, Kravitz HM: The long-term management of bipolar disorders with lithium, carbamazepine, and antidepressants. J Clin Psychiatry 46:58–60, 1985

Fink M: Convulsive Therapy: Theory and Practice. New York, Raven, 1979

Goodwin FK, Prange A, Post RM, et al: Potentiation of antidepressant effects by L-triiodothyronine in tricyclic non-responders. Am J Psychiatry 139:34–38, 1982

Guttmacher LB: Concise Guide to Somatic Therapies in Psychiatry. Washington, DC, American Psychiatric Press, 1988

Hyman SE, Arana GW: Handbook of Psychiatric Drug Therapy. Boston, MA, Little, Brown, 1987

Jabbari B, Brian GE, Marsh EE, et al: Incidence of seizures with tricyclic antidepressants. Arch Neurol 42:480–481, 1985

Jefferson JW, Greist JH, Ackerman DL, et al: Lithium Encyclopedia for Clinical Practice, 2nd Edition. Washington, DC, American Psychiatric Press, 1986

Jones KL, Lacro RV, Johnson KA, et al: Pattern of malformations in the children of women treated with carbamazepine during pregnancy. N Engl J Med 320:1661–1666, 1989

Kane J, Honigfeld G, Singer J, et al: Clozapine for the treatment-resistant schizophrenic— a double blind comparison with chlorpromazine. Arch Gen Psychiatry 45:789–796, 1988

Kocsis JH, Frances AJ, Voss C, et al: Imipramine treatment for chronic depression. Arch Gen Psychiatry 45:253–257, 1988

Kramlinger KG, Post RM: Adding lithium carbonate to carbamazepine: antimanic efficacy of treatment-resistant mania. Acta Psychiatr Scand 79:378–385, 1989

Kupfer DT, Carpenter LL, Frank E: Possible role of antidepressants in precipitating mania and hypomania in recurrent depression. Am J Psychiatry 145:804–808, 1988

Lerer B, Moore M, Meyendorf FE, et al: Carbamazepine versus lithium in mania. J Clin Psychiatry 48:89–93, 1987

Levenson DF, Simpson GM: Neuroleptic induced extrapyramidal symptoms with fever— heterogeneity of the "neuroleptic malignant syndrome." Arch Gen Psychiatry 43:839–848, 1986

Lipinsky JF, Zubenko G, Cohen BM, et al: Propranolol in the treatment of neuroleptic induced akathisia. Am J Psychiatry 141:412–415, 1984

Lusznat RM, Murphy DP, Nunn CMH: Carbamazepine vs lithium in the treatment and prophylaxis of mania. Br J Psychiatry 153:198–204, 1988

Mellinger GD, Balter MB, Uhlenhuth EH: Prevalence and correlates of the long-term regular use of anxiolytics. JAMA 251:375–379, 1984

Nair NPV, Suranyi-Cadotte B, Schwartz G, et al: A clinical trial comparing intramuscular haloperidol decanoate and oral haloperidol in chronic schizophrenic patients: efficacy, safety, and dosage equivalents. J Clin Psychopharmacol 6:30S–37S, 1986

Noyes R, Anderson DJ, Clancy J, et al: Diazepam and propranolol in panic disorder and agoraphobia. Arch Gen Psychiatry 41:287–292, 1984

Noyes R, Garvey MJ, Cook BL, et al: Benzodiazepine withdrawal: a review of the evidence. J Clin Psychiatry 49:382–389, 1988

Olajide D, Lader M: A comparison of buspirone, diazepam, and placebo in patients with chronic anxiety states. J Clin Psychopharmacol 75:148–152, 1987

Perry JC, Jacobs D: Overview: clinical applications of the Amytal interview in psychiatric emergency settings. Am J Psychiatry 139:552–559, 1982

Perry PJ, Alexander B, Liskow BI: Psychotropic Drug Handbook, 5th Edition. Cincinnati, OH, Harvey Whitney Books, 1988

Placidi GF, Lenzi A, Lazzerini F, et al: The comparative efficacy and safety of carbamazepine versus lithium. J Clin Psychiatry 47:490–494, 1986

Price LH, Charney DS, Heninger DR: Variability of response to lithium augmentation in refractory depression. Am J Psychiatry 143:1387–1392, 1986

Quitkin FM, Stewart JW, McGrath PJ, et al: Phenelzine versus imipramine in the treatment of probable atypical depression: defining syndrome boundaries of selective MAOI responders. Am J Psychiatry 145:306–311, 1988

Richelson E: Synaptic pharmacology of antidepressants: an update. McLean Hospital Journal 13:67–88, 1988

Rickels K, Feighner JP, Smith WT: Alprazolam, amitriptyline, doxepin, and placebo in the treatment of depression. Arch Gen Psychiatry 42:134–141, 1985

Rickels K, Fox IL, Greenblatt DJ, et al: Clorazepate and lorazepam: clinical improvement and rebound anxiety. Am J Psychiatry 145:312–317, 1988

Roose SP, Glassman AH, Giardina EGV, et al: Tricyclic antidepressants in depressed patients with cardiac conduction disease. Arch Gen Psychiatry 44:273–275, 1987

Rosebush P, Stewart T: A prospective analysis of 24 episodes of neuroleptic malignant syndrome. Am J Psychiatry 146:717–725, 1989

Santos JL, Cabranes JA, Vasquez C: Clinical response and plasma haloperidol levels in chronic and subchronic schizophrenia. Biol Psychiatry 26:381–388, 1989

Small JG, Klapper MH, Kellams JJ, et al: Electroconvulsive treatment compared with lithium in the management of manic states. Arch Gen Psychiatry 45:727–732, 1988

Tyrer P, Murphy S: The place of benzodiazepines in psychiatric practice. Br J Psychiatry 151:719–723, 1987

Self-assessment Questions

1. What is the mechanism of action of the antipsychotics?
2. What are the common indications for antipsychotics?
3. How are the antipsychotics used in the treatment of acute psychosis? in maintenance treatment?
4. What are the common extrapyramidal side effects that occur with antipsychotics? Describe the syndromes and discuss their clinical management.
5. What disorders can be treated with antidepressants? How is the term *antidepressant* a misnomer?
6. What is the putative mechanism of action of the TCAs? MAO inhibitors? newer agents?
7. Are blood levels of TCAs meaningful? When should they be obtained?
8. What are the common side effects of TCAs? MAO inhibitors? newer agents?
9. What agent is associated with the occurrence of priapism? Why is this worrisome?
10. What are the typical plasma level ranges for lithium carbonate for acute treatment of mania? prophylaxis?
11. What are the common side effects of lithium carbonate?
12. What is carbamazepine used to treat? What are its side effects?
13. Benzodiazepines may be used to treat several clinical conditions. What are these?
14. What are the advantages of benzodiazepines over the barbiturates? What are their pharmacokinetics?
15. What conditions are treated with psychostimulants?
16. What are the relative advantages and disadvantages of dextroamphetamine, methylphenidate, and pemoline?
17. Describe how ECT is administered. What is the purpose of atropine? succinylcholine? methohexital?
18. What conditions respond well to ECT?
19. What are the side effects of ECT?
20. Describe the "Amytal" interview. When is this technique useful?

Appendix

Brief Psychiatric Rating Scale

DIRECTIONS: Place an X in the appropriate box to represent level of severity of each symptom.

	Not Present	Very Mild	Mild	Moderate	Mod. Severe	Severe	Extremely Severe
SOMATIC CONCERN—preoccupation with physical health, fear of physical illness, hypochondriasis.	☐	☐	☐	☐	☐	☐	☐
ANXIETY—worry, fear, over-concern for present or future, uneasiness.	☐	☐	☐	☐	☐	☐	☐
EMOTIONAL WITHDRAWAL—lack of spontaneous interaction, isolation deficiency in relating to others.	☐	☐	☐	☐	☐	☐	☐
CONCEPTUAL DISORGANIZATION—thought processes confused, disconnected, disorganized, disrupted.	☐	☐	☐	☐	☐	☐	☐
GUILT FEELINGS—self-blame, shame, remorse for past behavior.	☐	☐	☐	☐	☐	☐	☐
TENSION—physical and motor manifestations of nervousness, over-activation.	☐	☐	☐	☐	☐	☐	☐
MANNERISMS AND POSTURING—peculiar, bizarre unnatural motor behavior (not including tic).	☐	☐	☐	☐	☐	☐	☐
GRANDIOSITY—exaggerated self-opinion, arrogance, conviction of unusual power or abilities.	☐	☐	☐	☐	☐	☐	☐
DEPRESSIVE MOOD—sorrow, sadness, despondency, pessimism.	☐	☐	☐	☐	☐	☐	☐
HOSTILITY—animosity, contempt, belligerence, disdain for others.	☐	☐	☐	☐	☐	☐	☐
SUSPICIOUSNESS—mistrust, belief others harbour malicious or discriminatory intent.	☐	☐	☐	☐	☐	☐	☐
HALLUCINATORY BEHAVIOR—perceptions without normal external stimulus correspondence.	☐	☐	☐	☐	☐	☐	☐
MOTOR RETARDATION—slowed weakened movements or speech, reduced body tone.	☐	☐	☐	☐	☐	☐	☐
UNCOOPERATIVENESS—resistance, guardedness, rejection of authority.	☐	☐	☐	☐	☐	☐	☐
UNUSUAL THOUGHT CONTENT—unusual, odd, strange, bizzare thought content.	☐	☐	☐	☐	☐	☐	☐
BLUNTED AFFECT—reduced emotional tone, reduction in formal intensity of feelings, flatness.	☐	☐	☐	☐	☐	☐	☐

	Not Present	Very Mild	Mild	Moderate	Mod. Severe	Severe	Extremely Severe
EXCITEMENT—heightened emotional tone, agitation, increased reactivity.	☐	☐	☐	☐	☐	☐	☐
DISORIENTATION—confusion or lack of proper association for person, place, or time.	☐	☐	☐	☐	☐	☐	☐

Global Assessment Scale (Range 1–100) _____

Source.   Reprinted with permission from Overall JE: The Brief Psychiatric Rating Scale (BPRS): recent developments in ascertainment and scaling. Psychopharmacol Bull 24:97–99, 1988.

Scale for the Assessment of Negative Symptoms (SANS)

0 = None   1 = Questionable   2 = Mild   3 = Moderate   4 = Marked   5 = Severe

AFFECTIVE FLATTENING OR BLUNTING

1   *Unchanging Facial Expression*
    The patient's face appears wooden, changes less than
    expected as emotional content of discourse changes.   0 1 2 3 4 5

2   *Decreased Spontaneous Movements*
    The patient shows few or no spontaneous movements,
    does not shift position, move extremities, etc.   0 1 2 3 4 5

3   *Paucity of Expressive Gestures*
    The patient does not use hand gestures, body position,
    etc., as an aid to expressing his ideas.   0 1 2 3 4 5

4   *Poor Eye Contact*
    The patient avoids eye contact or "stares through"
    interviewer even when speaking.   0 1 2 3 4 5

5   *Affective Nonresponsivity*
    The patient fails to smile or laugh when prompted.   0 1 2 3 4 5

6   *Lack of Vocal Inflections*
    The patient fails to show normal vocal emphasis
    patterns, is often monotonic.   0 1 2 3 4 5

7   *Global Rating of Affective Flattening*
    This rating should focus on overall severity of
    symptoms, especially unresponsiveness, eye contact,
    facial expression, and vocal inflections.   0 1 2 3 4 5

ALOGIA

8   *Poverty of Speech*
    The patient's replies to questions are restricted in
    amount, tend to be brief, concrete, and unelaborated.   0 1 2 3 4 5

515

0 = None   1 = Questionable   2 = Mild   3 = Moderate   4 = Marked   5 = Severe

9   *Poverty of Content of Speech*   0 1 2 3 4 5
    The patient's replies are adequate in amount but tend
    to be vague, overconcrete, or overgeneralized, and
    convey little information.

10 *Blocking*   0 1 2 3 4 5
    The patient indicates, either spontaneously or with
    prompting, that his train of thought was interrupted.

11 *Increased Latency of Response*   0 1 2 3 4 5
    The patient takes a long time to reply to questions;
    prompting indicates the patient is aware of the
    question.

12 *Global Rating of Alogia*   0 1 2 3 4 5
    The core features of alogia are poverty of speech and
    poverty of content.

AVOLITION-APATHY

13 *Grooming and Hygiene*   0 1 2 3 4 5
    The patient's clothes may be sloppy or soiled, and he
    may have greasy hair, body odor, etc.

14 *Impersistence at Work or School*   0 1 2 3 4 5
    The patient has difficulty seeking or maintaining
    employment, completing school work, keeping house,
    etc. If an inpatient, cannot persist at ward activities,
    such as OT, playing cards, etc.

15 *Physical Anergia*   0 1 2 3 4 5
    The patient tends to be physically inert. He may sit
    for hours and does not initiate spontaneous activity.

16 *Global Rating of Avolition-Apathy*   0 1 2 3 4 5
    Strong weight may be given to one or two prominent
    symptoms if particularly striking.

ANHEDONIA-ASOCIALITY

17 *Recreational Interests and Activities*   0 1 2 3 4 5
    The patient may have few or no interests. Both the
    quality and quantity of interests should be taken into
    account.

0 = None   1 = Questionable   2 = Mild   3 = Moderate   4 = Marked   5 = Severe

18 *Sexual Activity*   0 1 2 3 4 5
    The patient may show a decrease in sexual interest and
    activity, or enjoyment when active.

19 *Ability to Feel Intimacy and Closeness*   0 1 2 3 4 5
    The patient may display an inability to form close or
    intimate relationships, especially with the opposite sex
    and family.

20 *Relationships With Friends and Peers*   0 1 2 3 4 5
    The patient may have few or no friends and may prefer
    to spend all of his time isolated.

21 *Global Rating of Anhedonia-Asociality*   0 1 2 3 4 5
    This rating should reflect overall severity, taking into
    account the patient's age, family status, etc.

ATTENTION

22 *Social Inattentiveness*   0 1 2 3 4 5
    The patient appears uninvolved or unengaged. He may
    seem "spacy."

23 *Inattentiveness During Mental Status Testing*   0 1 2 3 4 5
    Tests of "serial 7s" (at least five subtractions) and
    spelling "world" backwards: Score: 2 = 1 error; 3 = 2
    errors; 4 = 3 errors.

24 *Global Rating of Attention*   0 1 2 3 4 5
    This rating should assess the patient's overall
    concentration, clinically and on tests.

Source.   Available from Nancy C. Andreasen, M.D., Ph.D., Department of Psychiatry, College of Medicine, The University of Iowa, Iowa City, IA 52242. Copyright 1984 Nancy C. Andreasen. Reprinted with permission.

Scale for the Assessment of Positive Symptoms (SAPS)

0 = None   1 = Questionable   2 = Mild   3 = Moderate   4 = Marked   5 = Severe

HALLUCINATIONS

1 *Auditory Hallucinations*　　　　　　　　　　0 1 2 3 4 5
   The patient reports voices, noises, or other sounds that
   no one else hears.

2 *Voices Commenting*　　　　　　　　　　　　0 1 2 3 4 5
   The patient reports a voice which makes a running
   commentary on his behavior or thoughts.

3 *Voices Conversing*　　　　　　　　　　　　0 1 2 3 4 5
   The patient reports hearing two or more voices
   conversing.

4 *Somatic or Tactile Hallucinations*　　　　　　0 1 2 3 4 5
   The patient reports experiencing peculiar physical
   sensations in the body.

5 *Olfactory Hallucinations*　　　　　　　　　　0 1 2 3 4 5
   The patient reports experiencing unusual smells which
   no one else notices.

6 *Visual Hallucinations*　　　　　　　　　　　0 1 2 3 4 5
   The patient sees shapes or people that are not actually
   present.

7 *Global Rating of Hallucinations*　　　　　　　0 1 2 3 4 5
   This rating should be based on the duration and
   severity of the hallucinations and their effects on the
   patient's life.

DELUSIONS

8 *Persecutory Delusions*　　　　　　　　　　　0 1 2 3 4 5
   The patient believes he is being conspired against or
   persecuted in some way.

0 = None   1 = Questionable   2 = Mild   3 = Moderate   4 = Marked   5 = Severe

9   *Delusions of Jealousy*   0 1 2 3 4 5
The patient believes his spouse is having an affair with
someone.

10 *Delusions of Guilt or Sin*   0 1 2 3 4 5
The patient believes that he has committed some
terrible sin or done something unforgiveable.

11 *Grandiose Delusions*   0 1 2 3 4 5
The patient believes he has special powers or abilities.

12 *Religious Delusions*   0 1 2 3 4 5
The patient is preoccupied with false beliefs of a
religious nature.

13 *Somatic Delusions*   0 1 2 3 4 5
The patient believes that somehow his body is
diseased, abnormal, or changed.

14 *Delusions of Reference*   0 1 2 3 4 5
The patient believes that insignificant remarks or
events refer to him or have some special meaning.

15 *Delusions of Being Controlled*   0 1 2 3 4 5
The patient feels that his feelings or actions are
controlled by some outside force.

16 *Delusions of Mind Reading*   0 1 2 3 4 5
The patient feels that people can read his mind or
know his thoughts.

17 *Thought Broadcasting*   0 1 2 3 4 5
The patient believes that his thoughts are broadcast so
that he himself or others can hear them.

18 *Thought Insertion*   0 1 2 3 4 5
The patient believes that thoughts that are not his
own have been inserted into his mind.

19 *Thought Withdrawal*   0 1 2 3 4 5
The patient believes that thoughts have been taken
away from his mind.

20 *Global Rating of Delusions*   0 1 2 3 4 5
This rating should be based on the duration and
persistence of the delusions and their effect on the
patient's life.

0 = None   1 = Questionable   2 = Mild   3 = Moderate   4 = Marked   5 = Severe

BIZARRE BEHAVIOR

21 *Clothing and Appearance*   0 1 2 3 4 5
    The patient dresses in an unusual manner or does
    other strange things to alter his appearance.

22 *Social and Sexual Behavior*   0 1 2 3 4 5
    The patient may do things considered inappropriate
    according to usual social norms (e.g., masturbating in
    public).

23 *Aggressive and Agitated Behavior*   0 1 2 3 4 5
    The patient may behave in an aggressive, agitated
    manner, often unpredictably.

24 *Repetitive or Stereotyped Behavior*   0 1 2 3 4 5
    The patient develops a set of repetitive action or
    rituals that he must perform over and over.

25 *Global Rating of Bizarre Behavior*   0 1 2 3 4 5
    This rating should reflect the type of behavior and the
    extent to which it deviates from social norms.

POSITIVE FORMAL THOUGHT DISORDER

26 *Derailment*   0 1 2 3 4 5
    A pattern of speech in which ideas slip off track onto
    ideas obliquely related or unrelated.

27 *Tangentiality*   0 1 2 3 4 5
    Replying to a question in an oblique or irrevelant
    manner.

28 *Incoherence*   0 1 2 3 4 5
    A pattern of speech which is essentially
    incomprehensible at times.

29 *Illogicality*   0 1 2 3 4 5
    A pattern of speech in which conclusions are reached
    which do not follow logically.

30 *Circumstantiality*   0 1 2 3 4 5
    A pattern of speech which is very indirect and delayed
    in reaching its goal idea.

31 *Pressure of Speech*   0 1 2 3 4 5
    The patient's speech is rapid and difficult to interrupt;
    the amount of speech produced is greater than that
    considered normal.

0 = None   1 = Questionable   2 = Mild   3 = Moderate   4 = Marked   5 = Severe

32 *Distractible Speech*   0 1 2 3 4 5
    The patient is distracted by nearby stimuli which
    interrupt his flow of speech.

33 *Clanging*   0 1 2 3 4 5
    A pattern of speech in which sounds rather than
    meaningful relationships govern word choice.

34 *Global Rating of Positive Formal Thought Disorder*   0 1 2 3 4 5
    This rating should reflect the frequency of abnormality
    and degree to which it affects the patient's ability to
    communicate.

INAPPROPRIATE AFFECT

35 *Inappropriate Affect*   0 1 2 3 4 5
    The patient's affect is inappropriate or incongruous,
    not simply flat or blunted.

Source.   Available from Nancy C. Andreasen, M.D., Ph.D., Department of Psychiatry, College of Medicine, The University of Iowa, Iowa City, IA 52242. Copyright 1984 Nancy C. Andreasen. Reprinted with permission.

Hamilton Rating Scale for Depression

For each item select the "cue" which best characterizes the patient.

1: DEPRESSED MOOD (Sadness, hopeless, helpless, worthless)
   0 Absent
   1 These feeling states indicated only on questioning
   2 These feeling states spontaneously reported verbally
   3 Communicates feeling states nonverbally—i.e., through facial expression, posture, voice, and tendency to weep
   4 Patient reports VIRTUALLY ONLY these feeling states in his spontaneous verbal and nonverbal communication

2: FEELINGS OF GUILT
   0 Absent
   1 Self-reproach, feels he has let people down
   2 Ideas of guilt or rumination over past errors or sinful deeds
   3 Present illness is a punishment. Delusions of guilt
   4 Hears accusatory or denunciatory voices and/or experiences threatening visual hallucinations

3: SUICIDE
   0 Absent
   1 Feels life is not worth living
   2 Wishes he were dead or any thoughts of possible death to self
   3 Suicide ideas or gesture
   4 Attempts at suicide (any serious attempt rates 4)

4: INSOMNIA EARLY
   0 No difficulty falling asleep
   1 Complains of occasional difficulty falling asleep—i.e., more than ¼ hour
   2 Complains of nightly difficulty falling asleep

5: INSOMNIA MIDDLE
   0 No difficulty
   1 Patient complains of being restless and disturbed during the night
   2 Waking during the night—any getting out of bed rates 2 (except for purpose of voiding)

6: INSOMNIA LATE
   0 No difficulty
   1 Waking in early hours of the morning but goes back to sleep
   2 Unable to fall asleep again if gets out of bed

7: WORK AND ACTIVITIES

    0 No difficulty

    1 Thoughts and feelings of incapacity, fatigue or weakness related to activities, work, or hobbies

    2 Loss of interest in activity, hobbies, or work—either directly reported by patient, or indirect in listlessness, indecision and vacillation (feels he has to push self to work or activities)

    3 Decrease in actual time spent in activities or decrease in productivity. In hospital, rate 3 if patient does not spend at least three hours a day in activities (hospital job or hobbies) exclusive of ward chores

    4 Stopped working because of present illness. In hospital, rate 4 if patient engages in no activities except ward chores, or if patient fails to perform ward chores unassisted

8: RETARDATION (Slowness of thought and speech; impaired ability to concentrate; decreased motor activity)

    0 Normal speech and thought

    1 Slight retardation at interview

    2 Obvious retardation at interview

    3 Interview difficult

    4 Complete stupor

9: AGITATION

    0 None

    1 "Playing with" hands, hair, etc.

    2 Hand wringing, nail biting, hair pulling, biting of lips

10: ANXIETY PSYCHIC

    0 No difficulty

    1 Subjective tension and irritability

    2 Worrying about minor matters

    3 Apprehensive attitude apparent in face or speech

    4 Fears expressed without questioning

11: ANXIETY SOMATIC

    0 Absent   Physiological concomitants of anxiety, such as:

    1 Mild

    2 Moderate   Gastrointestinal—dry mouth, wind, indigestion, diarrhea, cramps, belching

    3 Severe

    4 Incapacitating

Cardiovascular—palpitations, headaches

Respiratory—hyperventilation, sighing

Urinary frequency

Sweating

12: SOMATIC SYMPTOMS GASTROINTESTINAL
0 None
1 Loss of appetite but eating without staff encouragement. Heavy feelings in abdomen
2 Difficulty eating without staff urging. Requests or requires laxatives or medication for bowels or medication for G.I. symptoms

13: SOMATIC SYMPTOMS GENERAL
0 None
1 Heaviness in limbs, back or head. Backaches, headache, muscle aches. Loss of energy and fatigability
2 Any clear cut symptom rates 2

14: GENITAL SYMPTOMS
0 Absent   Symptoms such as: Loss of libido
1 Mild   Menstrual disturbances
2 Severe

15: HYPOCHONDRIASIS
0 Not present
1 Self-absorption (bodily)
2 Preoccupation with health
3 Frequent complaints, requests for help, etc.
4 Hypochondriacal delusions

16: LOSS OF WEIGHT
A: WHEN RATING BY HISTORY
0 No weight loss
1 Probable weight loss associated with present illness
2 Definite (according to patient) weight loss
B: ON WEEKLY RATINGS BY WARD PSYCHIATRIST, WHEN ACTUAL WEIGHT CHANGES ARE MEASURED
0 Less than 1 lb. weight loss in week
1 Greater than 1 lb. weight loss in week
2 Greater than 2 lb. weight loss in week

17: INSIGHT
0 Acknowledges being depressed and ill
1 Acknowledges illness but attributes cause to bad food, climate, overwork, virus, need for rest, etc.
2 Denies being ill at all

18: DIURNAL VARIATION
A.M. P.M.
0   0   Absent   If symptoms are worse in the morning
1   1   Mild   or evening note which it is and rate
2   2   Severe   severity of variation

19: DEPERSONALIZATION AND DEREALIZATION

0 Absent   Such as: Feelings of unreality
1 Mild   Nihilistic ideas
2 Moderate
3 Severe
4 Incapacitating

20: PARANOID SYMPTOMS

0 None
1
   Suspiciousness

2
3 Ideas of reference
4 Delusions of reference and persecution

21: OBSESSIONAL AND COMPULSIVE SYMPTOMS

0 Absent
1 Mild
2 Severe

22: HELPLESSNESS

0 Not present
1 Subjective feelings which are elicited only by inquiry
2 Patient volunteers his helpless feelings
3 Requires urging, guidance, and reassurance to accomplish ward chores or personal hygiene
4 Requires physical assistance for dress, grooming, eating, bedside tasks, or personal hygiene

23: HOPELESSNESS

0 Not present
1 Intermittently doubts that "things will improve" but can be reassured
2 Consistently feels "hopeless" but accepts reassurances
3 Expresses feelings of discouragement, despair, pessimism about future, which cannot be dispelled
4 Spontaneously and inappropriately perseverates "I'll never get well" or its equivalent

24: WORTHLESSNESS (Ranges from mild loss of esteem, feelings of inferiority, self-depreciation to delusional notions of worthlessness)

0 Not present
1 Indicates feelings of worthlessness (loss of self-esteem) only on questioning
2 Spontaneously indicates feelings of worthlessness (loss of self-esteem)

3 Different from 2 by degree. Patient volunteers that he is "no good," "inferior," etc.

4 Delusional notions of worthlessness—i.e., "I am a heap of garbage" or its equivalent

Source.   Reprinted with permission from Hamilton M: A rating scale for depression. J Neurol Neurosurg Psychiatry 23:56–62, 1960.

Hamilton Anxiety Rating Scale

Patient's Name

Date of First Report

Diagnosis

Date of This Report

Current Therapy

Instructions This checklist is to assist the physician in evaluating each patient
with respect to degree of anxiety and pathological condition.
Please fill in the appropriate rating.

0 None
1 Mild
2 Moderate
3 Severe
4 Severe, grossly disabling

Item		Rating	Item		Rating
Anxious Mood	Worries, anticipation of the worst, fearful anticipation, irritability.		Somatic (Sensory)	Tinnitus, blurring of vision, hot and cold flushes, feelings of weakness, picking sensation.	
Tension	Feelings of tension, fatigability, startle response, moved to tears easily, trembling, feelings of restlessness, inability to relax.		Cardiovascular Symptoms	Tachycardia, palpitations, pain in chest, throbbing of vessels, fainting feelings, missing beat.	
Fear	Of dark, of strangers, of being left alone, of animals, of traffic, of crowds.		Respiratory Symptoms	Pressure or constriction in chest, choking feelings, sighing, dyspnea.	
Insomnia	Difficulty in falling asleep, broken sleep, unsatisfying sleep and fatigue on waking, dreams, nightmares, night terrors.		Gastrointestinal Symptoms	Difficulty in swallowing, wind, abdominal pain, burning sensations, abdominal fullness, nausea, vomiting, borborygmi, looseness of bowels, loss of weight, constipation.	
Intellectual (Cognitive)	Difficulty in concentration, poor memory.		Genitourinary Symptoms	Frequency of micturition, urgency of micturition, amenorrhea, menorrhagia, development of frigidity, premature ejaculation, loss of libido, impotence.	
Depressed Mood	Loss of interest, lack of pleasure in hobbies, depression, early waking, diurnal swing.		Autonomic Symptoms	Dry mouth, flushing, pallor, tendency to sweat, giddiness, tension headache, raising of hair.	
Behavior at Interview	Fidgeting, restlessness or pacing, tremor of hands, furrowed brow, strained face, sighing or rapid respiration, facial pallor, swallowing, belching, brisk tendon jerks, dilated pupils, exophthalmos.		Somatic (Muscular)	Pains and aches, twitchings, stiffness, myoclonic jerks, grinding of teeth, unsteady voice, increased muscular tone.	
			Total Score		

Source.   Reprinted with permission from Hamilton M: The assessment of anxiety states by rating. Br J Med Psychol 32:50–55, 1959.

Abnormal Involuntary Movement Scale (AIMS)

		None	Minimal	Mild	Moderate	Severe
		0	1	2	3	4
FACIAL AND ORAL MOVEMENTS	1: Muscles of Facial Expression e.g., movements of forehead, eyebrows, periorbital area, cheeks; include frowning, blinking, smiling, grimacing	0	1	2	3	4
	2: Lips and Perioral Area e.g., puckering, pouting, smacking	0	1	2	3	4
	3: Jaw e.g., biting, clenching, chewing, mouth opening, lateral movement	0	1	2	3	4
	4: Tongue Rate only increase in movement both in and out of mouth, NOT inability to sustain movement	0	1	2	3	4
EXTREMITY MOVEMENTS	5: Upper (arms, wrists, hands, fingers) Include choreic movements (i.e., rapid, objectively purposeless, irregular, spontaneous), athetoid movements (i.e., slow, irregular, complex, serpentine). Do NOT include tremor (i.e., repetitive, regular, rhythmic)	0	1	2	3	4
	6: Lower (legs, knees, ankles, toes) e.g., lateral knee movement, foot tapping, heel dropping, foot squirming, inversion and eversion of foot	0	1	2	3	4
TRUNK MOVEMENTS	7: Neck, shoulders, hips e.g., rocking, twisting, squirming, pelvic gyrations	0	1	2	3	4
GLOBAL JUDGMENT	8: Severity of abnormal movements	0	1	2	3	4
	9: Incapacitation due to abnormal movements	0	1	2	3	4

10: Patient's awareness of abnormal movements Rate only patient's report	No awareness	0
	Aware, no distress	1
	Aware, mild distress	2
	Aware, moderate distress	3
	Aware, severe distress	4
11: Current problems with teeth and/or dentures	No	0
	Yes	1
12: Does patient usually wear dentures?	No	0
	Yes	1

Examination Procedures for AIMS

Either before or after completing the Examination Procedure observe the patient unobtrusively, at rest (e.g., in waiting room). The chair to be used in this examination should be a hard, firm one without arms.

1: Ask patient whether there is anything in his/her mouth (i.e., gum, candy, etc.) and if there is, to remove it.

2: Ask patient about the *current* condition of his/her teeth. Ask patient if he/she wears dentures. Do teeth or dentures bother patient *now*?

3: Ask patient whether he/she notices any movements in mouth, face, hands, or feet. If yes, ask to describe and to what extent they *currently* bother patient or interfere with his/her activities.

4: Have patient sit in chair with hands on knees, legs slightly apart, and feet flat on floor. (Look at entire body for movements while in this position.)

5: Ask patient to sit with hands hanging unsupported. If male, between legs, if female and wearing a dress, hanging over knees. (Observe hands and other body areas.)

6: Ask patient to open mouth. (Observe tongue at rest within mouth.) Do this twice.

7: Ask patient to protrude tongue. (Observe tongue at rest within mouth.) Do this twice.

*8: Ask patient to tap thumb, with each finger, as rapidly as possible for 10–15 seconds; separately with right hand, then with left hand. (Observe facial and leg movements.)

9: Flex and extend patient's left and right arms (one at a time). (Note any rigidity and rate on NOTES.)

10: Ask patient to stand up. (Observe in profile. Observe all body areas again, hips included.)

*11: Ask patient to extend both arms outstretched in front with palms down. (Observe trunk, legs, and mouth.)

*12: Have patient walk a few paces, turn, and walk back to chair. (Observe hands and gait.) Do this twice.

* Activated movements.

Source. Reprinted from Guy W: ECDEU: assessment manual for psychopharmacology (DHEW Publ No 76-338). Washington, DC, Department of Health, Education, and Welfare, Psychopharmacology Research Branch, 1976.

Simpson-Angus Rating Scale

1. **GAIT:** The patient is examined as he walks into the examining room; his gait, the swing of his arms, his general posture, all form the basis for an overall score for this item. This is rated as follows:
   0 Normal
   1 Diminution in swing while the patient is walking.
   2 Marked diminution in swing with obvious rigidity in the arm.
   3 Stiff gait with arms held rigidly before the abdomen.
   4 Stooped shuffling gait with propulsion and retropulsion.

2. **ARM DROPPING:** The patient and the examiner both raise their arms to shoulder height and let them fall to their sides. In a normal subject a stout slap is heard as the arms hit the sides. In the patient with extreme Parkinson's syndrome the arms fall very slowly.
   0 Normal, free fall with loud slap and rebound.
   1 Fall slowed slightly with less audible contact and little rebound.
   2 Fall slowed, no rebound.
   3 Marked slowing, no slap at all.
   4 Arms fall as though against resistance; as though through glue.

3. **SHOULDER SHAKING:** The subject's arms are bent at a right angle at the elbow and are taken one at a time by the examiner who grasps one hand and also clasps the other around the patient's elbow. The subject's upper arm is pushed to and fro and the humerus is externally rotated. The degree of resistance from normal to extreme rigidity is scored as follows:
   0 Normal
   1 Slight stiffness and resistance.
   2 Moderate stiffness and resistance.
   3 Marked rigidity with difficulty in passive movement.
   4 Extreme stiffness and rigidity with almost a frozen shoulder.

4. **ELBOW RIGIDITY:** The elbow joints are separately bent at right angles and passively extended and flexed, with the subject's biceps observed and simultaneously palpated. The resistance to this procedure is rated. (The presence of cogwheel rigidity is noted separately.) Scoring is from 0 to 4, as in the Shoulder Shaking test.
   0 Normal
   1 Slight stiffness and resistance.
   2 Moderate stiffness and resistance.
   3 Marked rigidity with difficulty in passive movement.
   4 Extreme stiffness and rigidity with almost a frozen shoulder.

5. **FIXATION OF POSITION OR WRIST RIGIDITY:** The wrist is held in one hand and the fingers held by the examiner's other hand, with the wrist moved to extension flexion and both ulner and radial deviation. The resistance to this procedure is rated as in Items 3 and 4.

   0 Normal
   1 Slight stiffness and resistance.
   2 Moderate stiffness and resistance.
   3 Marked rigidity with difficulty in passive movement.
   4 Extreme stiffness and rigidity with almost a frozen shoulder.

6. **LEG PENDULOUSNESS:** The patient sits on a table with his legs hanging down and swinging free. The ankle is grasped by the examiner and raised until the knee is partially extended. It is then allowed to fall. The resistance to falling and the lack of swinging form the basis for the score on this item:

   0 The legs swing freely.
   1 Slight diminution in the swing of the legs.
   2 Moderate resistance to swing.
   3 Marked resistance and damping of swing.
   4 Complete absence of swing.

7. **HEAD DROPPING:** The patient lies on a well-padded examining table and his head is raised by the examiner's hand. The hand is then withdrawn and the head allowed to drop. In the normal subject the head will fall upon the table. The movement is delayed in extrapyramidal system disorder, and in extreme Parkinsonism it is absent. The neck muscles are rigid and the head does not reach the examining table. Scoring is as follows:

   0 The head falls completely, with a good thump as it hits the table.
   1 Slight slowing in fall, mainly noted by lack of slap as head meets the table.
   2 Moderate slowing in the fall, quite noticeable to the eye.
   3 Head falls stiffly and slowly.
   4 Head does not reach examining table.

8. **GLABELLA TAP:** Subject is told to open his eyes wide and not to blink. The glabella region is tapped at a steady, rapid speed. The number of times patient blinks in succession is noted:

   0   0 to 5 blinks
   1   6 to 10 blinks
   2   11 to 15 blinks
   3   16 to 20 blinks
   4   21 or more blinks

9. **TREMOR:** Patient is observed walking into examining room and then is reexamined for this item:

   0 Normal
   1 Mild finger tremor, obvious to sight and touch.

2 Tremor of hand or arm occurring spasmodically.

3 Persistent tremor of one or more limbs.

4 Whole body tremor.

10. **SALIVATION:** Patient is observed while talking and then asked to open his mouth and elevate his tongue. The following ratings are given:

0 Normal

1 Excess salivation to the extent that pooling takes place if the mouth is open and the tongue raised.

2 When excess salivation is present and might occasionally result in difficulty in speaking.

3 Speaking with difficulty because of excess salivation.

4 Frank drooling.

Source. Reprinted with permission from Simpson GM, Angus JWS: A rating scale for extrapyramidal side effects. Acta Psychiatr Scand [Suppl] 212:11–19, 1970. Copyright 1970 Munksgaard International Publishers, Ltd.

"Mini-Mental State"

ORIENTATION

5   (   )   What is the (year) (season) (date) (day) (month)?
5   (   )   Where are we: (state) (country) (town) (hospital) (floor)?

REGISTRATION

3   (   )   Name 3 objects: 1 second to say each. Then ask the patient all 3 after you
            have said them. Give 1 point for each correct answer. Then
            repeat them until he learns all 3. Count trials and record.
            Trials _____

ATTENTION AND CALCULATION

5   (   )   Serial 7's. 1 point for each correct. Stop after 5 answers. Alternatively spell
            "world" backwards.

RECALL

3   (   )   Ask for the 3 objects repeated above. Give 1 point for each correct.

LANGUAGE

9   (   )   Name a pencil, and watch (2 points)
            Repeat the following, "No ifs, ands or buts." (1 point)
            Follow a 3-stage command:
                "Take a paper in your right hand, fold it in half, and put it on the
                floor"
                (3 points)
            Read and obey the following:
                CLOSE YOUR EYES (1 point)
            Write a sentence (1 point)
            Copy design (1 point)

_____   Total score
            ASSESS level of consciousness along a continuum ─────────────────
                                                    Alert   Drowsy   Stupor   Coma

INSTRUCTIONS FOR ADMINISTRATION OF MINI-MENTAL STATE EXAMINATION

ORIENTATION

(1) Ask for the date. Then ask specifically for parts omitted, e.g., "Can you also tell me what season it is?" One point for each correct.

(2) Ask in turn "Can you tell me the name of this hospital?" (town, county, etc.). One point for each correct.

REGISTRATION

Ask the patient if you may test his memory. Then say the names of 3 unrelated objects, clearly and slowly, about one second for each. After you have said all 3, ask him to repeat them. This first repetition determines his score (0–3) but keep saying them until he can repeat all 3, up to 6 trials. If he does not eventually learn all 3, recall cannot be meaningfully tested.

ATTENTION AND CALCULATION

Ask the patient to begin with 100 and count backwards by 7. Stop after 5 subtractions (93, 86, 79, 72, 65). Score the total number of correct answers.

If the patient cannot or will not perform this task, ask him to spell the word "world" backwards. The score is the number of letters in correct order, e.g. dlrow = 5, dlorw = 3.

RECALL

Ask the patient if he can recall the 3 words you previously asked him to remember. Score 0–3.

LANGUAGE

Naming: Show the patient a wrist watch and ask him what it is. Repeat for pencil. Score 0–2.

Repetition: Ask the patient to repeat the sentence after you. Allow only one trial. Score 0 or 1.

3-Stage command: Give the patient a piece of plain blank paper and repeat the command. Score 1 point for each part correctly executed.

Reading: On a blank piece of paper print the sentence "Close your eyes," in letters large enough for the patient to see clearly. Ask him to read it and do what it says. Score 1 point only if he actually closes his eyes.

Writing: Give the patient a blank piece of paper and ask him to write a sentence for you. Do not dictate a sentence, it is to be written spontaneously. It must contain a subject and verb and be sensible. Correct grammar and punctuation are not necessary.

Copying: On a clean piece of paper, draw intersecting pentagons, each side about 1 in., and ask him to copy it exactly as it is. All 10 angles must be present and 2 must intersect to score 1 point. Tremor and rotation are ignored.

Estimate the patient's level of sensorium along a continuum, from alert on the left to coma on the right.

Source.   Reprinted with permission from Folstein MF, Folstein SE, McHugh PR: "Mini-Mental State": a practical method for grading the cognitive state of patients for the clinician. J Psychiatr Res 12:189–198, 1975. Copyright 1975 Pergamon Press PLC.

Global Assessment Scale (GAS)

Rate the subject's lowest level of functioning in the last week by selecting the lowest range which describes his functioning on a hypothetical continuum of mental health-illness. For example, a subject whose "behavior is considerably influenced by delusions" (range 21–30) should be given a rating in that range even though he has "major impairment in several areas" (range 31–40). Use intermediary levels when appropriate (e.g., 35, 58, 63). Rate actual functioning independent of whether or not subject is receiving and may be helped by medication or some other form of treatment.

100
|
91 — No symptoms, superior functioning in a wide range of activities, life's problems never seem to get out of hand, is sought out by others because of his warmth and integrity.

90
|
81 — Transient symptoms may occur, but good functioning in all areas, interested and involved in a wide range of activities, socially effective, generally satisfied with life, "everyday" worries that only occasionally get out of hand.

80
|
71 — Minimal symptoms may be present but no more than slight impairment in functioning, varying degrees of "everyday" worries and problems that sometimes get out of hand.

70
|
61 — Some mild symptoms (e.g., depressive mood and mild insomnia) OR some difficulty in several areas of functioning, but generally functioning pretty well, has some meaningful interpersonal relationships and most untrained people would not consider him "sick."

60
|
51 — Moderate symptoms OR generally functioning with some difficulty (e.g., few friends and flat affect, depressed mood, and pathological self-doubt, euphoric mood and pressure of speech, moderately severe antisocial behavior).

50
|
41 — Any serious symptomatology or impairment in functioning that most clinicians would think obviously requires treatment or attention (e.g., suicidal preoccupation or gesture, severe obsessional rituals, frequent anxiety attacks, serious antisocial behavior, compulsive drinking).

40
|
31 — Major impairment in several areas, such as work, family relations, judgment, thinking, or mood (e.g., depressed woman avoids friends, neglects family, unable to do housework), OR some impairment in reality testing or communication (e.g., speech is at times obscure, illogical, or irrelevant), OR single serious suicide attempt.

30
|
21 — Unable to function in almost all areas (e.g., stays in bed all day), OR behavior is considerably influenced by either delusions or hallucinations, OR serious impairment in communication (e.g., sometimes incoherent or unresponsive) or judgment (e.g., acts grossly inappropriately).

20
|
11 — Needs some supervision to prevent hurting self or others, or to maintain minimal personal hygiene (e.g., repeated suicide attempts, frequently violent, manic excitement, smears feces), OR gross impairment in communication (e.g., largely incoherent or mute).

10
|
1 — Needs constant supervision for several days to prevent hurting self or others, or makes no attempt to maintain minimal personal hygiene.

Source. Reprinted with permission from Endicott J, Spitzer RL, Fleiss JL, et al: The Global Assessment Scale: a procedure for measuring overall severity of psychiatric disturbance. Arch Gen Psychiatry 33:766–771, 1976. Copyright 1976/78, American Medical Association.

Index

L

M